IMMUNOLOGY

FOURTH EDITION

IMMUNOLOGY

FOURTH EDITION

Ivan Roitt MA DSc(Oxon) Hon FRCP(Lond) FRCPath FRS

Emeritus Professor of Immunology
University College London Medical School
London, UK

Jonathan Brostoff MA DM(Oxon) DSc FRCP FRCPath

Reader in Clinical Immunology
Department of Immunology
University College London Medical School
London, UK

David Male MA PhD

Senior Lecturer in Neuroimmunology
Department of Neuropathology
Institute of Psychiatry
London, UK

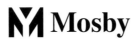 Mosby

London Baltimore Barcelona Bogotá Boston Buenos Aires Caracas Carlsbad, CA Chicago Madrid Mexico City Milan Naples, FL New York
Philadelphia St. Louis Seoul Singapore Sydney Taipei Tokyo Toronto Wiesbaden

Publisher:	Dianne Zack
Development Editor:	Louise Cook
Project Manager:	Peter Harrison
Design:	Pete Wilder
Layout:	Rob Curran
Cover Illustration:	Richard Prime and Nick Lloyd for The Picture Palace on Alias Power Animator®
Illustration Manager:	Lynda Payne
Illustration:	Richard Prime
Production:	Jane Tozer
Index:	A. Cottingham

Copyright © 1996 Times Mirror International Publishers Limited

Published by Mosby, an imprint of Times Mirror International Publishers Limited

Printed by Grafos SA, Arte sobre papel, Barcelona, Spain

10 9 8 7 6 5 4 3 2 1   1998   1997   1996

ISBN 0 7234 2178 1

For full details of all Times Mirror International Publishers Limited titles, please write to Times Mirror International Publishers Limited, Lynton House,   7–12 Tavistock Square, London WC1H 9LB, England.

A CIP catalogue record for this book is available from the British Library.

Library of Congress Cataloging-in-Publication Data has been applied for

PREFACE

The editors, contributors and publisher have joined forces once again to deliver a completely new top quality edition. We have emphasized making the material more accessible to aid understanding of this fascinating subject. We have looked carefully at which areas are central to immunology and have enlarged and divided some of the previous chapters. Now there are separate chapters on T-cell receptors and MHC molecules as well as antibodies and their receptors. We have also enlarged the section on immunity to infection and this has been divided into immunity to viruses and immunity to bacteria and fungi. Brand new diagrams explain these fast growing areas.

Several new features have been added to improve the style, continuity and presentation of the book to make it more 'user friendly'. A list of points now appears at the beginning of each chapter summarizing the main concepts and at the end of each chapter we pose a series of thought-provoking questions which should provide a basis for in-depth discussion. We have also used 'telegraph headings' to identify ideas which are expanded in the subsequent text.

Making science relevant to the practice of medicine is an important challenge for any textbook. In addition to the clinical chapters where the underlying basis of disease is presented by mechanism, we now have an updated and enlarged *Case Studies in Immunology* as a companion to this text. Immunology is relevant and indeed central to many disease processes in both animals and man and we are sure that this unique presentation of basic immunology with clinical case studies will provide enhanced understanding of the subject as a whole. Readers are also encouraged to look out for the appearance of an exciting new *CD-ROM* linked to this fourth edition which should greatly help the processes of learning and revision.

As always, it is our earnest hope that the style and presentation of the book will bring pleasure and understanding to our many readers at the undergraduate, graduate and clinical stages of their careers.

Ivan M Roitt
Jonathan Brostoff
David K Male

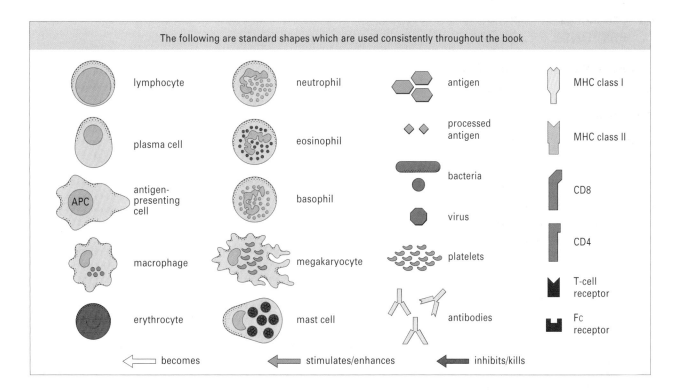

The following are standard shapes which are used consistently throughout the book

lymphocyte	neutrophil	antigen	MHC class I
plasma cell	eosinophil	processed antigen	MHC class II
antigen-presenting cell (APC)	basophil	bacteria	CD8
macrophage	megakaryocyte	virus	CD4
erythrocyte	mast cell	platelets	T-cell receptor
		antibodies	Fc receptor

⟵ becomes   ⟵ stimulates/enhances   ⟵ inhibits/kills

We owe a great debt of gratitude to Dianne Zack and to the senior project manager Peter Harrison who have coped admirably with all the changes we have made. We are also grateful to Pete Wilder for his input to the design of the whole project and we also wish to thank Steve McGrath for his invaluable editorial contribution. As with all previous editions, it is an enormous pleasure to acknowledge the vital support and encouragement, both intellectual and gastronomic, given by Fiona Foley throughout the gestation of this book.

CONTENTS

9. CELL-MEDIATED IMMUNE REACTIONS

Professor Graham Rook

10. DEVELOPMENT OF THE IMMUNE SYSTEM

Professor Peter Lydyard and Professor Carlo Grossi

11. REGULATION OF THE IMMUNE RESPONSE

Dr Anne Cooke

12. IMMUNOLOGICAL TOLERANCE

Professor Jacques Miller

13. COMPLEMENT

Professor Mark Walport

14. CELL MIGRATION AND INFLAMMATION

Dr David Male

15. EVOLUTION OF IMMUNITY

Dr John Horton and Professor Norman Ratcliffe

16. IMMUNITY TO VIRUSES

Professor Tony Nash

25. HYPERSENSITIVITY – TYPE IV

Professor Ross StC Barnetson, Dr David Gawkrodger and Associate Professor Warwick Britton

26. TRANSPLANTATION AND REJECTION

Professor Ian Hutchinson

27. AUTOIMMUNITY AND AUTOIMMUNE DISEASE

Professor Ivan Roitt

28. IMMUNOLOGICAL TECHNIQUES

Professor Michael Steward and Dr David Male

Appendices

Glossary
Index

CONTRIBUTORS

Professor Ross StC Barnetson
Department of Dermatology
University of Sydney
NSW 2006, Australia

Professor Peter C L Beverley
Imperial Cancer Research Fund
Tumour Immunology Unit
University College London Medical School
London, UK

Dr Janette E Bradley
Department of Medical Microbiology
Manchester Royal Infirmary
Manchester, UK

Associate Professor Warwick J Britton
Department of Clinical Immunology
Royal Prince Alfred Hospital
Camperdown
NSW 2050, Australia

Dr Jonathan Brostoff
Department of Immunology
University College London Medical School
London, UK

Dr Anne Cooke
Immunology Division
Department of Pathology
University of Cambridge
Cambridge, UK

Professor Marc Feldmann
Kennedy Institute of Rheumatology
Hammersmith
London, UK

Dr David Gawkrodger
Department of Dermatology
University of Sheffield
Royal Hallamshire Hospital
Sheffield, UK

Professor Carlo Enrico Grossi
Department of Immunology
University of Genoa
Genoa, Italy

Dr Tony Hall
Ciba–Geigy AG
CH-4002 Basel
Switzerland

Professor Frank C Hay
Division of Immunology
St George's Hospital Medical School
London, UK

Dr John Horton
Department of Biological Sciences
University of Durham
Durham, UK

Professor Ian V Hutchinson
School of Biological Sciences
University of Manchester
Manchester, UK

Professor Peter Lydyard
Department of Immunology
University College London Medical School
London, UK

Professor Jacques F A P Miller
Thymus Biology Unit
Walter and Eliza Hall Institute of Medical Research
Melbourne
Victoria 3050, Australia

Dr David K Male
Department of Neuropathology
Institute of Psychiatry
London, UK

Professor Tony Nash
Department of Veterinary Pathology
University of Edinburgh
Edinburgh, UK

Dr Michael J Owen
Lymphocyte Molecular Biology Laboratory
Imperial Cancer Research Fund
London, UK

Professor John H. L. Playfair
Department of Immunology
University College London Medical School
London, UK

Professor Norman Ratcliffe
School of Biological Science
University College of Swansea
Swansea, UK

Professor Ivan M Roitt
Institute of Biomedical Science
University College London Medical School
London, UK

Professor Fred S Rosen
Department of Pediatrics
Harvard University Medical School
Boston, USA

Professor Graham Rook
Department of Medical Microbiology
University College London Medical School
London, UK

Professor Michael Steward
Molecular Immunology Unit
London School of Hygiene and Tropical Medicine
London, UK

Dr Janice Taverne
Department of Immunology
University College London Medical School
London, UK

Professor Malcolm W Turner
Division of Cell and Molecular Biology
Institute of Child Health
University of London
London, UK

Professor Mark J Walport
Rheumatology Unit, Department of Medicine
Royal Postgraduate Medical School
Hammersmith Hospital
London, UK

Dr Olwyn MR Westwood
School of Life Sciences
Roehampton Institute
University of Surrey
London, UK

INTRODUCTION TO THE IMMUNE SYSTEM

The immune system has evolved to protect us from pathogens. Some, such as viruses, infect individual cells; others, including many bacteria, divide extracellularly within tissues or the body cavities.

The cells which mediate immunity include lymphocytes and phagocytes. Lymphocytes recognize antigens on pathogens. Phagocytes internalize pathogens and degrade them.

An immune response consists of two phases. In the first phase, antigen activates specific lymphocytes that recognize it; in the effector phase, these lymphocytes coordinate an immune response that eliminates the source of the antigens.

Specificity and memory are two essential features of adaptive immune responses. The immune system mounts a more effective response on second and subsequent encounters with a particular antigen.

Lymphocytes have specialized functions. B cells make antibodies; cytotoxic T cells kill virally infected cells; helper T cells coordinate the immune response by direct cell–cell interactions and the release of cytokines, which help B cells to make antibody; and macrophages kill parasites that have invaded them.

Antigens are molecules which are recognized by receptors on lymphocytes. B lymphocytes usually recognize intact antigen molecules, while T lymphocytes recognize antigen fragments on the surface of other cells.

Clonal selection involves recognition of antigen by a particular lymphocyte; this leads to clonal expansion and differentiation to effector and memory cells.

The immune system may break down. This can lead to immunodeficiency or hypersensitivity diseases or to autoimmune diseases.

Our environment contains a great variety of infectious microbes – viruses, bacteria, fungi, protozoa and multicellular parasites. These can cause disease, and if they multiply unchecked they will eventually kill their host. Most infections in normal individuals are short-lived and leave little permanent damage. This is due to the immune system, which combats infectious agents.

Since microorganisms come in many different forms, a wide variety of immune responses are required to deal with each type of infection. In the first instance, the exterior defences of the body present an effective barrier to most organisms, and very few infectious agents can penetrate intact skin (*Fig. 1.1*). However, many gain access across the epithelia of the gastrointestinal or urogenital tracts. Others can infect the nasopharynx and lung. A small number, such as malaria and hepatitis B, can only infect the body if they enter the blood directly.

The site of the infection and the type of pathogen largely determine which immune responses will be effective. The most important distinction is between pathogens which invade the host's cells and those which do not. All viruses, some bacteria and some protozoan parasites replicate inside host cells, and to clear an infection the immune system must recognize and destroy these infected cells. Many bacteria and larger parasites live in tissues, body fluids or other extracellular spaces, and the responses to these pathogens are quite different. During the course of an infection, however, even intracellular pathogens must reach their target cells by moving through the blood and tissue fluid. At this time they are susceptible to elements of the immune system which normally counter extracellular pathogens (see *Fig. 1.2*).

This chapter introduces the basic elements of the immune system and of immune responses, which are detailed in Chapters 2–20. There are various ways in which the immune system can fail, leading to immunopathological reactions, and these are outlined in the second half of the book. However, it is important to stress that the primary function of the immune system is to eliminate infectious agents and to minimize the damage they cause.

■ ADAPTIVE AND INNATE IMMUNITY

Any immune response involves, firstly, recognition of the pathogen or other foreign material, and secondly, mounting a reaction against it to eliminate it. Broadly speaking, the different types of immune response fall into two categories: innate (or non-adaptive) immune responses, and adaptive

Exterior defences

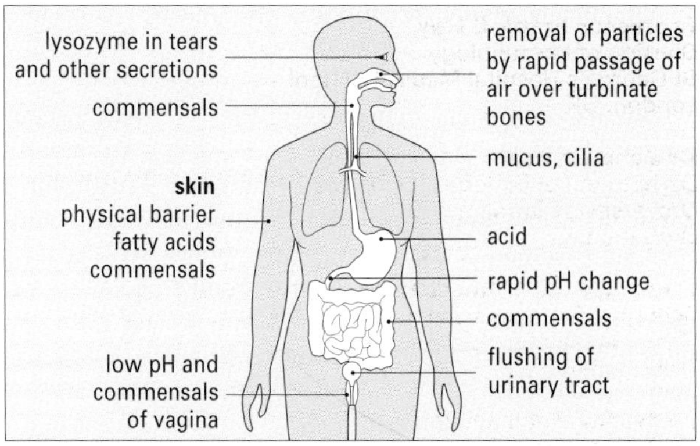

lysozyme in tears and other secretions

commensals

skin
physical barrier
fatty acids
commensals

low pH and commensals of vagina

removal of particles by rapid passage of air over turbinate bones

mucus, cilia

acid

rapid pH change

commensals

flushing of urinary tract

Fig 1.1 Most of the infectious agents that an individual encounters do not penetrate the body surface, but are prevented from entering by a variety of biochemical and physical barriers. The body tolerates a number of commensal organisms, which compete effectively with many potential pathogens.

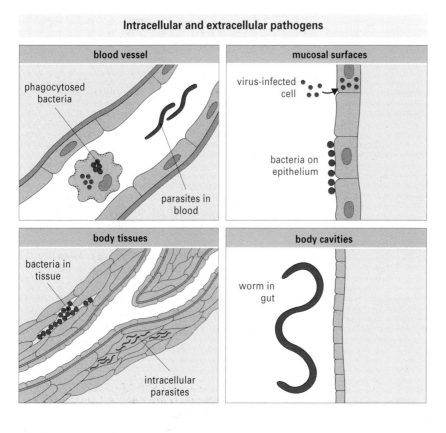

Fig. 1.2 The immune system must recognize and react against pathogens in a number of different locations. For example, viruses must invade cells to reproduce, while protozoa such as *Plasmodium* spp. (malaria) and *Trypanosoma cruzi* (Chagas' disease), and bacteria such as *Salmonella typhi*, all have intracellular phases. Some protozoan parasites (e.g. African trypanosomes) live in the blood, while many large multicellular parasites live in tissues or organs (e.g. tapeworms). Many bacteria colonize epithelial surfaces and may invade the host to multiply in tissues.

immune responses. The important difference between these is that an adaptive immune response is highly specific for a particular pathogen. Moreover, although the innate response does not alter on repeated exposure to a given infectious agent, the adaptive response improves with each successive encounter with the same pathogen: in effect the adaptive immune system 'remembers' the infectious agent and can prevent it from causing disease later. For example, diseases such as measles and diphtheria induce adaptive immune responses which generate a life-long immunity following an infection. The two key features of the adaptive immune response are thus specificity and memory.

Immune responses are produced primarily by leucocytes, of which there are several different types.

Phagocytes and innate immune responses – One important group of leucocytes is the phagocytic cells, such as the monocytes, macrophages and polymorphonuclear neutrophils. These cells bind to microorganisms, internalize them and then kill them. Since they use primitive non-specific recognition systems, which allow them to bind to a variety of microbial products, they are mediating innate immune responses. In effect they are acting as a first line of defence against infection.

Lymphocytes and adaptive immune responses – Another important set of leucocytes is the lymphocytes. These cells are central to all adaptive immune responses, since they specifically recognize individual pathogens, whether they are inside host cells or outside in the tissue fluids or blood. In fact there are several different types of lymphocyte, but they fall into

two basic categories – T lymphocytes (or T cells) and B lymphocytes (or B cells). B cells combat extracellular pathogens and their products by releasing antibody, a molecule which specifically recognizes and binds to a particular target molecule, called the antigen. The antigen may be a molecule on the surface of a pathogen, or a toxin which it produces. T lymphocytes have a wider range of activities. Some are involved in the control of B lymphocyte development and antibody production. Another group of T lymphocytes interacts with phagocytic cells to help them destroy pathogens they have taken up. A third set of T lymphocytes recognizes cells infected by virus and destroys them.

Interaction between lymphocytes and phagocytes – In practice there is considerable interaction between the lymphocytes and phagocytes. For example, some phagocytes can take up antigens and show them to T lymphocytes in a form they can recognize, a process which is called antigen presentation. In turn, the T lymphocytes release soluble factors (cytokines), which activate the phagocytes and cause them to destroy the pathogens they have internalized. In another interaction, phagocytes use antibodies released by B lymphocytes to allow them to recognize pathogens more effectively (*Fig. 1.3*). One consequence of these interactions is that most immune responses to infectious organisms are made up of a variety of innate and adaptive components. In the earliest stages of infection, innate responses predominate, but later the lymphocytes start to generate adaptive immune responses. They then 'remember' the pathogen, and mount more effective and rapid responses should the individual become reinfected with the same pathogen at a later date.

Interaction between lymphocytes and phagocytes

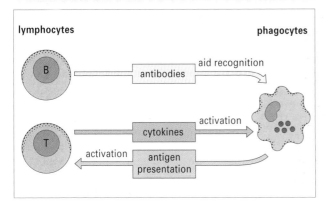

Fig. 1.3 B lymphocytes release antibodies, which bind to pathogens and their products and so aid recognition by phagocytes through Fcγ receptor binding. Cytokines released by T cells activate the phagocytes to destroy the material they have taken up. In turn, mononuclear phagocytes can present antigen to T cells, thereby activating them.

■ CELLS OF THE IMMUNE SYSTEM

Immune responses are mediated by a variety of cells, and by the soluble molecules which they secrete. Although the leucocytes are central to all immune responses, other cells in the tissues also participate, by signalling to the lymphocytes and responding to the cytokines released by T lymphocytes and macrophages. *Figure 1.4* lists the main cells and molecules involved in immune reactions.

Phagocytes internalize antigens and pathogenic microorganisms and degrade them

Mononuclear phagocytes – The most important group of long-lived phagocytic cells belongs to the mononuclear phagocyte lineage. These cells are all derived from bone marrow stem cells, and their function is to engulf particles, including infectious agents, internalize them and destroy them. For this purpose they are strategically placed where they will encounter such particles. For example, the Kupffer cells of the liver line the sinusoids along which blood flows, while the synovial A cells line the synovial cavity (*Fig. 1.5*). In the blood, cells belonging to this lineage are known as monocytes. In time, these migrate out into the tissues, where they develop into tissue macrophages. These cells are very effective at presenting antigens to T lymphocytes.

Polymorphonuclear neutrophils – A second important phagocytic cell is the polymorphonuclear neutrophil, often just called a neutrophil or PMN. Neutrophils constitute the majority of the blood leucocytes and develop from the same early precursors as monocytes and macrophages. Like monocytes, they too migrate into tissues, in response to certain stimuli, but neutrophils are short-lived cells, which engulf material, destroy it and then die.

Lymphocytes occur as two major types, B cells and T cells, which are responsible for specific recognition of antigens

Lymphocytes are wholly responsible for the specific immune recognition of pathogens, so they initiate adaptive immune responses. All lymphocytes are derived from bone-marrow stem cells, but T lymphocytes then develop in the thymus, while B lymphocytes develop in the bone marrow (in adult mammals).

Components of the immune system

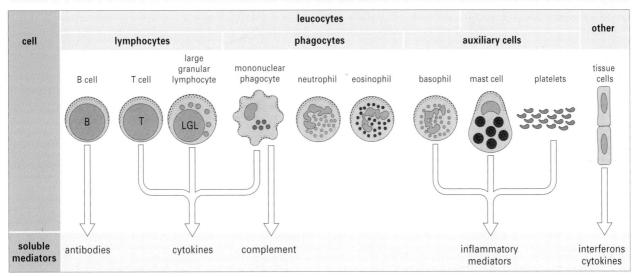

Fig. 1.4 The principal components of the immune system are shown, indicating which cells produce which soluble mediators. Complement is made primarily by the liver, although there is some synthesis by mononuclear phagocytes. Note that each cell produces and secretes only a particular set of cytokines or inflammatory mediators.

Phagocytes of the mononuclear phagocyte lineage

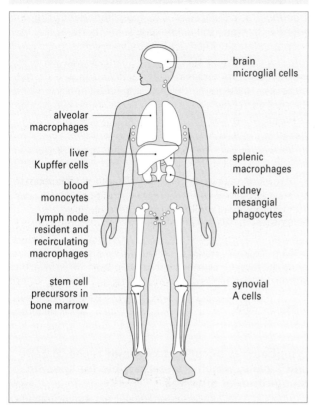

brain
microglial cells

alveolar
macrophages

liver
Kupffer cells

blood
monocytes

lymph node
resident and
recirculating
macrophages

stem cell
precursors in
bone marrow

splenic
macrophages

kidney
mesangial
phagocytes

synovial
A cells

Fig. 1.5 Many organs contain phagocytic cells derived from blood monocytes which are manufactured in the bone marrow. Monocytes pass out of the blood vessel and become macrophages in the tissues. Resident phagocytic cells of different tissues were previously referred to as the reticuloendothelial system, but they too appear to belong to the monocyte lineage.

B cells – Each B cell is genetically programmed to encode a surface receptor specific for a particular antigen. Having recognized its specific antigen, the B cells multiply and differentiate into plasma cells, which produce large amounts of the receptor molecule in a soluble form which can be secreted. This is known as antibody. These antibody molecules are large glycoproteins found in the blood and tissue fluids: because they are virtually identical to the original receptor molecule, they bind to the antigen that initially activated the B cells.

T cells – There are several different types of T cells, and they have a variety of functions. One group interacts with B cells and helps them to divide, differentiate and make antibody. Another group interacts with mononuclear phagocytes and helps them destroy intracellular pathogens. These two groups of cells are called T-helper (TH) cells. A third group of T cells is responsible for the destruction of host cells which have become infected by viruses or other intracellular pathogens – this kind of action is called cytotoxicity and these T cells are hence called T-cytotoxic (TC) cells. In every case, the T cells recognize antigens, but only in association with familiar markers on host cells. They use a specific receptor to do this, termed the T-cell antigen receptor (TCR). This is related, both in function and structure, to the surface antibody which B cells use as their antigen receptors. T cells generate their effects, either by releasing soluble proteins, called cytokines, which signal to other cells, or by direct cell–cell interactions. The principal functions of lymphocytes are summarized in *Figure 1.6*.

Cytotoxic cells recognize and destroy other cells that have become infected

Several cell types have the capacity to kill other cells, of which the TC cell is probably the most important.

Large granular lymphocytes – The group of lymphocytes known as large granular lymphocytes (LGLs) also has the capacity to recognize the surface changes that occur on a

Functions of lymphocytes

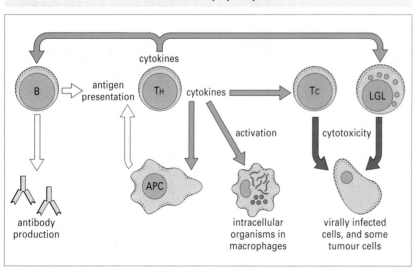

cytokines

B

antigen
presentation

TH

cytokines

TC

LGL

antibody
production

APC

activation

intracellular
organisms in
macrophages

cytotoxicity

virally infected
cells, and some
tumour cells

Fig. 1.6 B cells produce antibodies, while T helper (TH) cells are stimulated by antigen-presenting cells (APC) and B cells to produce cytokines, which control immune responses. Macrophages are activated to kill intracellular microorganisms. Cytotoxic T (TC) cells and large granular lymphocytes (LGL) can recognize and kill target host cells.

variety of tumour cells and virally infected cells. LGLs damage these target cells, but unlike Tc cells, they use recognition systems which are rather non-specific. This action is sometimes called natural killer (NK) cell activity. Both macrophages and LGLs may also recognize and destroy some target cells (or pathogens) which have become coated with specific antibody.

Eosinophil polymorphs – Also known as eosinophils, these are a specialized group of leucocytes which have the ability to engage and damage large extracellular parasites, such as schistosomes.

All of these cell types damage their different targets by releasing the contents of their intracellular granules close to them. Other molecules secreted by the cytotoxic cells, but not stored in granules, contribute to the damage.

Auxiliary cells control inflammation

A number of other cells mediate inflammation, the main purpose of which (see below) is to attract leucocytes and the soluble mediators of immunity towards a site of infection.

Basophils and mast cells – These have granules containing a variety of mediators that produce inflammation in surrounding tissues. These mediators are released when the cells are triggered. They can also synthesize and secrete a number of mediators which control the development of immune reactions. Mast cells lie close to blood vessels in all tissues, and some of the mediators act on cells in the vessel walls. Basophils are functionally similar to mast cells but are circulating.

Platelets – These can also release inflammatory mediators when activated during thrombogenesis or by means of antigen–antibody complexes.

■ SOLUBLE MEDIATORS OF IMMUNITY

A wide variety of molecules are involved in the development of immune responses. These include antibodies and cytokines, produced by lymphocytes, and a variety of other molecules that are normally present in serum. The serum concentration of a number of these proteins increases rapidly during infection and they are therefore called acute phase proteins. One example is C-reactive protein (CRP), so called because of its ability to bind to the C-protein of pneumococci. This promotes their uptake by phagocytes, a process known as opsonization (see *Fig. 1.10*). Molecules such as antibody, complement and C-reactive protein that promote phagocytosis are said to act as opsonins.

Complement proteins mediate phagocytosis, control inflammation and interact with antibodies in immune defence

The complement system is a group of about 20 serum proteins whose overall function is the control of inflammation. The components interact with each other, and with other elements of the immune system. For example, a number of microorganisms spontaneously activate the complement system, via the so-called alternative pathway, which is an innate, non-specific reaction. This results in a coat of complement molecules on the microorganism, leading to its uptake by phagocytes. The complement system can also be activated by antibodies bound to the pathogen surface (the 'classical pathway'), when it co-mediates a specific, adaptive response.

Complement activation is a cascade reaction, with each component sequentially acting on others, in a similar way to the blood-clotting system. Activation by either the classical or the alternative pathway generates peptides which have the following effects.

- Opsonization of microorganisms for uptake by phagocytes and eventual intracellular killing.
- Attraction of phagocytes to sites of infection (chemotaxis).
- Increased blood flow to the site of activation and increased permeability of capillaries to plasma molecules.
- Damage to plasma membranes on cells, Gram-negative bacteria, enveloped viruses or other organisms which have induced the activation. This in turn can produce lysis of the cell or virus and reduce the infection.
- Release of further inflammatory mediators from mast cells. These functions are outlined in *Figure 1.7* and detailed in Chapter 13.

Complement functions

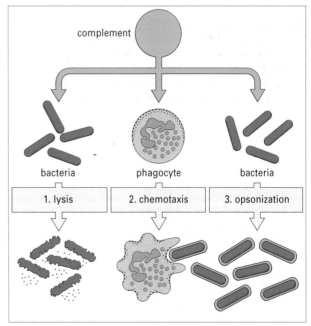

Fig. 1.7 1. The complement system has an intrinsic ability to lyse the cell membranes of many bacterial species. 2. Complement products released in this reaction attract phagocytes to the site of the reaction – chemotaxis. 3. Complement components coat the bacterial surface – opsonization – allowing the phagocytes to recognize the bacteria and engulf them. These reactions may be triggered by the intrinsic ability of the complement system to recognize microbial components or by antibodies bound to the microorganism.

Cytokines are diverse molecules which signal between lymphocytes, phagocytes and other cells of the body

Cytokine is the general term for a large group of molecules involved in signalling between cells during immune responses. All cytokines are proteins or peptides, some with sugar molecules attached (glycoproteins). The different cytokines fall into a number of categories, and those produced by lymphocytes are often called lymphokines. The principal sets of cytokines are outlined below.

Interferons (IFNs) – These are particularly important in limiting the spread of certain viral infections. One group of interferons (IFNα and IFNβ) is produced by cells which have become virally infected; another type, IFNγ, is released by certain activated T cells. IFNs induce a state of antiviral resistance in uninfected tissue cells (*Fig. 1.8*). They are produced very early in infection and are the first line of resistance to a great many viruses.

Interleukins (ILs) – These are a large group of cytokines (IL-1 to IL-15) produced mainly by T cells, although some are also produced by mononuclear phagocytes, or by tissue cells. They have a variety of functions, but most of them are involved in directing other cells to divide and differentiate. Each interleukin acts on a specific, limited group of cells which express the correct receptors for that interleukin.

Colony stimulating factors (CSFs) – These are involved in directing the division and differentiation of bone-marrow stem cells, and the precursors of blood leucocytes. The balance of different CSFs is partially responsible for the proportions of different cell types which will be produced. Some CSFs also promote further differentiation of cells outside the bone marrow.

Other cytokines – Of these tumour necrosis factors, TNFα and TNFβ and transforming growth factor-β (TGFβ) have a variety of functions, but are particularly important in mediating inflammation and cytotoxic reactions.

Antibody specifically binds to antigen and then mediates secondary effects

Antibodies (Ab), also called immunoglobulins (Ig), are a group of serum molecules produced by B lymphocytes. In fact, as discussed earlier, they are the soluble form of the B cells' antigen receptor. All antibodies have the same basic structure, but they are diverse in the region that binds to the antigen. In general, each antibody can bind specifically to just one antigen.

While one part of an antibody molecule (the Fab portion) binds to antigen, other parts interact with other elements of the immune system, such as phagocytes, or one of the complement molecules. In effect, antibodies act as flexible adaptors, linking various elements of the immune system to recognize specific pathogens and their products (*Fig. 1.9*).

The part of the antibody molecule that interacts with cells of the immune system, is termed the Fc portion. Neutrophils, macrophages and other mononuclear phagocytes have Fc receptors on their surface. Consequently, if antibody binds to a pathogen, it can link to a phagocyte via the Fc portion. This

Interferons (IFNs)

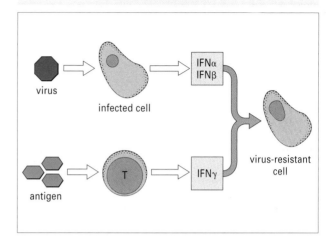

Fig. 1.8 When host cells become infected by virus, they may produce interferon. Different cell types produce interferon-α (IFNα) or interferon-β (IFNβ); interferon-γ (IFNγ) is produced by some types of lymphocyte (T) after activation by antigen. Interferons act on other host cells to induce a state of resistance to viral infection. IFNγ has many other effects as well.

Antibody – a flexible adaptor

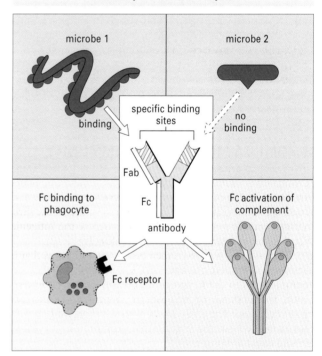

Fig. 1.9 When a microorganism lacks the inherent ability to activate complement or bind to phagocytes, the body provides antibodies as flexible adaptor molecules. The body can make several million different antibodies able to recognize a wide variety of infectious agents. Thus the antibody illustrated binds microbe 1, but not microbe 2, by its 'antigen-binding portion' (Fab). The Fc portion may activate complement or bind to Fc receptors on host cells, particularly phagocytes.

allows the pathogen to be ingested and destroyed by the phagocyte (phagocytosed) – the antibody acts as an opsonin. Phagocytes can recognize material using either activated complement (C3b) or antibody as the opsonin, but phagocytosis is most effective when both are present (*Fig. 1.10*).

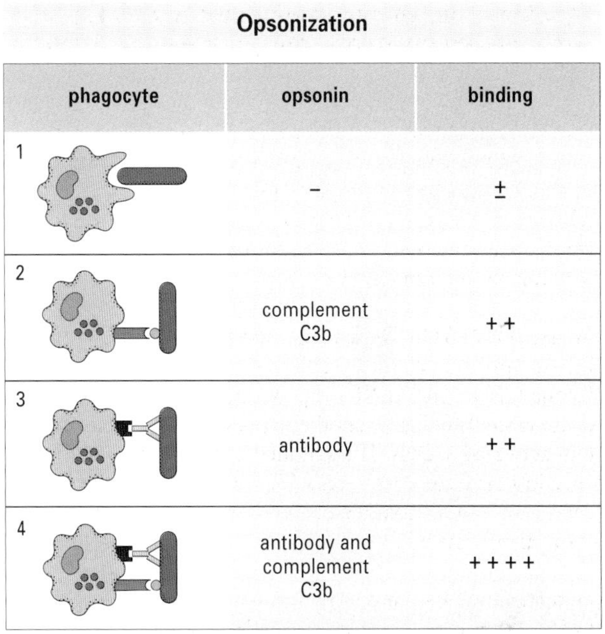

■ ANTIGENS

Originally the term antigen was used for any molecule that induced B cells to produce a specific antibody (*anti*body *gen*erator). Now however the term is much more widely used to indicate any molecule that can be specifically recognized by the adaptive elements of the immune system, that is by B cells or T cells, or both.

Antibody molecules do not bind to the whole of an infectious agent. Because of their specificity, each antibody molecule binds to one of the many molecules – antigens – on the microorganism's surface. There may be several different antibodies for a given pathogen, each binding to a different antigen on that pathogen's surface. Each antibody binds to a restricted part of the antigen called an epitope. A particular antigen can have several different epitopes or repeated epitopes (*Fig. 1.11*). Antibodies are specific for the epitopes rather than the whole antigen molecule.

The way in which a sufficient diversity of antibody molecules is generated to bind to all the different antigens encountered in a lifetime is explained in Chapter 6.

Antigen recognition is the foundation of all adaptive immune responses

T cells also recognize antigens, but they recognize antigens originating from within cells that are presented at the surface of the host cell as small polypeptide fragments. For example, a host cell that has been infected with a virus will express small fragments of viral proteins on its surface, thus making it instantly recognizable by cytotoxic T cells. The antigen fragments are presented on the surface of the cell by a specialized group of molecules. These are encoded in a set of genes known as the major histocompatibility complex (MHC), and are consequently called MHC molecules. The T cells use their antigen-specific receptors (TCRs) to recognize the antigenic peptides bound to these MHC molecules (*Fig. 1.12*).

The essential point to remember about antigen, is that it is the initiator and driving force for all adaptive immune responses. The immune system has evolved to recognize antigens, destroy them and eliminate the source of their production – bacteria, virally infected cells, etc. When antigen is eliminated, immune responses switch off.

■ IMMUNE RESPONSES

You will recall that there are two major phases of any immune response:
• Recognition of the antigen.
• A reaction to eradicate it.
In adaptive immune responses, lymphocytes are responsible for immune recognition, and this is achieved by clonal selection.

Opsonization

	phagocyte	opsonin	binding
1		–	±
2		complement C3b	+ +
3		antibody	+ +
4		antibody and complement C3b	+ + + +

Fig. 1.10 1. Phagocytes have some intrinsic ability to bind directly to bacteria and other microorganisms, but this is much enhanced if the bacteria have activated complement. 2. They will then have bound C3b so that the cells can bind the bacteria via C3b receptors. 3. Organisms which do not activate complement well, if at all, are opsonized by antibody (Ab) which can bind to the Fc receptor on the phagocyte. 4. Antibody can also activate complement and if both antibody and C3b opsonize the microbe, binding is greatly enhanced.

Antigens

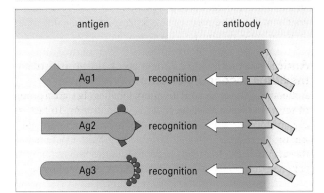

Fig. 1.11 Molecules that generate antibodies are called antigens. Antigen molecules each have a set of antigenic determinants, also called epitopes. The epitopes on one antigen (Ag1) are usually different from those on another (Ag2). Some antigens (Ag3) have repeated epitopes. Epitopes are molecular shapes recognized by antibodies and T-cell receptors of the adaptive immune system. Each antibody receptor recognizes one epitope rather than the whole antigen. Even simple microorganisms have many different antigens which may be protein, lipid or carbohydrate.

T-cell recognition of antigen

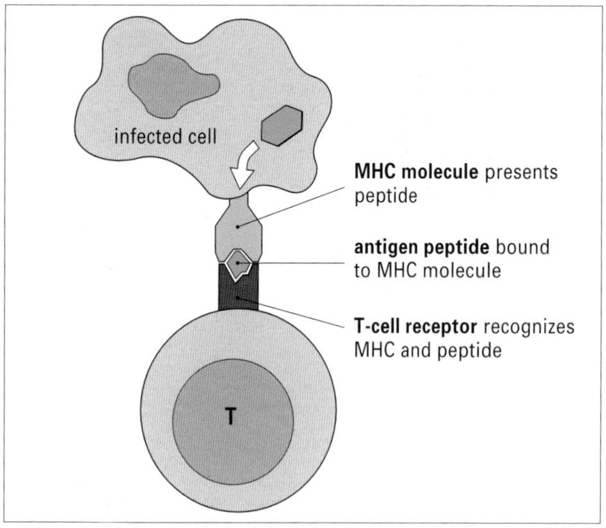

infected cell

MHC molecule presents peptide

antigen peptide bound to MHC molecule

T-cell receptor recognizes MHC and peptide

T

Fig. 1.12 T cells recognize antigens that originate within other cells, such as viral peptides from infected cells. They do this by binding specifically to antigenic peptides presented on the surface of the infected cells by molecules encoded by the major histocompatibility complex (MHC molecules). The T cells use their specific receptors (TCRs) to recognize the unique combination of MHC molecule plus antigenic peptide. Unlike B cells, which recognize just a portion of the antigen, the epitope that a T cell recognizes is made up of residues from the MHC molecule and the antigen peptide.

B-cell clonal selection

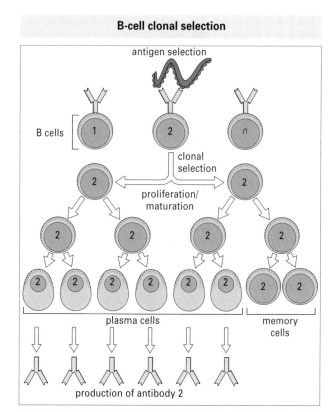

antigen selection

B cells

1   2   n

clonal selection

proliferation/ maturation

plasma cells

memory cells

production of antibody 2

Fig. 1.13 Each antibody-producing cell (B cell) is programmed to make just one antibody, which is placed on its surface as an antigen receptor. Antigen binds to only those B cells with the appropriate surface receptor – B cell 2 in this example. In this way these cells are stimulated to proliferate and mature into antibody-producing cells, and the longer-lived memory cells, all having the same antigen-binding specificity.

Clonal selection involves proliferation of cells that recognize a specific antigen

Each lymphocyte (whether a B cell or T cell) is genetically programmed to be capable of recognizing essentially only one particular antigen. The immune system as a whole can specifically recognize many thousands of antigens, so the lymphocytes recognizing any particular antigen must represent only a minute proportion of the total. How then is an adequate immune response to an infectious agent generated? The answer is that when an antigen binds to the few cells that can recognize it, they are induced to proliferate rapidly. Within a few days there are a sufficient number to mount an adequate immune response. In other words, the antigen selects for and generates the specific clones of its own antigen-binding cells (*Fig. 1.13*), a process called clonal selection. This operates for both B cells and T cells.

One might wonder how the immune system can 'know' which specific antibodies will be needed during an individual's lifetime. In fact, it does not. The immune system generates antibodies that can recognize an enormous range of antigens even before it encounters them. Many of these will never be called upon to protect the individual against infection. However, the tremendous number of infectious organisms, and their capacity to change their antigens through mutation, makes it necessary for all these different antibodies to be available, just in case they are ever needed.

Lymphocytes that have been stimulated, by binding to their specific antigen, take the first steps towards cell division. They express new receptors which allow them to respond to cytokines from other cells, which signal proliferation. The lymphocytes may also start to secrete cytokines themselves. They will usually go through a number of cycles of division, before differentiating into mature cells, again under the influence of cytokines. For example, proliferating B cells eventually mature into antibody-producing plasma cells. Even when the infection has been overcome, some of the newly produced lymphocytes remain, available for re-stimulation if the antigen is encountered once more. These cells are called memory cells, since they retain the immunological memory of particular antigen. It is memory cells that confer the lasting immunity to a particular pathogen.

Different immune effector mechanisms are available for handling the vast range of diverse pathogens

There are numerous ways in which the immune system can destroy pathogens, each way being suited to a given type of infection at a particular stage of its life cycle. These defence mechanisms are often referred to as effector systems.

Neutralization – In one of the simplest effector systems, antibodies can combat certain pathogens just by binding to them. For example, antibody to the outer coat proteins of some rhinoviruses (which cause colds) can prevent the viral particles from binding to and infecting host cells.

Phagocytosis – More often antibody is important in activating complement, or acting as an opsonin to promote ingestion by phagocytes. Phagocytic cells, which have bound to an opsonized microbe, engulf it by extending pseudopodia around it. These fuse and the microorganism is internalized (endocytosed) in a phagosome (*Fig. 1.14*). The phagocytes have several ways of dealing with this material. For example, macrophages reduce molecular oxygen to form microbicidal reactive oxygen intermediates (ROIs), which are secreted into the phagosome. Neutrophils contain lactoferrin, which chelates iron and prevents some bacteria from obtaining that vital nutrient. Finally, granules and lysosomes fuse with the phagosome, pouring enzymes into the phagolysosome, which digest the contents (*Fig. 1.15*). The mechanisms involved are described fully in Chapters 9 and 17.

Cytotoxic reactions and apoptosis – Cytotoxic reactions are effector systems directed against whole cells, that are in general too large for phagocytosis. The target cell may be recognized either by specific antibody bound to the cell surface, or by T cells using their specific TCRs. In cytotoxic reactions the attacking cells direct their granules towards the target cell, in contrast to phagocytosis where the contents are directed into the phagosome. The granules of cytotoxic T cells contain molecules called perforins which can punch holes in the outer membrane of the target. (In a similar way, antibody bound to the surface of a target cell can direct complement to make holes in its plasma membrane.) Some cytotoxic cells can also signal to the target cell to embark upon a programme of self-destruction – a process called apoptosis.

■ INFLAMMATION

The cells of the immune system are widely distributed throughout the body, but if an infection occurs it is necessary to concentrate them and their products at the site of infection. The process by which this occurs manifests itself as inflammation. Three major events occur during this response.

- Blood supply to the infected area is increased.
- Capillary permeability is increased due to retraction of the endothelial cells. This permits larger molecules than usual to escape from the capillaries, and thus allows the soluble mediators of immunity to reach the site of infection.
- Leucocytes migrate out of the venules into the surrounding tissues. In the earliest stages of inflammation, neutrophils are particularly prevalent, but in later stages monocytes and lymphocytes also migrate towards the site of infection.

Chemotaxis and cell migration – The process of cell migration is controlled by the adhesion of cells to the endothelium of inflamed tissues (pavementing). This occurs because molecules on the surface of the leucocytes interact with corresponding ones on the activated endothelium (*Fig. 1.16*).

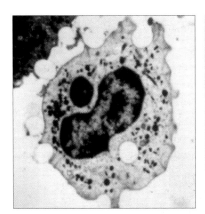

Fig. 1.14 Electronmicrograph study of phagocytosis. This micrograph shows a human phagocyte engulfing latex particles. ×3000 (Courtesy of Professor C. H. W. Horne.)

Phagocytosis

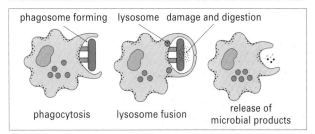

phagosome forming   lysosome   damage and digestion

phagocytosis   lysosome fusion   release of microbial products

Fig. 1.15 Phagocytes arrive at a site of inflammation by chemotaxis. They may then attach to microorganisms by way of their non-specific cell surface receptors. Alternatively, if the organism is opsonized with a fragment of the third complement component (C3b) and/or antibody, attachment will be through the phagocyte's receptors for C3b and/or Fc (see *Fig. 1.10*). If the phagocyte membrane now becomes activated, microbicidal oxygen metabolites are formed and the infectious agent is taken into a phagosome by pseudopodia extending around it. Once inside, lysosomes fuse with the phagosome to form a phagolysosome and the infectious agent is killed. Undigested microbial products may be released to the outside.

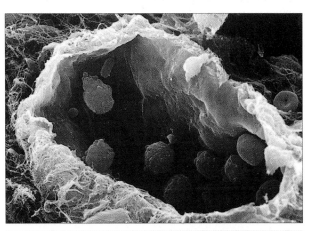

Fig. 1.16 Scanning electron micrograph showing leucocytes adhering to the wall of a venule in inflamed tissues. ×16 000. (Courtesy of Professor M. J. Karnovsky.)

Once in the tissues, cells migrate towards the site of infection by a process of chemical attraction known as chemotaxis.

Phagocytes will actively migrate up concentration gradients of certain (chemotactic) molecules. Particularly active is C5a, a fragment of one of the complement components (*Fig. 1.17*), which attracts both neutrophils and monocytes. When purified C5a is applied to the base of an ulcer *in vivo*, neutrophils can be seen sticking to the endothelium of nearby venules shortly afterwards. The cells then squeeze between the endothelial cells and move through the basement membrane of the microvessels to reach the tissues. The whole process is called diapedesis and is described more fully in Chapter 14.

■ DEFENCES AGAINST EXTRACELLULAR AND INTRACELLULAR PATHOGENS

It will be clear that there is a fundamental difference between immune responses to extracellular and intracellular pathogens. In dealing with extracellular pathogens, the immune system aims to destroy the pathogen itself and neutralize its products. In response to intracellular pathogens, there are two options. Either the T cells can destroy the infected cell – cytotoxicity – or they can activate the cell to deal with the pathogen for itself. This occurs, for example, when helper T cells release cytokines which activate macrophages to destroy organisms they have endocytosed.

Since many pathogens have both intracellular and extracellular phases of infection, different mechanisms are usually effective at different times. For example, the influenza virus travels through the blood stream to infect its target cells. Antibody is particularly effective at blocking this early phase of the infection. However, to clear an established infection, Tc cells must kill any cell that has become infected. Consequently, antibody is important in limiting the spread of infection, and preventing reinfection with the same virus, while Tc cells are essential to deal with infected cells (*Fig. 1.18*). These considerations play an important part in the development of effective vaccines.

Chemotaxis

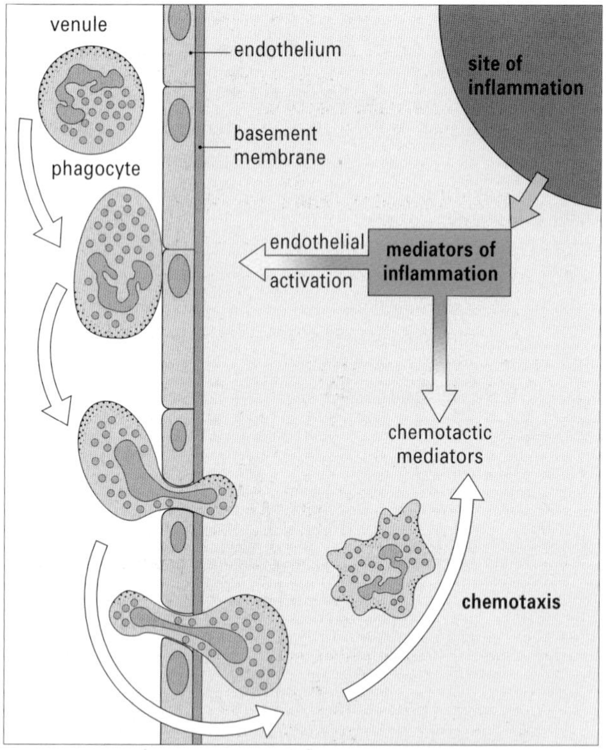

Fig. 1.17 At a site of inflammation, tissue damage and complement activation by the infectious agent cause the release of mediators of inflammation (e.g. C5a, a fragment of complement and one of the most important chemotactic peptides). These mediators diffuse to the adjoining venules, causing passing phagocytes to adhere to the endothelium. The phagocytes insert pseudopodia between the endothelial cells and dissolve the basement membrane. They then pass out of the blood vessels and move up the concentration gradient of the chemotactic mediators in the direction of the site of inflammation (chemotaxis).

Reaction to extracellular and intracellular pathogens

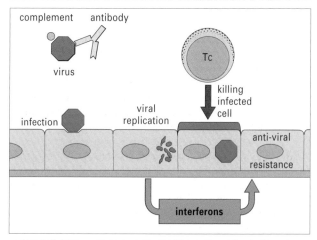

Fig. 1.18 Different immunological systems are effective against different types of infection, here illustrated as a virus infection. Antibodies and complement can block the extracellular phase of the life cycle, and promote phagocytosis of the virus. IFNs produced by infected cells can signal to uninfected cells, and induce a state of antiviral resistance in them. Viruses can only multiply within living cells; TC cells are effective at recognizing and destroying the infected cells before significant replication has occurred.

VACCINATION

One area in which immunological studies have had most immediate and successful application is in the field of vaccination. The principle of vaccination is based on two key elements of adaptive immunity, namely specificity and memory. Memory cells allow the immune system to mount a much stronger response on a second encounter with antigen. This secondary response is both faster to appear and more effective than the primary response.

The aim in vaccine development is to alter a pathogen or its toxins in such a way that they become innocuous without losing antigenicity. This is possible because antibodies and T cells recognize particular parts of antigens, the epitopes, and not the whole organism or toxin. Take, for example, vaccination against diphtheria. The diphtheria bacterium produces a toxin which destroys muscle cells. The toxin can be modified by formalin treatment so that it retains its epitopes but loses its toxicity; the resulting toxoid is used as a vaccine (*Fig. 1.19*). Whole infectious agents, such as the polio virus, can be attenuated so they retain their antigenicity but lose their pathogenicity.

Vaccination is discussed in more detail in Chapter 19.

IMMUNOPATHOLOGY

Up to this point, the immune system has been presented as an unimpeachable asset. It is certainly true that deficiencies in any part of the system leave the individual exposed to a greater risk of infection, although other parts of the system may partially compensate for such deficiencies. Clearly, strong evolutionary pressure from infectious microbes has lead to the development of the immune system in its present form. However, there are occasions when the immune system is itself a cause of disease or other undesirable consequences (*Fig. 1.20*).

In essence the system can fail in one of three ways.

Inappropriate reaction to self antigens: autoimmunity – Normally the immune system recognizes all foreign antigens and reacts against them, while recognizing the body's own tissues as 'self' and making no reaction against them. If the system reacts against self-components, autoimmune disease occurs. Examples of autoimmune disease are rheumatoid arthritis and pernicious anaemia (see Chapter 27).

Ineffective immune response: immunodeficiency – If any elements of the immune system are defective, the individual may not be able to fight infections adequately. These conditions are termed immunodeficiency. Some are hereditary deficiencies which start to manifest themselves shortly after birth, while others, such as acquired immunodeficiency syndrome (AIDS), develop later (see Chapter 21).

Overactive immune response: hypersensitivity – Sometimes immune reactions are out of all proportion to the damage that may be caused by a pathogen. The immune system may also mount a reaction to a harmless antigen, such as a food molecule. The immune reactions may cause more damage than the pathogen, or antigen, and in this case we speak of hypersensitivity (see Chapters 22–25). For example, molecules

Principle of vaccination

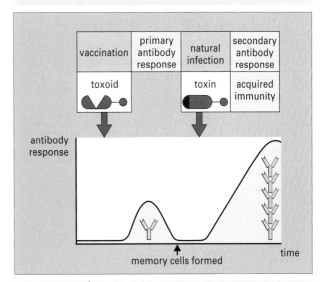

Fig. 1.19 The principle of vaccination is illustrated by immunization with diphtheria toxoid. Chemical modification of diptheria toxin produces a toxoid which has lost toxicity but retains its epitopes. Thus, a primary antibody response to these epitopes is produced following vaccination with toxoid. In a natural infection the toxin re-stimulates B memory cells, which produce the faster and more intense secondary antibody response to the epitope, so neutralizing the toxin.

Failure of the immune system

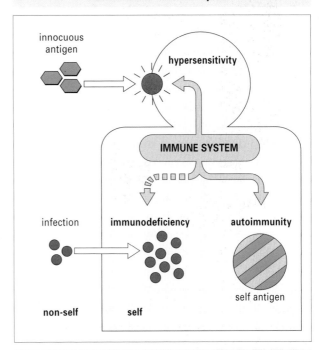

Fig. 1.20 There are three principal ways in which the immune system can fail – hypersensitivity, immunodeficiency and autoimmunity. The first two are due to an inappropriately large or small immune response, respectively. Autoimmunity is caused by a failure of self/non-self discrimination in immune recognition.

on the surface of pollen grains are recognized as antigens by particular individuals, generating the symptoms of hay fever or asthma.

Finally, there are occasions when the immune system acts normally, but the immune responses it produces are inconvenient in the context of modern medicine. The most important examples of this are in blood transfusion and graft rejection. In these cases it is necessary to match carefully the donor and recipient tissues so the immune system of the recipient does not attack the donated blood or graft tissue. These problems are, however, a small price to pay for an essential system of the body, which is absolutely vital to protect individuals against infection.

Critical Thinking

- Occasionally, individuals have a genetic defect that prevents their lymphocytes from developing. What effect do you think this would have?

- Why has the immune system evolved with so many different ways of dealing with pathogens?

- Individuals can make antibodies that do not recognize any known pathogen. What is the advantage of this?

- When we examine the immunological function of an individual, we often isolate lymphocytes or phagocytes from the blood. In simple terms, what are blood leucocytes actually doing?

CELLS INVOLVED IN THE IMMUNE RESPONSE

Many cells of different lineages are adapted to carry out specialized functions in the immune response.

B and T lymphocytes express specific antigen receptors and other surface molecules (markers) important for their different functions.

Antigen-presenting cells are required by T cells to enable them to respond to antigens. B lymphocytes recognize native antigens not processed and presented by other cells.

There are functional subpopulations of T lymphocytes which have helper, suppressor and cytotoxic activities.

New surface molecules appear on lymphocytes following activation by specific antigens.

Phagocytic cells with specific surface markers are found in the circulation (monocytes and granulocytes) and reside in tissues (e.g. Kupffer cells in the liver).

The cells of the immune system arise from pluripotent stem cells through two main lines of differentiation (*Fig. 2.1*):
- The lymphoid lineage produces lymphocytes.
- The myeloid lineage produces phagocytes (monocytes, macrophages and neutrophils) and other cells.

Lymphocytes can be T cells, B cells, or NK cells

The two main kinds of lymphocytes are called T cells and B cells. T cells develop from their precursors in the thymus, whereas mammalian B cells differentiate in the fetal liver and in the adult bone marrow. In birds, B cells differentiate in a uniquely avian organ, the bursa of Fabricius. These sites of lymphocyte differentiation are called the central or primary lymphoid organs. It is here that B- and T-cell precursors

acquire the ability to recognize antigens through the development of specific surface receptors.

A third population of lymphocytes do not express antigen receptors and are called natural killer (NK) cells. NK cells are derived from lymphoid cell progenitors in the bone marrow and can be functionally distinguished from T and B cells by their ability to lyse certain tumour cell lines (but not fresh tumours) *in vitro* without prior sensitization. These cells are morphologically large granular lymphocytes (LGLs).

Phagocytes can be monocytes/macrophages or polymorphonuclear granulocytes

The phagocytes are also of two basic kinds – monocytes/ macrophages and polymorphonuclear granulocytes. The latter

Origin of cells involved in the immune response

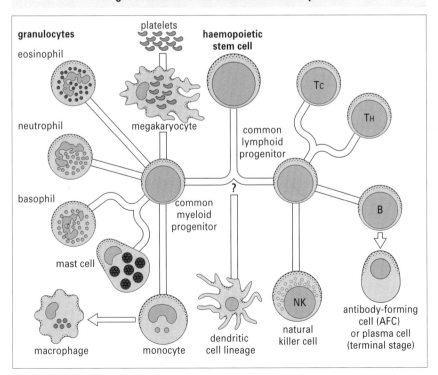

Fig. 2.1 All haemopoietic cells are derived from pluripotent stem cells which give rise to two main lineages; one for lymphoid cells and the other for myeloid cells. The common lymphoid progenitor has the capacity to differentiate into either T cells or B cells depending on the microenvironment to which it homes. In mammals, T cells develop in the thymus while B cells develop in the fetal liver and bone marrow. The precise origin of some antigen-presenting cells (APCs) is uncertain, although they do develop ultimately from the haemopoietic stem cells. NK cells also derive from the common lymphoid progenitor cell. The myeloid cells differentiate into the committed cells shown on the left. The collective name 'granulocyte' is used for eosinophils, neutrophils and basophils.

have a distinctive lobed, irregularly shaped (polymorphic) nucleus. They may be divided into neutrophils, basophils and eosinophils, on the basis of how the cytoplasmic granules respond to different types of staining agent when prepared for microscopy. The three types of cell also have distinct effector functions. The most numerous are the neutrophils, also called PMNs (polymorphonuclear neutrophils), which constitute the majority of leucocytes (white blood cells) in the bloodstream.

Accessory cells

In addition to lymphocytes and phagocytes, there are a number of accessory cells:
- Antigen-presenting cells (APCs) present antigen to T cells.
- Platelets are involved in blood clotting and inflammation.
- Mast cells have structural and functional similarities to basophil polymorphs.
- Endothelial cells express molecules capable of recognizing certain lymphocytes but not others, and thus control lymphocyte traffic and distribution.

■ LYMPHOCYTES

Lymphocytes are produced in the primary or central lymphoid organs (thymus and adult bone marrow) at a high rate (10^9 per day). Some of these cells migrate via the circulation into the secondary lymphoid tissues (the spleen, lymph nodes, tonsils, and mucosa-associated lymphoid tissue). The average human adult has about 10^{12} lymphoid cells and the lymphoid tissue as a whole represents about 2% of total body weight. Lymphoid cells represent about 20% of the leucocyte population in the adult circulation. Many mature lymphoid cells are long-lived, and may persist as memory cells for several years, or even for the lifetime of the individual.

Lymphocytes are morphologically heterogeneous

Lymphocytes in a conventional blood smear vary greatly both in size (6–10 μm in diameter) and morphology. Differences are seen in the nuclear to cytoplasmic ratio (N:C ratio), the nuclear shape, and the presence or absence of azurophilic granules.

Two distinct morphological types of resting lymphocytes can be distinguished in the circulation using light microscopy and a haematological stain such as Giemsa. The first is relatively small, is typically agranular and has a higher N:C ratio. The second type is larger, has a lower N:C ratio, contains intracytoplasmic azurophilic granules, and is known as the large granular lymphocyte (LGL). LGLs should not be confused with granulocytes (neutrophils, eosinophils and basophils) or with monocytes, which also have azurophilic granules (Fig. 2.2).

Resting blood T cells – These can show either of these morphological patterns. The majority (≥ 90%) of T helper (TH) cells and a proportion (≥ 65%) of cytotoxic T (TC) cells are of the smaller type (non-granular with a high N:C ratio). They also carry a cytoplasmic structure termed the 'Gall body', which consists of a cluster of primary lysosomes associated with a lipid droplet. The Gall body is easily identified by lysosomal enzyme cytochemistry and electron microscopy (Fig. 2.3).

The other morphological pattern is shown by up to 10% of TH cells and 35% of TC cells. These display LGL morphology, with primary lysosomes dispersed in the cytoplasm and a well-developed Golgi apparatus (Fig. 2.4).

The gamma/delta (γδ) or TCR-1+ lymphocyte population is another subset of T cells with LGL characteristics. These cells display a dendritic morphology in the lymphoid tissues (Fig. 2.5); when cultured *in vitro* they may adhere to the substrate, showing a variety of morphological changes (Fig. 2.6).

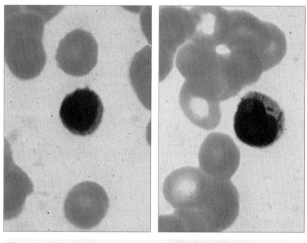

Fig. 2.2 Morphological heterogeneity of lymphocytes.
Left: The small lymphocyte has no granules, a round nucleus and a high N:C ratio. **Right:** The large granular lymphocyte has a lower N:C ratio, indented nucleus and azurophilic granules in the cytoplasm. Giemsa stain, ×1000.

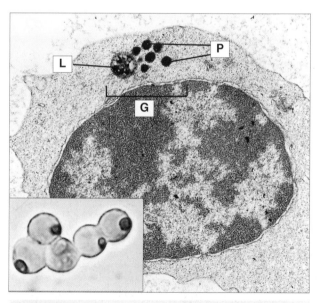

Fig. 2.3 Ultrastructure of a non-granular T cell. This electronmicrograph shows the Gall body (G) that is characteristic of the majority of resting T cells. It consists of primary lysosomes (P) and a lipid droplet (L). ×10 500. **Inset:** This structure is also seen as a single 'spot' following staining for non-specific esterases in light microscopy. ×400.

Resting blood B cells – These do not display Gall bodies or LGL morphology and their cytoplasm is predominantly occupied by scattered single ribosomes (*Fig. 2.7*). Occasionally, activated B cells are found with developing rough endoplasmic reticulum (*Fig. 2.8*).

NK cells – Like γδ T cells and some Tc cells, these are characterized by LGL morphology. They do, however, display a larger number of azurophilic granules than do granular T cells.

Lymphocytes can be identified by characteristic markers

Lymphocytes (and other leucocytes) express a large number of different molecules on their surfaces which can be used to distinguish ('mark') cell populations. Many of these cell markers can now be identified by specific monoclonal antibodies. A systematic nomenclature called the CD system has been developed, in which the term CD (cluster designation) refers to groups (clusters) of monoclonal antibodies, each cluster binding specifically to a particular cell marker. The CD system derives from analysis of monoclonal antibodies (mAb), produced mainly in mice, against human leucocyte antigens. The work is carried out in a number of laboratories worldwide, and a series of International Workshops determine the patterns of mAb binding on different leucocyte populations, and the molecular weights of the markers. Monoclonal antibodies with similar characteristics, defined by these criteria, are grouped together and given a CD number. However, it is now customary to use the CD number to indicate the marker molecule recognized by each group of monoclonal antibodies. (A list of CD markers is given in the Appendix.)

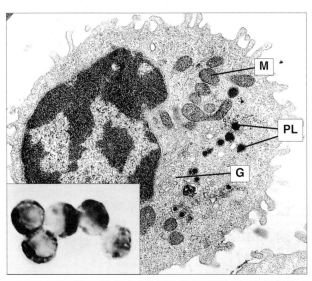

Fig. 2.4 Ultrastructure of T cells with granular morphology. These cells characteristically have electron-dense peroxidase-negative granules (primary lysosomes [PL]). These granules are dispersed in the cytoplasm with some close to the well-developed Golgi apparatus (G). There are many mitochondria (M) present. ×10 000. **Inset:** Cytochemical staining for acid phosphatase shows a granular pattern of staining under light microscopy. ×400.

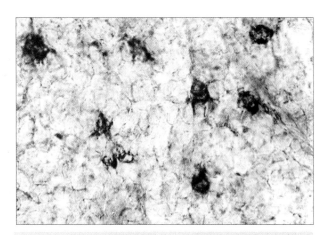

Fig. 2.5 Dendritic morphology of γδ TCR-1⁺ cells in the tonsil. This T-cell population is predominantly localized in the interfollicular T-cell-dependent zones in the lamina propria, and within the surface epithelium. Note the dendritic morphology of the cells. Anti-TCR-1 mAb and immunoperoxidase, ×900. (Courtesy of Dr A. Favre, from *Eur J Immunol* 1991:**21**;173, with permission.)

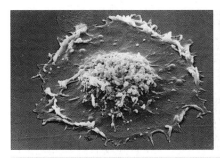 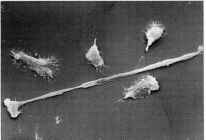 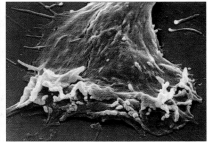

Fig. 2.6 Morphological changes in cloned γδ T cells *in vitro*. Left: Cells adhere to the substrate in a similar way to macrophages. ×6000. **Centre:** The cells become elongated with uropod formation, extending two polar filopodia. ×6000. **Right:** Adhesion plaques are formed at the terminal ends of the filopodia. ×20 000. (Courtesy of Dr G. Arancia and Dr W. Malorni, from *Eur J Immunol* 1991:**21**;173, with permission.)

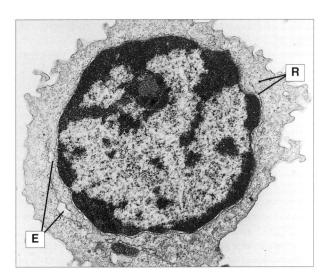

Fig. 2.7 Ultrastructure of a resting B cell. These cells have no Gall body or granules. Scattered ribosomes (R) and isolated profiles of rough endoplasmic reticulum (E) are seen in the cytoplasm. Development of the Golgi lysosomal system in the B cell occurs only on activation. ×11 500.

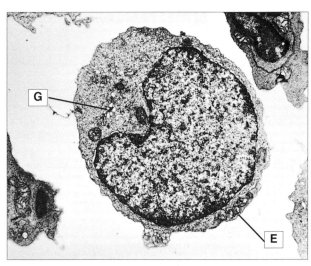

Fig. 2.8 The ultrastructure of a B-cell blast. The main feature of activated B cells is the development of the machinery for immunoglobulin synthesis. This includes rough endoplasmic reticulum (E), free polyribosomes and the Golgi apparatus (G), which is involved in glycosylation of the immunoglobulins. ×7 500.

Molecular markers can be further defined according to the information they offer about the cell. For example:

- Lineage markers are exclusive to a particular cell line, e.g. CD3, which is found only on T cells.
- Maturation markers are transiently expressed during cell differentiation, e.g. CD1, which is only found on cells developing in the thymus and is not present on peripheral T cells.
- Activation markers, e.g. the low affinity T-cell growth factor receptor (IL-2 receptor, CD25), which is only expressed when the cell is stimulated by antigen.

Although it is sometimes useful to define markers in this way, it is not always possible to do so. A maturation marker for one lineage is sometimes an activation marker for another. For example, B cells express MHC class II antigens during most of their lifetime, but human T cells only express these molecules following activation. Furthermore, 'activation' markers may already be present at low density on cells, which increase following activation. An example of this is CD11a (LFA-1) on monocytes.

Cell markers can be grouped into 'families'

Cell surface molecules exist as a number of different families which probably originate, in evolutionary terms, from a few ancestral genes. These families include the following major groups:

- The immunoglobulin superfamily contains molecules whose structural characteristics are similar to those of the immunoglobulins. This family includes CD2, CD3, CD4, CD8, murine Thy-1, and many more.
- The integrin family consists of heterodimeric molecules containing α and β chains. There are a number of integrin subfamilies; all members of a particular subfamily share a common β chain, but each has a unique α chain.

One subfamily (the β_2 integrins) uses CD18 as the β chain. This chain can be associated with CD11a, CD11b or CD11c – these combinations make up the lymphocyte function antigen LFA-1, Mac-1 (CR3) and p150,95 (CR4) surface molecules respectively – and are commonly found on leucocytes. A second subfamily (the β_1 integrins) has CD29 as the β chain, again associated with various other polypeptides, and includes the VLA (very late activation) markers.

- Selectins (E, L and P), expressed on leucocytes (L) or activated endothelial cells (E and P). They have lectin-like specificity for a variety of sugars expressed on heavily glycosylated membrane glycoproteins.
- Proteoglycans, typically CD44, which can bind to components of extracellular matrix.

Surface molecules (markers) may be demonstrated using fluorescent antibodies as probes (*Fig. 2.9*). This is exploited by the technique of flow cytometry, which can enumerate and separate cells on the basis of their size and fluorescence intensity (see Chapter 28), and which has revolutionized studies on lymphoid cell populations.

T cells

T cells can be distinguished by their different antigen receptors

Historically, human T cells were distinguished from B cells by their fortuitous ability to bind to sheep erythrocytes. (This is now known to be identified as the CD2 molecule on T cells.) However, the definitive T-cell lineage marker is the T-cell antigen receptor (TCR). There are presently two defined types of TCR; TCR-2 is a heterodimer of two disulphide-linked polypeptides (α and β); TCR-1 is structurally similar but consists of γ and δ polypeptides. Both receptors are associated with a set of five polypeptides, the CD3 complex, to

Immunofluorescent demonstration of T-cell markers

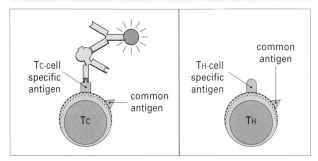

Fig. 2.9 Mouse antibodies directed towards a T-cell subset-specific antigen on a T cytotoxic (Tc) cell will bind to such cells, but not to T helper (TH) cells. The bound antibody is detected using antibodies to mouse immunoglobulin coupled to a fluorescent molecule. This provides a method for identifying and counting T-cell subsets.

give the T-cell receptor complex (TCR–CD3 complex; see Chapter 5). Approximately 90–95% of blood T cells express TCR-2(α,β), and the remaining 5–10% are TCR-1$^+$(γ,δ).

TCR-2$^+$ T cells are further distinguished by their expression of CD4 or CD8

TCR-2$^+$ T cells can be subdivided into two distinct non-overlapping populations: a subset which carries the CD4 marker and mainly 'helps' or 'induces' immune responses (TH), and a subset which carries the CD8 marker and is predominantly cytotoxic (Tc). Since CD4$^+$ T cells recognize their specific antigens in association with MHC class II molecules, whereas CD8$^+$ T cells recognize antigens in association with MHC class I molecules (See Chapter 5), the presence of CD4 or CD8 limits (restricts) the types of cell with which the T cells can interact. Most circulating TCR-1$^+$ cells do not express either the CD4 or the CD8 marker, although a few of them may be CD8$^+$.

There are functional subsets of TCR-2$^+$ CD4$^+$ cells

The CD4 set has been functionally divided into two further subsets:

- T cells that positively influence the response of T cells and B cells (the helper cell function) are CD29$^+$. Practically all the cells in this population also express a low molecular weight isoform of the CD45 leucocyte common antigen designated CD45R0.
- Cells that induce the suppressor/cytotoxic functions of CD8$^+$ cells (the suppressor/inducer function) express a different isoform of the CD45 molecule, designated CD45RA.

Over the last five years, CD45RA$^+$ and CD45R0$^+$ TH cells have been designated 'naïve' and 'memory' cells respectively. However, current opinion holds that the expression of CD45R0/CD29 by CD4$^+$ TH cells is more relevant to the state of activation of the cell.

TCR-2$^+$ CD4$^+$ lymphocytes can also be classified on the basis of cytokine secretion

Functional diversity of T cells has also been demonstrated by analysis of TH clones for cytokine secretion patterns. In mice, and in man, two groups of CD4$^+$ T-cell clones have been found. The TH1 subset secretes IL-2 and IFNγ, and the TH2 subset produces IL-4, IL-5, IL-6 and IL-10 (see Chapter 8). TH1 cells mediate several functions associated with cytotoxicity and local inflammatory reactions. Consequently these cells are important for combating intracellular pathogens, including viruses, bacteria and parasites. TH2 cells are more effective at stimulating B cells to proliferate and produce antibodies, and therefore function primarily to protect against free-living microorganisms (humoral immunity).

Other criteria have been used to subdivide the CD4$^+$ set. For example, one rare subset of CD4$^+$ cells expresses NK cell markers, does not produce the lymphokine IL-2, and does not proliferate in response to antigens and mitogens.

There are subsets of CD8$^+$ cells

CD8$^+$ (cytotoxic) T cells can also be subdivided into specific functional subsets according to a number of criteria and using a variety of monoclonal antibodies.

One subset expresses CD28 molecules and produces IL-2 in response to activation signals. Another subset responds to (but does not produce) IL-2 and expresses the heterodimeric CD11b/CD18 molecule. Interestingly, cells of the first subset have a distinct Gall body whereas cells of the second subset show LGL morphology. Granule contents are known to be involved in the cytotoxic function of both T cells and NK cells, but the function of the Gall body is not known.

TCR-1$^+$ T cells are relatively enriched in epidermal and mucosal surfaces

TCR-1$^+$ T cells are most abundant in the mucosal epithelia, and form only a minor subpopulation of circulating T cells. The majority of intraepithelial lymphocytes (IELs) are TCR-1$^+$ in mice and express CD8, a marker that is not found on most circulating TCR-1$^+$ cells. It has recently been shown that TCR-1$^+$ CD8$^+$ cells have a repertoire of T-cell receptors biased towards bacterial antigens, and current opinion is that these cells may play an important role in protecting the mucosal surfaces of the body. Recently, a small subset of double negative (CD4$^-$ CD8$^-$) cells expressing TCR-2 has also been described.

Division of the TCR-, CD4- and CD8-bearing cells into different functional subsets is shown in *Figures 2.10 and 2.11*.

T cells share some markers with other cell lineages

So far we have described the cell markers and antigen-specific receptors which define T-cell subsets. There are also a number of surface molecules, expressed on all T cells (pan T-cell markers), which are found on cells of other lineages. The receptors for sheep erythrocytes (CD2) are a good example. Under normal circumstances, *in vivo* the CD2 molecule, together with the TCR–CD3 complex and other membrane-bound glycoproteins, help to activate T cells by binding to the appropriate ligand. However, CD2 is also found on about 75% of CD3$^-$ NK cells. Another molecule, involved in T-cell activation, CD5, is expressed on all T cells and on a

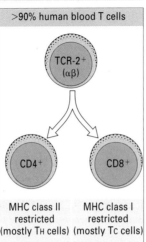

Major T-cell subsets

<10% human blood T cells	>90% human blood T cells

Fig. 2.10 T cells can be subdivided into different subsets based on the expression of one or other T cell receptor (TCR-1 or TCR-2). TCR-1⁺ cells are thought to have a restricted repertoire and to be mainly non-MHC restricted. TCR-2⁺ cells express either CD4 or CD8, which determines whether they see antigen in association with MHC class II or MHC class I molecules.

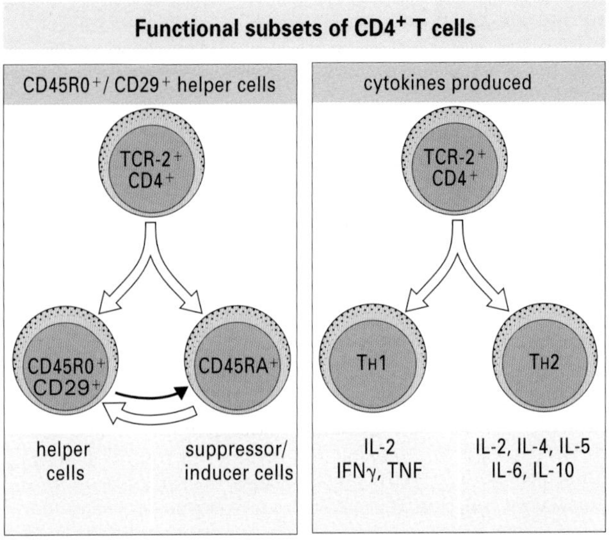

Functional subsets of CD4⁺ T cells

CD45R0⁺/ CD29⁺ helper cells	cytokines produced

Fig. 2.11 MHC class II restricted T cells have been divided into subsets on the basis of expression of isoforms of the CD45 and CD29 molecules (**left**). In addition, they can be subdivided into TH1 and TH2 populations based on their profiles of cytokine production (**right**).

subpopulation of B cells. Although CD5 can bind to CD72, it is debated whether this is the physiological ligand. CD7 is present on the majority of NK cells. A complete list of CD molecules on T cells, some of which are shared by other haemopoietic cells, is given in the Appendix.

Murine T cells express markers similar to those detected on human T cells. All murine T cells carry a molecule, Thy-1 or θ, with a molecular weight of 19–35 kDa; a human equivalent has been described but little studied.

Suppressor T cells

Although there is clear evidence for the existence of antigen-specific suppressor T cells (Ts), it is unlikely that they represent a functionally separate subset. There is evidence that both CD4⁺ and CD8⁺ T cells can suppress immune responses; this might operate through direct cytotoxicity of antigen-presenting cells , through 'suppressive' cytokines (see Chapter 8) or via the idiotype network.

A summary of major TCR-2⁺ cell markers in man and mouse is shown in *Figure 2.12*.

B cells

B cells are characterized by their surface immunoglobulins

B lymphocytes represent about 5–15% of the circulating lymphoid pool, and are classically defined by the presence of surface immunoglobulins. These immunoglobulin markers are made by the cells themselves, and are inserted into the surface membrane where they act as specific antigen receptors. The receptors can be detected on the surface of mature cells using fluorochrome-labelled antibodies specific for immunoglobulin of the species under investigation. Staining of cells in the cold results in the detection of the fluorescence

with a 'ring-like' (or patchy) appearance over the B cell (*Fig. 2.13*). Divalent antibodies to the surface immunoglobulin attach to and cross-link the surface receptors, producing 'patches' of immunoglobulin on the cell surface. When the cells are warmed up, most of these complexes are actively swept along the cell surface and are seen as a 'cap' over one pole of the cell (see *Fig. 2.13*). Capping is followed by

Surface markers of human and murine T cells

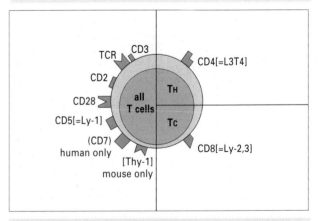

Fig. 2.12 The molecule CD7 has thus far only been detected in man, while Thy-1 is specific for the mouse. Other markers in square brackets are mouse equivalents of human markers. Most of these molecules belong to the immunoglobulin superfamily of adhesion molecules.

internalization and degradation of the immunoglobulin. Capping may also be seen with other surface glycoproteins, both on B cells and other cell types.

'B-cell receptor' complex
The majority of human B cells in peripheral blood express two immunoglobulin isotypes on their surface, IgM and IgD (see Chapter 4). On any given B cell, the antigen-binding sites of these isotypes are identical. Very few cells in the circulation express IgG, IgA or IgE, although these are present in larger numbers in specific locations in the body, for example, IgA-bearing cells in the intestinal mucosa. The surface IgM is associated with other molecules on the B cell surface to form the 'B-cell antigen receptor complex '(BCR). These 'accessory' molecules consist of disulphide-bonded heterodimers of Igα (CD79a, a 34 kDa molecule and product of the *mb*-1 gene) and Igβ (CD79b, a 39kDa molecule and product of the B29 gene). The heterodimers interact with the transmembrane segments of IgM and, like the separate molecular components of the TCR–CD3 complex, are involved in cellular activation.

Other B-cell markers and subsets
A number of other markers are expressed by both mouse and human B cells (*Fig. 2.14*). The majority of B cells carry MHC class II antigens, which are important for cooperative interactions with T cells. These class II molecules consist of I–A or I–E in the mouse and HLA-DP, DQ and DR antigens in man. Complement receptors for C3b (CR1, CD35) and C3d (CR2, CD21) are commonly found on B cells and are associated with activation and possibly 'homing' of the cells. Fc receptors for exogenous IgG (FcγRII, CD32) are also present, and play a role in negative signalling to the B cell.

CD19, CD20 and CD22 are the main markers currently used to identify human B cells. Other molecules that identify human B cells are CD72-78. The CD72 molecule has also been described for murine B cells (Lyb-2) together with B220, a high molecular weight (220 kDa) isoform of CD45 (Lyb-5). CD40 is an important molecule on B cells, and is involved in cognate interactions between T and B cells (see *Fig. 8.5*)

A marker originally found only on T cells (Ly1, CD5) has now been shown to be present on some B cells; it identifies a subset of B cells that is predisposed to autoantibody production. These cells (termed B1a cells) are found predominantly in the peritoneal cavity in mice, and there is some evidence for a separate differentiation pathway from 'conventional' B cells (B2 cells).

Some human B cells bind to (and form rosettes with) mouse erythrocytes (ME-R). This property, together with expression of the CD5 molecule, identifies a subset whose immunoglobulin repertoire is biased towards autoantigens including DNA, Fc of IgG, phospholipids and cytoskeletal components.

Natural killer (NK) cells
Natural killer (NK) cells account for up to 15% of blood lymphocytes and express neither TCR nor BCR antigen receptors.

Phenotypic markers of NK cells
Most surface antigens detectable on NK cells by monoclonal antibodies are shared with T cells or monocytes/macrophages. The major markers of human NK cells and their shared specificities are shown in *Figure 2.15*. Monoclonal antibodies to CD16 (FcγRIII) are commonly used to identify NK cells in purified lymphocyte populations. CD16 is involved in one of

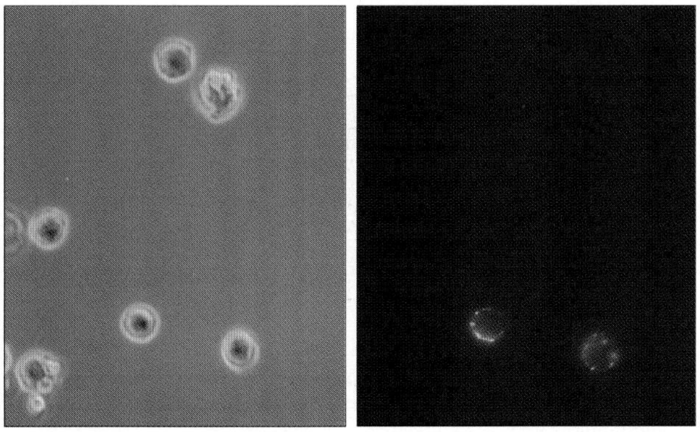

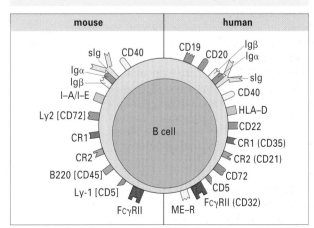

Surface markers of human and murine peripheral B cells

Fig. 2.14 Many of these molecules are homologous; they are shown in the same colour. Human equivalents to the mouse molecules are given in square brackets ([ ]). B220 was previously designated Lyb-5. Igα and Igβ chains associate with the surface immunoglobulin (sIg) to form the B-cell receptor complex. The CD numbers follow in brackets.

Fig. 2.13 B cells stained for surface immunoglobulin. Human blood B cells stained in the cold with fluoresceinated anti-human immunoglobulin show a patchy surface fluorescence viewed under ultraviolet light (**right**). Under phase contrast light microscopy (**left**) it can be seen that only 2 out of 6 in this field are B cells. The lower cell shows 'capping' of the fluorescent antibody.

Surface markers of human NK cells

marker	shared specificities
CD16 (FcγRIII)	minority of T cells, granulocytes, some macrophages
CD11b	granulocytes, monocytes, some T cells
CD38*	activated T cells, plasma cells, haemopoietic precursors
CD2*	all T cells
CD7	all T cells
CD8*	some T cells
CD56	minority of T cells
CD57	some T cells
IL-2R (β chain, p70)	activated T cells
p58 family	some T cells
CD94	some T cells
*expressed on 10–80% of NK cells.	

Fig. 2.15 None of these markers are lineage-specific.

Surface markers of murine NK cells

marker	shared specificities
Thy-1*	T cells
Lyb-5 (B220)	B cells
NK1	–
NK2	–
FcγRIII*	some T cells, granulocytes, some monocytes/macrophages
Asialo-GM1	–
CR3 (CD11b, MAC-1)	granulocytes, monocytes
Ly49	T cells
*expressed on some but not all murine NK cells	

Fig. 2.16 Although some molecules are shared by other cell types, some lineage-specific markers have been defined.

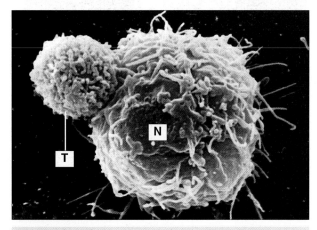

Fig. 2.17 An NK cell (N) attached to a target cell (T).
×4500. (Courtesy of Dr G. Arancia and K. Malorni, Rome.)

the activation pathways of NK cells, and is also expressed by neutrophils, some macrophages and some (mainly TCR-1⁺) T cells. On granulocytes, CD16 is linked to the surface membrane by a phosphatidylinositol glycan (PIG) linkage, whereas NK and TCR-1⁺ T cells express the transmembrane form of the molecule. The CD56 molecule, a homophilic adhesion molecule of the immunoglobulin superfamily, is another important marker of NK cells. The absence of CD3, but the presence of CD56 and/or CD16, is currently in use as a definitive marker for NK cells in man.

Resting NK cells also express the α chain of the IL-2 receptor, an intermediate affinity receptor of 70 kDa. Therefore, direct stimulation with IL-2 results in activation of NK cells. Interestingly, this 70 kDa receptor is also expressed on all T cells that display LGL morphology, namely TCR-1⁺ cells and a proportion of TCR-2⁺ CD8⁺ cells. All of these cells respond to IL-2 by acquiring non-specific cytotoxic functions, and are known collectively as lymphokine activated killer (LAK) cells. LAK cells kill fresh tumour cells and a broader spectrum of neoplastic targets in comparison to those lysed by resting NK cells.

A distinctive difference between human and murine NK cells is the presence in mouse cells of fewer, but much larger, azurophilic granules. A summary of phenotypic markers of murine NK cells is shown in *Figure 2.16.*

Functions of NK cells

The physiological function of NK cells is to recognize and kill certain tumour cells (*Fig. 2.17*) and virus-infected cells. The mechanism of this recognition is not fully understood. However, at least three families of apparently clonally-distributed surface molecules are known to be involved in protecting self cells from the cytotoxic action of NK cells. For example, the ligands of the p58 family are HLA-C gene products; engagement of these molecules by the NK cell receptor results in inhibition of self-cytotoxicity and protection of carrier cells. Modification of these HLA-C gene products by viruses or tumour-associated molecules (e.g. oncogene products) could prevent recognition by NK cells, leaving the aberrant cell vulnerable to attack.

NK cells are also able to bind and kill targets coated with IgG antibodies via their receptor for IgG (FcγRIII:CD16). This property is referred to as antibody-dependent cellular cytotoxicity (ADCC).

NK cells release interferon-γ (IFNγ) and other cytokines (e.g. IL-1 and GM–CSF) when activated, which may be important in the regulation of haemopoiesis and immune responses.

Activation of B and T cells

T and B cells are activated on binding their specific antigens. T cells need to 'see' antigen in the context of MHC molecules on antigen-presenting cells, whereas B cells can bind to free antigens, but generally need T-cell help to become activated. In addition to specific ligation of the antigen receptors on T and B cells, engagement of other surface molecules is required for effective T- and B-cell activation (see Chapter 8). Antigen-induced activation and proliferation normally occurs in the lymphoid tissues and can be visualized *in vitro* by culturing lymphocytes with an activating agent. Possible agents include:

- Antigen recognized by the surface antigen receptors.
- Monoclonal antibodies to CD3-TCR or to one of the epitopes of CD2.
- Lectins.

Lectins are carbohydrate-binding proteins derived from plants and bacteria. Some are able to activate lymphocytes by cross-linking the BCRs or TCRs, and are known as mitogens (proliferation-inducers). Mitogen stimulation of lymphocytes *in vitro* is believed to mimic stimulation by specific antigens fairly closely. T and B cells are activated by different mitogens. Phytohaemagglutinin (PHA) and Concanavalin A (Con-A) stimulate human and mouse T cells. Lipopolysaccharide (LPS) stimulates mouse B cells, while pokeweed mitogen (PWM) stimulates both human T cells and B cells (*Fig. 2.18*).

The use of these agents *in vitro* has shown that activation of T and B cells leads to the production of cytokines and cytokine receptors, which together drive the selected clones through their life cycle (proliferation) and ultimately to maturation and the production of effector or memory cells (see *Fig. 1.14* and *1.20*). The memory cells recirculate and ultimately lodge in the T- or B-dependent areas of lymphoid tissues where they remain, ready to respond if the same antigen is encountered again.

The activation signal is transmitted by 'second messengers'

The interaction of a resting lymphocyte with an antigen triggers a number of early biochemical events which result in the generation of 'second messengers' within the B cell or T cell. These messengers are responsible for changes at the level of the cell's DNA. Both T and B cells utilize a GTP-dependent component (or G-protein) to induce these signalling reactions, which work by stimulating phosphatidylinositol metabolism. This reaction generates two secondary messengers, inositol 1,4,5-trisphosphate (IP_3) and diacylglycerol. IP_3 triggers the release of Ca^{2+} from internal stores, and diacly-glycerol activates protein kinase C. Together with other kinases, protein kinase C phosphorylates a number of surface molecules leading to activation of specific genes. Soon after engagement of T lymphocytes with antigen, a number of surface molecules such as gp39 and receptors for cytokines such as IL-2, are expressed. Interaction with these molecules results in proliferation and maturation of the lymphocytes.

B-cell differentiation leads to the formation of plasma cells and memory cells

Following T- and B-cell activation by mitogen or antigen, distinctive differentiation features are observed at the ultrastructural level (see *Figs 2.8* and *2.19*). Ultimately, many B cell blasts mature into antibody-forming cells (AFCs), which progress *in vivo* to terminally differentiated plasma cells. Some B blasts do not develop rough endoplasmic reticulum cisternae. These cells are found in germinal centres and are named follicle centre cells or centroblasts and centrocytes. It seems more than likely that these are the B memory cells whose existence is inferred from the ability of the immune system to develop lasting immunity (*Fig. 2.20*).

Under light microscopy, the cytoplasm of the plasma cells is basophilic; this is due to the large amount of RNA being utilized for antibody synthesis in the rough endoplasmic reticulum (*Fig. 2.21*). At the ultrastructural level, the rough endoplasmic reticulum can often be seen in parallel arrays (*Fig. 2.22*). Plasma cells are seldom seen in the circulation, as they comprise less than 0.1% of the total lymphocyte population. They are normally restricted to the secondary lymphoid organs and tissues. Antibodies produced by a single plasma cell are of one specificity and immunoglobulin class. Immunoglobulins can be visualized in the plasma cell cytoplasm by staining with fluorochrome-labelled specific antibodies (*Fig. 2.23*). Plasma cells have a short life span, surviving for a few days only; they die from apoptosis (*Fig. 2.24*).

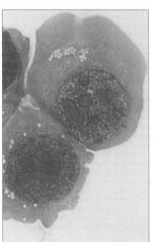
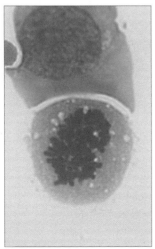

Fig. 2.18 Mitogen/antigen-induced lymphocyte blastogenesis. The human T cells and B cells shown here have been stimulated by pokeweed mitogen. **Left**: There is increased basophilia in the cytoplasm and an increase in the cell volume. **Right**: The chromosomes condense during cell division, and can be clearly seen during metaphase. Giemsa stain, ×2000.

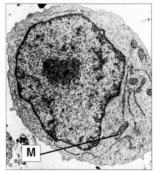
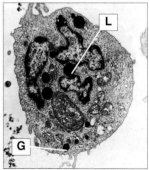

Fig. 2.19 The ultrastructure of T-cell blasts. T-cell blasts, developing after antigen or mitogen stimulation, are large cells with extended cytoplasm containing a variety of organelles, including mitochondria (M) and free polyribosomes. The blasts may be agranular (**left**) or granular (**right**) depending on the presence or absence of electron-dense granules (G). Note also the lipid droplets (L) in the granular blast. Studies on T-cell clones (i.e. populations derived from single activated cells) have shown that in humans all cytotoxic clones are granular. Studies in the mouse have shown that both cytotoxic and suppressor clones are granular, whereas those clones without these functions are agranular. ×3200.

Activation markers on lymphocytes

Activation of T and B cells triggers the *de novo* expression of certain surface molecules and also enhances the expression of others.

These activation markers include adhesion molecules, which allow a more efficient interaction with other cells, and receptors for growth and differentiation factors, required for continued cell proliferation and differentiation. For example, the IL-2 receptor (IL-2R) that is expressed following T cell activation is composed of three subunits. Resting T cells have the β unit, a low-affinity receptor of 55 kDa (CD25), and the γ unit; on activation the α subunit (70 kDa) is induced resulting in a heterotrimeric high affinity IL-2 receptor. The gp39 molecule is transiently induced on activated T cells, as are receptors for transferrin (CD71, important for proliferation), CD38 and CD69 are also expressed. These markers appear in the early phase of T-cell ontogeny, but disappear during intrathymic development (see Chapter 10). Class II MHC molecules are present on human T cells as late activation markers, but are absent from murine T cells. CD29 is expressed as a very late activation marker on T cells and by the cells designated as 'memory cells'. The memory function of the CD4⁺CD29⁺ cell population might therefore be explained as an activation-induced increase in various adhesion molecules, which facilitates interaction with other cells should the animal encounter the antigen again.

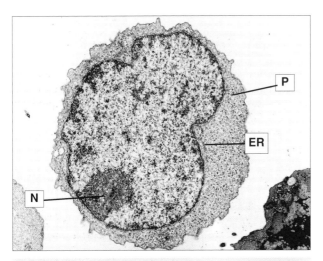

Fig. 2.20 A small follicle centre cell. This shows extended cytoplasm largely occupied by polyribosomes (P) and a few strands of rough endoplasmic reticulum (ER) but no stacks of cisternae (parallel arrays of ER). Note the large eccentric nucleolus (N) adjacent to the nuclear envelope. This cell, which may correspond to the memory B cell, is also seen as a tumour cell in certain lymphomas. ×8500.

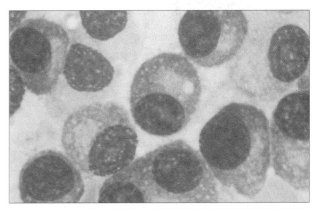

Fig. 2.21 Morphology of the plasma cell. The mature plasma cell has an eccentric nucleus and a large amount of basophilic cytoplasm, which is due to the abundant RNA required for protein synthesis. May–Grünwald–Giemsa stain, ×1500.

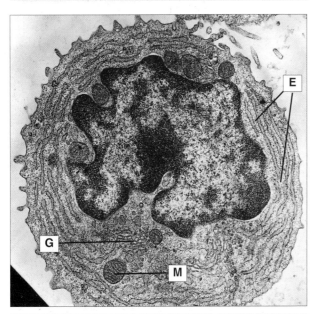

Fig. 2.22 The ultrastructure of the plasma cell. The plasma cell is characterized by parallel arrays of rough endoplasmic reticulum (E). In mature cells, these cisternae become dilated with immunoglobulins. Mitochondria (M) and a well-developed Golgi apparatus (G) are also seen. ×9500.

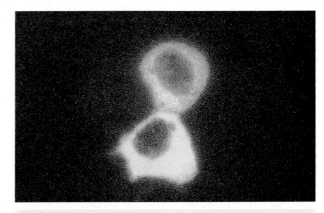

Fig. 2.23 The immunofluorescent staining of intracytoplasmic immunoglobulin in plasma cells. Fixed human plasma cells, treated with fluoresceinated anti-human–IgM (green) and rhodaminated anti-human–IgG (red) show extensive intracytoplasmic staining. As the distinct staining of the two cells shows, plasma cells normally only manufacture one class or subclass (isotype) of antibody. ×3000.

Activation markers on B cells include the high affinity IL-2R, and other receptors for growth and differentiation factors such as IL-3, IL-4, IL-5 and IL-6 (see Chapter 9). These receptors have all been cloned and sequenced. Transferrin receptors (CD71) and elevated levels of membrane class II MHC molecules are also detected. CD23 (FcεRII, a low-affinity IgE

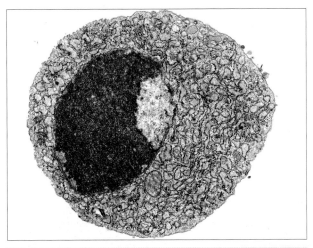

Fig. 2.24 Plasma cell death by apoptosis. Plasma cells are short-lived and then die by apoptosis (cell suicide). Note the nuclear chromatin changes, which are characteristic for apoptosis.

receptor) is present on murine and human activated B cells and is involved in driving B cells into proliferation. CD38, although not present on mature human B cells, is found on terminally differentiated plasma cells (as well as in the very early stages of B-cell development). PCA-1 molecules are only found at the plasma cell stage of human B-cell differentiation. Memory cells within the germinal centres of secondary follicles (see Chapter 10) do not express surface IgD or CD22.

Activation markers of NK cells include the class II MHC molecules.

MONONUCLEAR PHAGOCYTES

The mononuclear phagocyte system has two main functions, performed by two different types of bone-marrow derived cells:
- 'Professional' phagocytic macrophages, whose predominant role is to remove particulate antigens.
- Antigen-presenting cells (APCs), whose role is to take up, process and present antigen to T cells.

The network of phagocytic tissue macrophages, together with endothelial cells and polymorphs, was previously termed 'the reticuloendothelial system' (RES).
Phagocytic macrophages are found in many organs (*Fig. 2.25*) and can be visualized subsequent to intravenous injection of

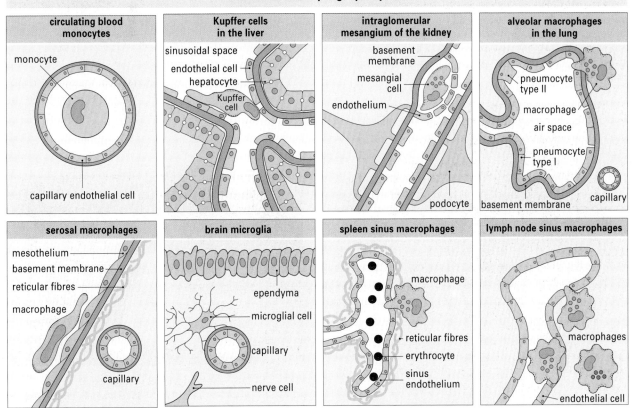

Fig. 2.25 The mononuclear phagocyte system includes blood monocytes, and phagocytes resident in tissues or fixed to the endothelial layer of blood capillaries. In the liver these resident macrophages are known as Kupffer cells, while in the kidney they are called the intraglomerular mesangial cells. Alveolar and serosal (e.g. peritoneal) macrophages are examples of 'wandering' macrophages. Brain microglia are cells which enter the brain around the time of birth and differentiate into fixed cells.

carbon particles which then become localized in these tissues This is shown in *Figure 2.26*.

Myeloid progenitor cells in the bone marrow differentiate into promonocytes and then into blood monocytes (see Chapter 10). Cells from this circulating pool migrate through the blood-vessel walls into the various organs and tissue systems to become macrophages. The human blood monocyte is large (10–18 μm diameter) relative to the lymphocyte. It usually has a horseshoe-shaped nucleus and often contains faint azurophilic granules (*Fig. 2.27*). Ultrastructurally, the monocyte possesses ruffled membranes, a well-developed Golgi complex and many intracytoplasmic lysosomes (*Fig. 2.28*). These lysosomes contain peroxidase and several acid hydrolases which are important in intracellular killing of microorganisms.

Monocytes/macrophages adhere strongly to glass and plastic surfaces, and actively phagocytose organisms or even tumour cells *in vitro*. Adherence and ingestion by monocytes occurs when the cells bind the microorganisms through specialized receptors. The receptors may bind to certain carbohydrates of the microbial cell wall, or to IgG and complement with which the microorganism has become coated.

Macrophage/monocyte cell markers

Human and murine monocyte/macrophages have mannosyl–fucosyl receptors (MFR) which bind to the sugars on the surface of microorganisms and of effete body cells, e.g. aged lymphocytes. Apoptotic cells are removed via phosphatidyl serine receptors on monocytes/ macrophages. These cells also express CD14, a receptor for lipopolysaccharide-binding protein (LBP) which is normally present in serum and which coats Gram-negative bacteria. There are also three distinct Fc receptors for IgG on human and murine macrophages:

- FcγRI (CD64) on human cells has a high affinity for IgG. This is homologous to the FcγRIIa receptor in the mouse.
- FcγRII (CD32) is of medium affinity and is equivalent to the FcγRIIb/1 receptor in the mouse.
- FcγRIII (CD16) or FcγRlo (mouse equivalent) is of low affinity and present on a subset of monocytes.

These Fc receptors probably have different functions, including triggering of extracellular killing, opsonization, and phagocytosis (see Chapter 1). Other receptors important in uptake of microorganisms include the complement receptor CR1 (C3b receptor, CD35) (see Chapter 13). Molecules involved mainly in adhesion and activation include the complement receptor CR3 (C3bi receptors, CD11b, MAC-1), present especially on activated macrophages, the leucocyte function antigen LFA-1 (CD11a), and p150,95 (CD11c). Both CD11b and CD11c are found in intracytoplasmic vesicles of macrophages and are rapidly expressed following activation. Class II MHC antigens are present on some monocytes/macrophages and are important in presentation of antigens to T cells. A low affinity receptor for the Fc of IgE (FcεRII; CD23) is also present on activated macrophages. Other molecules found on human macrophages include CD13, CD15, CD68 and VLA-4 (CD29/CD49d). It should be stressed that none of the markers mentioned above are lineage specific, although FcγRI is a particularly useful marker. Lineage specific markers in the mouse include F480 (160 kDa), sheep erythrocyte receptor (SER, not to be confused

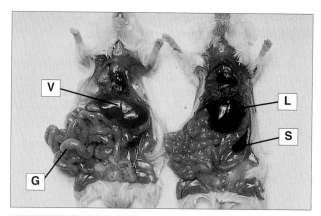

Fig. 2.26 Intravenously injected particles localize in the reticuloendothelial system. A mouse was injected intravenously with fine carbon particles and killed 5 minutes later. Carbon accumulates in organs rich in mononuclear phagocytes – lungs (L), liver (V), spleen (S) and areas of the gut wall (G). Normal organ colour is shown in the control mouse (**left**).

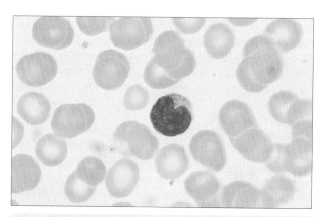

Fig. 2.27 Morphology of the monocyte. Blood monocytes have a characteristic horseshoe-shaped nucleus and are larger than most circulating lymphocytes. Giemsa stain, ×1200.

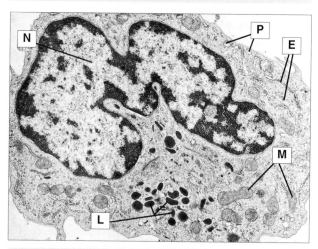

Fig. 2.28 The ultrastructure of the monocyte. This shows the horseshoe-shaped nucleus (N), the pinocytic vesicles (P), lysosomal granules (L), mitochondria (M) and isolated rough endoplasmic reticulum cisternae (E). ×8000. (Courtesy of Dr B. Nichols, from *J Cell Biol* 1971:**50**;498, with permission.)

with CD2) and erythroblast receptor (EbR). The main markers on human and mouse monocytes are summarized in *Figure 2.29*.

In addition to all of these molecules, monocytes and macrophages also have receptors for cytokines such as IL-2, IL-4, IFNγ and migration inhibition factor. The functions of monocytes and macrophages can therefore be enhanced by T-cell-derived cytokines through these receptors. Such activated monocytes/macrophages also generate cytokines themselves including IFNs, IL-1 and TNFα (see Chapter 9). Complement components and prostaglandins are also produced. Monocytes and, to a lesser extent, mature macrophages resemble neutrophils in that they contain peroxidase, which inactivates hydrogen peroxide.

■ ANTIGEN-PRESENTING CELLS

APCs are a heterogeneous population of leucocytes with exquisite immunostimulatory capacity. Some have a pivotal role in the induction of functional activity of TH cells; some communicate with other leucocytes. Cells other than leucocytes, such as endothelial or epithelial cells, can also acquire the ability to 'present' antigens when stimulated by cytokines.

APCs are found primarily in the skin, lymph nodes, spleen and thymus (*Fig. 2.30*). The archetypal APCs are the Langerhans' cells in the skin. These cells migrate as 'veiled cells' via the afferent lymphatics into the lymph node paracortex of the draining lymph nodes. Within the paracortex the cells interdigitate with many T cells (*Fig. 2.31*). This migration provides an efficient mechanism for carrying antigen from the skin to the TH cells located in the lymph nodes. These APCs are rich in class II MHC molecules, which are important for presenting antigen to TH cells.

Another specialized population of APCs, the follicular dendritic cells, are found in the secondary follicles of the B cell areas of the lymph nodes and spleen. They present anti-

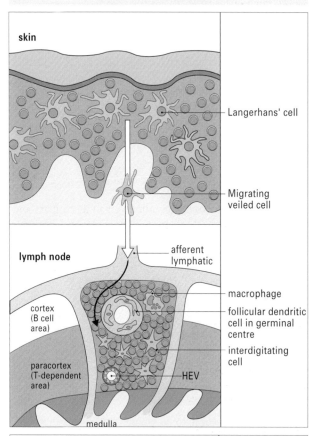

Antigen-presenting cells

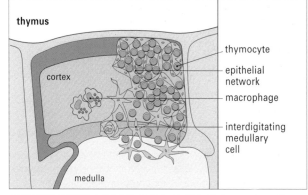

Fig. 2.30 Bone-marrow-derived antigen-presenting cells (APCs) are found especially in lymphoid tissues and in the skin. APCs are represented in the skin by Langerhans' cells, found in the epidermis and characterized by special granules (the tennis-racket shaped Birbeck granules). These cells, rich in MHC class II (mouse) or HLA-DR (human) determinants, are believed to carry antigens and migrate via the afferent lymphatics (where they appear as 'veiled' cells) into the paracortex of the draining lymph nodes. Here they interdigitate with T cells. These 'interdigitating cells', localized in the T-cell-dependent areas of the lymph node, present antigen to lymphocytes. Presentation to B cells is by follicular dendritic cells, which are found in the B-cell areas of the lymph nodes, and in particular in the germinal centres. Some macrophages located in the outer cortex and marginal sinus may also act as APCs. In the thymus, APCs occur as interdigitating medullary cells.

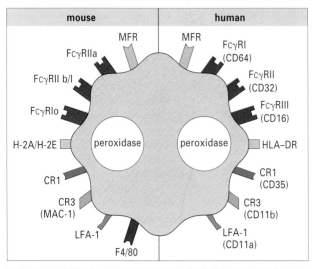

Summary of the main surface markers on murine and human monocytes/macrophages

Fig. 2.29 Equivalent molecules are shown in the same colour.

gen to B cells and lack class II MHC molecules, but instead express high levels of FcγR and the complement receptors CR1 (CD35) and CR2 (CD21) for interaction with immune complexes. Some of the markers found on different kinds of APCs are shown in *Figure 2.32*.

APCs are also present in the thymus, and are especially abundant in the medulla. They are rich in self antigens, including class II MHC molecules. The thymus is of crucial importance in the development and maturation of T cells, and it

appears that the interdigitating cells play a role in deleting T cells that react against self antigens. This process is referred to as 'negative selection' (see Chapter 12).

B cells are rich in class II MHC molecules (especially after 'activation') and are thus able to process and present antigen, especially when the B cell is specific for the antigen being presented (see Chapter 8).

Somatic cells other than immune cells do not normally express class II MHC molecules, but cytokines such as IFNγ and TNFα can induce these molecules on some cell types and thus allow them to present antigen. This induction of 'inappropriate' class II expression might contribute to the pathogenesis of autoimmune diseases and to prolonged inflammation.

■ POLYMORPHS AND MAST CELLS

Polymorphonuclear granulocytes (often referred to as 'granulocytes', or 'PMNs') are produced in the bone marrow at a rate of 80 million per minute and are short-lived (2–3 days) compared to monocytes/macrophages, which may live for months or years. Granulocytes make up 60–70% of the total normal blood leucocytes, and are also found in extravascular sites. Like monocytes, PMNs can adhere to endothelial cells lining the blood vessels, and extravasate (squeeze between them to escape from the blood vessel). This process is known as diapedesis. The adhesion is mediated by receptors on the granulocyte and ligands on the endothelial cells and is promoted by chemo-attractants such as IL-8 (see Chapter 14).

Granulocytes do not show any inherent specificity for antigens, but they play an important role in acute inflammation (usually synergizing with antibodies and complement) in protection against microorganisms. Their predominant role is phagocytosis. The importance of these cells is shown in individuals with reduced cell numbers, or with rare genetic defects which prevent extravasation in response to chemotactic stimuli. Both defects dramatically increase susceptibility to infection.

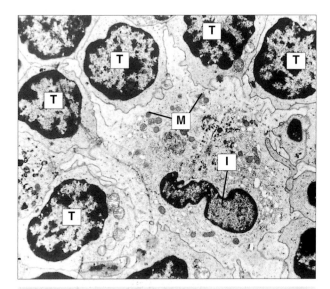

Fig. 2.31 The ultrastructure of an interdigitating cell (IDC) in the T cell area of the rat lymph node. Intimate contacts are made with the membranes of the surrounding T cells. The cytoplasm contains relatively few organelles and does not show the Birbeck granules characteristic of the skin Langerhans' cells. (T = T-cell nuclei; I = IDC nucleus; M = IDC membrane.) ×2000. (Courtesy of Dr B. H. Balfour.)

Markers on different antigen-presenting cells

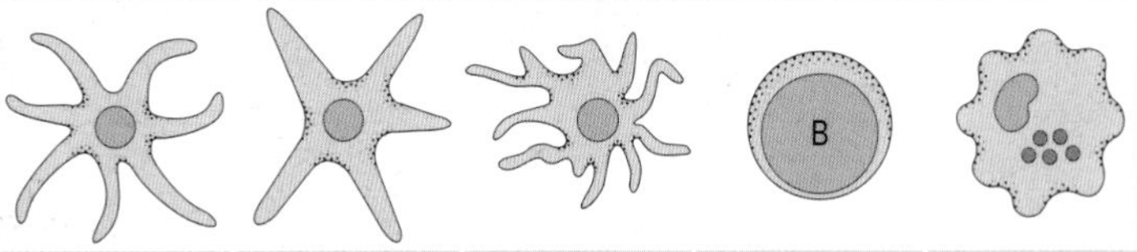

cell markers	cell type				
	Langerhans' cells	interdigitating cells	follicular dendritic cells	B cells	macrophages
MHC class II	+	+	–	+	(+)
FcγR	+	–	+	+	+
CR1 (CD35)	+	–	+	+	+
CR2 (CD21)	–	–	+	+	–
phagocyte function	–	–	–	–	+

Fig. 2.32 The Langerhans' cells (LCs), and the interdigitating cells derived from them, are rich in class II MHC for communicating with CD4+ T cells. LCs also possess receptors for IgG (FcγR) and for the complement protein C3b (CR1). Follicular dendritic cells located within the secondary follicles do not express class II MHC but have high levels of FcγR, CR1 and CR2 to enable them to trap immune complexes and interact with B cells. B cells and macrophages are also efficient as antigen-presenting cells and have been included for completeness.

Neutrophils

Neutrophils comprise over 90% of circulating granulocytes. They have a characteristic multilobed nucleus and are 10–20 μm in diameter (*Fig. 2.33*).

Chemotactic agents for neutrophils include protein fragments released when complement is activated (e.g. C5a), factors derived from the fibrinolytic and kinin systems, the products of other leucocytes and platelets, and the products of certain bacteria. Chemotactic stimuli result in neutrophil margination (adhesion to endothelial cells) and diapedesis. These events occur in three or more sequential steps:

- **Rolling** and **arrest** on endothelial cells mediated by selectins and their ligands (see above).
- **Activation** mediated by cytokines released by perivascular T cells and macrophages.
- **Firm adhesion** established by leucocyte integrins and their ligands expressed on activated endothelial cells (e.g. CR3/ICAM-1). This last event leads to extravasation of the activated leucocyte.

Neutrophils possess two main types of granules (*Fig. 2.34*). The primary (azurophilic) granules are lysosomes containing acid hydrolases, myeloperoxidase and muramidase (lysozyme). The secondary (specific) granules contain lactoferrin in addition to lysozyme. Ingested organisms are contained within vacuoles termed phagosomes, which fuse with the lysosomes to form phagolysosomes (*Fig. 2.35*).

Extracellular release of granules and cytotoxic substances by neutrophils can also occur when they are activated through their Fcγ receptors by immune complexes. This may be an important pathogenic mechanism in immune-complex diseases such as Type III hypersensitivity (see Chapter 24).

Eosinophils

Human blood eosinophils usually have a bilobed nucleus and many cytoplasmic granules (*Fig. 2.36*). They comprise 2–5% of blood leucocytes in healthy, non-allergic individuals. Although it is not their primary function, they appear to be capable of phagocytosing and killing ingested microorganisms.

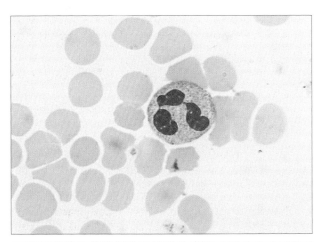

Fig. 2.33 Morphology of the neutrophil. This shows a neutrophil with its characteristic multilobed nucleus and neutrophilic granules in the cytoplasm. Giemsa stain, ×1500.

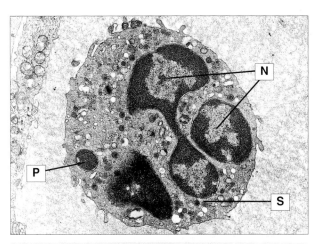

Fig. 2.34 The ultrastructure of the neutrophil. This mouse neutrophil lies within a skin blood vessel. The neutrophil cytoplasm contains primary (P) and secondary (S) granules of different electron opacity. (N = nucleus.) ×6000. (Courtesy of Dr D. McLaren.)

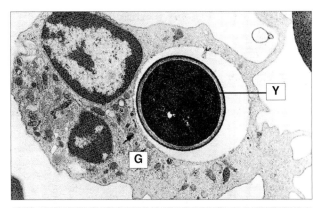

Fig. 2.35 A neutrophil that has phagocytosed a *Candida albicans* cell. Two lysosomal granules (G) can be seen fusing with the vacuole containing the yeast cell (Y). ×7000. (Courtesy of Dr H. Validimarsson.)

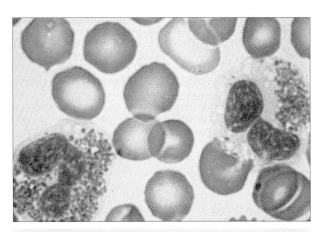

Fig. 2.36 Morphology of the eosinophil. The multilobed nucleus is stained purple and the cytoplasmic granules are stained red. Leishman stain, ×1800.

The granules in mature eosinophils are membrane-bound organelles with crystalloid cores that differ in electron opacity from the surrounding matrix (*Fig. 2.37*).

Certain stimuli will cause eosinophils to degranulate. Degranulation involves fusion of the intracellular granules with the plasma membrane, and release of the granule contents into the surrounding area. This type of reaction is the only way that these cells can use their granule armament against large targets, which cannot be phagocytosed. Eosinophils are thought to play a specialized role in immunity to parasitic worms using this mechanism (see Chapter 18).

Eosinophils are attracted by products such as eosinophil chemotactic factor of anaphylaxis (ECF-A), released from T cells, mast cells and basophils. They bind schistosomules (worm larvae) coated with IgG or IgE and degranulate, releasing a toxin known as 'major basic protein'. Eosinophils also release histaminase and aryl sulphatase, which inactivate the mast-cell products histamine and slow reactive substance of anaphylaxis (SRS-A). The effect of the eosinophil factors is thus to dampen down the inflammatory response and reduce granulocyte migration into the site of invasion.

Basophils and mast cells

Basophils are found in very small numbers in the circulation, constituting less than 0.2% of leucocytes, and are characterized by deep violet blue granules (*Fig. 2.38*). The mast cell, which is not found at all in the circulation, is often indistinguishable from the basophil in a number of its properties.

There are two different kinds of mast cell; the mucosal mast cell (MMC) associated with mucosal epithelia, and the connective tissue mast cell (CTMC). MMCs appear to be dependent on T cells for their proliferation, while the CTMCs are not. Both types can be visualized under light microscopy with Alcian blue staining (*Fig. 2.39*).

Mature blood basophils have randomly distributed granules surrounded by membranes (*Fig. 2.40*). The granules in both basophils and mast cells contain heparin, SRS-A and ECF-A.

The stimulus for eosinophil or mast-cell degranulation (*Fig. 2.41*) is often an allergen (an antigen causing allergic reaction). To be effective, an allergen must cross-link IgE molecules bound to the surface of the mast cell or basophil via its high-affinity Fc receptors for IgE (FcεRI). Characteristically, the degranulation of a basophil or mast cell is substantial, with all the gran-

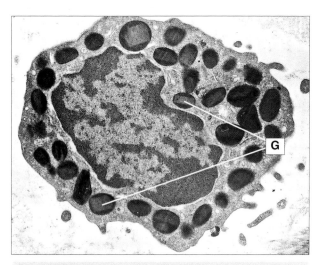

Fig. 2.37 The ultrastructure of a guinea-pig eosinophil. The mature eosinophil contains granules (G) with central crystalloids. ×8000. (Courtesy of Dr D. McLaren.)

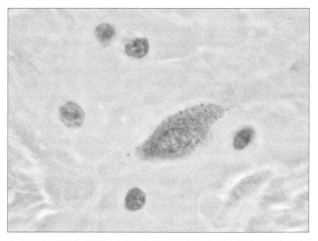

Fig. 2.39 Histological appearance of human connective tissue mast cells. This micrograph shows dark blue cytoplasm with purple granules. Alcian blue and safranin stain, ×600. (Courtesy of Dr T. S. Orr.)

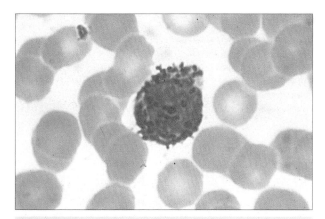

Fig. 2.38 Morphology of the basophil. This blood smear shows a typical basophil with its deep violet-blue granules. Wright's stain, ×1500.

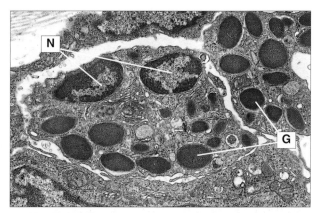

Fig. 2.40 The ultrastructure of the basophil. Basophils in guinea-pig skin showing the characteristic randomly distributed granules (G). (N = nucleus.) ×6000. (Courtesy of Dr D. McLaren.)

ules being released simultaneously. This is made possible by intracytoplasmic fusion of the granules, followed by rapid expulsion of their contents to the exterior (*Fig. 2.42*). Mediators such as histamine that are released by degranulation cause the adverse symptoms of allergy. On the positive side, they may also play a role in immunity against parasites. Granulocyte and mast-cell functional markers are summarized in *Figure 2.42*.

Platelets

Blood platelets, in addition to their role in blood clotting, are involved in immune responses and especially in inflammation. They are derived from megakaryocytes in the bone marrow and contain granules (*Fig. 2.43*). They express class I MHC products and receptors for IgG (FcγRII), and low-affinity receptors for IgE (FcεRII; CD23). In addition, megakaryocytes and platelets carry receptors for factor VIII and other molecules important for their function, such as the GpIIb/IIIa complex (CD41) and GpIb/GpIx complex (CD42). The GpIIb/IIIa complex is a cytoadhesin, and is responsible for binding to fibrinogen, fibronectin, and vitronectin. In addition, both this complex and the GpIb/GpIx complex are receptors for von Willebrand factor. There is an additional vitronectin receptor, CD51. Both receptors and adhesion molecules are important in activation of platelets. Following injury to endothelial cells, platelets adhere to the surface of the damaged tissue. The aggregated platelets release substances that increase permeability, as well as factors that activate complement and hence attract leucocytes.

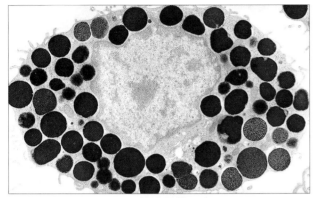

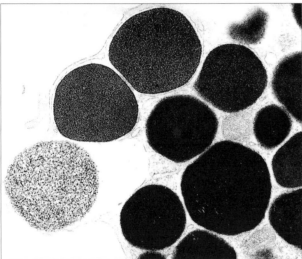

Fig. 2.41 Rat peritoneal mast cells. Upper: A non-degranulated cell with its electron-dense granules. ×6000. **Lower:** A granule leaving the cell. ×30 000. (Courtesy of Dr T. S. C. Orr.)

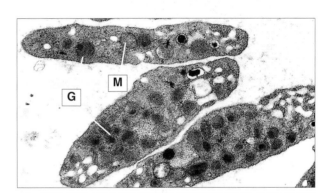

Fig. 2.43 The ultrastructure of a platelet. The cytoplasmic organelles, including granules (G) and mitochondria (M), are randomly dispersed. ×20 000. (Courtesy of Dr J. G. White.)

Human granulocyte and mast-cell functional markers

cell type	cell surface markers									granules		
	C5aR	CR1 (CD35)	CR3 (CD11b)	LFA-1 (CD11a)	VLA-4 (CD49d)	FcγRII (CD32)	FcγRIII (CD16)	FcεRI	FcεRII (CD23)	peroxidase	acid phosphatase	alkaline phosphatase
neutrophils	+	+	+	+	+	+	+	−	−	+	+	+
eosinophils	+	+	+	+	+	+	±	−	+	+	+	
basophils	+	+	+	+	+		+	+	−	+		
mast cells	+	+	+	+			+	+	−		+	+

Fig. 2.42 Neutrophils, eosinophils, basophils and mast cells all respond to C5a by chemotaxis and therefore must have a receptor for it. They all have receptors for C3 and express the adhesion molecules LFA-1 (CD11a) and VLA-4 (CD49d). They express FcγRII (CD32) and FcγRIII (CD16). Only basophils and mast cells have the high affinity receptor for IgE, (FcεRI). Several other glycoproteins, including CD13 and CD14 (weakly expressed), are found on some granulocytes. In addition, glycolipid molecules such as the Lex hapten (CD15) and lactosyl ceramide (CD17) are expressed by these cells. The granules in different cell types vary qualitatively in their enzyme content.

Critical Thinking

■ What are the functional subpopulations of T lymphocytes and how are they distinguished?

■ Why do we need so many different kinds of cells participating in the immune response?

■ What molecules are used by lymphocytes: (a) as antigen receptors; (b) for interaction between each other and other cells. What are the different families of molecules called?

FURTHER READING

Gordon JR, Burd PR, Galli SJ. Mast cells as a source of multifunctional cytokines. *Immunol Today* 1990;**11**:458.

Lloyd AR, Oppenheim JJ. Poly's lament: the neglected role of the polymorphonuclear neutrophil in the afferent limb of the immune response. *Immunol Today* 1992;**13**:169.

Playfair JHL. *Immunology at a Glance*. 5th ed. Oxford: Blackwell Scientific Publications, 1992.

Reth M, *et al*. The B-cell antigen receptor complex. *Immunol Today* 1991;**12**:201.

Roitt IM. *Essential Immunology*. 8th ed. Oxford: Blackwell Scientific Publications, 1994.

Romagnini S. Human TH1 and TH2 subsets: doubt no more. *Immunol Today* 1991;**11**:256.

Silverstein S, Unkeless J, eds. Innate Immunity. *Curr Opin Immunol* 1991;**3**:47.

Steinman RM. The dendritic cell system and its role in immunogenicity. *Ann Rev Immunol* 1991;**9**:271.

Lymphoid organs and tissues are either primary (central) or secondary (peripheral). Thymus and bone marrow are the primary lymphoid organs.

Lymphocytes differentiate from stem cells in the primary organs but migrate to, and function in, secondary organs and tissues.

The systemic lymphoid system includes the spleen and lymph nodes. The mucosal system includes all the lymphoid tissues associated with mucosal surfaces.

Peyer's patches are organized collections of lymphoid tissue present in the wall of the small intestine which process antigens present in the gut.

The peripheral lymphoid tissues are equipped with phagocytic cells and other accessory cells that assist the function of T and B lymphocytes located there.

Lymphocytes are not sessile – there is continuous lymphocyte traffic from the blood stream into lymphoid tissues and back again into the blood via the thoracic duct.

The cells involved in the immune response are organized into tissues and organs in order to perform their functions most effectively. These structures are collectively referred to as the lymphoid system.

■ LYMPHOID TISSUES CAN BE CLASSIFIED AS EITHER PRIMARY OR SECONDARY

The lymphoid system comprises lymphocytes, accessory cells (macrophages and antigen-presenting cells) and in some tissues, epithelial cells. It is arranged into either discretely capsulated organs or accumulations of diffuse lymphoid tissue. The major lymphoid organs and tissues are classified as either primary (central) or secondary (peripheral) (*Fig. 3.1*).

Primary lymphoid organs
Primary lymphoid organs are the major sites of lymphopoiesis (lymphocyte development). Here, lymphocytes differentiate from lymphoid stem cells, proliferate, and mature into functional cells. In mammals, T cells mature in the thymus, and B cells in the fetal liver and bone marrow (see Chapter 10). (Birds have a specialized site of B-cell generation, the bursa of Fabricius.) It is in the primary lymphoid organs that lymphocytes acquire their repertoire of specific antigen receptors to cope with antigenic challenges received during thir lifespans. The cells are selected for tolerance to autoantigens and are therefore capable of recognizing only non-self antigens when the cells are in the periphery.

Secondary lymphoid organs
Secondary lymphoid organs comprise the spleen, lymph nodes and mucosa-associated tissues, including the tonsils and Peyer's patches of the gut. Secondary lymphoid tissues provide an environment in which lymphocytes can interact with each other, with accessory cells, and with antigens. They also disseminate the immune response. Immune responses generated in secondary lymphoid tissues require phagocytic macrophages, antigen-presenting cells, and mature T and B cells.

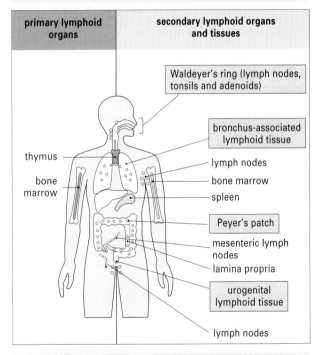

Major lymphoid organs and tissues

primary lymphoid organs	secondary lymphoid organs and tissues

Waldeyer's ring (lymph nodes, tonsils and adenoids)

bronchus-associated lymphoid tissue

thymus

lymph nodes

bone marrow

bone marrow

spleen

Peyer's patch

mesenteric lymph nodes

lamina propria

urogenital lymphoid tissue

lymph nodes

Fig. 3.1 Thymus and bone marrow are primary lymphoid organs. They are sites of maturation for T and B cells respectively. Cellular and humoral immune responses occur in the secondary (peripheral) lymphoid organs and tissues; effector and memory cells are generated here. Secondary lymphoid organs can be classified according to the body regions which they defend. The spleen responds predominantly to blood-borne antigens. Lymph nodes mount immune responses to antigens circulating in the lymph, absorbed either through the skin (superficial nodes) or from internal viscera (deep nodes). Tonsils, Peyer's patches and other mucosa-associated lymphoid tissues (blue boxes) respond to antigens which have penetrated the surface mucosal barriers. Note that bone marrow is both a primary and secondary lymphoid organ.

■ PRIMARY LYMPHOID ORGANS

The thymus is the site of T-cell development

The thymus in mammals is a bilobed organ, located in the thoracic cavity, overlying the heart and major blood vessels. Each lobe is organized into lobules which are separated from each other by connective tissue trabeculae (*Fig. 3.2*). Within each lobule the lymphoid cells (thymocytes) are arranged into an outer cortex and an inner medulla (*Fig. 3.3*). The tightly packed cortex contains the majority of relatively immature proliferating thymocytes; the medulla contains more mature cells, implying a differentiation gradient from cortex to medulla. Mature thymocytes in the medulla express CD44, which is not detected in cortical thymocytes. This receptor, which binds to hyaluronate and other connective tissue components, is found on all trafficking cells and is not expressed on sessile lymphocytes. There is a network of epithelial cells throughout the lobules which plays a role in the differentiation process from bone-marrow-derived stem cells to mature T lymphocytes.

Three types of epithelial cells are present in the thymic lobules.

At least three types of epithelial cells can be distinguished in the thymic lobules according to structure, function and phenotype. These are the epithelial nurse cells of the outer cortex, the cortical epithelial cells, which form an epithelial network, and medullary epithelial cells, mostly organized into clusters (see Chapter 10). In addition, interdigitating dendritic cells (IDCs) and macrophages (both derived from bone marrow) are found in thymic lobules, particularly at the corticomedullary junction. Traffic of cells into and out of the thymus occurs via high endothelial venules (HEVs) in this region. Epithelial cells, IDCs and macrophages express MHC molecules, which are crucial to T-cell development and selection.

Hassall's corpuscles are found in the thymic medulla. Their function is unknown but they appear to contain degenerating epithelial cells rich in high molecular weight cytokeratins.

The mammalian thymus involutes with age. In man, atrophy begins at puberty and continues throughout life. Thymic involution begins within the cortex and this region may disappear completely although medullary remnants persist. Cortical atrophy is related to corticosteroid sensitivity of the cortical thymocytes. Thus, all conditions associated with an acute increase in steroids, for example pregnancy and stress, promote thymic atrophy. However, it is conceivable that T-cell generation within the thymus continues into adult life, albeit at a low rate.

Sites of B-cell development
B cells develop in the bursa of Fabricius in birds

In birds, B cells differentiate in the bursa of Fabricius, hence the term 'B' cells. The bursa is a modified section of the dorsal wall of the cloaca, the common exit of the intestinal and genitourinary tracts in birds. It is composed of folds or plicae (like villi in the intestine) which are directed towards a central lumen (*Fig. 3.4*). Bursal follicles are organized into a cortex and a medulla and lie along the outer margins of the plicae, arranged in close contact with the surface epithelium.

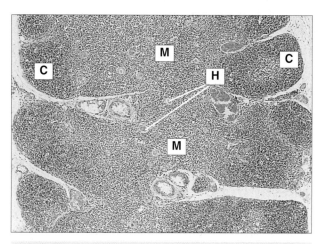

Fig. 3.3 Thymus section showing the lobular organization. This section shows the two main areas of the thymus lobule – an outer cortex of immature cells (C) and an inner medulla of more mature cells (M). Hassall's corpuscles (H) are found in the medulla. H&E stain.

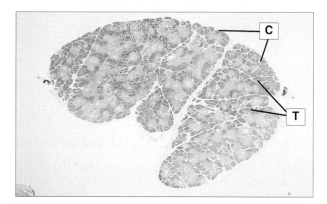

Fig. 3.2 Thymus section showing the lobular structure. This low power cross-section shows a fibrous capsule (C) with the thymocytes (developing T lymphocytes) organized into lobules separated from each other by connective tissue trabeculae (T). H&E stain, ×3.5.

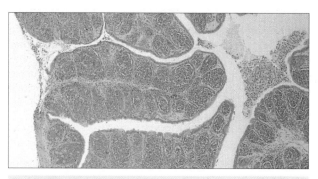

Fig. 3.4 Section of embryonic bursa of Fabricius showing the follicular structure. The avian bursa of Fabricius is a lymphoepithelial organ (like the thymus) and is found dorsal to the hindgut. The lumen of the bursa opens into the cloaca. Like the thymic lobules, bursal follicles are arranged into an outer cortex and inner medulla. The bursa, like the thymus, atrophies with age. H&E stain, ×10.

*Mammalian B cells develop in the fetal liver
and adult bone marrow*

Mammals have no bursa; instead, islands of haemopoietic cells in the fetal liver, and in the fetal and adult bone marrow, give rise directly to B lymphocytes. As well as being a site of B-cell generation, the adult bone marrow contains mature T cells and numerous plasma cells. Thus, in man, the bone marrow is also an important secondary lymphoid organ.

■ SECONDARY LYMPHOID ORGANS AND TISSUES

The generation of lymphocytes in primary lymphoid organs (lymphopoiesis) is followed by their migration into the peripheral secondary tissues. The secondary lymphoid tissues comprise well-organized encapsulated organs – the spleen and lymph nodes – and non-encapsulated accumulations that are found throughout the body. The bulk of the non-organized lymphoid tissue is found in association with mucosal surfaces and is called mucosa-associated lymphoid tissue (MALT).

Systemic organs and the mucosal system have different functions in immunity

The spleen is responsive to blood-borne antigens, and the lymph nodes protect the body from antigens that come from skin or internal surfaces via the lymphatic system. Responses to antigens encountered via these routes result in secretion of antibodies into the circulation and in local, cell-mediated responses. Patients who have had their spleen removed are much more susceptible to blood-borne infections

In contrast, the mucosal system protects the organism from antigens entering the body directly through mucosal epithelial surfaces. Thus, lymphoid tissues are found associated with surfaces lining the intestinal tract (gut-associated lymphoid tissues, or GALT), the respiratory tract (bronchus-associated lymphoid tissue, or BALT) and the genitourinary tract. The major effector mechanism at these sites is secretory IgA (sIgA), secreted directly onto the mucosal epithelial surfaces of the tract. It is perhaps not surprising that the bulk of the body's lymphoid tissues (>50%) are found associated with the mucosal system, especially the GALT, since this is a major pathway of entry for external antigens.

The systemic lymphoid organs
The spleen

The spleen lies in the upper left quadrant of the abdomen, behind the stomach, close to the diaphragm. Its outer layer consists of a capsule of collagenous bundles of fibres which penetrate into the parenchyma of the organ as trabeculae. These, together with a reticular framework, support the variety of cells found within the organ (*Fig. 3.5*). There are two main types of tissue; red pulp and white pulp (*Fig. 3.6*).

The white pulp – The white pulp consists of lymphoid tissue, the bulk of which is arranged around a central arteriole, and which is known as the periarteriolar lymphoid sheath (PALS). The PALS contain T- and B-cell areas; the T cells are found around the central arteriole; the B cells may be organized into either primary 'unstimulated' follicles (aggregates of virgin B cells), or secondary 'stimulated' follicles (which possess a germinal centre with memory cells) (*Figs 3.7 and 3.8*). The germinal centres also contain follicular dendritic cells and phagocytic macrophages. Specialized macrophages and a subset of B cells are found in the marginal zone – the area overlying the secondary follicles. Macrophages and the follicular dendritic cells present antigen to B cells in the spleen. B cells and other lymphocytes are free to leave and enter the PALS via capillary branches of the central arterioles that enter the

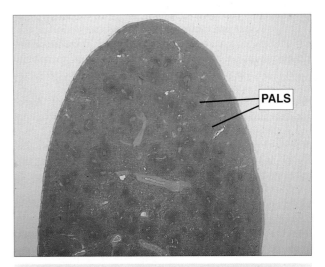

Fig. 3.6 Spleen section showing the tissue organization. This cross-section of the spleen shows the lymphoid tissue localized in the white pulp around the arterioles. The lymphoid tissue in the periarteriolar lymphoid sheaths (PALS) is easy to distinguish from the red pulp of the spleen. The red pulp is mainly involved in the destruction of aged erythrocytes and platelets, but also contains some lymphocytes, the majority of the plasma cells and a population of resident macrophages. H&E stain, × 7.

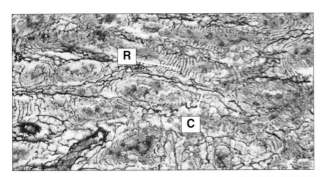

Fig. 3.5 Spleen section showing the connective tissue framework. This section is stained for reticulin and shows the architecture of the red pulp cords, and the ring fibres (R) that support the endothelial cells of the venous sinuses. These blood vessels have a discontinuous wall which allows free flow of plasma into their lumen, and selective passage of cells from the red pulp cords (C). × 125.

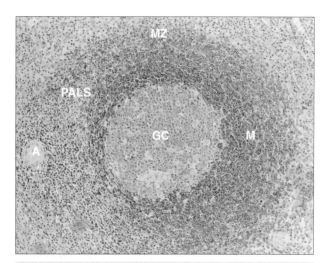

Fig. 3.7 Spleen section showing a white pulp lymphoid aggregate. A large secondary lymphoid follicle, with germinal centre (GC) and mantle (M), is surrounded by the marginal zone (MZ). Adjacent to the follicle, an arteriole (A) is surrounded by the periarteriolar lymphoid sheath (PALS) predominantly consisting of T cells. Note that the marginal zone is only present above the secondary follicle.

marginal zone. Some lymphocytes, especially maturing plasmablasts, can pass across the marginal zone via bridges into the red pulp.

The red pulp – This tissue consists of sinuses and cellular cords containing resident macrophages (*Fig. 3.9*), erythrocytes, platelets, granulocytes, lymphocytes and numerous plasma cells. Note that in addition to immunological functions, the spleen serves as a reservoir for platelets, erythrocytes and granulocytes. The spleen is also the site where aged platelets and erythrocytes are destroyed, a process carried out in the red pulp and referred to as 'haemocatheresis'. These functions are made possible by the vascular organization of the spleen. Central arteries surrounded by PALS end with arterial capillaries which open freely into the red pulp cords. Thus, circulating cells reach these cords and become trapped. Aged platelets and erythrocytes are recognized and phagocytosed by macrophages: blood cells that are not ingested and destroyed can re-enter the blood circulation by crossing the highly discontinuous walls of the venous sinuses, whereas plasma flows freely through the wall of the sinuses.

Lymph nodes and the lymphatic system
The lymph nodes form part of a network that filters antigens from the interstitial tissue fluid and lymph during its passage from the periphery to the thoracic duct (*Fig. 3.10*). Lymph nodes frequently occur at branches of the lymphatic vessels. Clusters of lymph nodes are strategically placed in areas such as the neck, axillae, groin, mediastinum and the abdominal cavity, which drain various superficial and deep regions of the body. Lymph nodes that protect the skin are superficial and termed somatic nodes. Deep lymph nodes, that protect the mucosal surfaces of the respiratory, digestive and genitourinary tracts, are termed visceral nodes.

Schematic organization of lymphoid tissue on the spleen

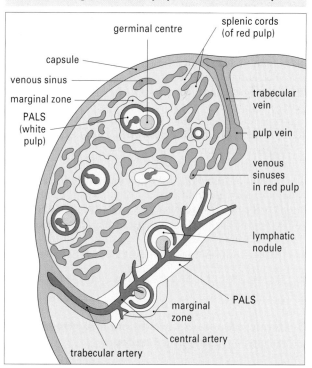

Fig. 3.8 The white pulp is composed of periarteriolar lymphoid sheaths (PALS), frequently containing germinal centres with mantle zones. The white pulp is surrounded by the marginal zone, which contains numerous macrophages, APCs, slowly recirculating B cells and NK cells. The red pulp contains venous sinuses separated by splenic cords. Blood enters the tissues via the trabecular arteries, which give rise to the many-branched central arteries. Some end in the white pulp, supplying the germinal centres and mantle zones, but most empty into or near the marginal zones. Some arterial branches run directly into the red pulp, mainly terminating in the cords. The venous sinuses drain blood into the pulp veins and then into the trabecular veins.

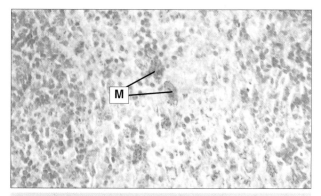

Fig. 3.9 Spleen section showing the red pulp macrophages. Microorganisms in the blood become trapped in the red pulp macrophages of the spleen, which are part of the reticuloendothelial system. This section shows intravenously injected mycobacteria phagocytosed by red pulp macrophages (M). Modified Ziehl-Neelsen stain ×125. (Courtesy of Dr I. Brown.)

Human lymph nodes are 2–10 mm in diameter, are round or kidney shaped, and have an indentation called the hilus where blood vessels enter and leave. Lymph arrives at the lymph node via several afferent lymphatic vessels, and leaves the node through one efferent lymphatic vessel at the hilus. A typical lymph node is surrounded by a collagenous capsule (*Fig. 3.11*). Radial trabeculae, together with reticulin fibres, support the various cellular components. The lymph node consists of a B-cell area (cortex), a T-cell area (paracortex), and a central medulla, which has cellular cords containing T cells, B cells, plasma cells and abundant macrophages (*Fig. 3.12*).

The paracortex contains many APCs (interdigitating cells) which express high levels of MHC class II surface antigens. The bulk of the lymphoid tissue is found in the cortex and paracortex. Some lymphoid tissue extends into the medulla, where it is organized into cords separated by lymph (medullary) sinuses which drain into the terminal sinus, the origin of the efferent lymphatic vessel (*Fig. 3.12*). Scavenger phagocytic cells are arranged along the lymph sinuses, especially in the medulla

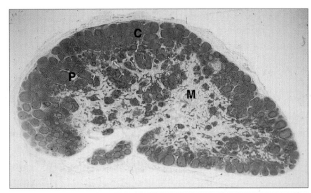

Fig. 3.11 Lymph node section. The lymph node is surrounded by a connective tissue capsule and is organized into three main areas – C, the cortex (B-cell area); P, the paracortex (T-cell area) and M, the medulla, which contains cords of lymphoid tissue (T- and B-cell area rich in plasma cells and macrophages). H&E stain, ×5. (Courtesy of Mr C. Symes).

The lymph node system

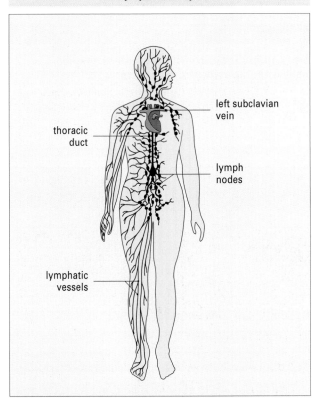

Fig. 3.10 Lymph nodes are found at junctions of lymphatic vessels and form a complete network, draining and filtering fluid derived from the blood in the tissue spaces. They are either superficial or visceral, draining the deep tissues and internal organs of the body. The lymph eventually reaches the thoracic duct which drains into the left subclavian vein and thus back into the circulation.

Schematic structure of the lymph node

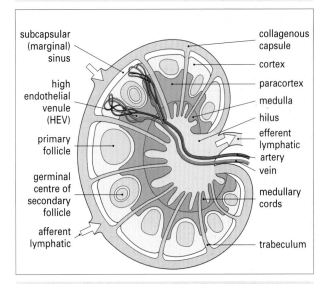

Fig. 3.12 Beneath the collagenous capsule is the subcapsular sinus, which is lined with phagocytic cells. Lymphocytes and antigens from surrounding tissue spaces or adjacent nodes, pass into the sinus via the afferent lymphatics. The cortex contains aggregates of B cells (primary follicles) most of which are stimulated (secondary follicles) and have a site of active proliferation, or germinal centre. The paracortex contains mainly T cells, many of which are associated with the interdigitating cells (antigen-presenting cells). Each lymph node has its own arterial and venous supply. Lymphocytes enter the node from the circulation through the specialized high endothelial venules (HEVs) in the paracortex. The medulla contains both T and B cells, as well as most of the lymph node plasma cells organized into cords of lymphoid tissue. Lymphocytes can only leave the node through the efferent lymphatic vessel.

(*Figs 3.13 and 3.14*). As the lymph passes across the nodes from afferent to efferent lymphatic vessels, particulate antigens are removed by the phagocytic cells and transported into the lymphoid tissue of the lymph node (*Fig. 3.14*).

The cortex contains aggregates of B cells as primary or secondary follicles, whereas T cells are localized primarily in the paracortex. Thus, if an area of skin or mucosa is challenged by a T-dependent antigen (see Chapter 8), the lymph nodes draining that particular area show active T-cell proliferation in the paracortex (*Fig. 3.15*). Further evidence for this localization of T cells comes from patients with congenital thymic aplasia (DiGeorge syndrome), who have fewer cells in the paracortex than normal. Similar observations are made in neonatally thymectomized, or congenitally athymic ('nude'), mice or rats (*Fig. 3.16*).

Germinal centres within secondary follicles are seen in antigen-stimulated lymph nodes. These are similar to the germinal centres seen in the B-cell areas of the splenic PALS and

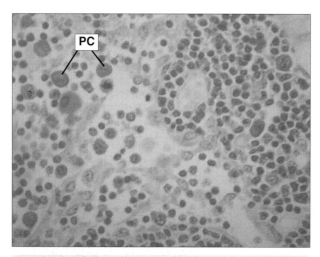

Fig. 3.13 Section of lymph node medulla. This section shows typical plasma cells (PC) in the medullary cords and sinuses. The plasma cell cytoplasm stains red with pyronin which binds to RNA. Macrophages are also abundant in this region. Methyl green pyronin stain, ×200.

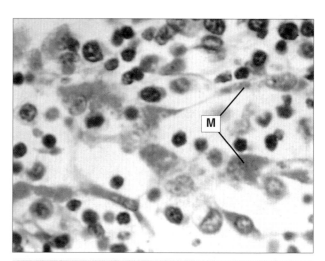

Fig. 3.14 Section of lymph node medulla showing phagocytic macrophages. The macrophages (M) line the medullary sinuses and can be seen following uptake of the red dye lithium carmine. Haematoxylin stain. ×330.

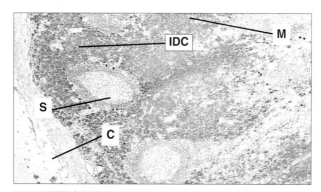

Fig. 3.15 Lymph node section showing paracortical expansion. A lymph node draining the skin area of a patient with chronic eczema. Antigens penetrating the skin are carried to draining lymph nodes by Langerhans' cells (antigen-presenting cells which are normally present in the epidermis). These cells are seen as veiled cells in the afferent lymphatics and they settle in the paracortex as interdigitating cells (IDCs). They are seen here stained brown with peroxidase-labelled monoclonal antibody. T-cell proliferation in response to specific antigen presented by IDCs results in paracortical expansion. M = medullary cord; C = capsule; S = secondary follicle. Haematoxylin counterstain, ×40.

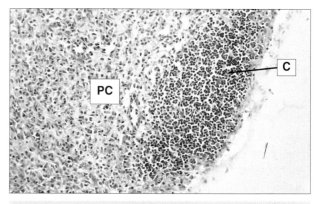

Fig. 3.16 Lymph node section from a congenitally athymic (nude) mouse showing paracortical depletion. A genetic defect in the nude mouse causes thymic aplasia and failure of T-cell development. This lymph node section from a 'T-less' mouse shows few cells in the T-dependent paracortex. (PC) There are, however, large numbers of interdigitating cells within the paracortex in this node. The cortex (C) is also poorly developed since T cells are required for the organization of the follicles. Compare the structure here with that visible in Fig. 3.15. H&E stain, ×125. (Courtesy of Dr H. Dockrell.)

of other peripheral lymphoid tissues. The large and small follicular centre cells are called centroblasts and centrocytes. Proliferating B cells within the germinal centres have a clearly defined nuclear shape (cleaved versus non-cleaved) which is useful in defining certain malignant lymphoproliferative disorders such as nodular lymphomas.

Germinal centres are surrounded by a mantle of lymphocytes (*Fig. 3.17*). B cells in these areas are rich in surface IgM and IgD; this can be detected by immunohistochemical staining (*Fig. 3.18*). In some secondary follicles, this thickened mantle or corona is more orientated towards the capsule of the node. Secondary follicles contain dendritic APCs, some macrophages, and a few CD4$^+$ T lymphocytes (*Fig. 3.19*). All these cells, taken together with specialized marginal sinus macrophages, appear to play a role in the development of B-

cell responses and, in particular, the development of memory B cells, which is probably the primary function of the germinal centres. (See Chapter 10 for a detailed description of the cellular organization of the germinal centre.)

The mucosal lymphoid system
Mucosa-associated lymphoid tissue (MALT)
Aggregates of non-encapsulated lymphoid tissue are found especially in the lamina propria and submucosal areas of the gastrointestinal, respiratory and genitourinary tracts (see *Fig. 3.1*). The lymphoid cells are either present as diffuse aggregates, or are organized into solitary or aggregated nodules containing germinal centres (secondary follicles). In man, the tonsils contain a considerable amount of lymphoid tissue, often with many large germinal centres (*Fig. 3.20*). Similar accumulations

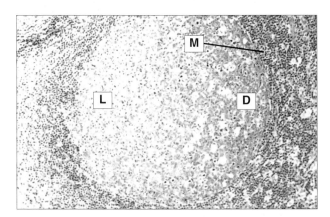

Fig. 3.17 Secondary lymphoid follicle section showing a germinal centre. This human lymph node germinal centre contains actively proliferating B cells. Zoning of the centre may be seen as a light part (L) and a more actively proliferating dark part (D), which contains tingible body macrophages. There is a well-developed mantle (M) or corona of small resting lymphocytes, which have much less cytoplasm than the lymphoblasts and appear more densely packed. Giemsa stain, ×40. (Courtesy of Dr K. McLennan.)

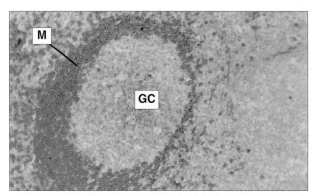

Fig. 3.18 Secondary lymphoid follicle showing the mantle (M) of lymphocytes around the germinal centre. Human lymph node germinal centre (GC) stained with anti-human IgD antibody labelled with horseradish peroxidase. Note that there are few IgD-positive cells in the centre itself; both areas contain IgM-positive cells. ×40. (Courtesy of Dr K. McLennan.)

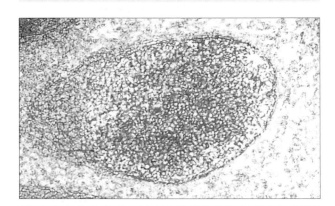

Fig. 3.19 Secondary lymphoid follicle section showing the reticular cell network. This lymph node follicle is stained with peroxidase-labelled monoclonal antibody to dendritic cells. Note the extension of the network into the mantle zone. Haematoxylin counterstain, ×40. (Courtesy of Dr K. McLennan.)

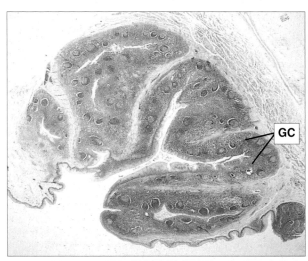

Fig. 3.20 Section of human tonsil showing MALT. This view shows the large number of germinal centres (GC) frequently found in tonsillar lymphoid tissue. H&E stain, ×4. (Courtesy of Mr C. Symes.)

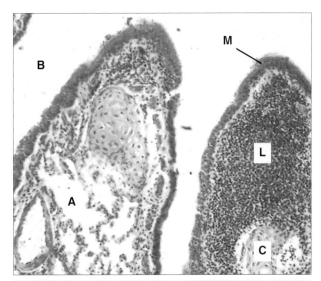

Fig. 3.21 Section of lung showing MALT. This section shows diffuse accumulation of lymphocytes in the bronchial wall. A = alveolar space; B = bronchial lumen; C = cartilage; L = lymphocytes; M = mucosal epithelium. H&E stain, ×40.

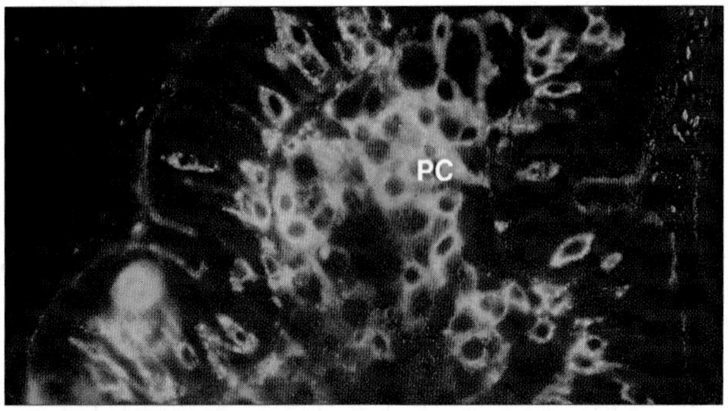

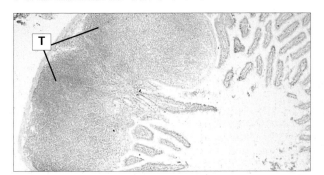

Fig. 3.22 Section of human jejunum showing MALT. Lymphoid cells in the epithelium and lamina propria fluoresce green (using anti-leucocyte monoclonal antibody, 2D1). Red cytoplasmic staining is obtained with anti-IgA antibody, which detects plasma cells (PC) in the lamina propria and IgA in the mucus. (Courtesy of Professor G. Janossy.)

Fig. 3.23 Section of mouse ileum showing Peyer's patches in the MALT. This shows the lymphoid tissue in the intestinal wall organized into Peyer's patches. The T-cell areas (T) are stained with peroxidase-labelled antibody to Thy-1 antigen on the T cells. Haematoxylin counterstain, × 40. (Courtesy of Dr E. Andrew.)

of lymphoid tissue are seen lining the bronchi (*Fig. 3.21*), and along the genitourinary tract. The respiratory epithelium contains dendritic cells similar to the Langerhans' cells found in the epidermis, for uptake, transport and processing of antigens.

Diffuse accumulations of lymphoid tissue are seen in the lamina propria of the intestinal wall (*Fig. 3.22*). The Peyer's patches of the lower ileum are particularly prominent in young animals and contain secondary follicles (*Fig. 3.23*). The intestinal epithelium overlying the Peyer's patches is specialized to allow the transport of antigens into the lymphoid tissue. This particular function is carried out by epithelial cells termed 'M' cells, so called because they have numerous microfolds on their luminal surface. M cells are able to absorb, transport and (possibly) process and present antigens to subepithelial lymphoid cells. Humoral immune responses at the mucosal level are mostly of the IgA isotype. Secretory IgA is an antibody that can traverse mucosal membranes and helps prevent entry of infectious microorganisms (*Fig. 3.24*).

Transport of IgA across the mucosal epithelium

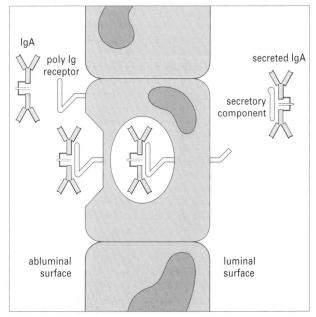

Fig. 3.24 Secretory IgA (sIgA) dimers secreted into the intestinal space by plasma cells bind to membrane receptors on the internal (abluminal) surface of the epithelial cells. The sIgA–receptor complex is then endocytosed and transported across the cell while still bound to the membrane of transport vesicles. These vesicles fuse with the plasma membrane at the luminal surface, releasing IgA dimers and secretory component derived from cleavage of the receptor. The dimeric IgA is probably protected from proteolytic enzymes outside the cell by the presence of this secretory component.

Mucosal lymphocytes

In addition to the organized lymphoid tissue that forms the MALT system, a large number of lymphocytes are found in the mucosa of the stomach, the small and large intestine, the upper and lower respiratory airways, and in the mucosa of several organs. The lymphocytes are found in the connective tissue of the lamina propria and within the epithelial layer:

- Lamina propria lymphocytes (LPLs) are predominantly activated T cells, but numerous activated B cells and plasma cells are also detected. These plasma cells secrete mainly IgA, which is transported across the epithelial cells and released into the lumen (see above).
- Intra-epithelial lymphocytes (IELs) are mostly T cells, and display phenotypic features distinct from those of LPLs (*Fig. 3.25*).

Phenotypic differences between human LPLs and IELs

cell type	TCR $\alpha\beta$	TCR $\gamma\delta$	CD4	CD8
lamina propria lymphocytes	>95%	<5%	70%	30%
intra-epithelial lymphocytes	60–90%	10–40%	<10%	70%

Fig. 3.25 In general, the phenotype of lamina propria lymphocytes (LPLs) is similar to that of cells circulating in the peripheral blood. A higher percentage of the intra-epithelial lymphocytes (IELs) are TCR $\gamma\delta$ cells, and more of this subset express CD8.

Although the phenotype of LPLs is similar to that of cells circulating in the peripheral blood, a higher percentage of IELs are TCR $\gamma\delta$ cells, most of which express CD8. This marker is not detected on the majority of TCR $\gamma\delta$ in the circulation. This expression of CD8 on $\gamma\delta$ IELs has been related to their state of activation.

Most LPL and IEL T cells belong to the CD45R0 subset of memory cells. They respond poorly to stimulation with antibodies to CD3, but may be triggered via other activation pathways (e.g. via CD2 or CD28).

The integrin α-chain HML-1 (CD103) is not present on resting circulating T cells, but is expressed following phytohaemagglutinin (PHA) stimulation. Antibodies to this molecule are mitogenic and induce expression of the low-affinity IL-2 receptor (CD25) on peripheral blood T cells. HML-1 is a novel α chain of the integrin family, which is coupled with a β_7 chain to form a αHML-1/β_7 heterodimer, an integrin expressed by IELs and other activated leukocytes.

IELs are known to release cytokines including IFNγ and IL-5. One function suggested for IELs is immune surveillance against mutated or virus-infected host cells.

■ LYMPHOCYTE TRAFFIC

The migration of lymphocytes from primary to secondary lymphoid tissues has already been described. Once in the secondary tissues the lymphocytes do not simply remain there; many move from one lymphoid organ to another via the blood and lymph (*Fig. 3.26*).

Lymphocytes leave the blood via high endothelial venules

Although some lymphocytes leave the blood through non-specialized venules, the main exit route in most mammals is

Lymphocyte traffic through the systemic lymphoid organs and tissues

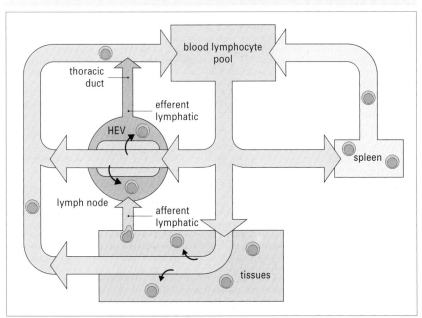

Fig. 3.26 The lymphocytes in a mature animal move through the circulation and enter the lymph nodes and MALT via the specialised endothelial cells of the post-capillary venules (HEVs). They leave through the efferent lymphatic vessels and pass through other nodes, finally entering the thoracic duct which empties into the circulation at the left subclavian vein (in humans). Lymphocytes enter the white pulp areas of the spleen in the marginal zones; they pass into the sinusoids of the red pulp and leave via the splenic vein.

through a specialized section of the post-capillary venules known as the high endothelial venule, or HEV (*Fig. 3.27*). In the lymph nodes these are found mainly in the paracortex, with some in the cortex and none in the medulla. Some lymphocytes, primarily T cells, arrive from the drainage area of the node through the afferent lymphatics; this is the main route by which antigen enters the nodes.

HEVs direct lymphocyte traffic

The HEVs are lined with cuboidal endothelial cells. These are activated cells which express a variety of adhesion molecules not found on the flat, resting endothelial cells of ordinary venules. One mechanism by which endothelial cells are activated is through locally produced cytokines such as IFNγ, IL-1, and TNF.

Endothelial cells may develop into HEVs at sites of chronic inflammatory reactions, for example in the skin and in the synovium, where HEVs are normally absent. This may in turn direct specific T-lymphocyte subsets to the area where the HEVs have formed. Molecules expressed by activated endothelial cells belong to the immunoglobulin superfamily, which includes ICAM-1 (CD54) and ICAM-2 (CD102), and VCAM-1 (CD106), or to the selectin family, which includes E-selectin (ELAM-1: CD62E) and P-selectin (CD62P). P-selectin is stored in Weibel-Palade bodies of endothelial cells, and is rapidly mobilized to the cell surface following activation (see Chapter 14). The molecule CD44, a 90 kDa protein expressed by all leucocytes, plays a major role in lymphocyte adhesion to HEVs. It is believed that several receptor–ligand interactions occur between lymphocytes and endothelial cells. These interactions not only direct lymphocytes to distinct specific target organs, but also mediate specific functions in the different phases of lymphocyte migration out of blood vessels (extravasation). These phases include cell margination, rolling over the endothelial surface, firm adhesion, attachment and diapedesis between endothelial cells (see Chapter 14) (*Fig. 3.28*).

Lymphocyte trafficking exposes antigen to a large number of lymphocytes

Lymphoid cells within lymph nodes return to the circulation by way of the efferent lymphatics, which pass via the thoracic duct into the left subclavian vein. About 1–2% of the lymphocyte pool recirculates each hour. Overall, this process allows a large number of antigen-specific lymphocytes to come into contact with their appropriate antigen in the microenvironment of the peripheral lymphoid organs. This is particularly important since lymphoid cells are monospecific, and there is only a limited number of lymphocytes capable of recognizing any particular antigen.

Under normal conditions there is continuous lymphocyte traffic through the nodes, but when antigen enters the lymph nodes of an animal already sensitized to that antigen there is a temporary shut down in the traffic, which lasts for approximately 24 hours. Thus, antigen-specific lymphocytes are preferentially retained in the lymph nodes draining the source of antigen. In particular, blast cells do not recirculate but appear to remain in one site.

One reason for considering the MALT as a system distinct from the systemic lymphoid organs, is that mucosa-associated lymphoid cells mainly recirculate within the mucosal lymphoid system. Thus, lymphoid cells stimulated in Peyer's patches pass via regional lymph nodes to the blood stream and then 'home' back into the intestinal lamina propria (*Fig. 3.29*). This specific recirculation is made possible because the lymphoid cells recognize adhesion molecules that are expressed specifically on endothelial cells of the mucosal post-capillary venules, and that are absent from lymph node HEVs. Thus, antigen stimulation at one mucosal area elicits an antibody response restricted to the MALT.

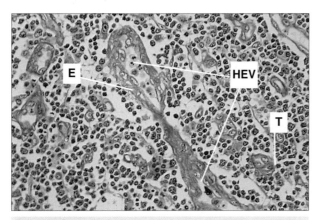

Fig. 3.27 Section of lymph nodes showing high endothelial venule (HEV). This section of lymph node paracortex shows the specialized high endothelial cells lining the HEV, through which lymphocytes leave the circulation and enter the node. E = endothelial cells; T = T-cell area. Giemsa stain (resin section), ×180. (Courtesy of Dr K. McLennan.)

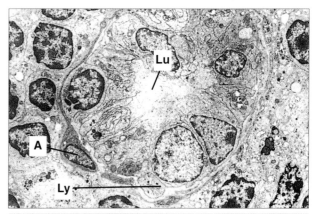

Fig. 3.28 Electron micrograph showing a high endothelial venule in the thymus-dependent area of a lymph node. A lymphocyte in transit from the lumen of the HEV can be seen close to the basal lamina. The HEV is partly surrounded by an adventitial cell. A = adventitial cell; Lu = lumen; Ly = lymphocyte. ×1600.

Lymphocyte circulation within the mucosal lymphoid system

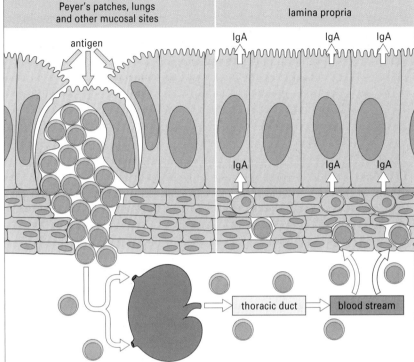

Fig. 3.29 Lymphoid cells which are stimulated with antigen in Peyer's patches (or the lungs, or another mucosal site) migrate via the regional lymph nodes and thoracic duct into the blood stream and thence to the lamina propria of the gut and probably other mucosal surfaces. Thus lymphocytes stimulated at one mucosal surface may become distributed throughout the MALT system.

Critical Thinking

■ Why is it that mammals need a highly specialized lymphoid system whilst the lower animals are able to survive without it?

■ Why is it important for lymphocytes to recirculate in the mucosal system and what molecules do they possess that enable them to do this?

■ What are the common features of the mucosal and systemic systems and how do they differ from one another? Is one more important than the other?

■ How does the lymphoid system differ from any other body system such as the respiratory or reproductive systems? (You may have to remind yourself of the different body systems in a physiology text book!)

■ What accessory cells do lymphoid tissues have and why? What are the functions of the primary and secondary lymphoid tissues?

FURTHER READING

Bros JD, Kapsenberg ML. The skin immune system. *Immunol Today* 1986;**7**:235.

Kuby J. *Cells and Organs of the Immune System.* New York: WH Freemanand Co, 1992:39–71.

Pardi R, Inverardi L, Bender JR. Regulatory mechanisms in leucocyte adhesion: flexible receptors for sophisticated travellers. *Immunol Today* 1992:**13**; 224.

Playfair JHL. *Immunology at a Glance.* 7th ed. Oxford: Blackwell Scientific Publications, 1992.

Roitt IM. *Essential Immunology.* 8th ed. Oxford: Blackwell Scientific Publications, 1994:Ch. 8;p.147.

Circulating antibodies recognize antigen in serum and tissue fluids.

There are five classes of antibody – IgG, IgA, IgM, IgD and IgE.

Immunoglobulins have a basic unit of two light chains and two heavy chains. The heavy chains differ between classes. IgA and IgM occur as oligomers of the four chain unit.

The chains are folded into discrete regions called domains. There are two domains in the light chain and four or five in the heavy chains, depending on their class.

Immunoglobulin fragments may be produced by proteolytic cleavage. These are useful experimentally and therapeutically. Papain generates two antigen binding **(Fab)** fragments and one **Fc** fragment from each IgG molecule whereas pepsin produces a large **F(ab')₂** fragment containing both antigen-binding sites.

Hypervariable regions form the antigen-binding sites. There are three such regions in the V domains of each light and heavy chain. The folding of the domains causes them to be clustered at the distal tips of the molecule, producing two antigen-binding sites for each four chain unit.

All antibodies are bifunctional. They exhibit one or more **effector functions** in addition to antigen binding. These biological activities (e.g. complement activation and cell binding) are localized to sites that are distant from the antigen binding sites (mostly in the Fc region).

Immunoglobulin receptor molecules are expressed by mononuclear cells, neutrophils, NK cells, eosinophils and mast cells. They interact with the Fc regions of different classes of immunoglobulins and promote activities such as phagocytosis, tumour cell killing and mast cell degranulation. Most of these Fc receptors are members of the **immunoglobulin superfamily** and have two or three extracellular immunoglobulin domains.

The recognition of foreign antigen is the hallmark of the specific adaptive immune response. Two distinct types of molecules are involved in this process – the immunoglobulins and the T-cell antigen receptors (TCRs) (*Fig. 4.1*). Diversity and heterogeneity are characteristic features of these molecules (see Chapter 6). There is evidence of extensive gene rearrangements which generate immunoglobulins or TCRs capable of recognizing many different antigens. T cell receptors are discussed in detail in Chapter 5.

Immunoglobulins are a group of glycoproteins present in the serum and tissue fluids of all mammals. Some are carried on the surface of B cells, where they act as receptors for specific antigens. Others (antibodies) are free in the blood or lymph. Contact between B cells and antigen is needed to cause the B cells to develop into antibody forming cells (AFCs), also called plasma cells, which secrete large amounts of antibody. ('Plasma cell' is the histological term for AFCs seen in blood and tissues.) The membrane-bound immunoglobulin on a precursor B cell has the same binding specificity as the antibody produced by the mature AFC.

■ IMMUNOGLOBULINS – A FAMILY OF PROTEINS

Five distinct classes of immunoglobulin molecule are recognized in most higher mammals, namely IgG, IgA, IgM, IgD and IgE. They differ in size, charge, amino acid composition and carbohydrate content.

In addition to the difference between classes, the immunoglobulins within each class are also very heterogeneous. Electrophoretically the immunoglobulins show a unique range of heterogeneity which extends from the γ to the α fractions of normal serum (*Fig. 4.2*).

Antigen recognition molecules

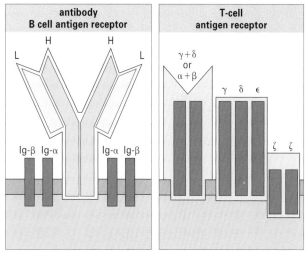

Fig. 4.1 The antigen receptors of T and B cells are probably derived from a common ancestor and both belong to the immunoglobulin superfamily. The primary immunoglobulin receptor consists of two identical heavy (H) chains and two identical light (L) chains. In addition, secondary components (Ig-α and Ig-β) are closely associated with the primary receptor and are thought to couple it to intracellular signalling pathways that activate IL-2 production. Circulating antibodies are structurally identical to the primary B cell antigen receptors, except that they lack the transmembrane and intracytoplasmic sections. The T-cell receptor has an antigen-binding portion consisting of an α and β chain (or a γ and δ chain) which are associated with four other transmembrane peptides (γ, δ, ε and ζ), structurally distinct from the chains of the receptor.

Immunoglobulins are bifunctional molecules

Each immunoglobulin molecule is bifunctional. One region of the molecule is concerned with binding to antigen while a different region mediates so-called effector functions. Effector functions include binding of the immunoglobulin to host tissues, to various cells of the immune system, to some phagocytic cells, and to the first component (Clq) of the classical complement system.

Immunoglobulin class and subclass depends on the structure of the heavy chain

The basic structure of all immunoglobulin molecules is a unit consisting of two identical light polypeptide chains and two identical heavy polypeptide chains, linked together by disulphide bonds (*Fig. 4.3*). The class and subclass of an immunoglobulin molecule are determined by its heavy chain type. Thus the four human IgG subclasses (IgG1, IgG2, IgG3 and IgG4) have heavy chains called γ1, γ2, γ3 and γ4 that differ slightly, although all are recognizably γ heavy chains.

The four subclasses of human IgG (IgG1–IgG4) occur in the approximate proportions of 66%, 23%, 7% and 4%, respectively. There are also subclasses of human IgA (IgA1 and IgA2), but none have been described for IgM, IgD or IgE. This range of immunoglobulin class and subclass is known as isotypic variation.

Immunoglobulin subclasses appear to have arisen late in evolution. Thus, the human IgG subclasses are different from the four known subclasses of IgG that have been identified in the mouse.

Each immunoglobulin class has a different set of functions

All immunoglobulins are glycoproteins, but the carbohydrate content ranges from 2–3% for IgG, to 12–14% for IgM, IgD, and IgE. The physicochemical properties of the immunoglobulins are summarized in *Figure 4.4*.

IgG – is the major immunoglobulin in normal human serum, accounting for 70–75% of the total immunoglobulin pool. IgG consists of a single four-chain molecule with a sedimentation coefficient of 7S and a molecular weight of 146 000. However, IgG3 proteins are slightly larger than the other subclasses; this is due to the slightly heavier γ3 chain. The IgG class, which is distributed evenly between the intravascular and extravascular pools, is the major antibody of secondary immune responses and the exclusive antitoxin class.

Maternal IgG also confers immunity in neonates. In man, IgG molecules of all subclasses cross the placenta and confer a high degree of passive immunity to the newborn. In species in which maternal immunoglobulin only reaches the offspring postnatally, for example the pig, IgG derived from the maternal milk selectively crosses the gastrointestinal tract.

IgM – accounts for approximately 10% of the immunoglobulin pool. The molecule is a pentamer of the basic four-chain structure. The individual heavy chains have a molecular weight of approximately 65 000 and the whole molecule has a molecular weight of 970 000. IgM is largely confined to the intravascular pool and is the predominant 'early' antibody, frequently seen in the immune response to antigenically complex infectious organisms.

IgA – represents 15–20% of the human serum immunoglobulin pool. In man more than 80% of IgA occurs as a monomer of the four-chain unit, but in most mammals the IgA in serum is mainly polymeric, occurring mostly as a dimer. IgA is the predominant immunoglobulin in seromucous secretions such as saliva, colostrum, milk, and tracheobronchial and genitourinary secretions.

Secretory IgA (sIgA), which may be of either subclass (IgA1 or IgA2) but mainly IgA2, exists mainly in the 11S, dimeric form and has a molecular weight of 385 000. It is abundant in seromucous secretions where it is associated with another protein, known as the secretory piece.

Distribution of the major human immunoglobulins

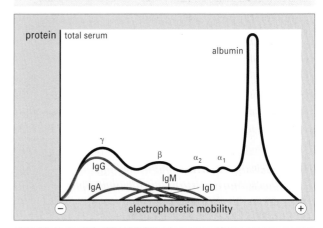

Fig. 4.2 Electrophoresis of human serum showing the distribution of the four major immunoglobulin classes. Serum proteins are separated according to their charges in an electric field, and classified as α1, α2, β, and γ, depending on their mobility. (The IgE class has a similar mobility to IgD but cannot be represented quantitatively because of its low level in serum.) IgG exhibits most charge heterogeneity, the other classes having a more restricted mobility in the β and fast γ regions.

The basic chain structure of immunoglobulins

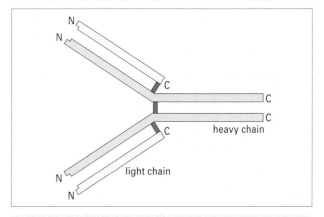

Fig. 4.3 The immunoglobulin unit consists of two identical light polypeptide chains and two identical heavy polypeptide chains linked together by disulphide bonds (red). Note the position of the amino- (N) and carboxy- (C) terminal ends of the peptide chains.

Physicochemical properties of human immunoglobulin classes

property	immunoglobulin type									
	IgG1	IgG2	IgG3	IgG4	IgM	IgA1	IgA2	sIgA	IgD	IgE
heavy chain	γ_1	γ_2	γ_3	γ_4	μ	α_1	α_2	α_1/α_2	δ	ϵ
mean serum conc. (mg/ml)	9	3	1	0.5	1.5	3.0	0.5	0.05	0.03	0.00005
sedimentation constant	7s	7s	7s	7s	19s	7s	7s	11s	7s	8s
mol. wt ($\times 10^3$)	146	146	170	146	970	160	160	385	184	188
half-life (days)	21	20	7	21	10	6	6	?	3	2
% intravascular distribution	45	45	45	45	80	42	42	trace	75	50
carbohydrate (%)	2–3	2–3	2–3	2–3	12	7–11	7–11	7–11	9–14	12

Fig. 4.4 Each immunoglobulin class has a characteristic type of heavy chain. Thus IgG possesses γ chains; IgM, μ chains; IgA, α chains; IgD, δ chains and IgE, ϵ chains. Variation in heavy chain structure within a class gives rise to immunoglobulin subclasses. For example, the human IgG pool consists of four subclasses reflecting four distinct types of heavy chain. The properties of the immunoglobulins vary between the different classes. Note that in secretions, IgA occurs in a dimeric form (sIgA) in association with a protein chain termed the secretory piece. Serum concentration of sIgA is very low, whereas the level in mucosal secretions can be very high.

IgD – accounts for less than 1% of the total plasma immunoglobulin but is present in large quantities on the membrane of many B cells. The precise biological function of this class is unknown, but it may play a role in antigen-triggered lymphocyte differentiation.

IgE – though scarce in serum, is found on the surface membrane of basophils and mast-cells in all individuals; it also sensitizes cells on mucosal surfaces such as the conjunctival, nasal and bronchial mucosa. This class of immunoglobulin may play a role in immunity to helminthic parasites, but in developed countries is more commonly associated with allergic diseases such as asthma and hay fever.

■ ANTIBODY STRUCTURE

The basic four-chain model for immunoglobulin molecules (*Fig. 4.5*) is based on two distinct types of polypeptide chain. The smaller (light) chain has a molecular weight of 25 000 and is common to all classes, whereas the larger (heavy) chain has a molecular weight of 50 000–77 000 and is structurally distinct for each class or subclass. The polypeptide chains are linked together by covalent and non-covalent forces.

All light chains have one variable and one constant region
The light chains of most vertebrates have been shown to exist in two distinct forms called kappa (κ) and lambda (λ). These are isotypes. Either of the light chain types may combine with any of the heavy chain types, but in any one immunoglobulin molecule both light chains are identical as are the two heavy chains.

Hilschmann, Craig and others in 1965 established that light chains consist of two distinct regions. The C-terminal half of the chain (approximately 107 amino acid residues) is constant except for certain allotypic and isotypic variations (see below) and is called the C_L (Constant:Light chain) region, whereas the N-terminal half of the chain shows much sequence variability and is known as the V_L (Variable:Light chain) region.

IgG has a 'typical' antibody structure
The IgG molecule may be thought of as a 'typical' antibody (*Fig. 4.5*). It has two intrachain disulphide bonds in the light

The basic structure of IgG1

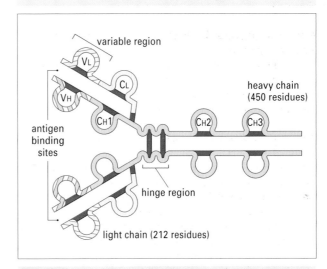

Fig. 4.5 The N-terminal end of IgG1 is characterized by sequence variability (V) in both the heavy and light chains, referred to as the V_H and V_L regions respectively. The rest of the molecule has a relatively constant (C) structure. The constant portion of the light chain is termed the C_L region. The constant portion of the heavy chain is further divided into three structurally discrete regions: C_H1, C_H2 and C_H3. These globular regions, which are stabilized by intrachain disulphide bonds, are referred to as 'domains'. The sites at which the antibody binds antigen are located in the variable domains. The hinge region is a segment of heavy chain between the C_H1 and C_H2 domains. Flexibility in this area permits the two antigen-binding sites to operate independently. There is close pairing of the domains except in the C_H2 region (see *Fig. 4.8*). Carbohydrate moieties are attached to the C_H2 domains.

Basic folding in the light chain

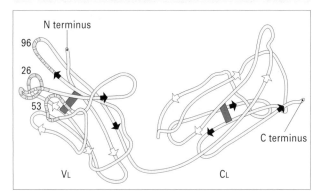

Fig. 4.6 The immunoglobulin domains in the light chain share a basic folding pattern with several straight segments of polypeptide chain lying parallel to the long axis of the domain. Light chains have two domains – one constant and one variable. Within each domain, the polypeptide chain is arranged in two layers, with many hydrophobic amino acid side-chains between the layers. One of the layers has four segments (arrowed white), the other has three (arrowed black); both are linked by a single disulphide bridge (red). Folding of the VL domains causes the hypervariable regions to become exposed in three separate but closely disposed loops. One numbered residue from each hypervariable region is identified.

chain – one in the variable region and one in the constant region (*Fig. 4.6*). There are four such bonds in the heavy (γ) chain, which is twice the length of the light chain. Each disulphide bond encloses a peptide loop of 60–70 amino acid residues; if the amino acid sequences of these loops are compared a striking degree of homology is revealed. Essentially this means that each immunoglobulin peptide chain is composed of a series of globular regions with very similar secondary and tertiary structure (folding). This is shown for the light chain in *Figure 4.6*.

The peptide loops enclosed by the disulphide bonds represent the central portion of a 'domain' of about 110 amino acid residues. In both the heavy and the light chains the first of these domains corresponds to the variable region, VH and VL respectively (*Fig. 4.7*). In the heavy chain of IgG, IgA and IgD there are three further domains, which make up the constant part of the chain, CH1, CH2 and CH3. In both μ and ε chains there is an additional domain immediately after CH1 (see *Fig. 4.11*). Thus, the C-terminal domains of IgM and IgE heavy chains (referred to as Cμ4 and Cε4) are homologous to the CH3 domain of IgG (Cγ3).

X-ray crystallography has provided structural data on complete IgG molecules, making it possible to construct both α-carbon backbone and computer-generated atomic models for this class of immunoglobulin (*Figs 4.8 and 4.9*). These show the Y-shaped structure that has also been visualized by electron microscopy.

Structure of IgG1

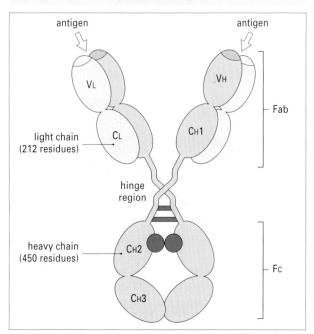

Fig. 4.7 A model of IgG1 indicating the globular domains of heavy (H) and light (L) chains. Note the apposition of the CH3 domains and the separation of the CH2 domains. The carbohydrate units (blue) lie between the CH2 domains. In this figure (and in *Fig. 4.11* onwards) the interchain disulphide bonds between H and L chains are not shown.

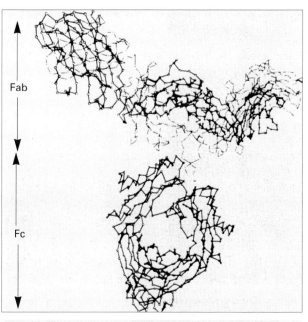

Fig. 4.8 Model of the α-carbon backbone of human IgG1. This model is based on X-ray crystallography studies which reveal that the polypeptide is folded into globular domains, forming a Y-shaped structure. The antigen-binding surfaces formed between the variable regions of the light and heavy chains are located at the tips of the arms. The model clearly shows the hinge region between the Fab and Fc regions, as well as suggesting weak interaction between the Cγ2 domains and strong interaction between the Cγ3 domains. (Courtesy of Professor R. Huber.)

Homologous domains of the light and heavy chains are paired in the Fab region (indicated in *Fig. 4.7*). The Cγ3 domains of the γ heavy chains are also paired, but the Cγ2 domains are separated by carbohydrate moieties.

Despite the structural similarities between domains there are striking differences at the level of domain interaction. For example, the variable domains associate with each other through their three segment layers, whereas the constant domains associate through the four-segment layers. (See *Fig. 4.6* for an explanation of the layers in light-chain domains.) The model of IgG1 shown in *Figure 4.7* is useful for all immunoglobulins; however, there are differences of detail between every class, and between subclasses.

IgG – With human IgG, the four subclasses differ only slightly in their amino acid sequences. Most of the differences are clustered in the hinge region and give rise to differing patterns of interchain disulphide bonds between the four proteins. The most striking structural difference is the elongated hinge region of IgG3 which accounts for its higher molecular weight and possibly for some of its enhanced biological activity (*Fig 4.10*).

IgM – Human IgM is usually found as a pentamer of the basic four-chain unit (*Fig. 4.11*). The μ chains of IgM differ from γ chains in amino acid sequence and have an extra constant region domain in place of the IgG hinge. The subunits of the pentamer are linked by disulphide bonds between the Cμ3 domains, and possibly by disulphide bonds between the C-terminal 18-residue peptide tailpieces. The complete molecule consists of a densely packed central region with radiating arms, as seen in electron micrographs.

Structure of human IgG3

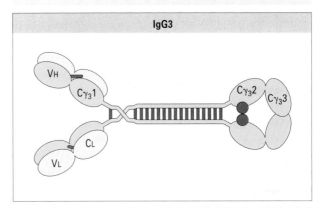

Fig. 4.10 Polypeptide chain structure of human IgG3. Note the elongated hinge region.

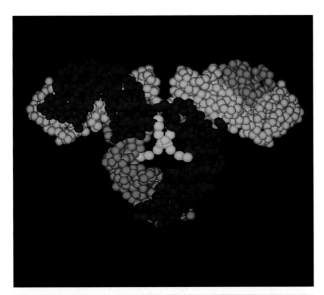

Fig. 4.9 Computer-generated model of the hinge-deleted human IgG1 protein Dob. Such proteins lack the flexibility characteristic of normal IgG molecules. Their rigidity permits structural determinations at a higher resolution. One heavy chain is shown in blue and one in red, with two light chains being depicted in green. Carbohydrate bound to the Fc portion of the molecule is shown in turquoise. The structure of this immunoglobulin was determined by David R. Davies *et al.* (*Proc Natl Acad Sci USA* 1977; **74**). The computer graphics were generated using the system developed by Richard J. Feldmann at the National Institutes of Health.

Structure of human IgM

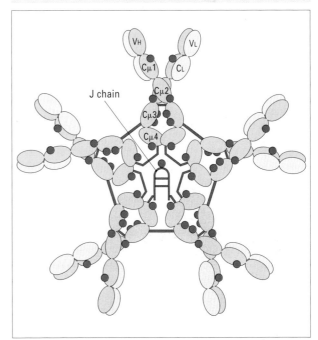

Fig. 4.11 IgM heavy chains have five domains with disulphide bonds cross-linking adjacent Cμ3 and Cμ4 domains. Also shown are the carbohydrate side-chains (blue) and possible location of the J chain. IgM does not have hinge regions, but flexion can occur about the Cμ2 domains.

Photographs of IgM antibodies binding to bacterial flagella show molecules adopting a 'staple' configuration (*Fig. 4.12*). This suggests that flexion readily occurs between the Cμ2 and Cμ3 domains, although note that this region is not structurally homologous to the IgG hinge. The dislocation resulting in the 'staple' configuration appears to be related to the activation of complement by IgM.

Two other features characterize the IgM molecule: an abundance of oligosaccharide units associated with the μ chain, and an additional peptide chain, the J (joining) chain, thought to assist the process of polymerization prior to secretion by the AFC. The J chain is a cysteine-rich peptide of 137 amino acid residues. One J chain is incorporated into the IgM structure by disulphide bonding to the 18-residue peptide tailpiece of the separate monomers. Binding is to the penultimate cysteine residues of the tailpieces. If J chains are not freely available, there is evidence that hexameric IgM becomes the preferred form.

IgA – The 472 amino-acid residues of the α-chain are arranged in four domains: VH, Cα1, Cα2 and Cα3 (*Fig. 4.13*). A feature shared with IgM is an additional C-terminal 18-residue peptide with a penultimate cysteine residue, which is able to bind covalently to a J chain to form dimers. Electron micrographs of IgA dimers show double Y-shaped structures, suggesting that the monomeric subunits are linked end-to-end through the C-terminal Cα3 regions (*Fig. 4.14*).

Secretory IgA (sIgA) exists mainly in the form of a molecule sedimenting at 11*s* (mol. wt 380 000). The complete molecule is made up of two units of IgA, one secretory component (mol. wt 70 000) and one J chain (mol. wt 15 000) (*Fig. 4.15*). It is not clear how the various peptide chains are linked together. In contrast to the J chain, secretory component is not synthesized by plasma cells but by epithelial cells. IgA held in dimer configuration by a J chain, and secreted by submucosal plasma cells, actively binds secretory component as it traverses epithelial cell layers. Bound secretory component facilitates the transport of sIgA into secretions, as well as protecting it from proteolytic attack.

IgA1 is the predominant subclass in serum, whereas IgA2 predominates in secretions. This may be because many microorganisms in the respiratory and gastrointestinal tracts release proteases that cleave IgA1.

IgD – Less than 1% of the total immunoglobulin in serum is IgD. This protein is more susceptible to proteolysis than IgG1, IgG2, IgA or IgM, and also has a tendency to undergo spontaneous proteolysis. There appears to be a single disulphide bond between the δ chains and a large amount of carbohydrate distributed in multiple oligosaccharide units (*Fig. 4.16*).

Structure of human IgA1

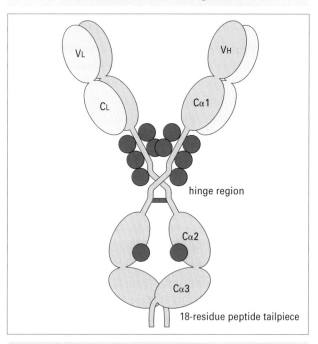

Fig. 4.13 This diagram shows the domain structure of IgA1 and the possible location of carbohydrate units (purple). Note the presence of the C-terminal 18-residue tailpiece (a feature shared with IgM) and a hinge region.

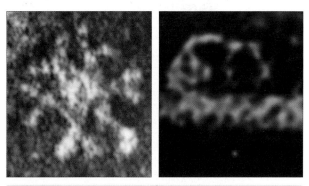

Fig. 4.12 Electron micrographs of IgM molecules. Left: In free solution, IgM adopts the characteristic star-shaped configuration. × 5 200 000. (Courtesy of Dr R. Dourmashkin.) Right: IgM bound to a single flagellum has adopted the crab-like, 'staple' configuration. × 5 200 000. (Courtesy of Dr A. Feinstein.)

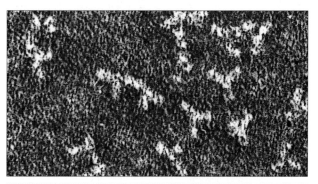

Fig. 4.14 Electron micrograph of a human dimeric IgA myeloma protein. The double Y-shaped appearance suggests that the monomeric subunits are linked end to end through the C-terminal Cα3 domain. × 1 600 000. (Courtesy of Dr R. Dourmashkin.)

IgE – The structure of IgE is shown in *Figure 4.17*. The higher molecular weight of the ε chain (72 500) is explained by the larger number of amino acid residues (approximately 550) distributed over five domains (VH, Cε1, Cε2, Cε3 and Cε4).

Sequence differences between antibody molecules may be isotypic, allotypic or idiotypic

Isotypic Variation – The genes for isotypic variants are present in all healthy members of a species. For example, the genes for γ1, γ2, γ3, γ4, μ, α1, α2, δ, ε, κ, and λ chains are all present in the human genome, and are therefore isotypes.

Structure of human secretory IgA (sigA)

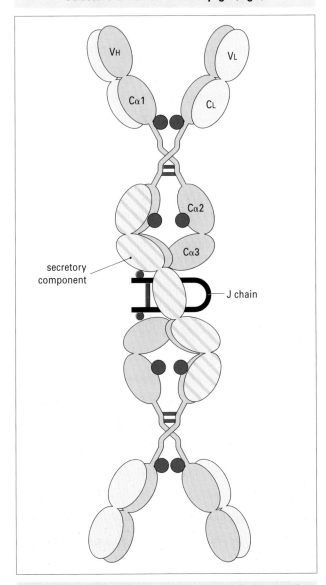

Fig. 4.15 The secretory component of sIgA is probably wound around the dimer and attached by disulphide bonds to the Cα2 domain of each IgA monomer. The J chain is required to join the two subunits.

Structure of human IgD

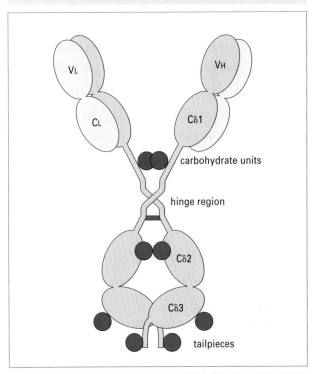

Fig. 4.16 This diagram of IgD shows the domain structure and a characteristically large number of oligosaccharide units. Note also the presence of a hinge region and short octapeptide tailpieces.

Structure of human IgE

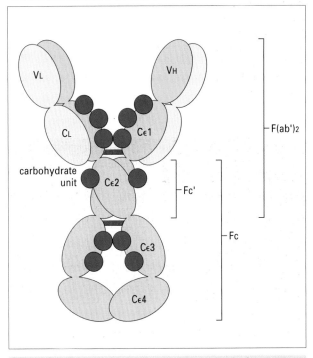

Fig. 4.17 IgE can be cleaved by enzymes to give the fragments F(ab')2, Fc and Fc'. Note the absence of a hinge region.

Allotypic Variation – This refers to genetic variation between individuals within a species, involving different alleles at a given locus. For example, the variant of IgG3 called G3m(b°) is characterized by a phenylalanine at position 436 of the γ3 heavy chain. It is not found in all people and is therefore an allotype. Allotypes occur mostly as variants of heavy chain constant regions.

Idiotypic Variation – Variation in the variable domain, particularly in the hypervariable regions, produces idiotypes, defined by their corresponding anti-idiotypes. These determine the binding specificity of the antigen binding site. Idiotypes are usually specific for individual B-cell clones (private idiotypes), but are sometimes shared between different B-cell clones (public, cross-reacting or recurrent idiotypes). The genetic basis of idiotypic variability is discussed in Chapter 6.

■ ANTIBODY EFFECTOR FUNCTIONS

The primary function of an antibody is to bind antigen. In a few cases this has a direct effect, for example by neutralizing bacterial toxin, or by preventing viral penetration of cells. In general, however, the interaction of antibody and antigen is without significance unless secondary 'effector' functions come into play (*Fig. 4.18*).

Activation of the complement system is one of the most important effector mechanisms of IgG1 and IgG3 molecules. The complement system is a complex group of serum proteins which mediate inflammatory reactions (see Chapter 13). Having bound to antigen, IgM, IgG1 and IgG3 may activate the complement enzyme cascade. IgG2 appears to be less effective in activating complement, while IgG4, IgA, IgD and IgE are ineffective.

The immunoglobulins display a complex pattern of interactions with various cell types (*Fig. 4.19*). These interactions are mediated by antibody receptors on the cell surfaces.

■ ANTIBODY RECEPTORS

There are three types of cell surface receptor for IgG

IgG receptors mediate several effector functions and have overlapping biological activities, which are triggered by cross-linking with the appropriate immunoglobulin. The major activities are phagocytosis, antibody dependent cellular cytotoxicity, mediator release and enhancement of antigen presentation.

Three groups of human IgG receptor are now recognized on cell surfaces: FcγRI (CD64), FcγRII (CD32) and FcγRIII (CD16). They are all characterized by extracellular domains showing significant homology with immunoglobulin V regions, i.e. they belong to the immunoglobulin superfamily, as does FcαR, a receptor specific for IgA molecules.

Properties and distribution of IgG receptors
Human FcγRI (CD64) binds monomeric IgG with high affinity (10^8–10^9 M^{-1}) and has a more restricted distribution than the other receptors.

FcγRII (CD32) is broadly distributed on cells and is frequently the only receptor to be expressed. It binds only complexed or polymeric IgG with a low affinity ($<10^7$ M^{-1}).

Major functions of human antibody classes and subclasses

effector function	immunoglobulin							
	IgG1	IgG2	IgG3	IgG4	IgM	IgA	IgD	IgE
complement fixation (classical pathway)	++	+	+++	–	+++	–	–	–
placental transfer	+	+	+	+	–	–	–	–
binding to staphylococcal protein A	+++	+++	–	+++	–	–	–	–
binding to streptococcal protein G	+++	+++	+++	+++	–	–	–	–

Fig. 4.18 These effector functions are associated with different parts of the Fc region. Placental transfer of IgG in man and intestinal transport in rodents are mediated by an MHC-I like receptor molecule.

Selected cell binding functions of human immunoglobulins

receptor		immunoglobulin									
		IgG1	IgG2	IgG3	IgG4	IgM	IgA1	IgA2	sIgA	IgD	IgE
mononuclear cells	FcγRI	++	–	+++	++	–	–	–	–	–	–
	FcγRIIa	+	(+)	++	–	–	–	–	–	–	–
	FcγRIIIa	+	–	+	–	–	–	–	–	–	–
	FcμR	–	–	–	–	+	–	–	–	–	–
	FcεRII	–	–	–	–	–	–	–	–	–	++
	FcαR	–	–	–	–	–	++	++	++	–	–
neutrophils	FcγRIIa	+	–	+	–	–	–	–	–	–	–
	FcγRIIIb	+	–	+	–	–	–	–	–	–	–
	FcαR	–	–	–	–	–	++	++	++	–	–
mast cells/ basophils	FcεRI	–	–	–	–	–	–	–	–	–	+++

Fig. 4.19 A complex family of receptor molecules able to bind immunoglobulin continues to be delineated (selected examples are listed here). FcμR is expressed by activated B cells but not by T cells or monocytes. FcεRII is also expressed on eosinophils, platelets, T cells and B cells.

FcγRIII (CD16) is extensively glycosylated and is expressed as a molecule with a range of molecular weights (50 000–80 000). FcγRIIIa is expressed on macrophages, NK cells and some T cells and interacts with complexed as well as monomeric IgG (affinity $3 \times 10^7 M^{-1}$). The GPI-linked FcγRIIIb is selectively expressed on granulocytes and has a low affinity for IgG ($<10^7 M^{-1}$).

IgG receptors are a diverse group

The three Fcγ receptors generate 12 different isoforms and genetic polymorphism has been described for both FcγRII and FcγRIII. In addition to this intrinsic heterogeneity, there is evidence that the receptors are expressed on cell surfaces as complexes in association with other chains. Two such chains have been identified to date in unrelated receptor complexes:
*   FcγRI is associated with disulphide-linked dimers of the γ chain also seen in FcεRI.
*   FcγRIIIa can associate with the same dimers of γ chains, or with dimers of ζ chains from the TCR complex, or with γ–ζ heterodimers.

In addition to preventing degradation of the FcγRIIIa complex in the endoplasmic reticulum, these associated chains appear to be essential for signal transduction. In the case of the GPI-anchored FcγRIIIb there appears to be no requirement for either γ or ζ chains (*Fig 4.20*).

Two distinct Fcε receptors bind to IgE

Two different receptors for IgE on cells are now known (*Fig. 4.21*). The high affinity receptor (FcεRI) is found on mast cells and basophils and is the 'classical' IgE receptor. This receptor is part of the immunoglobulin supergene family and quite distinct from the low affinity Fc receptor for IgE (FcεRII) found on leucocytes and lymphocytes. The low affinity receptor has not evolved from the immunoglobulin superfamily, but has substantial homology with several animal lectins such as mannose binding protein.

FcεRI is the high affinity IgE receptor

FcεRI has a tetrameric structure (see *Fig. 4.21*). The α-chain (45 kDa) is glycosylated and exposed on the cell surface. Antibodies against the α-chain can block IgE binding to the receptor and trigger histamine release from rat basophil leukaemia cells. The carbohydrate probably protects the α-chain from serum protease activity, as it does with many other cell-surface proteins. It is unlikely that the carbohydrate on the α chain plays a role in IgE-binding and IgE-mediated histamine release.

The single β chain (33 kDa) and the two disulphide-linked γ chains (9 kDa) are essential components of the αβγ₂ receptor unit. They are required for receptor expression on the cell surface, and may have a role in signal transduction.

The receptor interacts with the distal portion of the IgE heavy chain, that is, regions of the CH2 and/or CH3 domains. The interaction is highly specific and the binding constant for IgE is very high (approximately $10^{10} M^{-1}$). Neither the interaction of monovalent IgE with the receptor complex, nor the binding of substrate to a single IgE, appear to activate mast cells or basophils, since no histamine release occurs. It is the cross-linking of several surface-bound IgEs, by antigen or by other molecules, that stimulates degranulation.

The carbohydrate associated with IgE itself does not seem to be of importance in its interaction with FcεRI. Its role seems to be in the secretion of IgE from B cells. The high-affinity receptor was thought to be limited to mast cells and basophils, but some recent data suggest that receptors may also be found on Langerhans' cells.

FcεRII is the low affinity IgE receptor

The human lymphocyte FcεRII or CD23 antigen (45 kDa) shows the characteristics of a membrane-bound molecule, i.e. a transmembrane domain, but it is unusual in that it lies 'upside-down' in the cell membrane, the C-terminus being extracellular (see *Fig. 4.20*). Unlike other Fc receptors, FcεRII

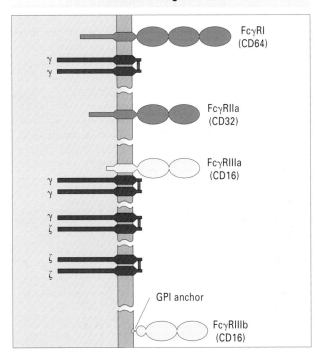

Selected phagocyte receptors interacting with immunoglobulins

Fig 4.20 The human Fcγ receptor structures shown are those for FcγRI (expressed by monocytes), FcγRIIa (expressed by monocytes and neutrophils), FcγRIIIa (expressed by moncytes and attached as a normal transmembrane protein) and FcγRIIIb (expressed by neutrophils and attached by a phosphatidyl inositol glycan [GPI] membrane anchor). Each receptor belongs to the immunoglobulin superfamily and expresses two or three extracellular immunoglobulin-like domains. Several of the receptors are now known to exist as complexes with various disulphide linked subunits. FcγRI and FcγRIIIa both associate with dimers of the γ chain originally described as part of the high affinity FcεRI complex (see *Fig. 4.21*). FcγRIIIa has also been shown to associate with dimers of the ζ-chain found in the TCR-CD3 complex. In the case of FcγRIIIa these subunits can associate as either homodimers (γ–γ or ζ–ζ) or as heterodimers (γ–ζ). They appear to be essential for surface expression and signal transduction. In FcγRI interactions, the receptor appears to bind a structural motif centred around Leu 235 in the CH2 domain, present in IgG1, IgG3 and IgG4.

is not a member of the immunoglobulin superfamily but belongs to a primitive superfamily of animal lectins.

Two forms of the human FcεRII have now been identified, cloned and sequenced. They differ only in the N-terminal cytoplasmic region, the extracellular domains being identical. The FcεRIIa is normally expressed on B cells, whereas expression of FcεRIIb is inducible on T cells, B cells, monocytes and eosinophils by the cytokine IL-4. Expression of FcεRIIb is often increased on B cells and monocytes of individuals with eczema, and on lymphocytes of hayfever sufferers.

■ ANTIBODY STRUCTURE AND FUNCTION

Antibody fragments generated by proteases offer insight into structure and function

The plant protease papain cleaves the IgG molecule in the hinge region between the Cγ1 and Cγ2 domains, to give two identical Fab (antigen binding) fragments and one Fc (crystallizable) fragment. These papain-generated fragments have been of enormous value in structure/function studies on the antibody molecule because they separated the Fab region, which binds to antigen, from the Fc region, which mediates effector functions such as complement fixation and monocyte binding. The Fc region is also important in placental transmission.

Papain also generates, after prolonged digestion, a degraded fragment of the Cγ3 region called the Fcᶦ fragment.

Some of these major points of enzymatic cleavage are shown in *Figure 4.22*.

Pepsin is another useful enzyme for structure/function studies, and generates two major fragments of IgG: the F(ab')₂ fragment, which broadly encompasses the two Fab regions linked by the hinge region, and the pFc' fragment, which corresponds to the Cγ3 domain of the molecule.

Many other enzymes are known to cleave the IgG molecule. Brief trypsin digestion of acid-treated Fc fragments yields the Cγ2 domain; isolation of this fragment has permitted structural and functional comparison with other subfragments such as pFc'.

Hypervariable sequences in the antigen-binding site allow antibodies to bind a range of antigens

Within the variable regions of both heavy and light chains, some short polypeptide segments show exceptional variability. Termed hypervariable regions, these segments are located near amino acid positions 30, 50 and 95 (*Fig. 4.23*). Because they create the antigen-binding site, hypervariable regions are sometimes referred to as complementarity determining regions (CDRs). The intervening peptide segments

Fc receptors for IgE

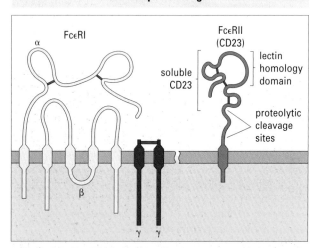

Fig. 4.21 The model for FcεRI proposes a tetramer consisting of one α chain with two disulphide-linked immunoglobulin-like loops. The β chain has two extracellular portions near two γ chains which are linked by disulphide bonds (red). The α-chain is crucial for IgE binding. The model for FcεRII is hypothetical, and is based on sequence data and the homology with animal lectins. Proteolytic cleavage can release several types of IgE-binding factors, including the 25 kDa soluble CD23 molecule, which contains the lectin binding domain. This cleavage is inhibited by IgE, accounting for the apparent increase of FcεRII expression on lymphocytes cultured in the presence of IgE.

Enzymic cleavage of human IgG1

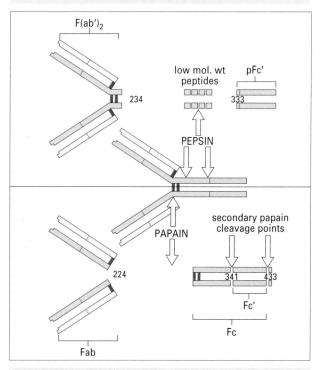

Fig. 4.22 Pepsin cleaves the heavy chain of human IgG1 at positions 234 and 333, to yield the F(ab')2 and pFc' fragments. Further action reduces the central fragment to low molecular weight peptides. Papain splits the molecule in the hinge region (at residue 224) yielding two Fab fragments and the Fc fragment. Secondary action on the Fc fragment at residues 341 and 433 gives rise to Fc'.

are called framework regions (FRs). In both light and heavy chain V regions there are three CDRs (CDR1–CDR3) and four FRs (FR1–FR4). (The basis of hypervariability is discussed more fully in Chapter 6.)

The variable regions of the light and heavy chains are folded in such a way that the regions of hypervariability are brought together to create the surface structure that binds antigen. These regions are, in the main, associated with bends in the peptide chain (see *Fig. 4.6*).

Many of the sites of effector functions in antibodies have now been identified

In contrast to the rapid progress made in localizing the antigen binding sites of antibodies, the precise structural locations of most effector functions have proved to be elusive. Enzymic subfragments and peptide inhibition studies provided provisional data, but further progress was slow until the technique of site-directed mutagenesis was introduced. This allowed researchers to selectively alter amino acids at different positions in the known peptide sequence, and thus to assess the importance of specific residues for particular functions.

An investigation of complement activation by IgG was one of the first to use this technique. Earlier studies had already suggested that the C1q subcomponent of C1 interacted with the Cγ2 domain of IgG. Site-directed mutagenesis was used to localize the binding site for C1q to three side chains in the Cγ2 domain, Glu 318, Lys 320 and Lys 322. This IgG sequence motif appears to be the common feature in interactions between C1q and IgG molecules.

In the case of IgM, complement activation seems to involve a different mechanism. Free circulating IgM in the star-shaped configuration is clearly incapable of activating complement, whereas IgM bound to antigen is a potent activator. Feinstein and colleagues suggested that the process of IgM binding to a polymeric or latticed antigen dislocates the F(ab')₂ units out of their original plane and leads to the so-called 'staple' configuration visualized by electron microscopy (see *Fig. 4.12*). These conformational changes would unveil a ring of C1q binding sites that are hidden in the star-shaped configuration of IgM by the close juxtaposition of the subunits. Candidate residues are His 430, Asp/Gly 432 and Pro 436, which occupy a structural location in the Cμ3 domain that is analogous to the proposed C1q binding site in the Cγ2 domain of IgG.

IgG molecules interact with a wide range of cellular Fc receptors. Site-directed mutagenesis studies suggest that the high affinity FcγRI receptor of monocytes interacts with a motif centred around a leucine residue at position 235 of the IgG heavy chain, between the Cγ2 domain and the hinge region (see *Fig. 4.20*). The localization of sites interacting with other Fc receptors will probably require similar experimental approaches.

Another genetic engineering approach has been used to study the sites on the IgE molecule that interact with mast-cells through the FcεRI receptor, or with B cells through the FcεRII receptor. Recombinant peptides containing ε-chain sequences were synthesized and then used to inhibit IgE-

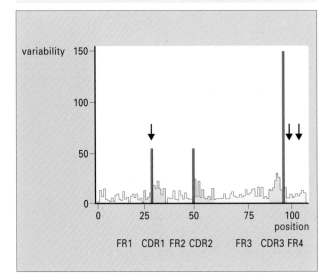

Amino acid variability in the variable region of immunoglobulin light chains

Fig. 4.23 Variability is calculated by comparing the sequences of many individual chains and, for any position, is equal to the ratio of the number of different amino acids found at that position, to the frequency of the most common amino acid. The areas of greatest variability, of which there are three in the VL domain, are the hypervariable regions. In some sequences studied, extra amino acids have been found, but these are excluded here to enhance comparison; their positions are indicated by arrows. The areas shaded orange denote regions of hypervariability (CDR), and the most hypervariable positions are shaded red. The four framework regions (FR) are shown in yellow. (Courtesy of Professor E. A. Kabat.)

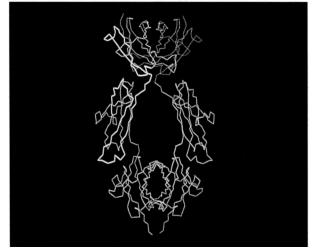

Fig. 4.24 Suggested location of the mast-cell receptor (FcεRI) binding site on human IgE. The Fc domains shown are (from top to bottom) Cε2, Cε3, and Cε4. The putative location of the peptide involved in binding is shown as a white segment extending from residue Gln 301 to residue Arg 376. (Reproduced from Helm *et al.* [1988] with permission.)

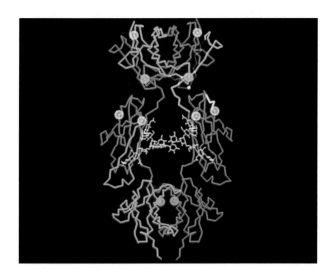

receptor interactions. In the case of FcεRI interactions, a 76-residue peptide spanning the Cε2–Cε3 junction appears to be critical (*Fig. 4.24*). In contrast, the FcεRII site appears to recognize a motif involving residues in the Cε3 domains of both chains (*Fig. 4.25*).

The interaction between protein A of *Staphylococcus aureus* and the Fc region of IgG has also been mapped in some detail. The data suggest a binding site spanning the Cγ2–Cγ3 junction in the Fc region.

Fig. 4.25 Suggested location of the B-cell binding site (FcεRII) on human IgE. Model of IgE Fc showing the Cε2 on top, the Cε3 in the middle and the Cε4 at the bottom. The residues Lys 367–Val 370 of both ε chains (arrowed in white) are believed to contribute to the critical structure of the binding site. (Reproduced from Vercelli *et al.* [1989], with permission.)

Critical Thinking

■ Antibody molecules are structurally diverse in their so-called constant regions. How does such diversity manifest itself and how is it advantageous to the host?

■ It is believed that immunoglobulins have evolved from a primordial protein equivalent to a single domain. How has genetic duplication to give a multi-domain protein assisted the evolution of a functionally potent molecule?

■ A large family of Fcγ receptors has been identified. From a knowledge of their common overall structure explain how interactions with immunoglobulins might be enhanced.

■ How is molecular biology helping to map the effector function sites of immunoglobulins? How is this approach superior to techniques used previously?

FURTHER READING

Burton DR. Antibody: the flexible adaptor molecule. *Trends Biochem Sci* 1990;**15**:64–69.

Capra D, Edmundson AB. The antibody-combining site. Sci Am 1977;**236**:50.

Conrad DH. The low affinity receptor for IgE. *Annu Rev Immunol* 1990;**8**:623–45.

Davies DR, Metzger H. Structural basis of antibody function. *Annu Rev Immunol* 1983;**1**:87–117.

Davis AC, Schulman MJ. IgM – molecular requirements for its assembly and function. *Immunol Today* 1989;**10**:118–22, 127–28.

Duncan AR, Winter G. The binding site for C1q on IgG. *Nature* 1988;**332**:738–40.

Duncan AR, Woof JM, Partridge LJ, Burton DR, Winter G. Localization of the binding site for the human high-affinity Fc receptor on IgG. *Nature* 1988;**332**:563–64.

Feinstein A, Richardson N, Taussig MJ. Immunoglobulin flexibility in complement activation. *Immunol Today* 1986;**7**:169–73.

Hahn GS. Antibody structure, function and active sites. In: Ritzmann SE, ed. *Physiology of Immunoglobulins: Diagnostic and Clinical Aspects*. New York: Alan Liss Inc, 1982.

Helm B, Marsh P, Vercelli D, Padlan E, Gould H, Geha R. The mast cell binding site on human immunoglobulin E. *Nature* 1988;**331**:180–83.

Möller G, ed. Immunoglobulin D: structure, synthesis, membrane representation and function. *Immunol Rev* 1977;**37**.

Möller G, ed. Immunoglobulin E. *Immunol Rev* 1978;**41**.

Möller G, ed. The B-cell antigen receptor complex. *Immunol Rev* 1993;**132**.

Nisonoff S. *Introduction to Molecular Immunology*. 2nd ed. Baltimore: Sinauer Associates Inc, 1984.

Perkins SJ, Nealis AS, Sutton BJ, Feinstein A. Solution structure of human and mouse immunoglobulin M by synchrotron X-ray scattering and molecular graphics modelling. *J Mol Biol* 1991; **221**:1345–66.

Ravetch JV, Kinet J–P. Fc receptors. *Annu Rev Immunol* 1991;**9**:457–92.

Shakib F, ed. The human IgG subclasses. Molecular analysis of structure, function, and regulation. Oxford: Pergamon Press, 1990.

Story CM, Mikulska JE, Simister NE. A major histocompatibility complex Class I-like Fc receptor cloned from human placenta: possible role in transfer of immunoglobulin G from mother to fetus. *J Exp Med* 1994;**180**:2377–81.

Turner MW. Structure and function of immunoglobulins. In: Glynn LE, Steward MW, eds. *Immunochemistry: An advanced textbook*. Chichester: John Wiley & Sons, 1977.

Underdown BJ, Schiff JM. Immunoglobulin A: strategic defence initiative at the mucosal surface. *Annu Rev Immunol* 1986;**4**:389–417.

Van de Winkel JGJ, Capel PJA. Human IgG Fc receptor heterogeneity: molecular aspects and clinical implications. *Immunol Today* 1993;**14**:215–21

Vercelli D, Helm B, Marsh P, Padlan E, Geha RS, Gould H. The B cell binding site on human immunoglobulin E. *Nature* 1989;**338**:649–51.

Williams AF, Barclay AN. The immunoglobulin superfamily – domains for cell surface recognition. *Annu Rev Immunol* 1988;**6**:381–405.

T-CELL RECEPTORS AND MHC MOLECULES

The T-cell antigen receptor (TCR) is a disulphide-linked heterodimeric (either αβ or γδ) glycoprotein that enables T cells to recognize a diverse array of antigens. It is associated at the cell surface with a complex of polypeptides known collectively as CD3.

The major histocompatibility complex (MHC) encodes two sets of highly polymorphic cell surface molecules, termed MHC class I and MHC class II. The αβ TCR recognises processed antigen as peptide fragments bound to MHC class I or class II molecules. Both MHC and peptide residues associate with the TCR.

A peptide binding cleft is formed by the folding of an MHC molecule. This accommodates peptides that have been processed by the cell, to be presented to T cells. Peptides of 8 or 9 residues can bind to class I molecules, whereas longer peptides can bind to class II molecules.

Binding pockets within the clefts are able to accommodate different peptides depending on the haplotype. Since MHC molecules are highly polymorphic, and since a cell can express several different MHC molecules, this explains how the cell can present many different antigenic peptides to a T cell.

■ T-CELL RECEPTORS

Antigen recognition by T lymphocytes is central to the generation and regulation of an effective immune response. Many important questions in immunology have centred on the nature of the receptor on T cells that mediates specific antigen recognition.

A T-cell receptor (TCR) was first defined and purified using specific antibodies directed against a clone-specific molecule on T cells. It was called the αβ TCR because it was a heterodimeric molecule comprising an α chain and a β chain linked by a disulphide bond. Independently, genes which might encode TCR chains were isolated from cDNA libraries, on the basis of their being expressed in some clones but not others. The amino acid sequence deduced from the nucleotide sequence of the genes matched the partial sequence obtained from α and β TCR proteins purified using monoclonal antibodies. Thus, the two different approaches had identified the same entity. In further experiments, a second TCR, called γδ, was isolated.

The CD3 complex associates with the αβ and γδ forms of the T-cell receptor

The αβ and γδ forms of the TCR are both associated physically with a series of polypeptides, collectively called CD3. This association is required for surface expression of the TCR complex at the cell surface. The CD3 components show no amino acid variability on different T cells and thus cannot generate the diversity associated with TCRs. Rather, the CD3 component of the TCR is most probably required for signal transduction following antigen recognition by the TCR heterodimer. CD3 comprises at least 5 invariant polypeptides, called γ, δ, ε, ζ and η. The organization of the TCR complex is shown schematically in *Figure 5.1*.

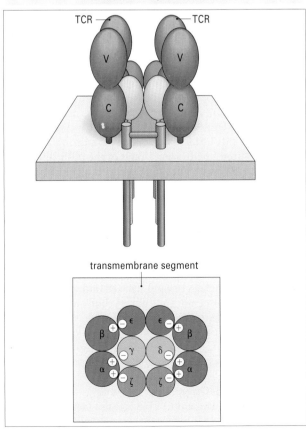

The T-cell receptor complex

TCR — TCR

V V

C C

transmembrane segment

ε ε
β + + β
γ δ
α + + α
ζ ζ

Fig. 5.1 The TCR α and β (or γ and δ) chains each comprise an external V and C domain, a transmembrane segment containing positively charged amino acids and a short cytoplasmic tail. The two chains are disulphide-linked on the membrane-side of their C domains. The CD3 γ, δ and ε chains comprise an external immunoglobulin-like C domain, a transmembrane segment containing a negatively charged amino acid and a longer cytoplasmic tail. A dimer of ζζ, ηη or ζη is also associated with the complex. Several lines of evidence support the notion that the TCR/CD3 complex exists at the cell surface as a dimer. The transmembrane charges are important for the assembly of the complex. A plausible arrangement which neutralizes opposite charges is shown.

The CD3 γ, δ and ε chains are the products of three closely linked genes and are clearly related in their primary sequences. The polypeptides are members of the immunoglobulin superfamily, each containing an external domain followed by a transmembrane region and a highly conserved cytoplasmic tail of 40 or more amino acids. An unusual feature of the transmembrane regions is that they each contain a negatively-charged amino acid, rather than being completely apolar.

The CD3 ζ and η polypeptides are products of a single gene and differ at their C-terminal ends due to differential splicing of the corresponding RNA. The CD3 ζη gene is on a different chromosome to the CD3 γδε gene complex and the ζη and γδε polypeptides are structurally unrelated. The ζ and η chains comprise a small extracellular domain of only nine amino acids, a transmembrane segment including a negatively-charged residue, and a large cytoplasmic tail. The cytoplasmic domain of CD3 η is 42 amino acids longer than that of CD3 ζ at the C terminus. The CD3 ζ and η chains exist as disulphide-linked dimers. Three dimeric forms (ζ–ζ, η–η and ζ–η) exist.

The stoichiometry of the TCR complex, and the way in which the CD3 chains are thought to interact with the αβ or γδ heterodimers, are discussed below.

CD3 is phosphorylated after engagement of the T-cell receptor

During T-cell activation, various components of the CD3 complex become phosphorylated on their intracytoplasmic portions. Murine and human CD3 γ chains are rapidly phosphorylated following mitogen or antigen stimulation. This phosphorylation is mediated by the enzyme, protein kinase C. Minor phosphorylation of the murine δ chain also occurs. Protein kinase C-mediated phosphorylation of CD3 is thought to play a role in the rapid downregulation of cell-surface TCR expression that follows occupancy of the TCR by antigen/MHC. This decrease in surface TCR levels may be involved in the desensitization of the T cells that occurs after initial antigen stimulation.

Immune activation of T cells also results in rapid and transient tyrosine phosphorylation of CD3 ζ, within a sequence called the antigen recognition activation motif (ARAM). The tyrosine kinase, p56^{lck}, is thought to be important in T-cell activation and recent studies suggest that p56^{lck} phosphorylates tyrosine residues within the ARAMs of ζ chains. Tyrosine phosphorylation on CD3 ζ is likely to form an early part of the signal transduction pathway that carries signals from the cell surface to the nucleus.

The αβ TCR heterodimer forms the recognition unit of the receptor

The αβ TCR comprises a disulphide-linked heterodimer of α (40–50 kDa) and β (35–47 kDa) subunits. The structural features of the αβ heterodimer are presented in *Figure 5.1*. Each polypeptide chain comprises two immunoglobulin-like domains of approximately 110 amino acids, anchored into the plasma membrane by a transmembrane peptide which has a short cytoplasmic tail. The difference in molecular weights of the human α and β chains is accounted for by the presence of extra N-linked carbohydrate on the α chain. The function of this carbohydrate is unknown

The amino acid sequence variability of the TCR resides in the N-terminal domains of the α and β polypeptides, which are homologous with the variable domains of immunoglobulins. This domain is encoded by rearranging V, D and J gene segments for β, and the V and J gene segments for α (see Chapter 6). Analysis of different TCR V domain sequences has revealed areas of relatively greater variability which correspond to immunoglobulin hypervariable regions, also known as complementarity-determining regions (CDRs).

The disulphide bond that links the α and β chains is in a peptide sequence between the constant domain and the transmembrane peptide. An unusual feature of both α- and β-chain transmembrane regions is the inclusion of positively-charged residues (see *Fig. 5.1*). These charged residues have been implicated in the assembly and intracellular transport of the TCR complex.

Structure of the receptor complex

The stoichiometry and subunit interactions of the components of the TCR complex have been the subject of extensive study. *In vitro* mutagenesis studies have shown that the charged residues within the transmembrane regions are essential for the assembly and surface expression of the TCR complex. This presumably involves the generation of ion pairs or hydrogen bonds within the lipid bilayer, between the basic amino acids in the TCR αβ peptides and the complementary acidic residues in the CD3 chains.

The immunoglobulin-like extracellular domains of the TCR (αβ or γδ) and CD3 (γ, δ and ε) polypeptides probably also form associations. In particular, the V domains of the αβ and γδ TCRs are thought to associate in much the same way as the VH/VL domains of immunoglobulin molecules, bringing the six TCR hypervariable regions together to form the antigen-binding site. In the case of T cells, this binding site must also bind sites on the MHC molecule that presents the antigen. There are, however, no structural data to support this contention, although the key residues involved in VH/VL interactions are conserved in TCR V domains.

The TCR–CD3 complex probably exists at the cell surface as a higher order structure. Stoichiometry measurements have revealed that CD3ε is found as two copies in the mature complex and that there is a 1:1 ratio of the αβ heterodimer and CD3ε molecules. This, together with measurements of the molecular weight of the solubilized TCR–CD3 complex point to a model for the TCR as an $(\alpha\beta)_2, \gamma, \delta, \varepsilon_2, \zeta_2$ structure. This divalent model, shown in *Figure 5.1*, exactly matches the transmembrane positive and negative charges.

The γδ TCR structurally resembles the αβ TCR

The overall structure of the γδ TCR is similar to that of its αβ counterpart, each chain being organized into external V and C domains, a transmembrane segment containing positively-charged residues and a short cytoplasmic tail.

The structure of γδ TCRs is more variable in humans than in the mouse. Human γ and δ chains can be disulphide linked, or can exist as monomers; the disulphide link correlates with the presence of the Cγ2 constant region exon rather than Cα1, because only Cγ2 possesses a cysteine. (See Chapter 6 for TCR gene organization.) TCR γ chains containing a Cγ2 constant region vary in molecular weight due to duplication or triplication of this second exon. The biological significance of these structural differences remains unclear. In the mouse, non-disulphide linked forms for the $\gamma\delta$ TCR have not been reported.

T cells with $\alpha\beta$ TCRs have a different distribution to those with $\gamma\delta$ TCRs

The two forms of TCR show quite distinct anatomical locations. The $\alpha\beta$ TCR is present on more than 95% of peripheral T cells and on the majority of TCR-expressing thymocytes. In contrast, T cells expressing the $\gamma\delta$ receptor often have defined anatomical locations. Although $\gamma\delta$ T cells form only a small proportion of T cells in the thymus and secondary lymphoid organs, they are abundant in various epithelia, such as the epidermis (in mice but not humans), intestinal epithelium, uterus and tongue.

The $\gamma\delta$ T cells in each epithelial tissue form distinct subsets which differ structurally in terms of which V regions are expressed. The expression of different V gene segments by distinct $\gamma\delta$ subsets may reflect their ontogeny. For example, $\gamma\delta$ T cells residing in mouse skin (dendritic epidermal cells or DECs) express exclusively the Vγ3 and Vδ1 regions (see Chapter 6), whereas intraepithelial lymphocytes (IELs) from the gut epithelium express Vγ5 almost exclusively (in combination with predominantly Vδ4, Vδ5, Vδ6 or Vδ7). It is thought that these populations may arise at distinct stages during intrathymic T-cell development.

▉ MAJOR HISTOCOMPATIBILITY COMPLEX (MHC) ANTIGENS

The genetic loci involved in rejection of foreign or non-self tissues form a region known as the major histocompatibility complex (MHC). The highly polymorphic cell surface structures involved in rejection are known as MHC antigens, because they were initially identified using alloantibodies produced by one inbred strain of mouse in response to immunization with cells of other strains differing genetically only at the MHC. Subsequently, specific antibodies to molecules encoded in subregions of the MHC, defined from crossovers in inbred strains, were used to map the MHC in detail. Similar techniques were used to define the human MHC, which is known as the human leucocyte antigen (HLA) system. The nomenclature reflects the way in which these molecules were characterized, i.e. as antigens that allowed alloantibodies to bind and destroy leucocytes. Thus, although they are known as antigens, they are only recognized as such when exposed to a non-self immune system, e.g. following organ transplantation.

The overall organization of the human and murine MHCs is presented in *Figure 5.2*. Three classes of molecules (I, II and III) have been identified as encoded within the murine and human MHCs. Class I and class II molecules represent distinct structural entities; that is, although multiple class I and class II genes exist within the MHC, all class I and class II gene products have similar overall structure. In contrast, the class III region contains a rather diverse collection of over 20 genes, including some that encode complement system molecules (C4, C2, factor B), and some that are involved in the processing of antigen. There are no established functional or structural similarities between class III gene products and the class I or class II molecules. Therefore, only those loci involved in triggering T lymphocytes – the class I and II genes and their gene products – are described in this chapter.

The structure of MHC class I molecules

A scheme for the structure of MHC class I molecules is presented in *Figure 5.3*. It comprises a glycosylated heavy chain (45 kDa) non-covalently associated with β_2-microglobulin (12 kDa), a polypeptide that is also found free in serum.

The MHC class I heavy chain has three extracellular domains

The class I heavy chain consists of three extracellular domains, designated α_1 (N-terminal), α_2 and α_3, a transmembrane region and a cytoplasmic tail. The three extracellular domains

Organization of murine and human MHCs

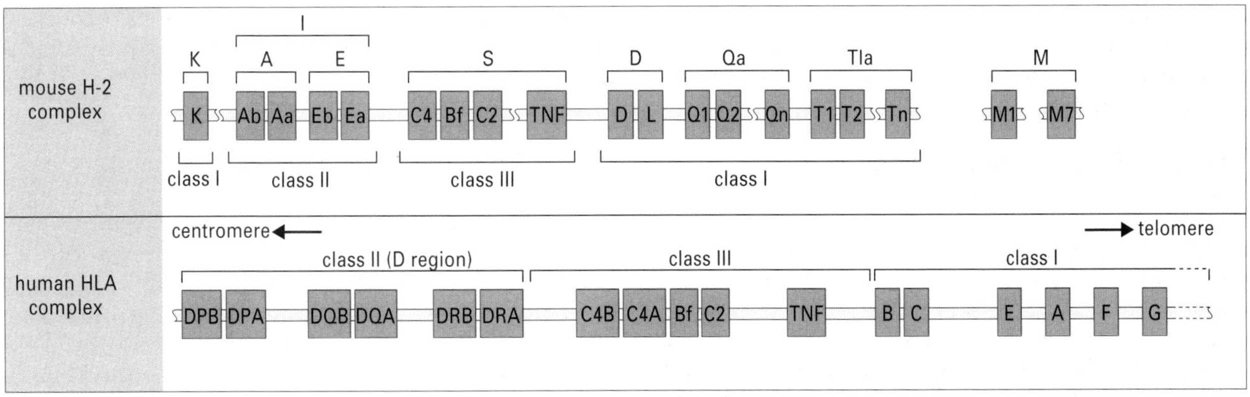

Fig. 5.2 Diagram showing the locations of subregions of the murine and human MHCs and the positions of the major genes within these subregions. The human organization pattern, in which the class II loci are positioned between the centromere and the class I loci, occurs in every other mammalian species so far examined. The regions span 3–4 Mbp of DNA.

each comprise about 90 amino acids and can be cleaved from the surface with the proteolytic enzyme papain. The α_2 and α_3 domains both have intrachain disulphide bonds enclosing loops of 63 and 86 amino acids respectively. The α_3 domain is homologous with immunoglobulin C domains. The extracellular portion of the class I heavy chain is glycosylated, the degree of glycosylation depending on the species and haplotype. The predominantly hydrophobic transmembrane region comprises 25 amino acid residues and traverses the lipid bilayer most probably in an α-helical conformation. The hydrophilic cytoplasmic domain, 30–40 residues long, may be phosphorylated *in vivo*.

β_2-microglobulin is essential for expression of MHC class 1 molecules

β_2-microglobulin (β_2m) is *non-polymorphic* in man, but is dimorphic in mice (a single amino acid change at position 85). It has the structure of an immunoglobulin C domain.

This molecule also associates with a number of other class I-related structures, for example the products of the CD1 genes on chromosome 1 in man, and the Fc receptor that mediates the uptake of IgG from milk in intestinal cells of neonatal rats. β_2m is essential for expression of all class I molecules at the cell surface – mutant mice lacking β_2m do not express class I.

Heavy chain α_1 and α_2 domains form the binding groove

The three-dimensional structures of the extracellular portion (α_1, α_2, α_3 domains and β_2m) of several human class I molecules have been elucidated by X-ray diffraction (*Fig. 5.4*). As predicted, the α_3 and β_2m domains have immunoglobulin-like folds. However, the β_2m-α_3 interaction, with the β_2m molecule sitting at an angle under the α_1 and α_2 domains, does not mirror the interaction of constant domains in antibodies.

The α_1 and α_2 domains constitute a platform of eight antiparallel β strands supporting two anti-parallel α helices (*Fig. 5.5*). The disulphide bond in the α_2 domain connects the N-terminal β strand to the α helix of the α_2 domain.

A long groove separates the α helices of the α_1 and α_2 domains. The original crystal structure of the HLA-A2 molecule revealed the presence of diffuse 'extra electron density' in the groove, suggesting that it was the binding site for

A model of an intact human MHC class I molecule

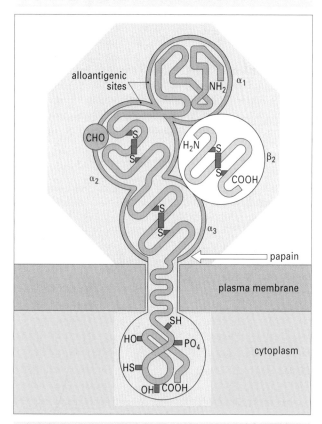

Fig. 5.3 The three globular domains (α_1, α_2 and α_3) are shown in green. The α_3 domain is closely associated with the non-MHC encoded peptide, β_2-microglobulin (grey). β_2-microglobulin is stabilized by an intrachain disulphide bond (red) and has a similar tertiary structure to an immunoglobulin domain. Alloantigenic sites (carrying determinants specific to each individual) occur on the α_1 and α_2 domains and there is a carbohydrate unit attached to the α_2 domain (CHO). Papain cleaves the molecule close to the outer margin of the plasma membrane.

The extracellular domains of an MHC class I molecule

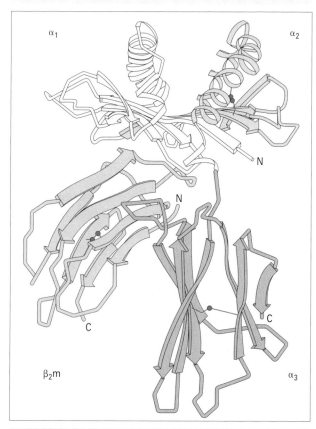

Fig. 5.4 The peptide backbone of HLA-A2 is shown. The three domains of the heavy chain each make interactions with β_2m. The groove formed by the α_1 and α_2 domains is clearly visible.

processed antigen. This contention is strengthened by the observation that the majority of polymorphic residues and T-cell epitopes on class I molecules are located in or near the groove (see *Fig. 5.5*).

Variations in amino acid sequence change the shape of the binding groove

Comparisons of the structures of HLA-A2 and HLA-Aw68 have further refined our understanding of the structural basis for the binding of peptide to class I antigens. The differences between HLA-A2 and HLA-Aw68 result from amino acid side-chain differences at 13 positions: six in α_1, six in α_2, and one (residue 245, which contributes to interactions with CD8) in α_3. Ten of the α_1 and α_2 differences are at positions lining the floor and side of the peptide-binding groove (*Fig. 5.6*). These differences give rise to dramatic differences in the shape of the groove and on the peptides that it will bind. Interestingly, the groove is not a smooth structure, but has a number of subsites formed from ridges and pockets with which amino acid side chains could interact (*Fig. 5.7*). For example, the side chains or ends of peptides could fit into two pockets that extend under the helix of the α_1 domain. Amino acid variations within the groove can vary the positions of the

pockets (see *Fig. 5.7*), providing a structural basis for differences in peptide binding affinity that in turn govern responsiveness versus non-responsiveness in the immune response.

The structure of MHC class II molecules
Class II molecules resemble class I molecules in their overall structure

The products of the class II genes (A and E in the mouse, DR, DQ and DP in humans) are heterodimers of heavy (α) and light (β) glycoprotein chains. The α chains have molecular weights of 30–34 kDa. The β chains range from 26–29 kDa, depending on the locus involved. A number of lines of evidence indicate that the α and β chains have the same overall structures. An extracellular portion comprising two domains (α_1 and α_2, or β_1 and β_2) is connected by a short

HLA-A2 and HLA-Aw68

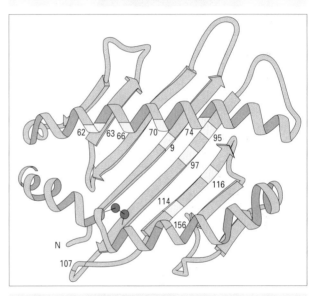

Fig. 5.6 HLA-A2 and HLA-Aw68 differ at 13 amino acid residues. Twelve of these are in the α_1 and α_2 domains. The ten amino acid differences that line the peptide groove are coloured yellow. (Modified from Parham [1989].)

The top surface of HLA-A2

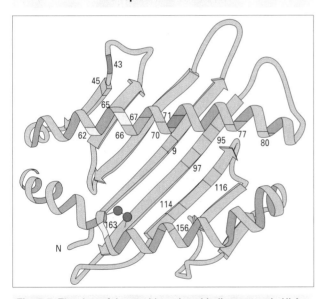

Fig. 5.5 The view of the peptide antigen-binding groove in HLA-A2 as 'seen' by the TCR. The α_1 and α_2 domains each consist of four antiparallel β strands followed by a long helical region. The domains pair to form a single eight-stranded β sheet topped by a helices. The locations of the most polymorphic residues are highlighted. Five residues on the central β strands of the α_1–α_2 β sheet point up between the two helical regions and may make contact with bound antigenic peptides. Six residues face into the site from the sides of the helices (pink). Three residues are on the top face of the helices and are candidates for making direct contact with the TCR (yellow). Residues coloured green are not in a position to affect the binding of antigenic peptides. (Modified from Bjorkman *et al.* [1987].)

HLA-Aw68 and HLA-A2

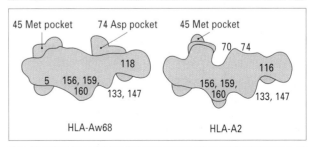

Fig. 5.7 Schematic outlines of the peptide-binding grooves of HLA-Aw68 and HLA-A2 are shown. The pockets into which residues of the bound antigenic peptides are thought to fit are labelled.

sequence to a transmembrane region of about 30 residues and a cytoplasmic domain of about 10–15 residues.

The α_2 and β_2 domains are similar to the class I α_3 domain and β_2m, possessing the structural characteristics of

immunoglobulin constant domains. The β_1 domain contains a disulphide bond generating a 64 amino acid loop. The difference in molecular weights of the class II α and β chains is primarily due to differential glycosylation. The α_1, α_2 and β_1 domains are N-glycosylated, and the β_2 domain is not.

The co-receptor molecule, CD4, binds to class II molecules. Mutagenesis studies using HLA-DR1 suggest that binding occurs to the β_2 domain. The association of CD4 and the TCR complex is thought to be important in recruiting p56^{lck}, which binds to the cytoplasmic portion of CD4 and initiates T-cell activation.

The MHC class II binding groove accommodates longer peptides

The three-dimensional structure of the HLA-DR1 molecule has been determined and is similar to that of class I HLA (*Fig. 5.8*). One major difference is that a dimer of the $\alpha\beta$ heterodimer is seen in the crystal forms of HLA-DR1. As with class I antigens, peptides are bound in an extended conformation. However, the class II groove is more open than that of class I, so that longer peptides can be accommodated (*Figs 5.9* and *5.10*). The structural features of the class II antigen

Ribbon diagrams of the extracellular domains of class I HLA-Aw68 and class II HLA-DR1

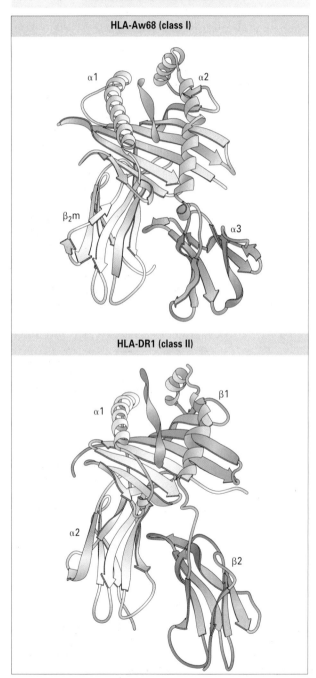

Fig. 5.8 Ribbon diagrams of the extracellular domains of class I HLA-Aw68 (**upper**) and class II HLA-DR1 (**lower**) histocompatibility antigens. The binding cleft is shown with a resident peptide. These diagrams emphasize the similarity in the three-dimensional structures of class I and class II antigens. Redrawn with permission from Stern LJ, *Structure,* **2**:245–51.

The peptide binding of class I (H–2K^b) and class II (HLA-DR1)

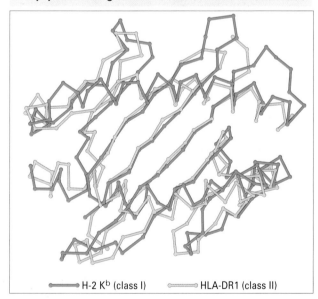

Fig. 5.9 The peptide binding of class I (H–2K^b) and class II (HLA-DR1) are shown as α-carbon atom traces in a top view of the peptide-binding clefts. The similarities between the two sites can clearly be seen, although there are also some differences. Some of these differences account for the difference in peptide length preference between class I (8-10 amino acid residues) and class II (>12 amino acid residues). Redrawn with permission from Stern LJ, *Structure,* **2**:245–51.

binding site have been illuminated by the determination of the crystal structure of HLA-DR1 complexed with an influenza virus peptide (see *Fig. 5.10*). Pockets were clearly visible within the peptide binding site that accommodate five side-chains of the bound peptide and explain the peptide specificity of HLA-DR1.

Hydrogen bonds with the main chain of the bound peptide

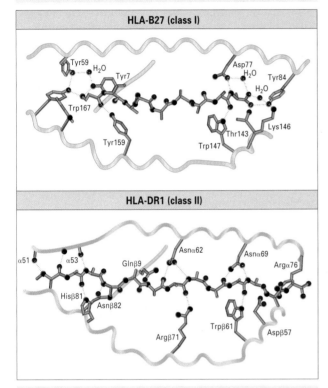

Fig. 5.10 The hydrogen bonds made by the main chain of a bound peptide with class I (HLA-B27) or class II (HLA-DR1) are shown. The major difference between the two hydrogen bonding patterns is the clustering of conserved class I peptide bonds at the ends of the peptide. In contrast, conserved class II peptide bonds are distributed throughout the length of the peptide. Redrawn with permission from Stern LJ, *Structure*, **2**:245–51.

■ GENOMIC ORGANIZATION OF THE MHC

Murine class I loci

The mouse MHC is called the H–2 locus. The regions encoding the class I and class II genes are given letter designations. For example, MHC class I molecules are encoded by the H–2K region. The MHC genes and gene loci are highly polymorphic – they vary between different strains both in the numbers of genes and in their structures. To indicate this, the MHC from different strains is given a superscripted letter. For example the Balb/c strain has the haplotype $H–2^d$.

The mouse MHC (H–2) has three class I loci, but the number of class I genes varies between haplotypes

There are about 30 class I genes in the murine haploid genome. This number varies among haplotypes of different inbred strains. Class I genes encode the classical, serologically defined H–2 loci, i.e. H–2K, H–2D and H–2L. Most of the remaining genes, which map to the Qa, Tla and M regions, are of unknown significance (*Fig. 5.11*), although it is possible to trigger T-cell activation via the Qa-2 molecule.

The organization of the H–2K region is similar in all strains that have been studied. It contains two class I genes, termed K and K2 (see *Fig. 5.11*). The H–2K gene encodes the H–2K antigen expressed on most cell types and recognized serologically, whereas the H–2K2 gene exhibits varied patterns of expression, depending on the strain.

$H–2^d$ and $H–2^b$ haplotypes have different numbers of class I genes in the H–2D/H–2L region (see *Fig. 5.11*). Five class I genes map to the D/L region of BALB/c ($H–2^d$) mice. Two of these genes encode the serologically detectable $H–2D^d$ and $H–2L^d$ antigens. Three additional class I genes are found in the region between the proximal $H–2D^d$ and distal $H–2L^d$ genes. These genes, called $D2^d$, $D3^d$ and $D4^d$ are of unknown function. Only one class I gene has been identified in the H–2D region of B10 mice ($H–2^b$).

Qa, Tla and M regions encode 'non-classical' MHC class I molecules

The Qa, TLa and M regions encode molecules which have a similar structure to the class I molecules described above. They are sometimes referred to as non-classical class I molecules. The Qa locus comprises about 200 kb of DNA

Genes within the murine class I region

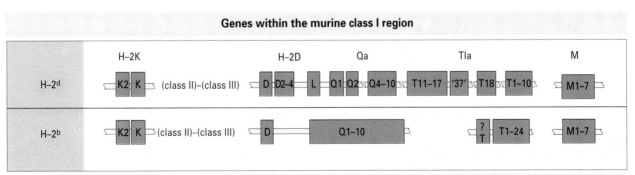

Fig. 5.11 The organization of the MHC class I region of two haplotypes, BALB/c ($H–2^d$) and B10 ($H–2^b$) is shown. The class II–class III region splits the H–2K and H–2D regions. The brackets denote gaps added to align alleles between the two haplotypes. The Tla region contains the largest number of class I genes, the functions of which are unknown.

distal to H–2D/L (see *Fig. 5.11*). This region encodes the serologically detectable specificities Qa-2, 3, 4 and 5 and encompasses a cluster of eight (BALB/c) to ten (B10) class I genes.

The murine Tla region, although defined initially as encoding the TL (thymus leukaemia) antigen, has subsequently been shown to contain the largest number of class I genes and the greatest number of differences in organization between the B10 and BALB/c haplotypes (see *Fig. 5.11*). The M region is located between the K and A regions and contains a number of new class I genes, termed M1–M7. These genes exhibit a low degree of polymorphism.

There are three human class I loci

The human class I region contains three loci, called HLA-A, HLA-B and HLA-C. Each locus encodes the heavy chain of a classical MHC class I antigen and the whole region extends over 1.5 million bases of DNA (*Fig. 5.12*). However, further analysis of this region has revealed multiple additional class I genes. The HLA-E, -F and -G genes may encode MHC class I proteins, and the HLA-G gene product has been demonstrated in extravillous cytotrophoblast-derived choriocarcinoma cell lines and in the tamarins (a group of New World

primates). Other class I genes that may be the human counterparts of the murine Qa, Tla and M genes reside near the HLA-G and HLA-A genes.

Murine class II genes are found in the H–2I region

The α and β chains of murine class II molecules are encoded by separate genes located in the I region of the H–2 complex (*Fig. 5.13*). The Ab and Aa genes encode the β and α chains of the A molecule. Eb and Ea genes likewise encode the two chains of the E molecule. (The gene nomenclature indicates first of all the locus and then the type of chain it encodes.) Several other class II a and b genes have been cloned, for which no protein product is known. One of these, Pb, is a pseudogene whereas two others, called Ob and Eb2, are potentially functional. These latter genes display a low level of polymorphism and are transcribed, but it is not known whether they are translated.

Almost the whole H–2I region has been mapped, and is linked to the class I H–2K subregion. Mice of the b, s, f and q haplotypes fail to express I–E class II products. The b and s haplotypes fail to transcribe the Ea gene but make normal cytoplasmic levels of Eβ chain. Mice of f and q haplotypes fail to make both Eα and Eβ chains.

Genes within the human class I region

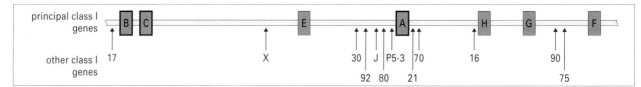

Fig. 5.12 The human class I region lies telomeric to the class II–class III region. In addition to the genes encoding the classical transplantation antigens (HLA-A, HLA-B and HLA-C), several other class I-like genes have been identified that may be the equivalent of the murine Tla/Qa region. Other non-class 1-like genes also reside in this region.

Genes within the human and murine class II regions

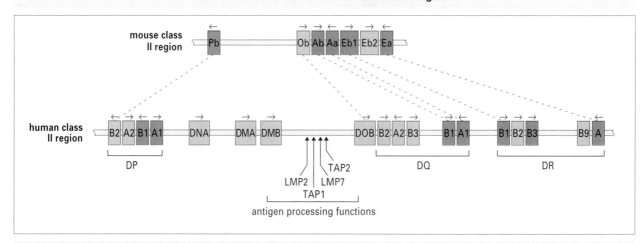

Fig. 5.13 The arrangement of the genes within the human and murine MHCs is shown. Homologous genes between the two species are indicated. Expressed class I and class II genes are coloured orange and pseudogenes are shown yellow.

Human class II genes are located in the HLA–D region

The HLA-D region encodes at least six α and ten β chain genes for MHC class II molecules (see *Fig. 5.13*). Three loci, DR, DQ and DP, encode the major expressed products of the human class II region, but additional genes have also been identified. The DR family comprises a single α gene (DRA) and up to nine β genes (DRB1–9) including pseudogenes. Several different gene arrangements occur within this locus. The DQ and DP families each have one expressed gene for α and β chains, and an additional pair of genes which may or may not be functional.

As with their murine counterparts, the DR, DQ and DP α chains associate in the cell primarily with β chains of their own loci. The DPA1 and DPB1 gene products associate to generate the HLA-DP class II molecules detected using specific antibodies. Similarly, DQA1 and DQB1 encode the HLA-DQ antigens.

The organization and length of the DRB region varies in different haplotypes (*Fig. 5.14*), with different numbers of β chains expressed. The DRB2 locus is a pseudogene. The DRB1, DRB3 and DRB4 loci are usually expressed. The DPA2, DPB2 and DQB3 genes are generally pseudogenes and are therefore not expressed. In contrast, the DNA, DOB, DQB2 and DQA2 genes may be functional.

The class II region also contains genes that encode proteins involved in antigen presentation that are not expressed at the cell surface. These genes and their gene products are discussed in Chapter 7.

The order of all the known HLA class II genes has been established using long-range genetic mapping techniques. The region spans about 1000 kb of DNA and the order and orientation of the various loci is similar to that of the homologous loci in the murine class II region.

MHC polymorphism is concentrated in and around the peptide-binding cleft

A hallmark of the MHC is the extreme degree of polymorphism (structural variability) of the molecules encoded within it. Polymorphism is not evenly spread throughout the MHC. The class I-like Qa, Tla and M antigens are much less polymorphic than the classical class I and class II antigens. A list of specificities, with the allelic variants detected for HLA class I and class II antigens, is shown in Appendix I.

Within a particular class I or class II molecule, the structural polymorphisms are clustered in particular regions of the molecule. The amino acid sequence variability in class I antigens is clustered in three main regions of the α_1 and α_2 domains. The α_3 domain appears to be much more conserved.

In class II molecules, the extent of variability depends on the subregion and on the polypeptide chain. For example, most polymorphism occurs in DRβ and DQβ chains while DPβ chains are slightly less polymorphic. DQα is polymorphic whereas DRα chains are virtually invariant and DRα chains are represented by two alleles. In outbred populations where individuals have two MHC haplotypes, hybrid class II molecules, with one chain from each haplotype, can be produced. This generates additional structural diversity in the expressed molecules.

Most of the polymorphic amino acids in class I and class II antigens are clustered on top of the molecule in the large groove that acts as the peptide binding site. Thus, variation is almost exclusively centred in the base of the antigen-binding groove or pointing in from the sides of the α helix region. The implications of this concentration of polymorphic residues for T-cell antigen recognition are discussed more fully in Chapter 7.

The number of DRB loci varies with different haplotypes

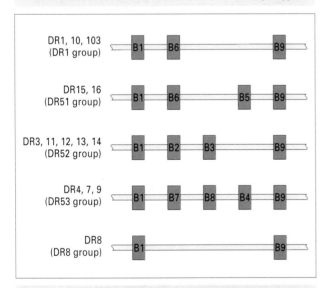

Fig. 5.14 The number of DRB loci varies with different haplotypes. Thus individuals of haplotype HLA-DR1, -DR10 and -DR103 have the arrangement shown in the top line. Not all these loci produce mRNA for DRβ chains.

Critical Thinking

■ The peptide-binding groove on a class I molecule accommodates a peptide of 8–10 amino acid residues. Is there any reason why we could not have evolved with MHC molecules that accommodate antigenic peptides of 3 or 30 residues?

■ The determination of the three-dimensional structure of class I and class II molecules has given rise to a detailed understanding of the means by which they bind peptides. It has been suggested that immune responses could be enhanced or inhibited by treatments with peptides that bind to MHC molecules. How would the information about MHC/peptide binding help us to develop such therapeutic peptides?

■ Unlike the B-cell receptor, the T-cell receptor is generally of low affinity and recognizes antigen only when it is complexed to class I or class II molecules. Accessory molecules on the cell surfaces are also a key part of the interactions of T cells with target cells. These molecules perform several functions. What processes other than antigen recognition occur when a T cell contacts a virally infected target?

■ The peptide-binding groove of a class II molecule may accommodate longer peptides than the class I molecule. What advantage might this have?

FURTHER READING

Bjorkman PJ, Parham P. Structure, function and diversity of Class I major histocompatibility complex molecules. *Ann Rev Biochem* 1990;**59**:253–88.

Bjorkman PJ, Saper MA, Samraoui B, Bennett WS, Strominger JL, Wiley DC. The structure of the human Class I histocompatibility antigen HLA-A2. *Nature* 1987;**329**:506–12.

Bjorkman PJ, Samraoui B, Bennett WS, Strominger JL, Wiley DC. The foreign antigen binding site and T-cell recognition regions of Class I histocompatibility antigens. *Nature* 1987;**329**:512–16.

Bodmer JG, Marsh, SE, Albert ED, *et al*. Nomenclature for factors of the HLA system, 1994. *Tissue Antigens* 1994;**44**:1–18.

Boulot G, Bentley GA, Karjalainen K, Msriuzza RA. Crystallization and preliminary X-ray diffraction analysis of the β-chain of a T-cell antigen receptor. *J Mol Biol* 1994;**235**:795.

Brenner MB, MacLean J, Dialynas DP, *et al*. Identification of a putative second T-cell receptor. *Nature* 1986;**322**:145–49.

Brown JH, Jardetzky TS, Gorga JC, *et al*. Three-dimensional structure of the human class II histocompatibility antigen HLA-DR1. *Nature* 1993;**364**:33–39.

Clevers H, Alarcon B, Wileman T, Terhorst C. The T-cell receptor/CD3 complex: a dynamic protein ensemble. *Annu Rev Immunol* 1988;**6**:629–62.

Garratt TPJ, Saper MA, Bjorkman PJ, Strominger JL, Wiley DC. Specificity pockets for the side chains of peptide antigens in HLA-w68. *Nature* 1989;**342**:692–96.

Green NM. The semiotics of charge. *Nature* 1991;**351**:349.

Hass W, Pereira P, Tonegawa S. Gamma/delta cells. *Ann Rev Immunol* 1993;**11**:637–685.

Koop BF, Hood L. Striking sequence similarity over almost 100 kilobases of human and mouse T-cell receptor DNA. *Nature Genetics* 1994;**7**:48–53.

Lefranc M-P, Rabbitts TH. The human T-cell receptor γ (TRG) genes. *Trends Biochem Sci* 1989;**14**:214–18.

Madden DR, Gorga JC, Strominger L, Wiley DC. The structure of HLA-B27 reveals nonamer self-peptides bound in an extended conformation. *Nature* 1991;**353**:321–25.

Manolios N, Letourneur F, Bonifacino JS, Klausner RD. Pairwise cooperative and inhibitory interactions describe the assembly and probable structure of the T-cell antigen receptor. *EMBO J* 1991;**10**:1643–51.

Neefjes JJ, Momburg F, Hämerling GJ. Selective and ATP-dependent translocation of peptides by the MHC-encoded transporter. *Science* 1993;**261**:769–71.

Nisonoff S. *Introduction to Molecular Immunology*. 2nd ed. Baltimore: Sinauer Associates Inc, 1984.

Powis SH, Trowsdale J. Human major histocompatibility complex genes. *Behring Inst Mitt* 1994;**94**:17–25.

Raulet DH. How γδ T cells make a living. *Curr Biol* 1994;**4**:246–251

Salter RD, Benjamin RJ, Wesley PK, *et al*. A binding site for the T-cell co-receptor CD8 on the α₃ domain of HLA-A2. *Nature* 1990;**345**:41–46.

Stern LJ, Wiley DC Antigenic peptide binding by class I and class II histocompatibility proteins. *Structure* 1994;**2**:245–51.

Stern LJ, Brown JH, Jardetzky TS, *et al*. Crystal structure of the human class II MHC protein HLA-DR1 complexed with an influenza virus peptide. *Nature* 1994;**368**:215–21.

Weiss A, Littman DR. Signal transduction by lymphocyte antigen receptor. *Cell* 1994;**76**:263–74.

Williams AF, Barclay AN. The immunoglobulin superfamily – domains for cell surface recognition. *Ann Rev Immunol* 1988;**6**:381–405.

THE GENERATION OF DIVERSITY   6

The immune system is able to recognize and respond to many antigens by generating great diversity in the antibodies produced by the B cells, and in the antigen receptors expressed by T cells.

Immunoglobulins are composed of heavy and light chains, the light chains being either κ or λ. The number of possible antigen-binding sites is the product of the number of heavy and light chains.

Immunoglobulin light chains are encoded by V and J gene segments; heavy chains are also encoded by V and J segment genes with additional diversity provided by the D gene segment.

Diversity is achieved by the recombination of a limited number of V, D and J gene segments to produce a vast number of variable domains

Immunoglobulin heavy and light chains undergo structural modifications after antigen stimulation, called somatic mutation. This does not occur with T-cell receptors.

The TCR is generated by four different sets of genes: α and β genes are expressed in the majority of peripheral T cells; γ and δ genes are expressed in a subpopulation of thymic T cells and in a minor population of peripheral T cells.

Diversification of the TCR receptor also occurs by recombination between V, D, and J gene segments, with minor variations in detail for each locus.

Recombination of V, D and J gene segments for both immunoglobulin and T-cell receptors is controlled, at least in part, by two recombination activating genes (RAG-1 and RAG-2).

In addition to simple combinations of V, D and J regions, diversity in the TCR and immunoglobulins depends upon N-region diversification, joining-site variation and multiple D regions.

Immunoglobulin class switching involves recombination of VDJ genes with various C region genes and differential RNA splicing

The ability of the immune system to recognize antigens depends on the antibodies generated by B cells, and on the antigen receptors expressed by T cells. Although the ways in which T cells and B cells recognize antigen are quite different, both cell populations are capable of recognizing a wide range of antigens. In spite of the differences between antibodies and T-cell receptors, the cellular and molecular processes which generate diversity are very similar for each type of molecule. This chapter is concerned with the ways in which the immune system generates a great diversity of antibodies and T-cell antigen receptors (TCRs), of different antigenic specificities.

Antibodies are remarkably diverse and provide enough different combining sites to recognize the millions of antigenic shapes in the environment. Each class of antibody also has a characteristic effector region so that, for instance, IgE can bind to Fc receptors on mast cells, whereas IgG can bind to phagocytes. It has been estimated that an individual produces more different forms of antibody than all the other proteins of the body put together. In fact, we produce more types of antibody than there are genes in our genome. How can all this diversity be generated? Ideas about the formation of antibodies have changed considerably over the years, but it is perhaps surprising how close Ehrlich came with his side-chain hypothesis at the beginning of this century (*Fig. 6.1*). His idea of antigen-induced selection is close to our present view of clonal selection, except that he placed several different receptors on the same cell.

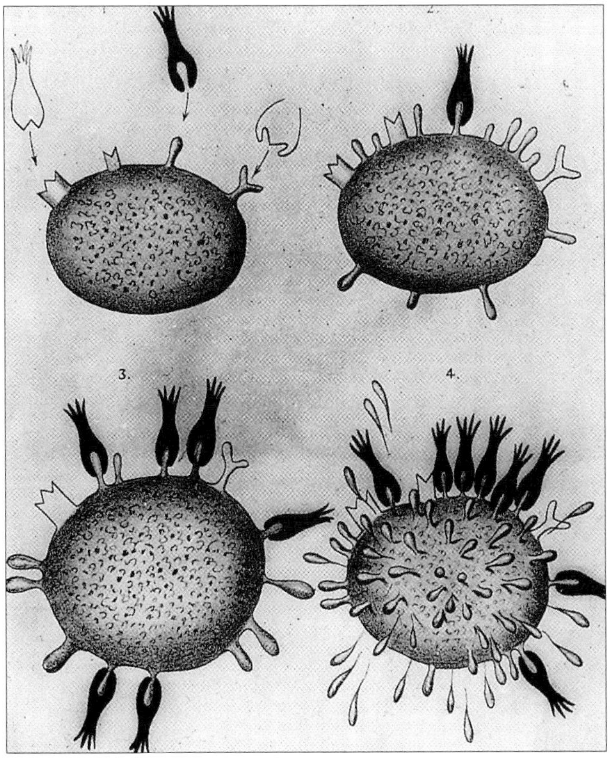

Fig. 6.1 Ehrlich's side-chain theory. Ehrlich proposed that the combination of antigen with a preformed B-cell receptor (now known to be antibody) triggered the cell to produce and secrete more of those receptors. Although the diagram indicates that he thought a single cell could produce antibodies to bind more than one type of antigen it is evident that he anticipated both the clonal selection theory and the idea that the immune system could generate receptors before contact with antigen.

■ THEORIES OF ANTIBODY FORMATION

After Ehrlich the situation became more complicated. The problem was that many new organic compounds were now being synthesized and Landsteiner was showing that the immune system could react with the production of specific antibody for each new compound. It was not thought possible that the immune system could, by natural selection, have maintained genes for all these antibodies directed at novel, artificial compounds. This led to the development of the instructive hypothesis, which proposes a flexible antibody molecule that is acted on by antigen to form a complementary binding site. With the spectacular progress in molecular biology in the 1950s and 1960s the instructive hypothesis became untenable, as it became clear that the mechanism for the proposed 'instruction' simply did not exist. The circle turned and selective theories came back into favour, with both Jerne and Burnet putting forward the idea of clonal selection. Each lymphocyte produces one type of immunoglobulin only, and the antigen selects and stimulates cells carrying that immunoglobulin type.

This still left the problem of antibody diversity. One solution was to postulate the existence of a separate gene for each antibody specificity. This immediately presented a problem. Looking at the structure of a light chain, half the chain is variable in amino acid sequence but the other half is constant; similarly with heavy chains, a quarter of the chain is variable while the rest is constant. How, if there

are so many genes, is it possible to maintain this constancy of sequence in the constant regions? Dreyer and Bennett proposed a solution to this problem by suggesting that the constant and variable portions of the chains are coded for by separate genes, with one or only a few genes coding for the constant (c) region and many genes coding for the variable (v) region. At this point, the theory only had to account for the multiple variable regions! A solution to this aspect of the diversity problem was suggested by the idea of somatic mutation, which proposes that relatively few germ line genes give rise to many mutated genes during the lifetime of the individual. It was also suggested that a number of gene segments could recombine to give a complete V gene. This gave three possible solutions to the problem of generating diversity:

- Multiple V region genes in the germ line.
- Somatic recombination between elements forming a V region gene.
- Somatic mutation.

It is now known that mammals use all three mechanisms to generate diversity (*Fig. 6.2*). Interestingly, sharks rely on having a large number of antibody genes, and do not use somatic recombination, while birds have small numbers of antibody genes that undergo a very high level of gene conversion (see Chapter 15). As will be discussed later, further diversity is introduced by random pairing of heavy and light chains, and by subtle variations in V, D J recombination.

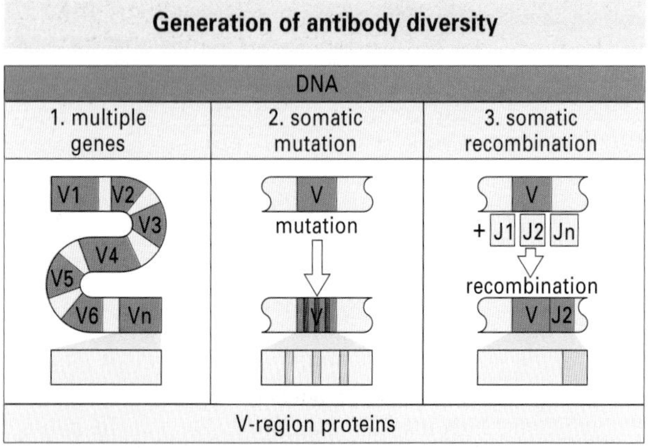

■ IMMUNOGLOBULIN VARIABILITY

Immunoglobulins are composed of heavy and light chains, the light chains being either κ or λ. Since virtually any light chain can combine with any heavy chain, the number of possible antigen-binding sites is the product of the number of heavy and light chains. Part of the variability in

Generation of antibody diversity

Fig. 6.2 Three mechanisms are proposed by which the immune system could generate different V regions on the immunoglobulin H and L chains.
1. Multiple genes. There are a large number of separate genes (V1–Vn), each encoding one V region domain.
2. Somatic mutation. A primordial V gene mutates during B cell ontogeny to produce different genes in different B cell clones.
3. Somatic recombination. A number of gene segments (J1–Jn) recombine to join the main part of the V region gene. This occurs during B cell ontogeny and results in a protein containing elements encoded by different gene segments. All three mechanisms are involved in the generation of antibody diversity in mammals.

Chromosome location of MHC and antigen receptor genes

peptide	mouse	human
IgH	12	14
λ	16	22
κ	6	2
TCRα	14	14
TCRβ	6	7
TCRγ	13	7
TCRδ	14	14
MHC	17	6
β₂-microglobulin	2	15

Fig. 6.3 The numbers refer to the chromosomal location of the genes for the various peptides in man and mouse. Note that all of the loci are completely separate, with the single exception of the T cell receptor (TCR) δ chain which lies within the TCR α loci.

immunoglobulin structure is derived from the interaction of these separate polypeptide chains. For example, if there are 10^4 different light chains each capable of binding with any of 10^4 different heavy chains, then 10^8 different antibody specificities are theoretically possible. Separate diversification mechanisms exist for each of the chains, as they are encoded on separate chromosomes (*Fig. 6.3*).

Polymorphic forms of immunoglobulins derive from variation in many parts of the molecule (*Fig. 6.4*). We will discuss idiotypic variability – relating to variability at the antigen-binding site –first.

Kabat and Wu analysed the variable regions from the amino acid sequences of many light and heavy chains. For a source of identical antibodies, they relied on myelomas (monoclonal B-cell tumours that produce antibody). They found that the variability in λ light chains was concentrated in three hypervariable regions, surrounded by relatively invariant framework residues. These hypervariable regions, later shown to be the regions that make contact with the antigen, are known as complementarity-determining regions (CDRs).

Initially they studied the mouse, a species in which less than 5% of the antibodies possess λ light chains, and diversity is correspondingly less. (This is due to the very small number of Vλ genes in the mouse.) Thus, out of 19 λ light chain sequences examined, 12 were found to be identical, with the other 7 differing from each other and the prototype sequence by only a few residues (*Fig. 6.5*).

Variability in the heavy chain is similarly concentrated in three hypervariable regions, with background variability on each side of the CDRs (*Fig. 6.6*). The heavy chain frameworks (the sequences between the CDRs) can be arranged into groups on the basis of similarity, or identity, of framework sequences (*Fig. 6.7*).

Variability of immunoglobulin structure

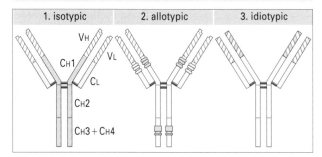

Fig. 6.4 All immunoglobulins have the basic four-chain structure. There are three types of immunoglobulin variability.
1. Isotypic variation is present in the germ line of all members of a species, producing the heavy (μ, δ, γ, ε, α) and light chains (Igκ, λ) and the V region frameworks (subgroups).
2. Allotypic variation is intraspecies allelic variability.
3. Idiotypic variation refers to the diversity at the antigen-binding site (paratope) and in particular relates to the hypervariable segments.

Variability of λ light chains

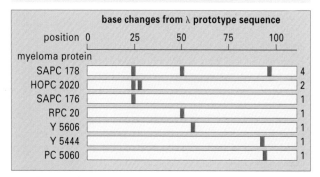

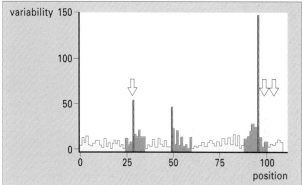

Fig. 6.5 The amino acid sequences of seven mouse λ1 myeloma proteins are represented. Positions in yellow indicate identity to the prototype sequence (MOPC 104E), positions in red indicate differences. The number of base changes in the DNA required to produce the given alteration in amino acid structure is given on the right. Below is a Kabat and Wu plot of light chain variability, calculated as the number of different amino acids at a given position divided by the frequency of most common amino acid (compare with Chapter 4). Arrows indicate extra amino acids in some sequences.

Variability of heavy chains

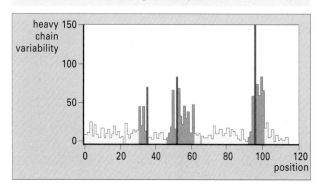

Fig. 6.6 This Kabat and Wu plot shows variability concentrated in three regions of the variable region of heavy chains.

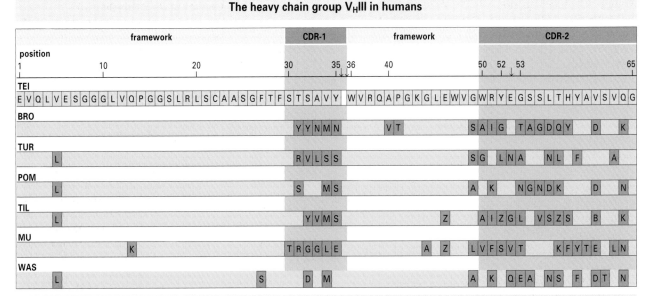

Fig. 6.7 The 65 N-terminal amino acids of six human myelomas falling into the VHIII group are compared diagrammatically to the prototype sequence TEI. Amino acids identical to those in TEI are shown in yellow; amino acids which differ from those at the same position in TEI are dark pink. The majority of differences within a single group occur within the complementarity-determining regions CDR-1 and CDR-2. The third hypervariable region is not shown.

■ IMMUNOGLOBULIN GENE RECOMBINATION

Light chain genes recombine V and J segments to make a gene for the Vλ domain

With the advent of recombinant DNA techniques in the 1970s it became possible to attempt analysis of the genes responsible for coding for antibodies. Because of its lesser heterogeneity, work started on the murine λ1 system (in the mouse there are 4 isotypes of λ, arranged sequentially at the λ gene locus, designated λ1–λ4). It was found that two separate segments of DNA code for the constant and variable regions. In cells not producing antibody, these gene segments are far apart on the chromosomes, but in antibody-forming cells they are brought closer together. However even in a fully differentiated B cell the two gene segments do not join directly, but remain about 1500 base pairs apart. Between the V and C segments, and joined onto the V segment in rearranged chromosomes, is a short section of DNA known as the J (joining) segment. (The J segment should not be confused with the J chain present in IgM and dimeric IgA.)

Structure of the λ chain system – The Vλ gene segment codes for the V region of the antibody light chain, up to and including amino acid 95; the Jλ gene segment codes for the rest of the V region (*Fig. 6.8*). In the mouse, but not in man, the total number of gene segments contributing to the λ light chain system is limited compared with the other immunoglobulin or T-cell receptor (TCR) loci. Three Vλ segments, and four Jλ – Cλ clusters have been described (see *Fig. 6.8*). One of these J segments,

Jλ4, is a pseudogene. Recombination nearly always takes place within a V–J–C cluster so that only four combinations are possible – Vλ2.Jλ2, VλX.Jλ2, Vλ1.Jλ3 and Vλ1.Jλ1 (see *Fig. 6.8*). Each V segment is preceded by a signal or leader sequence, a short hydrophobic sequence responsible for targeting the λ chain to the endoplasmic reticulum. The leader sequence is cleaved in the endoplasmic reticulum and the antibody molecule is then processed through the intracellular secretory pathway.

Structure of the κ chain system – This system has more V genes and is more heterogeneous, even though there is only one constant region gene (*Fig. 6.9*). In an embryonic or non-lymphoid cell the Vκ segment genes, of which there are about 350, are at some distance from the Cκ gene on the chromosome. The Vκ gene segments in the mouse appear to be organized in sets, each set comprising about seven genes. In between and closer to the C gene are five Jκ genes, one of which is a pseudogene and is never expressed.

During differentiation of lymphoid cells there is a rearrangement of the DNA such that one of the V genes is joined to a J gene. The number of possible κ chain variable regions that can be produced in this way is approximately 1400 (350 × 4). Following rearrangement, there is still an intron (a non-coding intervening sequence) between the J genes and the gene for the C region. This whole stretch of DNA (from the leader to the end of the C gene, including introns) is then transcribed into heterogeneous nuclear RNA, (hnRNA) i.e. unprocessed mRNA. A process of RNA splicing then removes the introns, leaving mRNA that can be translated into protein.

Heavy chain genes recombine V, D and J gene segments to make a gene for the V$_H$ domain

The heavy chain variable region is also encoded by V and J segment genes. Additional diversity is provided by a third gene segment, the D (diversity) segment gene (*Fig. 6.10*). The D segment is highly variable both in the number of codons and in the sequence of base pairs. In antibodies binding dextran this section comprises two amino acids; in those binding phosphorylcholine up to eight amino acids are inserted; in anti-levan antibodies this section is completely missing. More than one D segment may join to form an enlarged D region. The D region may be read

λ chain production in the mouse

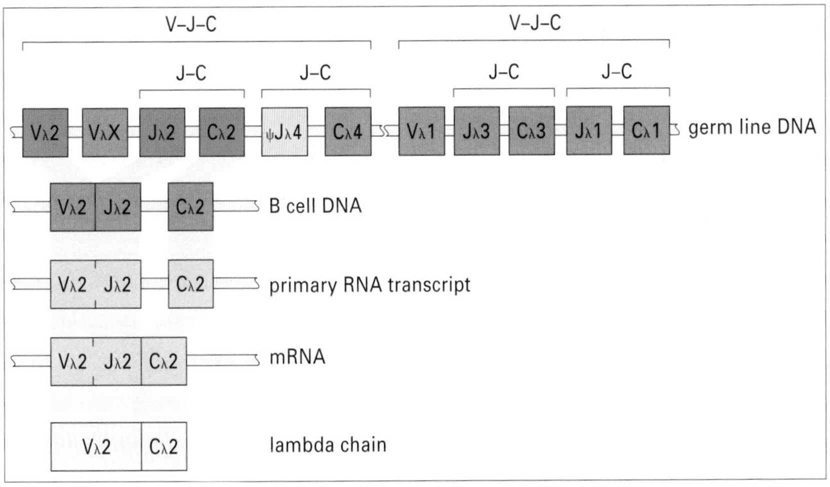

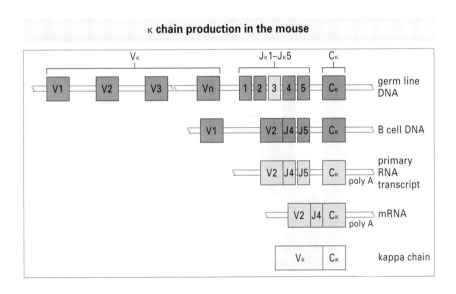

Fig. 6.8 During B-cell differentiation one of the germ line Vλ genes recombines with its J-associated segment to form a V–J combination. The rearranged gene is transcribed into a primary RNA transcript complete with introns (non-coding segments occurring between the genes), exons (which code for protein) and a poly-A tail. This is spliced to form messenger RNA (mRNA) with loss of the introns, and then translated into protein. Gene segments that encode the final polypeptide are indicated in a darker shade, B cell DNA is in light brown; RNA is in green; and immunoglobulin peptides are in yellow.

κ chain production in the mouse

Fig. 6.9 During differentiation of the pre-B cell one of several Vκ genes on the germ line DNA (V1–Vn) is recombined and apposed to a Jκ segment (Jκ1–Jκ5). The B cell transcribes a segment of DNA into a primary RNA transcript that contains a long intervening sequence of additional J segments and introns. This transcript is processed into mRNA by splicing the exons together, and is translated by ribosomes into kappa (κ) chains. Note that the J3 gene lacks the necessary base sequences to allow it to recombine and is therefore effectively an intron. The rearrangement illustrated is only one of the many possible recombinations.

V–D–J recombination in the mouse

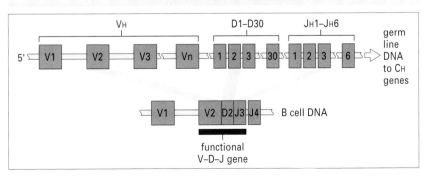

Fig. 6.10 The heavy chain gene loci combine three segments to produce the exon (V–D–J gene) which codes for the V$_H$ domain. One of several hundred V genes recombines with one of thirty D segments and one of six J segments, to produce a functional V–D–J gene in the B cell. The rearrangement illustrated is only one of the many thousands possible.

in three possible reading frames without generating stop codons, so adding to diversity. So far, thirty germ line D segments have been identified, with 100–200 different VH segments, six functional J segments and three J pseudogenes. However, solution analysis indicates that there may in fact be more than 1000 murine VH segments. The recombination junction of V, D, and J segments in the heavy chain is largely responsible for variability in the complementarity-determining region, CDR-3, which forms an essential part of the antigen-binding site. In some systems, such as the family of anti-dextran antibodies, the differences between antibodies are nearly all situated in this region.

V regions are rearranged and expressed in a programmed manner during early fetal life

When animals are immunized with selected antigens during fetal life or soon after birth, the ability to respond to each antigen develops in a precise order, suggesting a programmed pattern of development. We now know that the V regions nearest to the J regions are utilized first, and it is interesting that VH1, the nearest V gene, is a single conserved sequence. In all primate species examined, only a single copy is present and no sequence variation occurs within a species. Between humans and other primates, only 2% of the nucleotides vary.

This fetal repertoire is over-represented in autoantibodies, indicating that autoimmunity might, in part, be the result of dysregulation of these early sequences. There is similar over-representation of particular V segments in tumours of early B cells, 20 V segments being present in 85% of chronic lymphocytic leukaemias.

Recombination sequences flanking the V, D and J genes direct joining of the gene segments

The recombination of gene segments is a key feature of the generation of a functional gene for both light and heavy chain variable regions. The precise mechanism by which this recombination occurs is unknown, but specific base sequences that appear to act as joining signals have been identified (*Fig. 6.11*).

A signal sequence is found downstream (3') of V and D segment genes. It consists of a heptamer CACAGTG or its analogue, followed by a spacer of unconserved sequence, and then a nonamer ACAAAAACC or its analogue. Immediately upstream (5') of all germ line D and J segments is a corresponding signal sequence of a nonamer and then a heptamer, again separated by an unconserved sequence. The heptameric and nonameric sequences following a VL, VH or D segment are complementary to those preceding the JL, D or JH segments with which they recombine. If the heptamers and nonamers combine there are two sections of unpaired bases, one 12 bases long and the other 22–24 bases long, corresponding to either one or two turns of the DNA helix. It is thought that the recombinase that joins the gene segments together recognizes this structure.

The recombination process is controlled at least in part by two recombination activating genes (RAG-1 and RAG-2). It has not been confirmed whether these genes encode

the recombinase enzyme, or a factor that regulates recombinase activity. However, it has been shown that mice whose RAG-1 and RAG-2 genes have been 'knocked out' lack mature T and B cells, because of a failure to produce

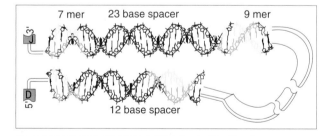

Recombination sequences

kappa chain	heavy chain

- ▪ exons
- ☐ introns: unpaired sequences
- ▨ cytosine
- ☐ adenosine
- ▨ guanosine
- ▱ thymosine

Fig. 6.11 It was proposed that the recombinational events involved in V–J splicing (κ light chains) (**upper left**) and V–D–J splicing (heavy chains) (**upper right**) were facilitated by the base sequences of the introns following the 3' end of V and D matching up with the bases preceding the 5' end of the J and D. Base pairing between these sequences appose the exons. Note that individual base-pair sequences may vary slightly but the heptamer – spacer – nonamer pairing patterns remain. It is thought that enzymes related to those involved in DNA repair effect the join. It now appears that hairpin joining sometimes occurs between the cut ends of the double stranded DNA (**lower**) which code for the heavy chains, after V and J DNA regions have been brought close together. This indicates that recombination may involve recognition of double stranded heptamer and nonamer regions

the T-cell receptors and immunoglobulins respectively. Interleukin-7 (IL-7), a cytokine produced by bone marrow stromal cells, has been shown to influence levels of RAG-1 and RAG-2 expression.

The place at which V and J segment genes join may vary slightly

Slight variations in the positions at which recombination takes place generate additional diversity. For example, the 95th residue of the κ light chain is usually encoded by the last codon of the V segment gene; the 96th is frequently encoded by the first Jκ triplet. Sometimes, however, the 96th amino acid is encoded by a composite triplet formed by the second and third, or third base alone, of the first Jκ triplet, with the other bases of the triplet coming from the intron 3' to the V segment gene (*Fig. 6.12*). This will lead to variations in amino acid sequence. Obviously, to produce a functional light chain the correct reading frame must be preserved; if the gene segments join out of phase, non-functional antibodies are produced.

Light chain diversity created by variable recombination

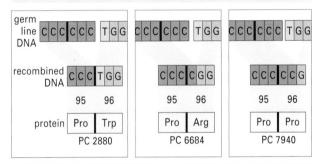

Fig. 6.12 The same Vκ21 and J1 sequences of the germ line create three different amino acid sequences in the proteins PC2880, PC6684 and PC7940 by variable recombination. PC2880 has proline and tryptophan at positions 95 and 96, caused by recombination at the end of the CCC codon. Recombination one base down produces proline and arginine in PC6684. Recombination two bases down from the end of Vκ21 produces proline and proline in PC7940.

On the heavy chain, similar imprecision in joining occurs between the D and JH segment genes and can extend over as many as 10 nucleotides (*Fig. 6.13*). Furthermore, a few nucleotides may be inserted between D and JH and between VH and D by means of the enzyme, terminal deoxynucleotidyl transferase, without the need for a template. The addition of these N-nucleotides ('N' because they are non-template encoded) is called N-region diversity. In mice, terminal deoxynucleotidyl transferase activity increases with age, giving rise to long N-segments in adult animals. Thus, the recombinational variability of the D region can be so great that no recognizable D gene segment remains.

Severe combined immune deficiency (SCID) mice do not generate functional T or B cells because of a defect in V–(D)–J recombination.

■ SOMATIC MUTATION

Immunoglobulin heavy and light chain genes undergo structural modifications after antigen stimulation

The idea that somatic mutations could occur during the lifetime of an individual and thus increase the diversity of antibodies has been strongly argued for many years. As seen earlier (see *Fig. 6.5*) most sequences in the murine λ1 light chain system are identical, with a few variations in the complementarity-determining regions giving eight sequences in all. However, only one Vλ1 gene segment has been found per haploid genome, and this corresponds to the main shared prototype sequence; thus, all variant sequences must be generated by somatic mutations produced by single base changes. Somatic mutants have also been identified in κ light chains and in heavy chains.

Further support for this idea has come from studies focusing on the family of antibodies binding the antigen phosphorylcholine. VH segments from nineteen such antibodies have been fully sequenced. Ten of these have an identical ('prototype') sequence, and the other nine differ from this sequence by one to eight residues. The germ line genome contains only the 'prototype' sequence, indicat-

Heavy chain diversity created by variable recombination

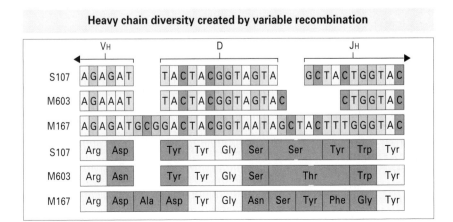

Fig. 6.13 The DNA sequence (upper) and amino acid sequence (lower) of three heavy chains of anti-phosphorylcholine are shown. Variable recombination between the germ line, V, D, and J regions causes variation (orange) in amino acid sequences. In some cases (e.g. M167) there appear to be additional inserted codons. However, these are in multiples of three, and do not alter the overall reading frame.

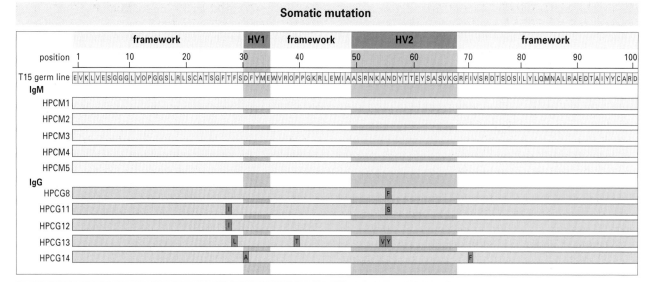

Fig. 6.14 The amino acid sequences of five IgM and five IgG hybridoma anti-phosphorylcholine antibody V$_H$ regions are compared to the primary amino acid structure of the T15 germ line DNA. Positions corresponding to the germ line sequence are shown in yellow; points at which different amino acids occur are shown in pink. Areas of hypervariability (HV1, HV2) are also indicated. Mutations have only occurred in the IgG molecules and the mutations are seen in both hypervariable and framework segments.

ing that the other sequences must have arisen by somatic mutation (*Fig. 6.14*). Strikingly, all the mutated forms were in the IgA and IgG classes, suggesting that the mutations were associated with immunoglobulin class switching. Presumably those somatic variants with a better fit for antigen are selected for; as is seen in the variants binding phosphorylcholine, which are of higher affinity than the germ-line encoded antibodies.

There is some evidence that the region of DNA encoding the variable region may be particularly susceptible to mutation. For example, examination of the nucleotide sequences of two anti-phosphorylcholine antibodies (T15 idiotype) shows them to have numerous mutations from the germ line sequence (3.8% of bases are mutated in the protein M167). These mutations are found in both introns and exons of the V region, but not in adjoining sequences, implying that the whole V region is particularly mutable (*Fig. 6.15*).

Antibody diversity thus arises at several levels. First there are the multiple V genes recombining with J and D segments. The imprecision with which recombination occurs achieves further variation. Note that the structures of the first and second hypervariable regions are coded for entirely by germ line genes, while variability in the third complementarity-determining region is largely the result of recombination. Additionally, point mutations occur throughout the variable region, giving fine variations in specificity. As virtually any light chain may pair with any heavy chain the combination binding of heavy and light chains amplifies the diversity enormously (*Fig. 6.16*). Somatic hypermutation probably contributes less than 5% of total sequence variability, but up to 90% of B cells express V$_H$ genes which have undergone somatic mutation.

Mutations in the DNA of two V$_H$ T15 genes

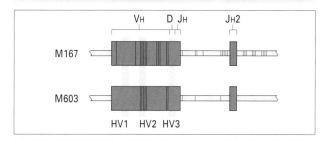

Fig. 6.15 DNA of two anti-phosphorylcholine antibodies with the T15 idiotype. Black lines indicate positions where the genome has mutated from the germ line sequence. There are large numbers of mutations in the introns and the exons of both genes, but particularly in the second hypervariable region, HV2. By comparison, no mutations are detectable in genes coding for the constant regions.

Five mechanisms for the generation of antibody diversity

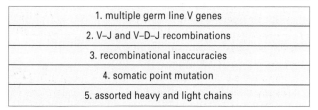

1. multiple germ line V genes
2. V–J and V–D–J recombinations
3. recombinational inaccuracies
4. somatic point mutation
5. assorted heavy and light chains

Fig. 6.16 Since each mechanism can occur with any of the others, the potential for increased diversity multiplies at each step of immunoglobulin production.

■ IMMUNOGLOBULIN DIVERSITY IN OTHER VERTEBRATES

Sharks have a limited repertoire of immunoglobulins

The development of an extensive antibody repertoire has been of great importance in vertebrate evolution, and the various groups have arrived at different solutions to the problem. In the elasmobranchs, which include the sharks and skates, the heavy chain genes are developed along the pattern of the mouse λ light chains. A basic unit of VH–DH1–DH2–JH–CH is multiply repeated but, as recombination can occur only within each repeat unit, there is no scope for recombination between different gene segments. This results in a rather limited repertoire.

Birds use gene conversion to diversify a limited genetic repertoire

In contrast to sharks, chickens possess extremely limited numbers of genes coding for immunoglobulins. In the light chain system there is only one V, one J and one C segment gene. The heavy chains are similarly restricted with single V and J segments. Although there are about 15 DH segments, these are all very similar in sequence and add little to diversity. Despite this great limitation chickens can mount a wide range of antibody responses and produce sequentially diverse antibody molecules.

Upstream of the VL gene is a region containing 25 sequences similar to VL , but which lack a leader exon, a promoter region, and the characteristic heptamer–spacer–nonamer sequences needed for V–J rearrangement. These pseudogenes are not wasted, but are used in a process of gene conversion in which sections of the pseudogene are inserted into the viable VL region. This is a continuous process which carries on after the B cells have left the bursa; multiple conversion events can occur during the lifetime of the B cell.

Similar processes occur with the heavy-chain gene locus, where up to 100 VH pseudogenes act to increase the diversity by similar conversion mechanisms.

Rabbits may use gene conversion to diversify their antibody repertoire

Rabbit immunoglobulins have always presented a puzzle, particularly in the way in which allotypes are regulated. Although the rabbit has many VH genes, the VH gene nearest to the D segment is used in most rabbit B cells. Recent evidence suggests that the rabbit may also use a gene conversion mechanism to diversify this single VH gene.

Pseudogenes may be involved in human diversification

Several V and J segment genes are also in the form of pseudogenes. Whether gene conversion is involved in generating human V regions is a matter of speculation and interest.

■ HEAVY CHAIN CONSTANT REGION GENES

All classes of immunoglobulin use the same set of variable region genes. When a mature antibody-forming cell switches antibody class, all that changes is the constant region of the heavy chain. This has been shown by the analysis of double myelomas, where 2 monoclonal antibodies are present in the serum at the same time. IgM and IgG antibodies from a patient with multiple myeloma have been found to have identical light chains and VH regions; only the constant regions are switched, from μ to γ. Similarly, IgM and IgD are often found on the surface of a lymphocyte at the same time; again, although the classes are different the antigen-binding specificities are identical.

All the constant region genes are arranged downstream from the J segment genes. In the mouse there is one gene for each of the IgM, IgE and IgA (μ, ε and α) isotypes and one γ gene for each of the four different IgG isotypes (γ1, γ2a, γ2b and γ3) (*Fig. 6.17*). In human beings the constant region genes are more complicated, and it appears that one section of this region has undergone gene duplication and diversification. The ordering of genes is μ, δ, [γ 3, γ 1, ε1

Constant region genes in the mouse

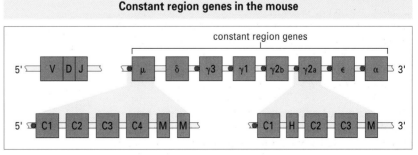

Fig. 6.17 The constant region genes of the mouse are arranged 6.5 kb downstream from the the recombined V–D–J segment. Each C gene (except Cδ) has one or more switching sequences at its start (red circles) which correspond to a sequence at the 5' end of the μ gene. This allows any of the C genes to recombine with V–D–J. δ genes appear to use the same switching sequences as μ but the μ gene transcript is lost in RNA processing to produce IgD. The C genes (expanded below for μ and γ2α) contain introns separating the exons for each domain (C1, C2, etc.). The γ genes also have a separate exon coding for the hinge (H), and all the genes have one or more exons coding for membrane-bound immunoglobulin (M).

Maturation of the immune response and class switching

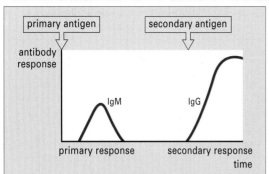

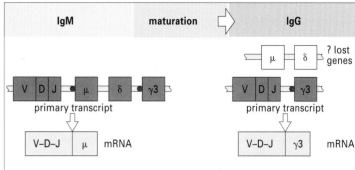

Fig. 6.18 Following a primary antigen injection there is an antibody response that consists mostly of IgM; the response following a secondary challenge is mostly IgG. The underlying mechanism for the class switch is shown (right). In the primary response the V–D–J region is transcribed with a μ gene. After removal of introns during processing, mRNA for secreted IgM is produced. During maturation (involving T-cell help and possibly activation of a mutation mechanism for the V–D–J segment) another C gene (Cγ3 in this case) is brought up to exchange with the μ gene at its switch region (red). The μ and δ genes are probably lost; transcription and processing produce mRNA for IgG3 heavy chain.

α1],γ, [γ2, γ4, ε , α2]. The two sets within square brackets indicate the possible area of reduplication. The genes ε1 and γ are pseudogenes, and not expressed. Upstream to the μ genes is a switch sequence (S) which is repeated upstream to each of the other constant region genes (*Fig. 6.18*).

Class switching may be achieved by gene recombination or by differential splicing of mRNA

Class switching is important in the maturation of the immune response and may be accompanied or preceded by somatic mutation. Initially a complete section of DNA that includes the recombined VH region and runs through to the δ and μ constant regions, is transcribed; two mRNA molecules are then produced by differential splicing, each with the same VH but having either μ or δ constant regions. It is suggested that much larger stretches of DNA are sometimes also transcribed together, with differential splicing giving other immunoglobulin classes sharing VH regions (*Fig. 6.19*). This has been observed in cells simultaneously producing IgM and IgE.

More often, class switching appears to be mediated by a recombination between S recombination sites, allowing a looping out and deletion of DNA, bringing another C region close to the VDJ gene. A further possibility has been suggested involving exchange between chromosomes (*Fig. 6.20*).

Membrane and secreted immunoglobulins are produced by differential splicing of RNA transcripts of heavy chain genes

Membrane-bound immunoglobulin (antigen receptor) is identical to secreted immunoglobulin (antibody), except for an extra stretch of amino acids at the C terminus of each heavy chain. Membrane immunoglobulins are therefore slightly larger than their secreted counterparts. Their additional amino acids traverse the cell membrane and anchor the molecule in the lipid bilayer. In membrane IgM, for example, a section of hydrophobic (lipophilic) amino acids are sandwiched between hydrophilic amino acids, which lie on either side of the membrane (*Fig. 6.21*). The hydrophobic residues are thought to form a stretch of α helix within the membrane. Membrane immunoglobulins only exist as the basic four-chain unit, and do not polymerize further.

Isotype switching by differential RNA splicing

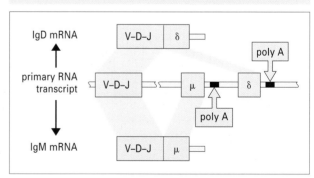

Fig. 6.19 Single B cells produce more than one antibody isotype from a single long primary RNA transcript. A transcript containing μ and δ is shown here. Polyadenylation can occur at different sites, leading to different forms of splicing, producing mRNA for IgD (top) or IgM (bottom). Even within this region there are additional polyadenylation sites which determine whether the translated immunoglobulin is the secreted or membrane-bound form.

Lost genes

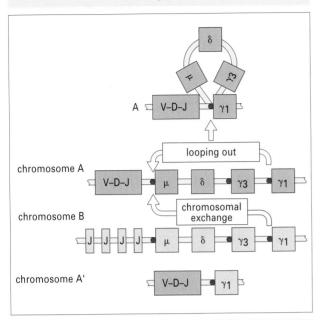

Fig. 6.20 A and B are chromatids of the chromosome section of the Ig genes. A contains the rearranged V–D–J segment. In the looping out hypothesis, a section of C genes (μ, δ, γ3) loop out and are lost. In the chromosome exchange hypothesis, similarities in the switching sequences permit unequal somatic recombination between maternal and paternal chromosomes. Thus, the A chromosome recombines with another part of the unrearranged B chromosome. The loss of gene segments gives rise to the IgM–IgG1 switch, shown as A'. The 'lost' C genes are on the other, non-functional chromosome B' (not shown), which now contains two copies of several C genes.

Membrane and secreted IgM: mouse

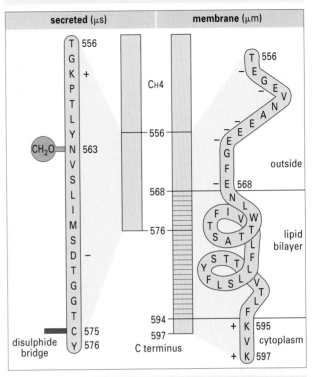

Fig. 6.21 C-terminal amino acid sequences for both secreted and membrane-bound IgM are identical up to residue 556. Secreted IgM has 20 further residues. Residue 563 (asparagine) has a carbohydrate unit attached to it while residue 575 is a cysteine involved in the formation of interchain disulphide bonds. Membrane IgM has 41 residues beyond 556. A stretch of 26 residues between 568 and 595 contains hydrophobic amino acids sandwiched between sequences containing charged residues. This hydrophobic portion may traverse the cell membrane as two turns of α-helix. A short, positively-charged section lies inside the cytoplasm.

Membrane and secreted IgM

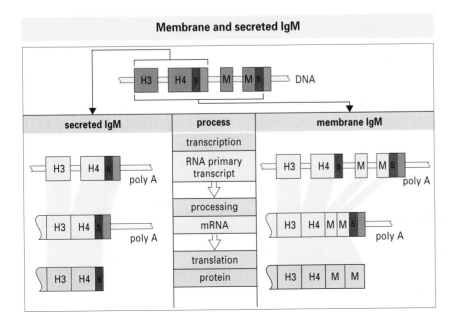

Fig. 6.22 Part of the DNA coding for IgM is shown diagrammatically. The exons for the μ3 and μ4 domains (H3 and H4) and the transmembrane segment of membrane IgM (M) are indicated. The 3' untranslated sequence is present at the end of the H4 and second membrane segments (S = secreted C-termini). The DNA can be transcribed in two ways. If transcription stops after H4 the transcript with a poly-A tail is processed to produce mRNA for secreted IgM. If transcription runs through to include the membrane segments, processing removes the codons for the terminal amino acids and the stop signal of H4, so that translation yields a protein with a different C terminus.

Production of the two forms of immunoglobulin occurs by differential transcription of the germ line C region gene (*Fig. 6.22*). It is thought that the poly-A sequence is important in determining which RNA transcript is produced, but exactly how this is controlled is uncertain.

■ REGULATION OF IMMUNOGLOBULIN PRODUCTION

Evidently the way in which cells regulate immunoglobulin production is complicated. The first step is the heavy chain rearrangement of D to J, followed by addition of V; μ chain stimulates the κ locus to attempt V–J rearrangement, followed by the lambda locus if necessary. It is postulated that this occurs repeatedly in both maternal and paternal chromosomes until a functionally recombined gene is produced or the genetic material is exhausted and the cell is aborted. Once the V regions of that cell are determined they remain essentially unaltered, except for any somatic mutation. However, there is still switching in the CH genes to produce different isotypes, and a change to production of secreted immunoglobulin following cell activation. A compilation of facts and hypotheses is shown in *Figure 6.23*.

Immunoglobulin chains are translated and targeted to the endoplasmic reticulum

Before the antibody is synthesized, it is necessary to splice the introns out of the primary RNA transcript. The beginning and end of each intron have particular forms of RNA base sequences, referred to as donor and acceptor junctions. It is thought that these junctions interact with each other and with ribonucleoproteins in the nucleus to remove the introns and splice the joins back together again to form mRNA. Of course, it is essential that this is done accurately so that the reading frame of the mRNA is unaltered.

Messenger RNA for immunoglobulins is translated and the nascent peptides targeted to the endoplasmic reticulum, after which the heavy and light chains associate (*Fig. 6.24*). The membrane-bound and secreted forms of immunoglobulins are processed differently to arrive at their correct locations, by mechanisms which have not yet been fully elucidated.

■ GENES OF THE T-CELL ANTIGEN RECEPTOR

The antigen–MHC binding portion of the TCR is generated by four different sets of genes. The α and β gene sets are expressed in the majority of peripheral T cells, whereas the γ and δ genes are expressed in a subpopulation of thymic T cells, and also in a minor population of peripheral T cells. These chains become associated with the γ, δ, ε and ζ chains of the CD3 molecule to form the complete TCR (see Chapter 5).

The general arrangement of TCR genes is remarkably similar to that of immunoglobulin heavy chains.

Interestingly, the δ genes for the TCR lie in the middle of the α genes, with their own sets of D, J, and C segments (*Fig. 6.25*).

Diversification of the TCR gene occurs by recombination between V, D, and J segments, with minor variations in detail for each locus

The α chain is superficially simple, except for the complication of the δ chain embedded between V and J loci. As in the κ locus, a complete variable region is produced by rearrangement of a Vα segment to a Jα segment. Diversity is markedly increased by the unusually large number of J segments.

The β locus includes two sets of D, J, and C genes. Most of the Vβ genes are grouped together, but one (Vβ14) is present at the extreme 3' end of the locus. The

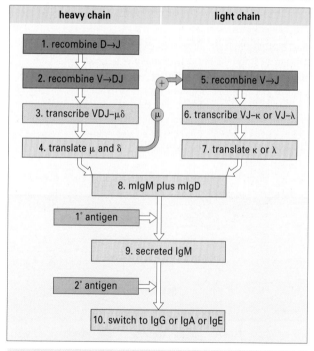

Summary scheme of immunoglobulin production

heavy chain	light chain
1. recombine D→J	
2. recombine V→DJ	5. recombine V→J
3. transcribe VDJ–μδ	6. transcribe VJ–κ or VJ–λ
4. translate μ and δ	7. translate κ or λ
8. mIgM plus mIgD	
1° antigen	
9. secreted IgM	
2° antigen	
10. switch to IgG or IgA or IgE	

Fig. 6.23 Stages of immunoglobulin production. Pre-B cells attempt to recombine heavy chain D and J segments, and then combine this with a V segment to make a functional heavy chain V–D–J. This is transcribed with μ and δ genes and translated to produce membrane μ and δ chains. The μ chain induces recombinations in the light chain loci. In each case the cell attempts to make functional chains using either the maternal or paternal chromosome, until it is either successful or runs out of unrearranged gene sets. Failure to make a functional immunoglobulin leads to clonal abortion. Virgin B cells express membrane IgM and IgD. After a primary antigen stimulation the cell can produce secreted IgM; after stimulation by a T-dependent antigen, and with T cell help, the cell can switch classes to produce either IgG, IgA or IgE. This step is often accompanied by somatic mutation of the V domains.

tandem duplication of Dβ, Jβ and Cβ must have occurred early in the evolution of mammals since it is present in both mice and humans. Extensive diversity is generated in the joining process as not only are V–D–J arrangements possible, but also V–J and V–D–D–J joins. The D segments are used in all three reading frames, adding even further to β chain diversity.

The arrangement of the γ-chain loci in mice and in humans is rather different. The murine locus bears a striking similarity to the antibody light-chain locus, with four Cγ genes (including a pseudogene), each associated with one J gene, and one to four Vγ genes. There are no D genes. In man there are eight Vγ genes, followed upstream (5') by three Jγ and the first Cγ; then there are two additional Jγ genes before Cγ2. Imprecise joining of V with J, together with insertions in the joins, is important in generating diversity.

The δ locus was discovered during studies on the α locus. Although relatively simple, with only five Vδ, two Dδ and six Jδ genes, it has been calculated that 1014 different δ chains could be generated by imprecision in joining, insertion of additional residues and use of the D genes in all three reading frames.

The mechanisms for TCR gene recombination appear to be similar to those of B cells, since the genes have similar patterns of heptamer(12 or 23 bases)–nonamer sequences flanking them. Similar or identical rearrange-

Production of secreted immunoglobulin

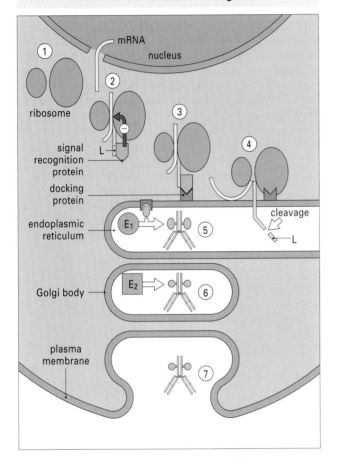

Fig 6.24 Messenger RNA for a secreted heavy chain leaves the nucleus and enters the cytoplasm where it is bound by a ribosome (1). The leader sequence (L) is translated and binds to signal recognition protein (SRP) which blocks further translation (2). The SRP-ribosome complex migrates to the endoplasmic reticulum (ER) where the SRP binds to the docking protein at a vacant site on the ER (3). Translation may now proceed and the synthesizing chain traverses the membrane into the ER (4). The leader sequence is removed and the chain combines with other H and L chains to form the immunoglobulin subunit (5). Enzymes (E1) add carbohydrate (blue) as the ER pinches off to form the transport vesicle (6). In the Golgi body further enzymes (E2) modify the carbohydrate before the completed molecule is secreted to the outside by reverse pinocytosis (7).

T-cell receptor genes

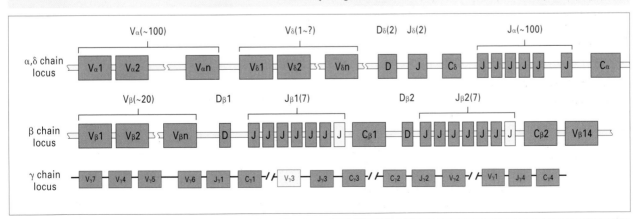

Fig. 6.25 The mechanism of recombination of the TCR genes is similar to that of the immunoglobulin heavy chain. The genes of the murine T-cell receptor αβ and γδ polypeptides are shown. The δ chain gene loci are embedded within the α locus, and tandem duplication has occurred in the β chain locus. The last of each set of Jβ genes and the Vγ3 are pseudogenes.

ment enzymes operate in B and T cells; experiments have shown that transfected TCR Dβ and Jγ genes can rearrange appropriately in B cells. N-region development is particularly marked and contributes extensively to the diversity.

Although somatic mutation is an important mechanism in generating immunoglobulin diversity, it does not occur in TCR genes. This may be linked with the need to maintain tolerance to self and recognition of MHC by T cells.

■ MAGNITUDE OF DIVERSITY

Diversity depends on the simple combinations of V, D and J regions plus N-region diversification, joining-site variation and multiple D regions. The precise distance between the end of germ line V and germ line J is variable; it corresponds to about 6–15 amino acid residues for Vβ and 3–7 residues for Vα. Hunkapiller and Hood have estimated that it is possible to make about 4.4×10^{13} different forms of Vβ and 6.5×10^{12} forms of Vα. These authors estimate that if only 1% of the sequences coded for viable proteins, this would still give 2.9×10^{22} receptors. Making the assumption that 99% of these are rejected owing to coding for autoantigens or other defects, this would still give 2.9×10^{20} possible murine TCRs. Since fewer than 10^9 thymocytes leave the thymus in the lifetime of a mouse, this raises the question: how random is the generation of receptors? A similar problem arises with immunoglobulins, where the potential repertoire is many orders of magnitude greater than the numbers of B cells ever produced.

Critical Thinking

■ How can a finite genome cope with an almost infinite number of antigens?

■ What is somatic mutation and how can this assist or hinder the immune response?

■ Compare antibody and MHC polymorphism within an individual and the population at large.

■ How might microbes have affected the evolution of the immune system?

■ If an animal lacked the recombination activating genes (RAG-1 and RAG-2), what effect would you expect this to have on the generation of diversity and on the immune system as a whole?

■ Following antigen stimulation, how do the genetic modifications to the antibody-forming genes bring about the maturation in antibody affinity seen in the immune response? How might advantageously mutated antibody genes be selected? What happens to clones with disadvantageous mutations?

FURTHER READING

Appasamy PM, Kenniston TW Jr, Weng Y *et al.* Interleukin 7-induced expression of specific T cell receptor gamma variable regions in murine fetal liver culture. *J Exp Med* 1993; **178**: 2201.

Austen BM, Westwood OMR. *Protein Targeting & Secretion.* Oxford: IRL Press, 1991.

Blackwell TK, Alt FW. Mechanism and developmental program of immunoglobulin gene rearrangement in mammals. *Ann Rev Genet* 1989;**23**:605.

Brack C, Hirama M, Lenhard-Schuller R, Tonegawa S. A complete immunoglobulin gene is created by somatic recombination. *Cell* 1978;**15**:1.

Chang B, Casali P. The CDR-1 sequences of a major proportion of human germline Ig VH genes are inherently susceptible to amino acid replacement. *Immunology Today* 1994; **15**: 367.

Davis MM, Bjorkman PJ. T-cell antigen receptor genes and T-cell recognition. *Nature* 1988;**334**:395.

Haas W, Pereira P, Tonegawa S. Gamma/Delta cells. *Ann Rev Immunol 1993;***11**:637.

Harriman W, Volk H, Defanoux N, Wabl M. Immunoglobulin class switch recombinations. *Ann Rev Immunol* 1993;**11**:385.

Hunkapiller T, Hood L. Diversity of the immunoglobulin gene superfamily. *Adv Immunol* 1990;**44**:1.

Leiden JM. Transcriptional regulation of T cell receptor genes. *Ann Rev Immunol* 1993;**11**:539.

Lewis SM. The mechanism of V(D)J joining: lessons from molecular, immunological and comparative analyses. *Adv Immunol* 1994;**56**:27.

Owen MJ, Lamb JR. *Immune Recognition.* Oxford: IRL Press. 1988.

Pascual V, Capra JD. Human immunoglobulin heavy-chain variable region genes: organization, polymorphism and expression. *Adv Immunol* 1991;**49**:1.

Antibodies are highly specific for the three-dimensional conformation of the epitope.

Antibody affinity is a measure of the strength of the bond between an antibody's combining site and a single epitope. The functional affinity or avidity of the interaction also depends on the number of binding sites on the antibody and their ability to react with multiple epitopes on the antigen.

T cells recognize cell-bound antigen in association with MHC class I or class II molecules. Peptide fragments from processed antigen bind to grooves of MHC antigens.

MHC class I and class II molecules present peptides derived, respectively, from endogenous and exogenous antigens. This is reflected by the intracellular site at which processed antigen accesses and binds to the MHC molecules.

Peptides that bind to MHC class I molecules are produced in the cytoplasm, probably due to the activity of an intracellular organelle called a proteasome. Peptides are transported across the endoplasmic reticulum by an 'ABC' family transporter. The ternary complex of class I heavy chain/β_2-microglobulin/peptide moves to the cell surface.

Peptides that bind to class II molecules are derived from endocytosed exogenous antigen which has been processed in an endosomal/lysosomal compartment. Class II molecules complexed with invariant (Ii) chain are transported through the Golgi complex to an acidic endosomal compartment, where dissociation of Ii and peptide loading occurs.

Peptide—MHC molecule complexes on the cell surface can be recognized by a specific T-cell receptor. However, a variety of additional interactions involving accessory molecules are required for T-cell activation.

Antibody and the T-cell antigen receptor (TCR) have many features in common. They both have variable (V) and constant (C) domains, and the processes of gene recombination which produce the variable domains (from V, D and J gene segments) are similar (see Chapter 6). Nevertheless, the ways in which B cells and T cells recognize antigens are quite different. Antibody recognizes antigens in solution or on cell surfaces, but always in their native conformation, whereas the T-cell receptor only recognizes antigen in association with MHC molecules on cell surfaces. Antigens recognized by T cells have often been degraded or processed in some way, so that the determinant recognized by the TCR is only a small fragment of the original antigen.

Another difference between antibody and the TCR is that antibody may be produced in two forms – as the B-cell antigen receptor or as secreted antibody – whereas the TCR is always an integral membrane protein. Secreted antibody is essentially a bifunctional molecule; the V domains are primarily concerned with antigen binding and the C domains interact with receptors on host tissues or complement.

This chapter describes the ways in which the domains of antibodies and TCRs form antigen-binding sites, and how they interact with specific antigens or antigen–MHC complexes. These interactions underlie the specificity of the adaptive immune response.

■ ANTIGEN–ANTIBODY BINDING

Antibodies form multiple non-covalent bonds with antigen

X-ray crystallography studies of antibody V domains show that the hypervariable regions (see Chapter 6) are clustered at the end of the Fab arms (see Chapter 4); particular residues in these regions interact specifically with antigen (*Fig. 7.1*).

The framework residues do not usually form bonds with the antigen. However, they are essential for producing the folding of the V domains and maintaining the integrity of the binding site.

The binding of antigen to antibody involves the formation of multiple non-covalent bonds between the antigen and amino acids of the binding site. Considered individually, the attractive forces (hydrogen bonds, and electrostatic, Van der Waals and hydrophobic forces) are weak by comparison with covalent bonds. However, the large number of interactions results in a large total binding energy.

The antibody-combining site

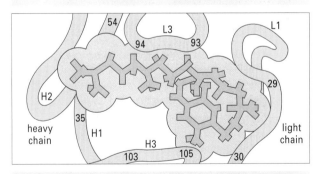

Fig. 7.1 The antigen molecule nestles in a cleft formed by the heavy and light chains, called the antibody-combining site. The example shown is based on X-ray crystallography studies of human IgG (the myeloma protein NEW) binding γ-hydroxyl vitamin K. The antigen makes contact with 10–12 amino acids in the hypervariable regions of both heavy and light chains. The numerals refer to amino acids identified as actually making contact with the antigen.

The conformations of target antigen and binding site are complementary

The strength of a non-covalent bond is critically dependent on the distance (d) between the interacting groups. The force is proportional to $1/d^2$ for electrostatic forces, and to $1/d^7$ for Van der Waals forces. Thus the interacting groups must be close (in molecular terms) before these forces become significant *(Fig. 7.2)*. In order for an antigenic determinant (epitope) and the antibody combining site (paratope) to combine (see *Fig. 7.1*), there must be suitable atomic groupings on opposing parts of the antigen and antibody, and the shape of the combining site must fit the epitope, so that several non-covalent bonds can form simultaneously. If the antigen and the combining site are complementary in this way, there will be sufficient binding energy to resist thermodynamic disruption of the bond. However, if electron clouds of the antigen and antibody overlap, steric repulsive forces come into play which are inversely proportional to the twelfth power of the distance between the clouds: $F \propto 1/d^{12}$. These forces play a vital role in determining the specificity of the antibody molecule for a particular antigen, and its ability to discriminate between antigens, since any variation from the ideal complementary shape will cause a fall in the total binding energy through increased repulsive forces and decreased attractive forces *(Fig. 7.3)*.

An examination of the interaction between lysozyme and the Fab of an antibody to lysozyme has shown that the antigen epitope and the binding site have complementary surfaces. These surfaces extend beyond the hypervariable regions. In total 17 amino acid residues on the antibody contact 16 residues on the lysozyme molecule *(Fig. 7.4)*. All of the hypervariable regions contribute to the antibody-binding site, although the third hypervariable region, formed by the V–D–J junction in the heavy chain gene, appears to be most important. This may be related to the greater variability generated by recombination of the V, D and J segments.

Antibody affinity indicates the strength of a single antigen–antibody bond

The strength of the bond between an antigen and an antibody is known as the antibody affinity. It is the sum of the attractive and repulsive forces described above *(Fig. 7.5)*. Interaction of the antibody-combining site with antigen can be investigated thermodynamically. To measure the affinity of a single combining site it is necessary to use a monovalent antigen, or even a single isolated antigenic determinant (a hapten). Since the non-covalent bonds between antibody and epitope are dissociable, the overall combination of an antibody and antigen must be reversible; thus the Law of Mass Action can be applied to the reaction and the equilibrium constant, K, can be determined. This is the affinity constant *(Fig. 7.6)*.

Antibody avidity indicates the overall strength of interaction between antibody and antigen

Since each antibody unit of four polypeptide chains has two antigen-binding sites, antibodies are potentially multivalent in their reaction with antigen. In addition, antigen can also be monovalent (e.g. haptens) or multivalent (e.g. microorganisms). The strength with which a multivalent antibody binds a multivalent antigen is termed avidity, to differentiate it from the affinity of a single antigenic determinant for an individual combining site. The avidity of an antibody for its antigen is dependent on the affinities of the individual com-

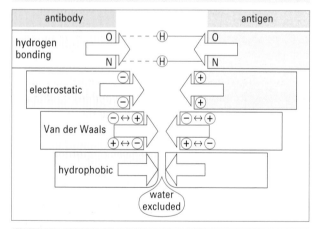

Intermolecular attractive forces

Fig. 7.2 The forces binding antigen to antibody require the close approach of the interacting groups. Hydrogen bonding results from the formation of hydrogen bridges between appropriate atoms. Electrostatic forces are due to the attraction of oppositely charged groups located on two protein side chains. Van der Waals bonds are generated by the interaction between electron clouds (here represented as induced oscillating dipoles). Hydrophobic bonds (which may contribute up to half the total strength of the antigen–antibody bond) rely on the association of non-polar, hydrophobic groups so that contact with water molecules is minimized. The distance between the interacting groups that gives optimum binding depends on the type of bond.

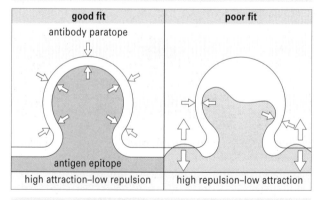

Good fit and poor fit

Fig. 7.3 A good fit between the antigenic determinant and the binding site of the antibody will create ample opportunities for intermolecular attractive forces to be created and few opportunities for repulsive forces to operate. Conversely, when there is a poor fit the reverse is true. When electron clouds overlap high repulsive forces are generated which override any small forces of attraction.

bining sites for the determinants on the antigen. It is greater than the sum of these affinities if both antibody binding sites can combine with the antigen. This is because all the antigen–antibody bonds must be broken simultaneously before the antigen and antibody dissociate *(Fig. 7.7)*. In normal physiological situations avidity is likely to be more relevant than affinity since naturally occurring antigens are multivalent. However, the precise measurement of hapten–antibody affinity is more likely to give an insight into the immunochemical nature of the antigen–antibody reaction.

Kinetics of antibody–antigen reactions

Measurements of antibody affinity relate to equilibrium conditions. Affinity indicates the tendency of the antibodies to form stable complexes with the antigen. However, for many biological activities of antibodies, it is possible that the kinetics of the reaction may also be significant.

Kinetics measures the forward rate (on-rate) constant $K_{1,2}$ (mol^{-1}s^{-1}) and the reverse rate (off-rate) constant $K_{2,1}$ (s^{-1}). At equilibrium the ratio of the two constants gives the equilibrium constant or affinity of the antibody. It has been claimed that differences in affinity are a result primarily of differences in off-rates, but more recently it has been shown that affinity can also be influenced by differences in on-rates.

Recent work has suggested that B-cell selection and stimulation during a maturing antibody response depend both upon selection for the ability of antibodies to bind to antigens rapidly (kinetic selection) and selection for the ability to bind antigens tightly (thermodynamic selection).

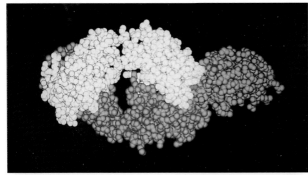

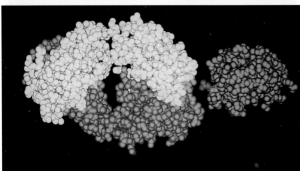

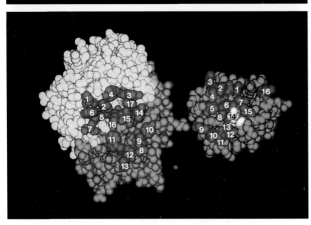

Fig. 7.4 The Fab–lysozyme complex. Upper: Lysozyme (green) binds to the hypervariable regions of the heavy (blue) and light (yellow) chains of the Fab fragment of antibody D1.3. Centre: The separated complex with Glu 121 visible (red). This residue fits into the centre of the cleft between the heavy and light chains.
Lower: The same molecules rotated 90° to show the contact residues which contribute to the antigen–antibody bond.
(Courtesy of Dr R. J. Poljak, from *Science* 1986;**233**:747–53, with permission.)

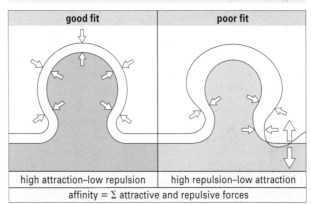

Fig. 7.5 The affinity with which antibody binds antigen is the sum of the attractive and repulsive forces between them. A high affinity antibody implies a good fit and conversely, a low affinity antibody implies a poor fit.

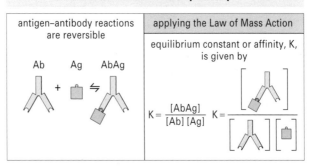

Fig. 7.6 All antigen–antibody reactions are reversible. The Law of Mass Action can therefore be applied, and the antibody affinity (given by the equilibrium constant, K) can be calculated. (Square brackets refer to the concentrations of the reactants.)

ANTIBODY SPECIFICITY AND AFFINITY

Antigen–antibody reactions can show a high level of specificity. For example, antibodies to a virus like measles will bind to the measles virus and confer immunity to this disease, but will not combine with, or protect against, an unrelated virus such as polio. The specificity of an antiserum is equal to the sum of the actions of every antibody in the antiserum. The antibody population may contain many paratopes, each reacting with a different epitope, or even with different parts of the same epitope *(Fig. 7.8)*. However, when some of the epitopes of an antigen, A, are shared by another antigen, B, then a proportion of the antibodies directed to A will also react with B. This phenomenon is termed cross-reactivity.

Antibodies recognize the overall conformation of antigens

There is evidence that an antibody recognizes the overall configuration of an epitope rather than particular chemical residues *(Fig. 7.9)*. Antibodies are capable of expressing remarkable specificity, and are able to distinguish between small differences in the primary amino acid sequence of protein antigens, as well as differences in charge, optical configuration and steric conformation *(Fig. 7.10)*. One consequence of this specificity is that many antibodies will bind only to native antigens, or to fragments of antigens that retain sufficient tertiary structure to permit the multiple interactions required for bond formation.

Affinity and avidity

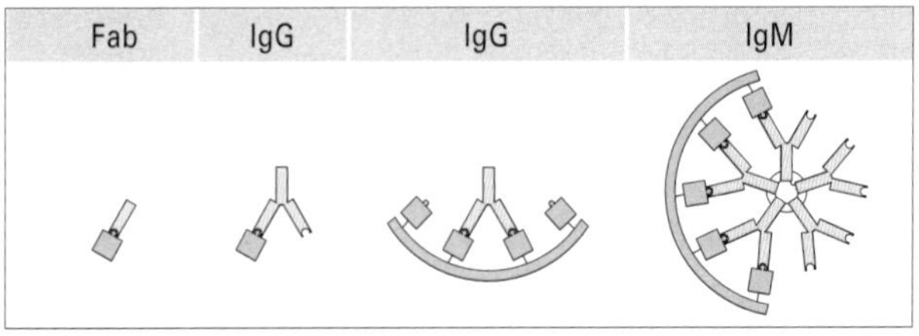

antibody	Fab	IgG	IgG	IgM
effective antibody valence	1	1	2	up to 10
antigen valence	1	1	n	n
equilibrium constant (L/M)	10^4	10^4	10^7	10^{11}
advantage of multivalence	–	–	10^3-fold	10^7-fold
definition of binding	affinity	affinity	avidity	avidity
	intrinsic affinity		functional affinity	

Fig. 7.7 Multivalent binding between antibody and antigen (avidity or functional affinity) results in a considerable increase in stability as measured by the equilibrium constant, compared to simple monovalent binding (affinity or intrinsic affinity, here arbitrarily assigned a value of 10^4 L/M). This is sometimes referred to as the 'bonus effect' of multivalency. Thus there may be a 10^3-fold increase in the binding energy of IgG when both valencies (combining sites) are utilized and a 10^7 increase when IgM binds antigen in a multivalent manner.

Specificity, cross-reactivity and non-reactivity

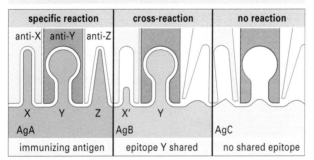

Fig. 7.8 Antiserum specificity results from the action of a population of individual antibody molecules (anti-X, anti-Y, and anti-Z) directed against different epitopes (X, Y, Z) on different antigen molecules. Antigen A (AgA) and antigen B (AgB) have epitope Y in common. Antiserum raised against AgA (anti-XYZ) not only reacts specifically with AgA but cross-reacts with AgB (through recognition of epitopes Y and X'). The antiserum gives no reaction with AgC because there are no shared epitopes.

Specificity and cross-reactivity

radical (R)	sulphonate	arsonate	carboxylate
	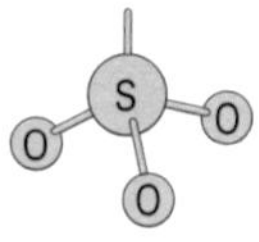 tetrahedral	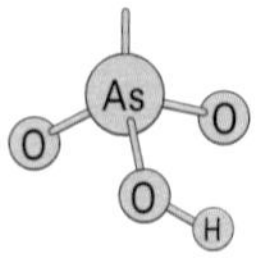 tetrahedral	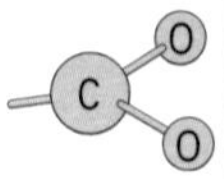 planar
ortho 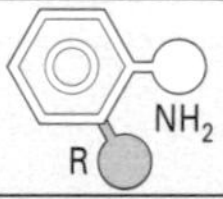	+ +	–	–
meta 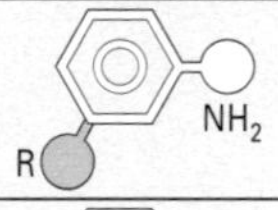	+ + +	+	±
para 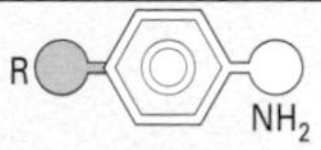	±	–	–

Fig. 7.9 Antiserum raised to the meta isomer of aminobenzene sulphonate (the immunizing hapten), is mixed with ortho and para isomers of aminobenzene sulphonate, and also with the three isomers (ortho, meta, para) of two different but related antigens: aminobenzene arsonate and aminobenzene carboxylate. The antiserum reacts specifically with the sulphonate group in the meta position but will cross-react (though more weakly) with sulphonate in the ortho position. Further, weaker cross-reactions are possible when the antiserum is reacted with either the arsonate group or the carboxylate group in the meta, but not in the ortho or para position. Arsonate is larger than sulphonate and has an extra hydrogen atom, while carboxylate is the smallest. These data suggest that an antigen's configuration is as important as the individual chemical groupings that it contains.

This specificity can create a problem when one wishes to produce antibodies for immunological assays. It is often easier to synthesize short polypeptide antigens of known primary structure than it is to purify sufficient amounts of the native antigen for immunization. However, antibodies to the synthetic polypeptides often do not bind well or predictably to the antigen in its native form.

Configurational specificity

antiserum	antigen		
	lysozyme	isolated 'loop' peptide	reduced 'loop
anti-lysozyme	+ +	+	–
anti-'loop' peptide	+	+ +	–

Fig. 7.10 The lysozyme molecule possesses an intrachain bond (red) which produces a loop in the peptide chain. Antisera raised against whole lysozyme (anti-lysozyme) and the isolated loop (anti-'loop' peptide), are able to distinguish between the two. Neither antiserum reacts with the isolated loop in its linear, reduced form. This demonstrates the importance of tertiary structure in determining antibody specificity.

Designer antibodies are produced by modifying antibody genes

Molecular biology has paved the way for the production of monoclonal antibodies (mAbs) of defined specificity, affinity and immunoglobulin isotype. It is possible to make antibody genes which have, for example, mouse V domains on human C regions. This allows immunologists to develop antibodies of a particular specificity in the mouse and then to attach that specificity to a human antibody. The resulting mAb is of low antigenicity in man and can be used in patients. Working at an even smaller scale, sets of complementarity determining regions (CDRs) from one species can be grafted into a framework V domain from another. It is even possible to alter individual residues in the combining site to increase the affinity of that antibody *(Fig. 7.11)*.

Polyfunctional binding sites can accommodate dissimilar epitopes

Over the past few years, research has suggested that an antibody molecule may be complementary to several different antigens. The binding of these antigens is competitive and appears to occur at different positions in the combining site *(Fig. 7.12)*.

The specificity of a population of antibodies is not due to each antibody reacting exclusively with the inducting antigen. However, if a large number of different polyfunctional antibodies all have a site which can combine with a particular antigen A, the net reactivity of these antibodies is high to A but low to all other antigens. Thus specificity can be a population phenomenon, i.e. an average characteristic of all the antibodies in an antiserum *(Fig. 7.13)*.

Designer antibodies

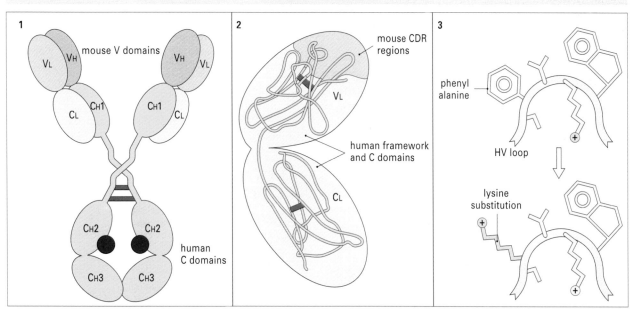

Fig. 7.11 It is possible to splice the genes for a mouse V domain onto human C genes, and to transfect this into a cell which then makes chimeric mouse/human antibodies (1). Alternatively, just the required CDR regions can be spliced into another framework (2). The affinity of a binding site can also be modified by point mutation of the DNA of the hypervariable loops – here illustrated as a Phe → Lys change (3).

High-affinity antibody is often more effective than low-affinity antibody

Binding affinity is not merely a matter of theoretical interest, since affinity and avidity affect the physiological and pathological properties of the antibodies. High-affinity antibody is superior to low-affinity antibody in a number of biological reactions *(Fig. 7.14)*. In experimental animals, antigen–antibody complexes containing low affinity antibody persist in the circulation, localize on the glomerular basement membrane of the kidney and impair renal function. High-affinity complexes are more rapidly removed from the circulation, localize in the mesangium of the kidney, and have little effect on renal function.

Antibody affinity to most T-dependent antigens increases during an immune response, and a similar effect can be produced by certain immunization protocols. For example, high affinity antibody subpopulations are potentiated following immunization with antigen and IFNγ *(Fig. 7.15)*. A number of adjuvants are capable of enhancing levels of antibody but few have this characteristic of also potentiating affinity. As affinity markedly influences the biological effectiveness of antibodies, IFNγ may be an important adjuvant for vaccine use.

Determination of antibody affinity

A number of methods are available for the determination of affinity and avidity. In each procedure a system is set up in which antigen and antibody are allowed to come to equilibrium: Ab + Ag $\rightleftharpoons$ Ab–Ag. The quantities of free antigen and complexed antigen are then measured without disturbing the equilibrium. There are several ways of doing this. Some separate the free antigen from bound antigen by physical methods such as dialysis, gel filtration, centrifugation and selective precipitation. Others use changes in the fluorescent properties of the complexed antigen or antibody.

Data from these systems is analyzed by applying the Law of Mass Action to give the equilibrium (affinity) constant, K:

$$K = \frac{[AbAg]}{[Ab][Ag]}$$

where [Ab–Ag] is the concentration of complexed antigen, [Ag] is the concentration of free antigen and [Ab] is the concentration of free antigen-binding sites at equilibrium. When half the binding sites are occupied by antigen, [Ab] = [Ab–Ag], so it follows that K = 1/[Ag]. In other words, a

Polyfunctional binding sites

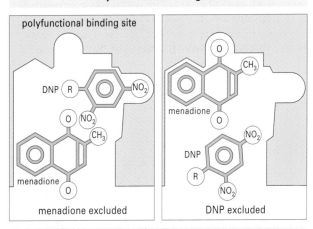

Fig. 7.12 The antibody-combining site may bind more than one antigenic determinant. For example, antibody 460 has two different sites in the binding cleft which are 1.2–1.4 nm apart. The antibody binds the hapten menadione or the hapten DNP. The binding is competitive, that is, the binding of one excludes binding of the other. Binding sites capable of binding more than one antigenic determinant are termed polyfunctional binding sites.

Antiserum specificity

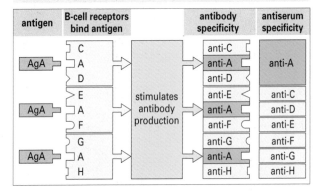

Fig. 7.13 Specificity as a population phenomenon. A single antigen (AgA) may bind to the antibody molecules of different B cells which are specific not only for A but also for other antigens (C, D, E, F, etc.). The B-cell receptors thus possess polyfunctional binding sites. Each B cell stimulated by AgA produces antibody specific not only to AgA, but also to the other antigens. Since all the B cells stimulated are AgA specific, but not all are specific to the other antigens, the concentration of antibody would be high to AgA but low to the other antigens.

Advantages of high-affinity antibody

haemagglutination
haemolysis
complement fixation
passive cutaneous anaphylaxis: - bactericidal activity - toxin neutralization - opsonic activity
immune elimination of antigen
membrane damage
virus neutralization
protective capacity against bacteria and viruses
enzyme inactivation
in vivo destruction of D⁺ erythrocytes

Fig. 7.14 Biological reactions in which high-affinity antibody is superior to low-affinity antibody.

high-affinity antibody (one with a high K) only requires a low antigen concentration to achieve binding of antigen to half its combining sites, whereas a low-affinity antibody requires a much higher concentration of antigen to achieve this.

The range of antibody affinities in an antiserum does not follow a normal distribution

When enzymes interact with their substrate, the equilibrium constant (K) for the reaction at different substrate concentrations is invariant. The reaction between antigen and antiserum does not follow this pattern. Instead, K is heterogeneous within the antibody population. For many years it was assumed that the range of antibody affinities seen in any particular antiserum would have a Gaussian (normal) distribution. This assumption has turned out to be false. Nevertheless, as a good approximation, average affinity of a population of antibodies in a serum (K_0) is defined as the reciprocal of the free antigen concentration at equilibrium when half of the total antigen binding sites are occupied: $K_0 = 1/[Ag_{free}]$. When the equilibrium constant for the reaction between an antiserum and antigen is analyzed, a non-Gaussian range of K values (affinities) is obtained *(Fig. 7.16)*.

Affinity heterogeneity is difficult to assess experimentally

No precise mathematical description of affinity heterogeneity is possible, because we are not sure whether the distribution of affinities in a particular serum is normal, skewed, biphasic or polyphasic. Sophisticated computer analyses of binding curves have been used to define heterogeneity, but have been based on the assumptions that the distribution is normal. A simple experimental approach to getting an assessment of heterogeneity, which does not rely on such assumptions, has been described. In this technique, an appropriate dilution of the antibody and serial dilutions of free antigen in solution are added to antigen-coated microtitre plates. (The free antigen blocks binding to the antigen on the plates.) The percentage inhibition at each concentration of free antigen is calculated and the molar concentration for 50% inhibition determined ($I_{0.5}$). The percentile inhibition contributed at each concentration of free antigen is calculated and the values used to analyse heterogeneity by histogram. A mathematical value describing heterogeneity (the Shannon index) can be calculated from these values. High values indicate a large spread of affinities, and low values indicate the converse.

■ THE STRUCTURE OF ANTIGENS

The number of different antibodies which may be produced to an antigen is high, because antigens are three-dimensional structures and present many different configurations to the B cells. Different antibodies to an antigen often bind to epitopes which overlap on the antigen surface. In this way different antibodies can bind to a particular antigenic region of the molecule, without binding to exactly the same epitope.

Immunodominant epitopes occur on exposed, flexible parts of the antigen

Although it is possible to produce antibodies to almost any part of an antigen, this does not normally happen in an

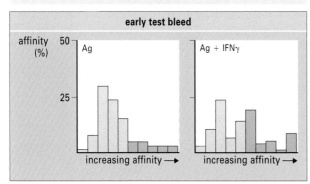

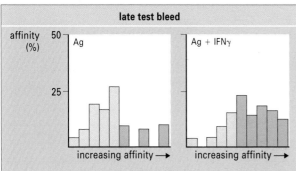

Fig. 7.15 Mice were immunized either with antigen alone (Ag) or with antigen plus 30 000 units of IFNγ (Ag + IFNγ). The affinity of the antibodies was measured either early or late after immunization. Mice receiving IFNγ show more high affinity antibody (darker bars) in both the early and late bleeds than those mice that received antigen alone.

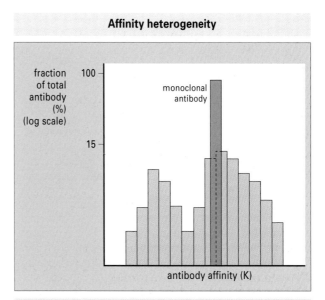

Fig. 7.16 This histogram shows a typical distribution of antibody affinities (K) in an antiserum to an antigenic determinant, compared to the single affinity with which a monoclonal antibody binds its antigenic determinant. Note that the antibody affinities in antiserum do not have a normal distribution.

immune response. It is usually found that certain areas of the antigen are particularly antigenic, and that the majority of antibodies bind to these regions. These regions, which are referred to as the immunodominant regions of the antigen, are often at exposed areas on the outside of the antigen, particularly where there are loops of polypeptide that lack a rigid tertiary structure.

In some cases, the immunodominant regions of the antigen correspond to the most mobile surface areas of the molecule. This observation has led immunologists to suspect that the interaction between antibody and antigen is not a rigid fit with perfect complementarity between the shape of the antibody and antigen. There may be some flexibility, both in the antigen epitope and the hypervariable loops of the antibody, which allows the optimum binding energy to be achieved. This proposal has been amply confirmed by X-ray crystallographic analysis of the complex between Fab and the antigen neuraminidase. The various factors involved in complementarity have been summarized elsewhere (see *Figs 7.2, 7.3* and *7.4*)

■ T CELL–ANTIGEN RECOGNITION

T cells recognize cell-bound antigen in association with MHC molecules. MHC class I and class II molecules act as guidance systems for T cells. This is known as MHC restriction.

The key experiment that demonstrated the principle of MHC restriction involved the murine cytotoxic T cell response to virally infected target cells (*Fig. 7.17*). It showed that cytotoxic T (Tc) cells from an animal infected with a virus are primed to kill cells of the same H–2 haplotype infected with that virus, but will not kill cells of a different haplotype infected by the same virus.

One advantage conferred by this dual recognition system is that by recognizing viral antigen only in association with MHC antigen, receptors on Tc cells do not become blocked with free virus. Most importantly, T cells can distinguish between intra- and extracellular antigens.

Similar principles of MHC-restricted recognition apply to helper T (TH) cells, which recognize antigen on cells such as macrophages and B cells in association with MHC class II molecules. In this case, the class II region molecules act as recognition signals between antigen-presenting cells (such as macrophages) and the TH cell.

■ ANTIGEN PROCESSING AND PRESENTATION

Antigens are processed before they are presented to T cells

Antibody responses and cell-mediated immune reactions are generally directed against different determinants on the antigen. For example, mouse B cells recognize an epitope at the N terminus of glucagon, whereas T cells recognize determinants near the C terminus (*Fig. 7.18*). This is because antigens are not presented by MHC antigens as intact proteins, but rather as processed peptides at the cell surface. The cells that process antigen in this way may be either specialized antigen-presenting cells (APCs), which are capable of stimulating T-cell division, or may be virally infected cells within the body which then become a target for Tc cells.

Antigen processing involves degrading the antigen into peptide fragments. Thus, the vast majority of epitopes recognized by T cells are fragments from a peptide chain, and are often inaccessible for immune recognition in the intact

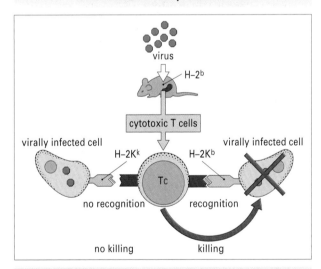

MHC restriction of cytotoxic T cells

Fig. 7.17 Killing of virally infected target cells and haplotype restricted killing. A mouse of the H–2^b haplotype is primed with virus, and the Tc cells thus generated are isolated. These T cells are tested for their ability to kill H–2^b and H–2^k cells infected with the same virus. The Tc cells kill H–2^b cells but not H–2^k cells. The T cell is recognizing a specific structure resulting from the association between the class I H–2K (or H–2D) product and viral antigen (e.g. a virus/H–2K complex). As a control measure, both groups are treated with anti-viral antibody, which is not haplotype-restricted but recognizes budding virus: infected cells of both haplotypes are killed by anti-viral antibody and complement.

T-cell and B-cell epitopes are distinct

glucagon	N 1	17 18	29
antibody response	+++		+
lymphocyte stimulation	–		+++
DTH response	+		+++

Fig. 7.18 The immune responses to two peptides of the antigen glucagon are shown. Antibody (a B-cell response) is primarily directed to epitopes at the N terminus, while the C-terminal peptide 18–29 stimulates T-cell responses, including lymphocyte stimulation *in vitro* and the delayed type hypersensitivity (DTH) response *in vivo*.

protein. Only a minority of peptide fragments from a protein antigen are able to bind to a particular MHC molecule. Furthermore, different MHC molecules bind different sets of peptides. For example, studies using a viral antigen that is recognized by mouse strains of several different haplotypes (that is, having different MHC molecules) showed that TH cells from each haplotype recognized a distinct peptide from that antigen *(Fig. 7.19)*. This depended largely on the ability of a particular peptide to bind to a particular MHC class II.

Antigens are partially degraded into peptides before binding to MHC molecules

The processing of antigens to generate peptides that can bind to MHC molecules occurs in intracellular organelles *(Fig. 7.20)*. For the purposes of laboratory studies, the internal degradation by APCs can be circumvented by the use of synthetic peptides. This ability, to use 'ready-made' peptides of known sequences has enabled workers to identify epitopes recognized by T cells with different specificities *(Fig. 7.21)*. The relative importance of different amino acids within a defined epitope can also be investigated by amino acid replacements at different sites. Using defined peptides, direct binding to both MHC class I and class II antigens has also been demonstrated. A comparison of the effects of an amino acid substitution on MHC binding and T-cell reactivity has enabled conclusions to be drawn on which amino acids contact the MHC molecule and which contact the T-cell receptor. For example, a peptide representing residues 52–61 of hen egg-white lysozyme is rec-

T-cell antigenic peptides in the γ repressor protein

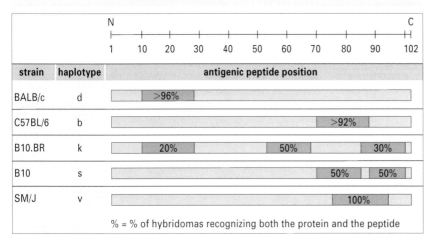

strain	haplotype	antigenic peptide position
BALB/c	d	>96%
C57BL/6	b	>92%
B10.BR	k	20% 50% 30%
B10	s	50% 50%
SM/J	v	100%

% = % of hybridomas recognizing both the protein and the peptide

Fig. 7.19 Diversity of antigenic peptides in relation to MHC class II. Mice were immunized with λ repressor protein. T-cell hybridomas generated from mouse cells were tested against a panel of overlapping peptides which spanned the entire protein. Positions of antigenic peptides are shown in dark blue. One peptide was always immunodominant, although more than one peptide was antigenic in some mouse strains. Adapted from data by Roy *et al.* (1989).

Antigen processing

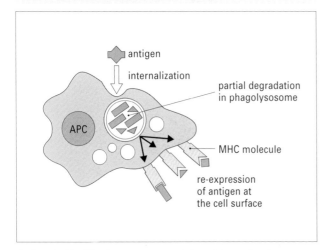

Fig. 7.20 Exogenous antigens are internalized by antigen-presenting cells and are then degraded by proteolytic enzymes in specialized intracellular compartments. Antigenic peptides associate with class II MHC molecules that cross the endocytic pathway on their way to the cell surface.

T-cell peptides in proteins

peptide	amino acid sequence
myoglobin	69–78 102–118 132–145
flu haemagglutinin	109–119 130–140 302–313
hepatitis B surface Ag	38–52 95–109 140–154
hepatitis B pre-S	120–132
FMDV VPI	141–160
rabies spike precursor	32–44

Fig. 7.21 The table shows peptides that are known to stimulate T cells. The peptides come from a number of proteins. Synthetic peptides corresponding to the entire amino acid sequence of a protein antigen can be used to stimulate specific T cells. Usually, only one or a few peptides from a protein are stimulators.

ognized by H–2-IA^k restricted T cells. This peptide binds to IA^k molecules, and functional data have implicated three amino acid residues within this peptide as interacting with MHC class II, and yet another three residues as contacting the TCR.

■ STRUCTURE AND ASSEMBLY OF MHC MOLECULE/PEPTIDE COMPLEXES

The peptide-binding site on an MHC molecule has a variety of pockets, clefts, ridges, intrusions and depressions. Its precise topology depends partly on the nature of the amino acids within the groove, and thus varies from one haplotype to the next. Peptide binding depends on the nature of the side chains of that peptide and their complementarity with the MHC molecule's binding groove. Some amino acid side chains of the peptide are oriented out of the groove and are available to contact the TCR (see Chapter 4).

Peptide/MHC association occurs in specific intracellular organelles and interaction of peptides with class I and class II antigens occurs at different sites within the cell.

Peptides are held in the MHC molecules' binding cleft by characteristic anchor residues

It is now possible to purify and sequence peptides that have been generated by a cell and then bound by MHC molecules at the cell surface. These peptides include not just foreign pep-tides from internalized antigens or viral particles, but also self molecules produced within the cell or endocytosed from extracellular fluids. Self peptides eluted from MHC class I molecules have been purified and sequenced. They were shown to be nine amino acids in length. This contrasts with the size of synthetic peptides (12–15 amino acids) that is known to be optimal. These 'natural' peptides were more precisely defined than expected. A number of peptides bound by particular MHC molecules were sequenced, and characteristic residues were identified – one at the C terminus and another close to the N terminus of the peptide. These characteristic motifs distinguish sets of binding peptides for different class I molecules (*Fig. 7.22*). They are thought to act as anchoring residues for the peptide within the groove.

Analysis of the three-dimensional structures of several class I molecules has generated a particularly clear picture of the peptide residing in the binding groove. It is an extended (not α-helical) chain of nine amino acids with its ends tethered at opposite ends of the groove. Some of the side chains extend into the pockets formed within the variable region of the class I heavy chain. This picture is consistent with the characteristic motifs found at the ends of peptides eluted from class I molecules.

Three-dimensional structural analysis has revealed a similar peptide-binding cleft in class II antigens. This cleft also incorporates a number of binding pockets. Consistent with this observation, peptides eluted from class II molecules also contain characteristic anchor residues *(Fig. 7.23)*.

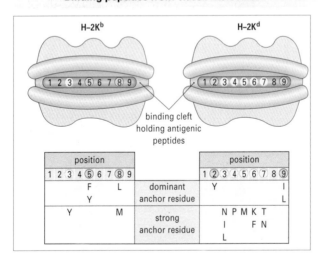

Binding peptides from class I molecules

position											position								
1	2	3	4	⑤	6	7	⑧	9			1	②	3	4	5	6	7	8	⑨
				F			L		dominant anchor residue		Y							I	
				Y														L	
				Y			M		strong anchor residue			N	P	M	K	T			
												I			F	N			
												L							

Fig. 7.22 Allele-specific motifs in peptides eluted from MHC molecules. Class I molecules from either H–2K^b or H–2K^d haplotypes were immunoprecipitated. Peptides bound to these molecules were purified and sequenced. Amino acid residues that were commonly found at a particular position are classified as dominant anchor residues. Residues that are fairly common at a site are shown as 'strong'. Positions for which no amino acid is shown could be occupied by several different amino acids with equal frequency. The one-letter amino acid code is used. The diagram represents the MHC class I binding cleft, viewed from above with anchor positions of each haplotype highlighted.

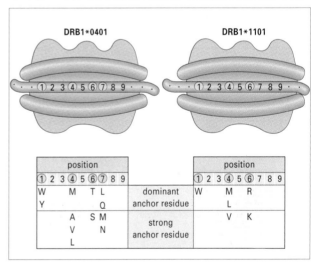

Allele-specific motifs in peptides eluted from MHC class II molecules

position											position								
①	2	3	④	5	⑥	⑦	8	9			①	2	3	④	5	⑥	7	8	9
W			M		T	L			dominant anchor residue		W			M		R			
Y						Q								L					
			A		S	M			strong anchor residue					V		K			
			V			N													
			L																

Fig. 7.23 HLA-DR molecules of two haplotypes (DRB1*0401 and DRB1*1101) were purified and incubated with a library of peptides (generated in phage M13). After multiple rounds of selection, peptides that bound effectively to the class II molecules were identified and sequenced. Residues whose frequency was higher than 20% are shown as dominant anchor residues. Other fairly common residues are shown as 'strong'. Data abstracted from Hammer *et al.* (1993). Note that the binding site on class II molecules accommodates longer peptides than that on class I.

Class I molecules associate with endogenously-synthesized peptides

A number of studies have shown that class I restricted T cells (Tc cells) recognize endogenous antigens synthesized within the target cell, whereas class II restricted T cells (TH cells) recognize exogenous antigen. Manipulation of the location of a protein determines whether it elicits a class I or class II restricted response. For example, influenza virus haemagglutinin (HA), a glycoprotein associated with the membranes of the host cell, normally elicits only a weak Tc cell response. However, influenza HA can be generated in the cytoplasm by deleting the cDNA sequence coding for the N-terminal signal peptide to HA. When this is done there is a strong Tc cell response to HA. Similarly, the introduction of ovalbumin into the cytoplasm of a target cell (using an osmotic shock technique) generates Tc cells recognizing ovalbumin, whereas addition of exogenous ovalbumin generates exclusively a TH cell response.

Proteasomes degrade cytoplasmic antigens, generating peptides

Cytoplasmic antigens are processed into peptides by cytoplasmic proteases prior to transport of the peptides into the rough endoplasmic reticulum (RER) of the cell. This is the organelle on which membrane proteins, including class I and class II antigens, are synthesized and assembled. Once within the RER, peptides are thought to associate efficiently with newly synthesized class I molecules. The assembly of the MHC heavy chain and β_2 microglobulin (β_2m) may be driven by peptide since 'empty' class I MHC complexes are unstable – the heavy chain and β_2m rapidly dissociate at physiological temperatures.

There is now a better understanding of the proteins that process and transport cytoplasmic peptides bound by class I molecules. Remarkably, some of these proteins are encoded within the MHC. Cytoplasmic antigens are thought to be processed, at least in part, by an organelle known as a proteasome. Proteasomes are multicatalytic proteinase complexes expressed ubiquitously, and are found throughout the animal kingdom. Two genes encoding components of the human and murine proteasomes have been mapped within the class II region of the MHC.

Transmembrane transporters move peptides into the ER for loading onto class I MHC molecules

Two genes encoding members of the so-called 'ABC' superfamily of transmembrane transporters have also been discovered in the class II region of the MHC. ABC family proteins transport a variety of substrates, including peptides, across cellular membranes in an ATP-dependent manner.. The positions of the murine and human MHC-encoded transporter and proteasome genes are shown in *Fig. 7.24.*

Viral or other proteins synthesized in the cytoplasm are processed by proteasome complexes. Peptides are transported into the RER by the ABC transporter. Some peptides associate with and stabilize class I–β_2m complexes. Only peptides that fulfil the steric requirements for fitting into the peptide–binding groove will bind. We do not know if the peptides transported into the RER are exclusively nonapeptides, or if larger peptides can bind to class I molecules and be trimmed after binding. The ternary complex is transported to the cell surface via the Golgi complex (*Fig. 7.25*). Class I molecules lacking bound peptide dissociate and are degraded intracellularly.

Class II molecules are loaded with exogenous peptides in an endosomal compartment

Class II α and β chains are found in the RER complexed to a polypeptide called the invariant chain (Ii). This protein is encoded by a non-MHC gene. The $\alpha\beta$–Ii complex is transported through the Golgi complex to an acidic endosomal or lysosomal compartment, where Ii is released. The $\alpha\beta$ complex spends 1–3 hours in this compartment before reaching the cell surface. Experiments suggest that the dissociation of Ii from the $\alpha\beta$ complex in the acidic environment of the endosomal/lysosomal compartment permits binding of peptide.

How do antigenic peptides derived from exogenous peptides meet class II molecules in the appropriate compartment? The answer to this question lies in the intracellular traffic routes of MHC molecules. Following synthesis in the RER, both are transported through the Golgi compartment, class I in association with antigenic peptide, and class II bound to the invariant chain. Class II molecules segregate from class I in the *trans*-Golgi network. They then join the

MHC genes involved in antigen processing and presentation

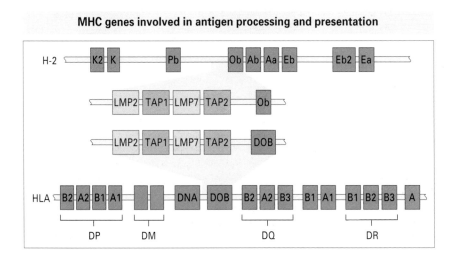

Fig. 7.24 Genes encoding a peptide transporter (TAP) and components of a multisubunit organelle called a proteasome (LMP) are located in the murine and human class II regions.

Assembly of endogenous peptides with MHC class I antigens

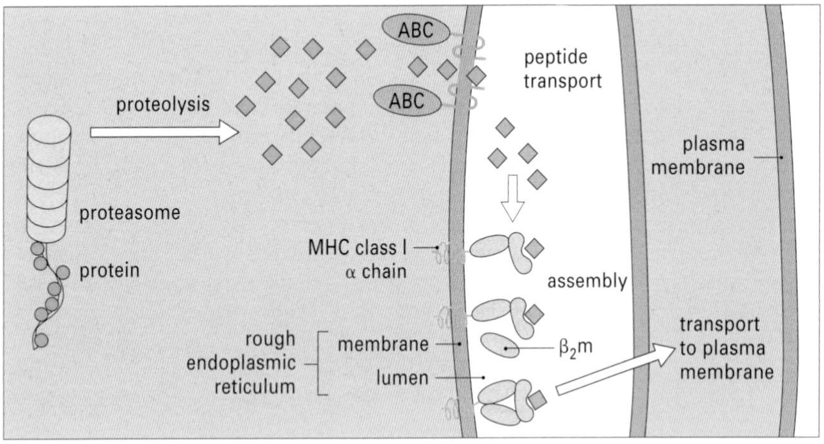

proteolysis

proteasome

protein

rough
endoplasmic
reticulum

MHC class I
α chain

membrane

lumen

β₂m

ABC

ABC

peptide
transport

assembly

plasma
membrane

transport
to plasma
membrane

Fig. 7.25 Proposed assembly pathway of antigen–MHC–complex. Cytoplasmic antigens are processed by proteasomes, two subunits of which are encoded by the MHC genes LMP-2 and LMP-7. Peptides are transported by two members of the 'ABC' superfamily of transporters, also encoded within the MHC (TAP-1 and TAP-2). Antigenic peptides associate with class I heavy chains and β₂m in the RER. Stabilized class I molecules are then transported to the cell surface (*Fig. 7.26*).

endosomal/lysosomal compartment *en route* to the plasma membrane. These vesicles are distinct from conventional endosomes and lysosomes and appear to be specialized for the transport and loading of class II molecules (*Fig. 7.26*).

The intracellular distribution of class I and class II molecules reflects the dichotomy in presentation of antigen from endogenous and exogenous origin. Further work is required to determine whether other antigen-presenting cells, such as macrophages, dendritic cells and Langerhans cells, use this mechanism for peptide–class II interaction.

The class II region also contains genes for an intracellular protein involved in the antigen-presentation pathway for class II molecules. The HLA-DMA and -DMB genes encode a heterodimeric protein with sequence homologies to both class I and class II molecules. This protein appears to function intracellularly to promote class II-peptide association.

■ ROLE OF ACCESSORY MOLECULES

The specificity of T-cell interactions with target cells clearly derives from the interaction of the TCR with class I or class II antigen loaded with peptide. However, measurements of the interaction of soluble TCR with soluble MHC molecules have revealed affinities in the micromolar range. This is probably not enough to activate T cells directly, and interactions between accessory molecules are required to increase the overall avidity.

Three important accessory molecules are CD2, which interacts with the LFA-3 ligand on the target cell; LFA-1, which interacts with its ligands ICAM-1 and ICAM-2, and CD28, which interacts with B7-1 and B7-2 ligands on APCs. The CD4 and CD8 accessory molecules have a weak affinity for MHC class II and class I molecules, respectively. Both molecules associate with the TCR–MHC–peptide complex. The low affinity of the interaction means that CD4 and CD8 are unlikely to contribute to the avidity of the T cell for its target cell. However, they may stimulate intracellular events that are important in the activation process. These aspects of T-cell activation are discussed more fully in Chapter 8.

Proposed routes of intracellular trafficking of MHC molecules involved in antigen presentation

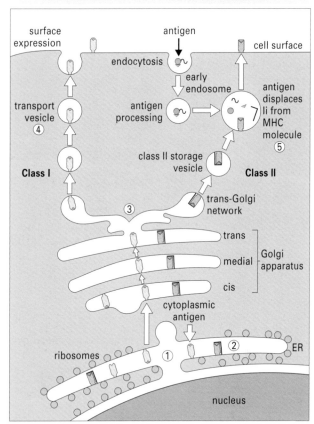

surface
expression

transport
vesicle
④

Class I

③

antigen

endocytosis

early
endosome

antigen
processing

class II storage
vesicle

trans-Golgi
network

trans

medial

cis

cytoplasmic
antigen

cell surface

antigen
displaces
li from
MHC
molecule
⑤

Class II

Golgi
apparatus

ribosomes

①

②

ER

nucleus

Fig. 7.26 Newly synthesized class I molecules are loaded with peptide (1). Class II molecules associate with li in the RER (2). li prevents loading with peptide and contains sequences that enable the class II molecule to exit the RER. Class I and class II molecules segregate after transit through the Golgi (3). Class I molecules go directly to the cell surface (4). Class II molecules enter an acidic compartment, where they are loaded with peptide derived from exogenous antigen (5).

Critical Thinking

■ What do you understand by the term epitope? How big is an epitope? Can epitopes overlap? Where on a protein antigen would you expect to find epitopes? What types of amino acid residue are usually found in epitopes?

■ If you have a monoclonal antibody against a structurally-defined antigen, how could you determine which part of the antigen is recognized by the antibody?

■ Is antibody specificity a clearly defined characteristic of a particular antibody, or does it depend on the context in which the antibody acts physiologically, or is used experimentally?

■ Is a monoclonal antibody more specific for an antigen than a polyvalent antiserum? Does it have a higher affinity than an antiserum?

■ Peptides presented by class I or class II antigens are distinguished not by their structures but by the different intracellular sites at which they access the MHC antigen. What are the advantages to the immune system of this system?

■ How does knowledge of antigen presentation pathways help in the design of peptide-based vaccines?

FURTHER READING

Bierer BE, Sleckman BP, Ratnofsky SE, Burakoff SJ. The biologic roles of CD2, CD4 and CD8 in T-cell activation. *Annu Rev Immunol* 1989;**7**:579–99.

Bhat TN, Bentley GA, Boulot G, *et al*. Bound water molecules and conformational stabilisation help mediate an antigen-antibody association. *Proc Nat Acad Sci USA* 1994;**91**:1089.

Burton DR. Structure and function of antibodies. In: Calabi F, Neuberger MS, eds. *Molecular Genetics of Immunoglobulin*. Amsterdam, Elsevier Science Publishers, 1987.

Cresswell P. Questions of presentation. *Nature* 1990;**343**:593.

DeFranco AL (1993) Structure and function of the B cell antigen receptor. *Ann Rev Cell Biol* 1993;**9**:377–410.

Demotz S, Grey HM, Appella E, Sette A. Characterization of a naturally processed MHC class II-restricted T-cell determinant of hen egg lysozyme. *Nature* 1989;**342**:682.

Falk K, Rötzschke O, Stevanovic S, Jung G, Rammensee H-G. Allele-specific motifs revealed by sequencing of self-peptides eluted from MHC molecules. *Nature* 1991;**351**:290–96.

Germain RN. MHC-dependent antigen processing and peptide presentation: providing ligands for T lymphocyte activation. *Cell* 1994;**76**:287–99.

Germain RN. Seeing double! *Curr Biol* 1993;**3**:586–89.

Germain RM, Margulies DH. The biochemistry and cell biology of antigen processing and presentation. *Annu Rev Immunol* 1993;**11**:403–50.

Getzoff ED, Tainer JA, Lerner RA. The chemistry and mechanism of antibody binding to protein antigens. *Adv Immunol* 1988;**43**:1.

Hammer J, Valsasnini P, Tolba K, *et al*. Promiscuous and allele-specific anchors in HLA-DR-binding peptides. *Cell* 1993;**74**:197–203.

Hunt DG, Henderson RA, Shabanowitz J, *et al*. Characterization of peptides bound to the class I MHC molecule HLA-A2.1 by mass spectrometry. *Science* 1995;**255**:1261–63.

Jardetzky TS, Lane WS, Robinson RA, Madden DR, Wiley DC. Identification of self peptides bound to purified HLA-B27. *Nature* 1991;**353**:326–29.

Lanzavecchia A. Receptor-mediated antigen uptake and its effect on antigen presentation to class II-restricted T lymphocytes. *Annu Rev Immunol* 1990;**8**:773.

Neefijies JJ, Stollorz V, Peters PJ, Geuze HJ, Ploegh HL. The biosynthetic pathway of MHC class II but not class I molecules intersects the endocytic route. *Cell* 1990;**61**:171.

Roche PA, Cresswell P. Invariant chain association with HLA-DR molecules inhibits immunogenic peptide binding. *Nature* 1990;**345**:615.

Roy S, Scherer MT, Briner TJ, Smith JA, Gefter ML. Murine MHC polymorphism and T cell specificities. *Science* 1989;**244**:572–75.

Rudensky A, Presotn HP, Hong SC, *et al*. Sequence analysis of peptides bound to MHC class II molecules. *Nature* 1991;**353**:622–27.

Teyton L, O'Sullivan D, Dickson PW, *et al*. Invariant chain distinguishes between the exogenous and endogenous antigen presentation pathways. *Nature* 1990;**348**:39–44.

Townsend A, Öhlen C, Bastin J, Ljunggren H-G, Foster L, Kärre K. Association of class I major histocompatibility heavy and light chains induced by viral peptides. *Nature* 1989;**340**:443.

Tulp A, Verwoerd D, Dobberstein B, Ploegh HL, Pieters, J. Isolation and characterization of the intracellular MHC class II compartment. *Nature* 1994;**353**:622–27.

van der Merwe PA, McNamee PM, Davies EA, Barclay AN, Davis SJ. Topology of the CD2-CD48 cell-adhesion molecule complex: implications for antigen recognition by T cells. *Curr Biol* 1995;**5**:74–84.

CELL COOPERATION IN THE ANTIBODY RESPONSE

Immune activation to stimulate antibody production involves cell interaction between T cells and APC, and later between these primed T cells and B cells.

T-cell activation involves antigen-specific interaction, cell adhesion molecules, and cytokines. The most potent co-stimulatory molecule is B7 (CD80 or CD86). In the absence of appropriate co-stimulation, antigen recognition by naive T cells may result in clonal anergy.

Lymphocyte proliferation is indirect, occurring via the induction of receptors for lymphocyte growth factors following cell activation. Lymphocyte growth factors (e.g. IL-2) are chiefly produced by T cells.

Two types of antigens induce antibody responses – T-dependent and T-independent. T-dependent antigens induce secondary immune responses characterized by IgG production and affinity maturation.

Cytokines are intercellular signalling proteins intimately involved in most biological processes – cell growth, activation, inflammation, immunity, repair, fibrosis, chemotaxis. Cytokines include proteins also known as interferons, interleukins, colony-stimulating factors and other growth factors.

Cytokines act at low molarity because they act on very high affinity receptors.

The organized lymphoid tissues, such as lymph nodes and spleen, consist of closely packed cells, as are the cells at an inflammatory site. This alone suggests that lymphoid cells do not function in isolation. Indeed, it is now known that they interact in a well organized sequence of events:

- T cells are activated when they recognize antigen presented to them by an antigen presenting cell.
- TH cells interact with B cells that present antigen fragments to them.
- Activated B cells proliferate and differentiate into antibody-forming cells.
- Antibody is produced and various immune responses follow.

In this chapter the principles of the cell interactions in the immune system are described, together with some of the consequences, such as affinity maturation and immunological memory, and some of the critical molecules involved, including cytokines.

■ ANTIGEN PRESENTATION TO T CELLS

Antigen processing

The pioneering studies of Ada and Nossal showed that only a very small proportion (<1%) of injected antigen is involved in the immune response, the rest being rapidly degraded and excreted. This suggests that antigen presentation is the rate-limiting step in immune reactions.

Antigen processing refers to the degradation of antigen into peptide fragments, which become bound to MHC class I or class II molecules (see Chapter 7). These are the critical fragments involved in the triggering of T cells, whose receptors recognize sequences of amino acids in peptides in the MHC groove, rather than the protein shapes, ('conformational' determinants), recognized by B-cell immunoglobulins. A store of antigen complexed with antibody and complement is maintained in the germinal centres of lymph nodes, adherent to dendritic follicular cells, and is used to trigger B cells.

Interaction with antigen-presenting cells is essential for T-cell activation

The interaction between T cells and the heterogeneous group of cells collectively termed 'antigen-presenting cells' (APCs) is the most extensively studied example of cell interaction in the immune system. It is the first such interaction to occur after antigen challenge, and its outcome largely dictates the subsequent course of events: if a sufficient number of CD4+ T-helper (TH) cells are triggered, then the activation of B cells or the development of delayed hypersensitivity almost certainly follows. If TH cells are not triggered, or are subject to a form of immunological tolerance known as 'clonal anergy' (see Chapter 12), then no other immunological events follow.

There are various types of APC

A wide spectrum of cells can present antigen, depending on how and where the antigen first encounters cells of the immune system (*Fig. 8.1*). Interdigitating dendritic cells (IDCs), which are found in abundance in the T-cell dependent areas of lymph nodes and spleen, are considered to be the most effective cells for the initial activation of resting CD4+ T cells. IDCs express high levels of MHC class II antigens, which interact with T-cell receptor (TCR) and CD4 on CD4+ (helper) T cells. However, macrophages and B lymphocytes can also expresss MHC class II, so this alone cannot explain the greater effectiveness of IDCs in antigen presentation.

IDCs are considered to be the major APC involved in primary immune responses because they induce T-cell proliferation more effectively than any other APC. Indeed, cell proliferation is a key step, as it multiplies the numbers of antigen-specific T cells, but it is only one facet of effective T cell triggering – macrophages may be just as effective as IDCs in inducing primary T-helper function, even though they are less efficient than IDCs at inducing proliferation. Similarly, blood monocytes (the most widely studied APC in humans) have the capacity to induce both proliferation and the helper function in T cells.

Localization of antigen in lymph nodes in association with APCs

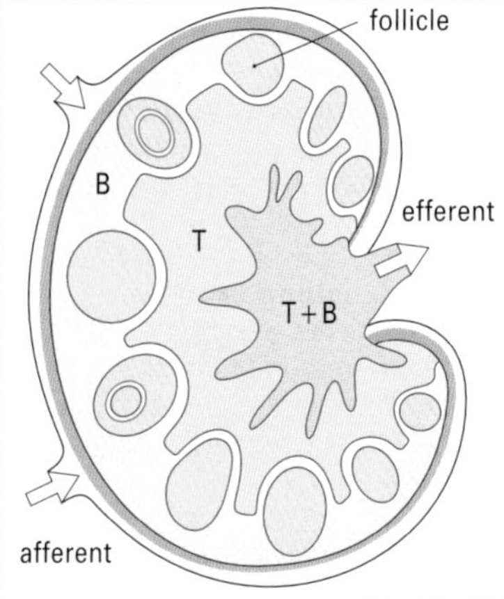

area	antigen-presenting cells	antigen	persistence of antigen
subcapsular (marginal) sinus	marginal zone macrophages	polysaccharides Ficoll (T_{ind})	+ + + +
follicles and B cell areas	follicular dendritic cells	immune complexes that fix complement	+ + +
medulla	classical macrophages	most antigens	+
T cell areas	interdigitating dendritic cells	most antigens	+ +

Fig. 8.1 A lymph node represented schematically (above, left) shows afferent and efferent lymphatics, follicles, the outer cortical B cell area and the paracortical T cell area. Different antigen-presenting cells predominate in these areas (though the demarcation is not absolute) and selectively take up different types of antigen which then persist on the surface of the cells for variable periods. Thus many polysaccharides are preferentially taken up by marginal zone macrophages and may persist for months or years, whereas antigens on recirculating macrophages in the medulla may last for only a few days or weeks. Note that recirculating 'veiled' cells (Langerhans' cells), which are thought to arise from the skin, change their morphology to become interdigitating dendritic cells within the lymph node. Both these cell types, and the follicular dendritic cells, have long processes which are in intimate contact with lymphocytes.

B cells also act as APCs – they can bind to a specific antigen, internalize it and then degrade the antigen into peptides, which become associated with MHC class II molecules. Thus, if antigen concentrations are very low, the specific, high-affinity receptors (IgM or IgD) on B cells make them the most effective APCs, because other APCs simply cannot capture enough antigen. Thus for secondary responses, where the number of antigen-specific B cells is high, B cells may be a major type of APC. The properties and functions of APCs are summarized in *Figures 8.2 and 8.3*.

Multiple cell surface molecules interact during antigen presentation to T cells

The TCR complex recognizes a specific peptide lodged in the peptide binding groove of the MHC molecule. This interaction dictates immunological specificity, since a peptide associated with an MHC molecule of one particular haplotype forms a unique structure to be recognized by the TCR. However, other molecules are involved in this interaction. Evidence for this came from experiments in which complementary DNA (cDNA) encoding human MHC molecules was transfected into mouse fibroblasts. The mouse cells expressed human MHC molecules and were able to act as human APCs, but with relatively low efficiency compared to cells expressing other 'co-stimulatory' molecules (*Fig. 8.4*). One such molecule, intercellular adhesion molecule-1 (ICAM-1), is known to interact with lymphocyte functional antigen-1 (LFA-1), present on all immune cells. Thus, if mouse cells are made to express both human MHC and human ICAM-1, their capacity to act as

human APCs is augmented. The known co-stimulatory molecules are shown in *Figure 8.4*, interacting with ligands on the surface of a T cell.

The most potent costimulatory molecules known are termed B7-1 (CD80) and B7-2 (CD86). These proteins are constitutively expressed on IDC, but are expressed and can be upregulated on monocytes, B cells and probably other APCs. They are the ligands for CD28 as well as its homologue CTLA-4, a molecule that is expressed on T cells and upregulated during T cell activation. CD28 stimulation has been shown to prolong and augment the production of IL-2 (which causes T-cell proliferation), and other cytokines.

The CD2 molecule on T cells is also involved in T-cell activation, in conjunction with the TCR. CD2 is a receptor for lymphocyte functional antigen-3 (LFA-3), which is widely distributed on cells and is present on all APCs. (The presence of LFA-3 on sheep red cells is responsible for the sheep red cell rosetting reaction [the E rosette], that was widely used to purify T cells before the advent of monoclonal antibodies.)

Molecules such as ICAM-1 and B7, that reinforce the signal from TCR and induce positive activation of T cells, have been termed the 'second signal'. T cells cannot respond without this signal, and if they recognize their antigen in a non-stimulating manner they become inactivated, producing a state of immunological tolerance. This tolerance is specific, only affecting TH cells that respond to a particular antigen, and is known as clonal anergy.

Apart from the cell-surface interactions, cytokines, acting locally, are also involved in T-cell activation. Interest has focused on IL-1 and IL-6, molecules produced by cer-

Antigen presentation

mononuclear phagocytes

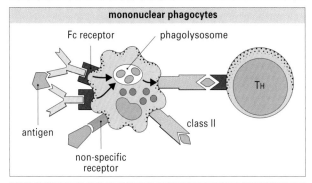

B cells

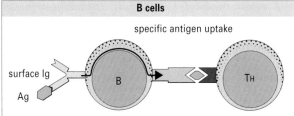

dendritic cells

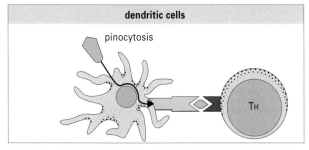

Fig. 8.2 Mononuclear phagocytes (top), B cells (centre) and dendritic cells (bottom) can all present antigen to MHC class II restricted T-helper (T$_H$) cells. Macrophages take up antigen via non-specific receptors or as immune complexes, process it and return fragments to the cell surface in association with class II molecules. Activated B cells can take up antigen via their surface immunoglobulin and present it to T cells alongside the class II molecules. Dendritic cells constitutively express class II MHC molecules, and take up antigen by pinocytosis.

Antigen-presenting cells

	phago-cytosis	type	location	class II expression
phagocytes (monocyte/ macrophage lineage)	+	monocytes	blood	(+)→ + + + inducible
		macrophages	tissue	
		marginal zone macrophages	spleen and lymph node	
		Kupffer cells	liver	
		microglia	brain	
non-phagocytic constitutive antigen-presenting cells	–	Langerhans' cells	skin	+ + constitutive
		interdigitating dendritic cells (IDCs)	lymphoid tissue	
		follicular dendritic cells	lymphoid tissue	–
lymphocytes	–	B cells and T cells	lymphoid tissues and at sites of immune reactions	– → + + inducible
facultative antigen-presenting cells	+	astrocytes	brain	inducible
		follicular cells	thyroid	inducible
	–	endothelium	vascular and lymphoid tissue	– → + + inducible
		fibroblasts	connective tissue	
		other types in appropriate tissue		

Fig. 8.3 Many APCs are unable to phagocytose antigen, but can take it up in other ways, such as pinocytosis. Endothelial cells, not normally considered APCs, that have been induced to express class II molecules by IFNγ are also capable of acting as APCs, as can certain epithelial cells. Another example of this phenomenon, is the thyroid follicular cell, which acts as an APC in the pathogenesis of Graves' autoimmune thyroiditis.

Critical molecules involved in antigen presentation

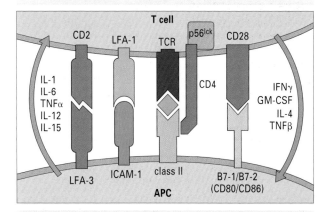

Fig. 8.4 The molecules involved in the interaction between T cells and APCs. The various cytokines and their direction of action are also shown. Note that other cell surface molecules, as yet uncharacterized, may also be important in antigen presentation.

tain APCs, including macrophages. T cells do not always require stimulation by these molecules – if they are already dividing, it is not necessary. However, in resting T cells IL-1 and IL-6 induce the expression of receptors for the T-cell growth factor, IL-2. IL–12 is also of importance in T cell activation, helping enhance IFNγ production.

While the interaction between CD4$^+$ T cells and APCs is reasonably well studied, that between CD8$^+$ T cells and APCs is less understood. It is known that CD4$^+$ cells help in the activation of most CD8$^+$ T cells. Since a single inter-digitating dendritic cell (IDC) can bind many T cells, it has been proposed that activation takes place in a cluster of CD4$^+$ and CD8$^+$ T cells gathered on the surface of one or more IDCs.

■ B–T CELL INTERACTION

Interaction of B cells and T cells also involves multiple surface molecules

Antigen specific T cell populations can be obtained by growing and cloning T cells with antigens, APCs and IL-2. It is thus possible to directly visualize B and T cell clusters interacting *in vitro*. The T cells become polarized, with T-cell receptors concentrated to the B-cell side. The B cells also become polarized and express most of the class II antigen in proximity to the T cells. The interactions in these clusters suggest an intense exchange of information, and lead to two important events in the B-cell life cycle: induction of proliferation, and differentiation into antibody-forming cells.

The interaction between T cells and B cells is a two-way process, in which B cells present antigen to T cells, and also receive signals from the T cells for division and differentiation. The central, highly specific interaction is that between the MHC class II–antigen complex and the TCR; it is augmented by interactions between LFA-3 and CD2, and ICAM-1 and LFA-1 (*Fig. 8.5*). A number of other cell surface molecules are also involved. The B7-1 and B7-2 surface antigens on B cells interact with CD28, which causes stabilization of mRNA for IL-2 and other cytokines in the T cells and thereby prolongs the delivery of the activation signals. Additionally, CD5 on T cells binds CD72 on the B cell surface, further promoting the interaction between the cells.

It is now recognized that CD40 delivers the most potent activating signal to B cells, more potent even than signals transmitted via surface immunoglobulin. Activated T cells transiently express a ligand that interacts with CD40.

IL-1 and IL-6 released by some B cells enhance expression of IL-2 receptor on T cells. However, since only some B cells make these cytokines, it is likely that most B cells can only efficiently activate preprimed or memory T cells.

Different T-cell subsets activate B cells in different ways

Recent work has indicated that CD4$^+$ T cells (in mice and in humans) can be divided into different subsets depending on their cytokine profile:

- CD4$^+$ T cells that produce IL-2 and IFNγ but not IL-4 are designated TH1 and are chiefly responsible for delayed type hypersensitivity responses. They can also help B cells to produce IgG2a, but not much IgG1 or IgE, in the mouse.
- CD4$^+$ T cells that produce IL-4 and IL-5, but not IL-2 or IFNγ are designated TH2. They are very efficient helper cells for antibody production, especially of IgG1 and IgE.
- Many T cells, especially in humans, are intermediate in their cytokine profile, and are known as TH0 cells.

T cell cytokine secretion and action is important for B cell activation

During the T–B cell interaction, T cells can secrete a number of cytokines that have a powerful effect on B cells. These include IL-2, a proliferation inducer for B cells as well as for T cells, IL-4 which acts early in B cell activation of proliferation, IL-5 which in the mouse (but not man) is a powerful B cell activator, and IL-6 which is a strong signal for B cell differentiation (*Fig. 8.6*). T cells also produce TNFα and TNFβ. These molecules have also been reported to be important for B cell growth. Despite this long catalogue of molecules that act to trigger B cells, there are other signals which remain to be identified.

B–T interaction may either activate or inactivate (anergize)

The above description of B–T interaction suggests that the only possible outcome is activation of the B cell. However, this is not the case. We have already seen that the APC–T cell interaction may yield two, diametrically opposing results, namely activation, or inactivation (clonal anergy) of T cells. In the same way, B cells frequently become anergic. This is important because affinity maturation of B cells during the immune response, due to rapid mutation in the genes encoding the antibody variable regions, could easily result in high-affinity autoantibodies. Clonal anergy in the periphery is an important device for silencing these potentially damaging clones. However, the molecular details of this process are unknown.

Cell surface molecules involved in the interactions between B cells and TH cells

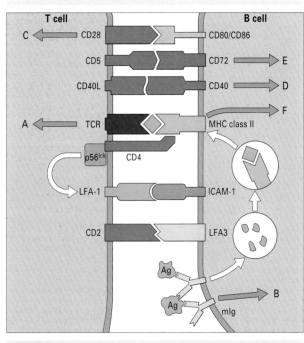

Fig. 8.5 Membrane-immunoglobulin (mIg) takes up antigen (Ag) into an intracellular compartment where it is degraded and peptides combine with MHC class II molecules. Other arrows show the discrete signal-transduction events that have been established. A and B are the antigen-receptor signal-transduction events involving tyrosine phosphorylation and phosphoinositide breakdown. The antigen receptors also regulate LFA-1 affinity for ICAM-1, possibly through the signal transduction events. In the T cell, CD28 also sends a unique signal to the T cell (C). In the B cell stimulation via CD40 is the most potent activating signal (D). Additionally, class II MHC molecules and CD72 appear to induce distinct signalling events (E and F). Not shown is the exchange of soluble interleukins and binding to the corresponding receptors on the other cell. (Adapted, with permission, from DeFranco, *Nature* 1991;**351**: 603.

The respective roles of IgM and IgD (the B-cell antigen receptors) in this process are not understood, as each receptor appears to be capable of transmitting signals for both functions.

T-independent antigens do not require T-cell help to stimulate B cells

The immune response to most antigens depends on both T cells and B cells recognizing that antigen. This type of antigen is called T-dependent (T_{dep}). There are, however, a small number of antigens capable of activating B cells without T-cell help, referred to as T-independent antigens (T_{ind}). T_{ind} antigens have a number of properties in common (*Fig. 8.7*). In particular, they are all large polymeric molecules with repeating antigenic determinants. Many possess the ability, at high concentrations, to activate B-cell clones that are specific for other antigens, a phenomenon known as polyclonal B cell activation; however, at lower concentrations they

only activate B cells specific for themselves. Many T_{ind} antigens are particularly resistant to degradation.

Primary antibody responses to T_{ind} antigens *in vitro* are generally slightly weaker than those to T_{dep} antigens, they peak fractionally earlier and generate mainly IgM. However, the secondary responses to T_{dep} and T_{ind} antigens differ greatly. The secondary response to T_{ind} antigens is very similar to the primary response; the secondary response to T_{dep} antigens is far stronger than the primary, and has a large IgG component (*Fig. 8.8*). It seems therefore that T_{ind} antigens do not induce the maturation of response seen with T_{dep} antigens that leads to class switching to IgG and increase in antibody affinity. Memory induction to T_{ind} antigens is also relatively poor.

The mechanism by which T_{ind} antigens trigger B cells without requiring TH cells is not fully understood. It is likely that their polymeric structure enables T_{ind} antigens to crosslink B-cell receptors; this process would be facilitated

---

Stages in B-cell activation and development

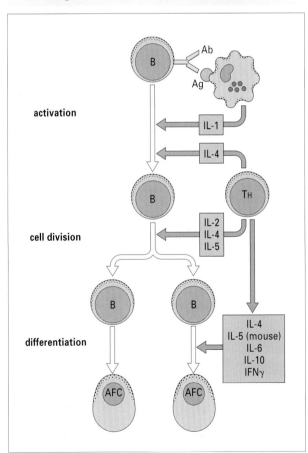

Fig. 8.6 B cells are activated by antigen on antigen-presenting cells (APCs) such as macrophages, in the presence of IL-4 and IL-1. This causes expression of receptors for IL-2 and other cytokines. IL-2, IL-4 and IL-5 (in the mouse) drive cell division. Only one cycle of cell division is illustrated although many cycles will usually occur. Differentiation into antibody-forming cells (AFCs) is effected by IL-4, IL-5 (in mouse), IL-6, IL-10 and IFNγ.

T-independent antigens

antigen	polymeric	polyclonal activation	resistance to degradation
lipopolysaccharide (LPS)	+	+ + +	+
Ficoll	+ + +	−	+ + +
dextran	+ +	+	+ +
levan	+ +	+	+ +
poly-D amino acids	+ + +	−	+ + +
polymeric bacterial flagellin	+ +	+ +	+

Fig. 8.7 The major common properties of some of the main T-independent (T_{ind}) antigens are listed. T_{ind} antigens induce the production of cytokines IL-1, TNF and IL-6 by macrophages. (Note: both poly-L amino acids and monomeric bacterial flagellin are T_{dep} antigens, demonstrating the role of antigen structure in determining T_{ind} properties.)

Comparison of secondary immune responses to T_{dep} and T_{ind} antigens *in vitro*

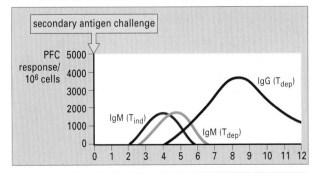

Fig. 8.8 The secondary response to T_{dep} antigens is stronger and induces a greater number of IgG-producing cells, as measured by plaque-forming cells (see Chapter 28).

by their resistance to degradation.

Many T_{ind} antigens are products of bacteria, for example, the endotoxin, dextrans and levans found in bacterial cell walls, and the polymerized flagellin found in flagella.

There are potential survival advantages for an organism whose immune response to bacteria does not depend on complex cell interactions and may therefore be more rapid. Many bacterial antigens bypass T-cell help because they are able to induce the production of cytokines IL-1, IL-6 and TNFα by macrophages. The short-lived response and lack of IgG may be due to the lack of IL-2, IL-4 and IL-5, normally produced by T cells in response to T_{dep} antigen. T_{ind} antigens often activate a subset of B cells expressing CD5.

T cells and B cells recognize different parts of antigens

In the late 1960s and early 1970s, studies with chemically modified proteins by Mitchison and others led to significant advances in our understanding of the different functions of T and B cells.

To induce an optimum secondary antibody response to a hapten (a small chemical group that is immunogenic only if bound to a protein carrier), an experimental animal must be immunized and re-challenged using the same hapten–carrier conjugate. Challenge with the same hapten on a different carrier fails to produce a full secondary response. This is known as the carrier effect. However, challenge using a different hapten carrier conjugate produces a full secondary response if the animal has previously been primed to the second carrier protein alone, or has received spleen cells from a donor primed to the second carrier (*Fig. 8.9*). If the experiment is repeated, using spleen cells from which all T cells have been removed, the secondary response disappears. This shows that the TH cells recognized the carrier, while the B cells recognized the hapten, i.e. T cells and B cells recognize different parts of antigens.

One consequence of this system is that a B cell recognizing a certain epitope can receive help from T cells specific for a number of different carrier peptides from the same antigen, provided that the B cell can present those peptides to each T cell.

In an immune response *in vivo* it is thought that the interactions between T cells and B cells that drive B cell division and differentiation involve T cells that have already been stimulated by contact with the antigen on other APCs (e.g. dendritic cells) (*Fig. 8.10*). It is also clear that two processes are required to activate a B cell to respond to a T_{dep} antigen.

These results have led to the basic scheme for cell interactions in the antibody response set out in *Figure 8.10*. It is proposed that antigen entering the body is processed by cells that present the antigen in a highly immunogenic form to the TH cells and B cells. The T cells recognize determinants on the antigen different to those recognized by the B cells. The T cells deliver help to appropriate B cells, which are stimulated to differentiate and divide into antibody-forming cells. Thus the two processes are required to activate a B cell:

- Antigen interacting with B cell Ig receptors
- Stimulating signal(s) from TH cells.

The classic experiments on T/B cooperation discussed in this section are underpinned by more recent information on how immune cells interact at the cellular level, showing that T cell stimuli are needed for optimal growth and differentiation of B cells (see *Fig. 8.5*).

Activation of lymphocytes and APCs

In immune responses, activation of T cells, B cells, and APCs takes place in different parts of the immune system and at varying times.

APCs

Activation of APCs is rapid and can be induced by the immunogenic entity itself, in the case of bacteria, or by the adjuvant component of a vaccine. However, the majority of APC activation is stimulated by cytokines produced by T cells. The best known macrophage-activating factors are

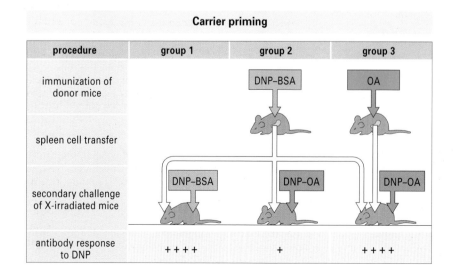

Carrier priming

procedure	group 1	group 2	group 3
immunization of donor mice		DNP–BSA	OA
spleen cell transfer			
secondary challenge of X-irradiated mice	DNP–BSA	DNP–OA	DNP–OA
antibody response to DNP	+ + + +	+	+ + + +

Fig. 8.9 Three groups of X-irradiated mice were given antigen-primed spleen cells and challenged with antigen: 1. Mice that received DNP–BSA primed cells and were then challenged with DNP–BSA gave a strong antibody response to DNP. 2. Mice that received DNP–BSA primed cells and were then challenged with DNP–OA, gave a weak antibody response (no carrier effect). 3. Mice that received DNP–BSA primed cells and OA-primed cells, and were then challenged with DNP–OA, gave a strong response to DNP. This shows that the need for carrier priming can be circumvented by supplying carrier-primed spleen cells.

IFNγ (interferon-γ), GM-CSF (granulocyte–macrophage colony stimulating factor), and TNFα (tumour necrosis factor). (As these names illustrate, the cytokine nomenclature, based on the first workable assay for the molecule, is rarely a good description of its actual functions.) When APCs are activated, they express more MHC class I and II, more Fc receptors and more adhesion (co-stimulatory) molecules, including B7-1 and B7-2, CD11a/b/c, and ICAM-1. They also produce numerous cytokines (e.g. IL-1, IL-6, TNFα) and enzymes.

Lymphocytes

Activation of lymphocytes leads to two partially competing processes: cell proliferation, and differentiation into effector cells. Cells at the end stage of differentiation, such as plasma cells, may become so specialized that they lose surface molecules such as class II and become unable to respond to regulatory signals or to proliferate.

The fate of lymphocytes responding to antigen is varied. Some can persist for a long time as memory cells. The lifespan of memory cells can be over 40 years in man – this figure has been arrived at by studying chromosome abnormalities (e.g. crosslinking of DNA, which would prevent mitosis) found in the blood cells of Hiroshima survivors. Others have a shorter lifespan (which explains why moderate antigenic stimulation does not lead to lymphoid enlargement) that is nevertheless sufficient for generating effective cell-mediated and antibody responses.

Antigen-specific activation of lymphocytes involves the specific receptors on T and B cells

The TCR complex can transmit messages to the interior of the cell (see Chapter 5). Molecules involved are CD3 (γ, δ, ε), the ζ and η chains, and the enzyme p56^{lck} that is attached to the intracellular portion of CD4 and CD8 (the name p56^{lck} signifies a lymphocyte-specific kinase of 56kDa). B cells are now also recognized to have a family of molecules that are attached to the surface IgM and IgD, and that are also involved in signal transduction (see Chapter 4).

It is still not clear exactly what is an effective antigenic signal. For a T cell, interaction at a single TCR is not sufficient, but exactly how many interactions are necessary may depend on what other lymphocyte stimulatory signals are present, and the type and activation state of the T cell being stimulated. Murine T-cell hybrids (derived from the fusion of a normal T cell with a T-cell tumour cell), are known to be easily triggered. To stimulate a T-cell hybrid, an effective APC (e.g. a macrophage) must carry over 60 MHC class II–antigen complexes. A weak APC, such as a class II transfected fibroblast, needs 5000 such complexes. This would suggest that, in normal circumstances, a few tens to a few hundred TCR need to be activated for effective triggering. This type of information is not available for T$_{dep}$ antigens and B cells; for T$_{ind}$ antigens, binding to a single receptor is not sufficient for triggering, but binding to tens or hundreds probably is.

T and B cell activation have been studied using mitogens, a class of molecule that can activate lymphocytes in a non-antigen-specific manner. The majority of T cells can be stimulated by the mitogens phytohaemagglutinin (PHA), extracted from red kidney beans, and concanavalin A (Con A), extracted from castor beans. The mechanism by which they do so has been extensively studied, and it is known that these molecules bind to T cell surface molecules involved in activation – TCR and CD2, for example.

Superantigens are another group of molecules that can activate T cells non-specifically. Most are of bacterial origin, and they include the staphylococcal enterotoxins (responsible for some types of acute food poisoning), toxic shock syndrome toxin (responsible for tampon-sepsis induced shock), exfoliative dermatitis toxin, and some viral proteins. Superantigens bind to MHC class II on APCs and are recognized by TCRs, but not in the same way that MHC class II–antigen complexes are recognized. They bind only to the Vβ chain of the TCR, but this is sufficient to activate the T cells (*Fig. 8.11*). Depending on experimental conditions, the effects are the same as with antigen: either an immune response is induced, or clonal anergy occurs.

Cell cooperation in the antibody response

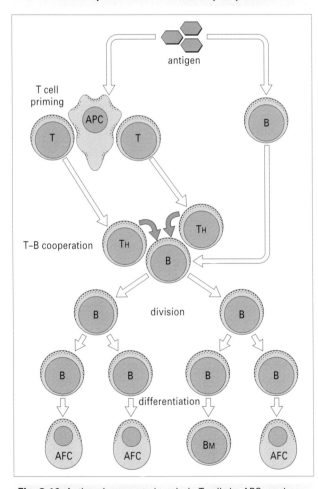

Fig. 8.10 Antigen is presented to virgin T cells by APCs such as dendritic cells. B cells also take up antigen and present it to the T cells, receiving signals from the T cells to divide and differentiate into antibody-forming cells (AFCs) and memory B cells (BM).

Co-stimulatory signals are needed for activation

Interaction at the TCR or membrane immunoglobin alone cannot mediate a positive activation signal for T or B cells. It may be sufficient for a negative or tolerogenic signal, but even that is doubtful. Lymphoid activation is currently believed to involve a number of interactions, each with a potential signalling function. Costimulatory signals are the name given to interactions that do not involve antigen-specific receptors.

These interactions may involve either secreted molecules, such as cytokines, or cell-surface molecules, which increase binding affinity and are collectively known as adhesion molecules. Adhesion molecules are not just responsible for binding: their cytoplasmic domains are also involved in signalling. Experimental deletion of the intracytoplasmic domain of (e.g.) CD2 has been shown to interfere with activation, but leaves the adhesion function unaltered.

Cytokines such as IL-1 and IL-6, made by certain APCs, are co-stimulatory signals for T-cell activation. One curious anomaly is that no-one has yet been able to demonstrate production of these cytokines by the APCs considered most active in primary T-cell activation, the interdigitating dendritic cells.

It is likely that there are other co-stimulatory cytokines. For example IL-7 is more potent than IL-1 or IL-6 in inducing T cells to express IL-2 receptor, but it is not known whether IL-7 is produced by any APCs.

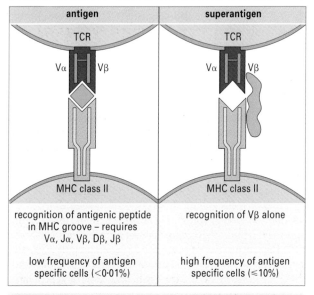

Differences between antigen and superantigen

recognition of antigenic peptide in MHC groove – requires Vα, Jα, Vβ, Dβ, Jβ

low frequency of antigen specific cells (<0·01%)

recognition of Vβ alone

high frequency of antigen specific cells (≤10%)

Fig. 8.11 Antigenic peptides must normally be processed in order to trigger the TCR. However, superantigens such as staphylococcal enterotoxins are not processed, but bind directly to class II and Vβ. Each superantigen activates a distinct set of Vβ-expressing T cells. This depends on which Vβ gene segment the T cell is using to encode its receptor.

■ CYTOKINES

Cytokines regulate important biological processes

Cytokines are proteins (usually glycoproteins) of relatively low molecular mass (rarely more than 8–25 kDa) and often consisting of just a single chain. They regulate all the important biological processes – cell growth, cell activation, inflammation, immunity, tissue repair, fibrosis and morphogenesis. Some cytokines (e.g. IL-8) are also chemotactic for specific cell types, and are now termed 'chemokines'.

Although cytokines are considered to be a 'family', this is a functional rather than a structural concept; these proteins are not all chemically related. However, there are pairs of cytokines that share about 30% of their sequences, e.g. IL-1α and IL-1β, TNFα and TNFβ, EGF and TGFα. There are also subfamilies that are highly (about 80%) homologous. IFNα, with about 20 members, is an example of a large subfamily. The properties of the best studied cytokines are summarized in *Figure 8.12*.

Interferons are antiviral cytokines

These proteins were first characterized by antiviral assays, but they are also potent immune regulators and growth factors. They fall into three groups: IFNα, the largest (20 variants), made by leucocytes in response to viruses or nucleic acids; IFNβ, a single protein made by fibroblasts in response to viruses or nucleic acids; and IFNγ, a single protein made by lymphocytes (T and LGL) in response to immune stimuli. The interferons all have antiviral activity (IFNγ much less than IFNα or IFNβ). The inhibition of cell growth by IFNα or IFNβ is clinically useful in certain rare cancers such as renal cell cancer and hairy cell leukaemia.

IFNγ is produced by activated T cells and natural killer (NK) cells. A degree of immune activation leads to the production of IFNγ and an increase in APC function (partly by inducing class II molecules), and the potential to activate T cells further. Thus, IFNγ acts as a positive feedback signal. IFNγ also activates macrophages in general, and probably enhances their capacity to act as APCs. The properties of IFNγ are summarized in *Figure 8.13*. IFNγ is probably responsible for regulating APC function in many cell types, including astrocytes, microglia, endothelium, and thymocytes. Excessive production of IFNγ can play a part in the induction of autoimmunity, as demonstrated in experimental animal models and transgenic mice.

Interleukins

Interleukins (represented by the abbreviations IL-1 to IL-15) were first given this name in 1981. They were defined as molecules made by leucocytes, and which acted on leucocytes. Although subsequent research has revealed that some of these molecules are also made by non-leucocytes, and that many also act on non-leucocytes, the nomenclature has stuck. The main targets for interleukin action vary from T and B cells to fibroblasts and endothelium. A summary of the most important properties of these molecules follows.

The main features of the best-studied cytokines

cytokine	mol. wt	cell source(s)	main cell target(s)	main actions
IFNγ	40–50 000 (dimer)	T cells, NK cells	lymphocytes, monocytes, tissue cells	immunoregulation, B cell differentiation, some antiviral action
IL-1α IL-1β	33 000 (precursor) 17 500 (mature)	monocytes, dendritic cells, some B cells, fibroblasts, epithelial cells, endothelium, astrocytes, macrophages	thymocytes, neutrophils, T and B cells, tissue cells	immunoregulation, inflammation, fever
IL-2	15 000	T cells NK cells	T cells, B cells, monocytes	proliferation, activation
IL-3	15 000	T cells	stem cells, progenitors	pan-specific colony stimulating factor
IL-4	15 000	T cells	B cells, T cells	division and differentiation
IL-5	20 000	T cells	B cells, eosinophils	differentiation
IL-6	20 000	macrophages, T cells, fibroblasts, some B cells	T cells, B cells, thymocytes, hepatocytes	differentiation, acute phase protein synthesis
IL-8 (family)	8000	macrophages, skin cells	granulocytes, T cells	chemotaxis
TNFα	50 000 (trimer)	macrophages, lymphocytes	fibroblasts, endothelium	inflammation, catabolism (cachexia), fibrosis; production of other cytokines (IL-1, IL-6, GM-CSF) and adhesion molecules
TNFβ (lymphotoxin)	50 000 (trimer)			

Fig. 8.12 Summary of the main features of the best-studied cytokines. In some cases the molecular weight is derived from study of cDNA sequences. Only the most important targets and actions are shown.

IL-1 – Previously known as endogenous pyrogen, lymphocyte activating factor and catabolin, IL-1 is made by many cells (e.g. endothelial cells, B cells, fibroblasts) but most abundantly by macrophages. It stimulates T and B cells, and induces inflammatory responses, for example the production of prostaglandins and degradative enzymes such as collagenase. This is believed to be of special importance for the destruction of cartilage and bone. IL-1 travels to the brain where it induces fever, and acts to augment corticosteroid release. In the liver it induces the production of acute phase proteins, liberated in response to injury. Virtually all cells of the body have receptors for IL-1 and can respond to it (*Figs 8.14 and 8.15*).

IL-2 – Previously known as T-cell growth factor, IL-2 is produced by T cells (chiefly CD4+, but also CD8+) and by LGLs. It acts on a restricted range of cells, chiefly T cells (all types) for which it is the most powerful growth factor and activator (*Fig. 8.16*). It also acts on LGLs and

B cells to induce growth and differentiation, and it activates macrophages and oligodendrocytes. IL-2 is used in experimental cancer therapy, especially for renal cell cancer. The benefit here may be related to the activation of many cells that can produce a cytotoxic anti-cancer effect, e.g. lymphokine-activated killer (LAK) cells.

IL-3 – Previously known as multispecific haemopoietin, IL-3 stimulates the growth of precursors of all the haemopoietic lineages (red cells, granulocytes, macrophages and probably lymphocytes). A minor population of T cells (CD4-CD8-, with the αβ TCR) also grows in response to IL-3.

IL-4 – Previously known as B-cell activating or differentiating factor-1, IL-4 acts on B cells to induce activation and differentiation, leading in particular to the production of IgG1 and IgE. It also acts on T cells as a growth and activation factor and promotes TH2 cell differentiation.

Actions of IFNγ

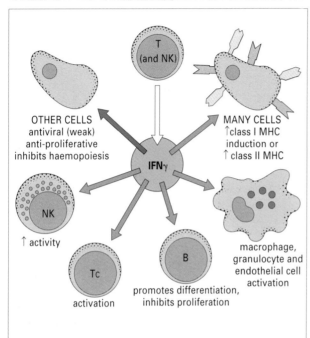

Fig. 8.13 IFNγ has numerous immunoregulatory actions. Its antiviral and antiproliferative activities are less potent than those of IFNα and IFNβ. Furthermore, it is not as effective as IFNα at inducing natural killer (NK) cells. It is, however, the most potent inducer of macrophage activation, and of class II molecules on tissue cells. In this and other functions it synergizes with TNFα and TNFβ.

On macrophages, it induces MHC class II expression, but inhibits production of pro-inflammatory cytokines such as IL-1 and TNFα. Excess IL-4 plays a part in allergic disease, causing high IgE production.

IL-5 – In man IL-5 is chiefly a growth and activation factor for eosinophils. In the mouse it also acts on B cells to induce growth and differentiation. IL-5 is responsible for the eosinophilia of parasitic disease.

IL-6 – Previously known as B-cell differentiating factor or hepatocyte stimulating factor, IL-6 is produced by many cells, including T cells, macrophages, B cells, fibroblasts and endothelial cells. It acts on most cells, but is particularly important in inducing B cells to differentiate into antibody-forming cells (AFCs). In the liver it stimulates the production of acute phase proteins. IL-6 is considered to be an important growth factor for multiple myeloma, a malignancy of plasma cells.

IL-7 – was initially described as a pre-B-cell growth factor, made by bone marrow stroma. IL-7 made by thymic stroma acts on thymocytes and is a T-cell growth and activation factor, and a macrophage activation factor.

IL-8 – belongs to a large family (over 30 members) of low molecular weight (about 8 kDa) cytokines. They are produced by most cells of the body, especially macrophages and endothelial cells, and are involved in inflammation and cell migration. IL-8 in particular is a powerful inducer of neutrophil chemotaxis (see Chapter 14). The related RANTES induces chemotaxis of memory T cells and monocytes.

Actions of IL-1 on non-immune cells

tissue/cell type	prostaglandin synthesis	proliferation	protein synthesis	other effects
brain	+	astrocyte tumours	–	fever, somnolence, anorexia
synovial cells	+	–	collagenase	proteolytic enzyme release
bone/osteoclasts	–	–	collagenase	–
cartilage/ chondrocytes	+	–	collagenase, plasminogen activator	–
muscle cells	+	–	–	proteolytic enzyme release
fibroblasts	+	+	collagenase	–
endothelium	+	+	procoagulant activity	boosts macrophages and neutrophil adhesion
epithelial cells	–	+	type IV collagen	–
liver/ hepatocytes	–	–	acute phase proteins	–

Fig. 8.14 IL-1 acts on many cell types other than those of the immune system in its role as an inflammatory mediator. On many cell types IL-1 induces the production of other cytokines, for example TNF, GM–CSF and IL-6, which in turn have a secondary effect on skin cells. The classic effect of IL-1 is as a pyrogen, which accounts for its effect in the brain. It also induces prostaglandin synthesis in cells of the musculoskeletal system. Proliferative effects are seen especially in astrocyte tumours, but also in vascular endothelium and fibroblasts. Protein synthesis, of enzymes such as collagenase for example, are a characteristic feature of IL-1 induced reactions, as is the production of acute phase proteins by hepatocytes.

IL-10 – Also known as cytokine synthesis inhibitory factor, IL-10 inhibits the production of IFNγ, inhibits antigen presentation and macrophage production of IL-1, IL-6 and TNFα, and is important in B-cell activation.

IL-12 – acts in a contrasting way to IL-10, in that it favours TH1 type responses, with macrophage and NK cell activation and induces IFNγ production.

IL-13 – has structural and functional similarites to IL-4 and promotes B-cell division.

Haemopoiesis involves many cytokines and cell surface molecules

Haemopoiesis is regulated by a wide spectrum of cytokines. Stem cell factor, IL-1 and IL-6 are involved in activating resting stem cells (self-renewing cells) to enter the cell cycle. IL-3 is involved in the growth of precursors of all haemopoietic lineages. GM–CSF promotes development of the precursors of granulocytes and macrophages. As cells differentiate, lineage-specific cytokines play a major role; erythropoietin (EPO) for the red cells, macrophage colony stimulating factor (M–CSF) for macrophages, granulocyte colony stimulating factor (G–CSF) for granulocytes.

Recently, a platelet generating factor, thymopoietin, has been cloned. GM–CSF, M–CSF and G–CSF also act on mature cells as activation factors, especially the former.

Less is known about inhibitory cytokines

Only a few cytokines are currently known which have inhibitory properties in the immune system. IL-10 has already been described. Transforming growth factor-β (TGFβ) is a family of five closely related molecules that stimulate connective tissue growth and collagen formation, but are inhibitory to virtually all immune and haemopoietic functions, especially before cell activation. IFNα, IFNβ and IFNγ can interfere with immune cell proliferation. IFNα and IFNβ inhibit class II induction by IFNγ. IFNγ can interfere with B cell class II induction by IL-4. IL-13 shares many of the inhibitory properties of IL-4. By inducing the differentiation of cells, including some leukaemic lines, IL-6 inhibits their proliferation.

Cytokine receptors have high affinity

Cytokines are effective at very low concentrations, often at a few pg/ml (10^{-12} gm/ml). This is due to their mode of action, involving binding to high-affinity receptors on cell surfaces, which transmit cytokine signals to the nucleus.

Actions of IL-1 on cells of the immune system

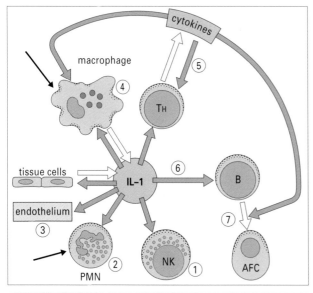

Actions of IL-2

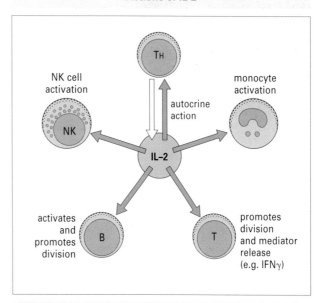

Fig. 8.15 IL-1 is produced by many cell types in response to damage, infection or antigens. It influences many cells and processes: 1. NK cell cytocidal activity increases. 2. PMNs are metabolically activated and move towards the site of IL-1 production by chemotaxis (black arrow). 3. In the endothelium, adhesion molecules and procoagulants are induced, and permeability is increased. 4. Prostaglandin production and cytocidal activity increase in macrophages. Chemotaxis is also stimulated (black arrow). 5. TH cell proliferation, IL-2 receptor expression and cytokine production are all enhanced. 6. B-cell proliferation and differentiation into AFCs is stimulated and regulated (7) by other cytokines.

Fig. 8.16 IL-2 is generated by TH cells. In addition to its essential role in promoting T-cell division and the release of mediators such as IFNγ, IL-2 also potentiates B-cell growth. The activation of monocytes and natural killer (NK) cells is important in amplifying the immune response. In patients with renal cell carcinoma, autologous NK precursors can be activated *in vitro* by high doses of IL-2 (1000 IU/ml) to produce lines of so-called lymphokine-activated killer (LAK) cells which are used in experimental cancer therapy.

While developments in biochemistry, and especially in gene cloning, have helped reveal the structure of many cytokine receptors, our knowledge of how they transmit signals is less advanced. This is probably because, for many receptors, only the cytokine binding chain has been elucidated. The associated chains that transmit the signals are, for the most part, yet to be defined.

Whereas the cytokine proteins do not have any structural resemblances, many cytokine receptors belong to families with distant similarities in their extracellular domains (*Fig. 8.17*). The haemopoietin family is the largest of these groups. Members share two main characteristics: four invariant amino acids, consisting of two doublets of tryptophan and serine near the transmembrane domain, and certain conserved cysteines. Receptors for erythropoietin (EPO), G–CSF, GM–CSF, IL-3, IL-4, IL-2 (β chain), IL-5, IL-6 and IL-7, all belong to this family.

Receptors for IL-1, IL-6 and M–CSF belong to the immunoglobulin superfamily, which includes many other important molecules, such as MHC, TCR and the immunoglobulins themselves.

Receptors for nerve growth factor (NGF) and TNF, as well as some surface antigens (e.g. CD40), belong to another family.

In contrast, the intracytoplasmic domains of cytokine receptors are not homologous, suggesting that there are many mechanisms of signal transduction to the cell. Our understanding of the receptors for IL-2 and IL-6 is more advanced; the IL-2 receptor is schematically represented in *Figure 8.18*. The IL-6 receptor has a cytokine binding chain whose affinity is augmented by a transmembrane protein called gp130 that is involved in signal transduction. There are two distinct receptors for TNF; they have homologous binding domains but differ in their intracytoplasmic segments (*Fig. 8.19*).

There is now evidence that certain chains involved in signalling are shared between several receptors. Thus IL-3, GM–CSF and IL-5 share a common β chain. The protein gp 130, first identified with IL-6, is also involved in

the receptors for CNTF (ciliary neurotrophic factor), LIF (leukaemia inhibitory factor), oncostatin M and IL-11. The IL-2 receptor γ-chain is also involved in IL-4, IL-7 and probably IL-9 and IL-15 signalling.

Cytokine antagonists are of two types

Two groups of cytokine inhibitory proteins have been described. Firstly, the receptor antagonists, which bind the receptor but do not activate the cell. for example, the IL-1 receptor antagonist (IL-1ra) is a protein of 18 kDa produced by IgG-adherent monocytes and keratinocytes. The protein binds to IL-1 receptor but has no agonist activity. It has been shown to protect mice after a lethal injection of *Escherichia coli* endotoxin (lipopolysaccharide – LPS). (This provided direct evidence that the lethal effects of LPS could be mediated partly through the action of IL-1.)

The great majority of cytokine inhibitors belong to the second group, which act by binding not the receptor, but the cytokine itself. Sequencing studies have shown that these soluble serum inhibitors of cytokines are fragments generated by enzymic cleavage from the extracellular domain of the cytokine receptors (*Fig. 8.20*). Among the soluble receptors detected in serum are those for IL-2 (p55

Cytokine receptor families

family	members	features
immunoglobulin	M–CSF, IL-6, IL-1	Ig-V or Ig-C like domains, IL-6 also has some haemopoietin features
haemopoietin	IL-2β, IL-3, 4, 5, 6, 7, EPO, GM–CSF, G–CSF	Trp–Ser ×2, conserved cysteines
TNF/NGF	TNF, NGF, CD40	4 cysteine-rich (6 cys) regions in extracellular domain

Fig. 8.17 Some cytokine receptors show sequence homology with others, which allows grouping into families. The IL-6 receptor has features of two families.

Structure of high affinity IL-2 receptor

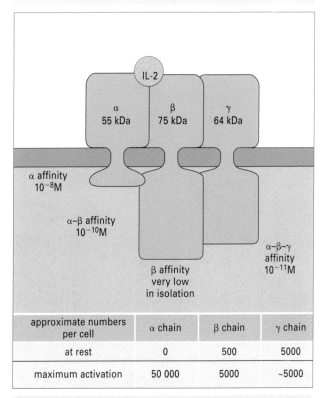

approximate numbers per cell	α chain	β chain	γ chain
at rest	0	500	5000
maximum activation	50 000	5000	~5000

Fig. 8.18 The high affinity IL-2 receptor consists of three chains, each of which alone can bind IL-2 only weakly. Resting T cells do not express the α-chain, but following activation, they may express up to 50 000/cell (maximum). Some of these associate with the β-chain to form the high affinity IL-2 receptor.

low affinity chain only), IL-4, IL-6 (not known to be inhibitory), IL-7, IFNγ and both TNF receptors. There are also soluble forms of receptors for hormones, for example growth hormone, and for adhesion molecules such as ICAM-1. The soluble TNF-receptor is known to be an important inhibitor of TNF.

Intracellular pathways of activation involve multiple pathways

T-cell activation appears to use similar mechanisms to those seen in other cell types. TCR ligation causes the activation of phospholipase C, leading to the generation of inositol triphosphate (IP_3) and diacyl glycerol (DAG). IP_3 leads to release of Ca^{2+} from intracellular stores while DAG is involved in the activation of protein kinase C (PKC). The activation process involves a complex series of phosphorylations of components of the TCR (CD3) as well as CD4 (or CD8) and the leucocyte common antigen CD45, which is associated with CD4 and is itself a phosphatase. In addition to PKC, three other kinases ($p56^{lck}$, associated with CD4 or CD8, $p59^{fyn}$ and ZAP 70) are involved in these steps.

Lymphocyte proliferation requires cytokines

Lymphocyte proliferation is a complex and indirect process. For example, stimulation of a T cell by an APC does not automatically lead to lymphocyte proliferation.

Effective interaction at the TCR leads to the production of the p55-α chain of the receptor for the T-cell growth factor (IL-2), which together with the existing p75 β and γ chains forms a high affinity receptor. In all T cells TCR activation also induces the production of cytokines. In most CD4+ and some CD8+ T cells, there is transient production of IL-2 for 1–2 days. During this time, the interaction of IL-2 with the high affinity IL-2 receptor results in T-cell growth and activation (*Fig. 8.21*).

IL-4 is a weaker growth factor for T cells, and its production is also inducible. Surface IL-4 receptor is also augmented by TCR activation. IL-7 is also a growth factor for T cells and it is likely that these three T-cell growth factors and other less understood ones such as IL-11, IL-12 and IL-15 permit the fine tuning of the growth and activation of T cells during an immune response. The transient expression of the high-affinity IL-2 receptor for only a week or so after stimulation of the TCR helps to limit T-cell growth.

■ ANTIBODY RESPONSES *IN VIVO*

The earliest studies on antibody responses followed the development of specific antibodies in animals immunized with T_{dep} or T_{ind} antigens. With our improved knowledge of B-cell development and maturation, it is now possible to understand the features of immune responses *in vivo* in terms of the underlying cellular events. Features of antibody responses *in vivo* that are related to the cellular events described above include:
- The enhanced secondary response.
- Isotype switching.
- Affinity maturation.
- The development of memory.

However, some of these events can only be understood by viewing the B cell population as a whole, rather than as a

TNF receptors

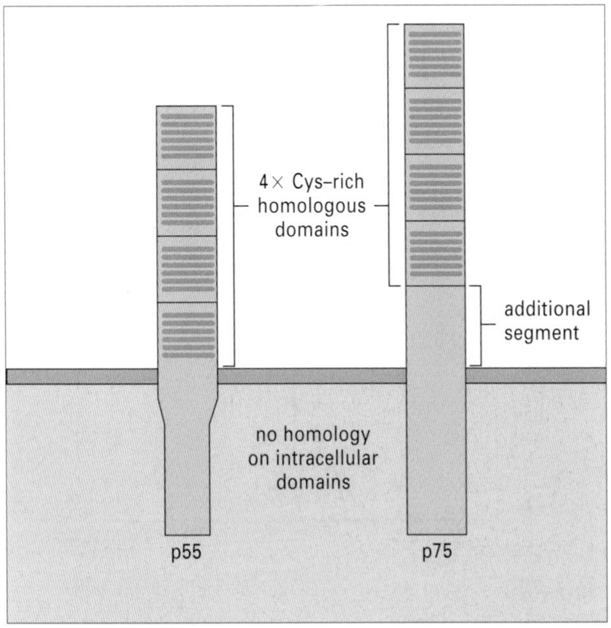

4× Cys–rich homologous domains

additional segment

no homology on intracellular domains

p55   p75

Fig. 8.19 There are two receptors for TNF, each of which binds both TNFα and TNFβ (lymphotoxin) with high affinity. Their extracellular domains are homologous, each with four sub-domains of 40 amino acids, containing six cysteines. They are believed to have evolved by gene duplication. In contrast the intracytoplasmic domains are not homologous, suggesting that their mechanism of signal transduction is distinct.

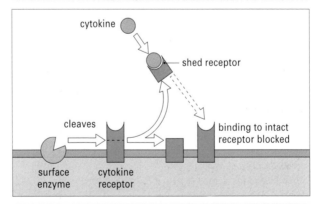

Soluble cytokine receptors

cytokine

shed receptor

cleaves

binding to intact receptor blocked

surface enzyme   cytokine receptor

Fig. 8.20 Enzyme cleavage of the extracellular domain of a receptor (for example, TNF, IFNγ, IL-6 or IL-2 [p55] receptor) releases the binding fragment. For TNF (and probably others) this soluble receptor retains its high-affinity binding properties. It is capable of neutralizing the ligand by blocking its access to intact receptors in the membrane.

collection of individual cells. The elements of the antibody response *in vivo* are detailed below.

The enhanced secondary response

Following primary antigenic challenge there is an initial lag phase when no antibody can be detected. This is followed by phases in which the antibody titre rises logarithmically to a plateau and then declines. The decline occurs because the antibodies are either naturally catabolized, or are bound to antigen and cleared from the circulation (*Fig. 8.22*).

An examination of the responses following primary and secondary antigenic challenge shows that the responses differ in four major respects.

Time course – The secondary response has a shorter lag phase and an extended plateau and decline.

Antibody titre – The plateau levels of antibody in the secondary response are much greater (typically by a factor of ten or more) than plateau levels in the primary response.

Antibody class – IgM antibodies make a major contribution to the primary response, whereas the secondary response consists almost entirely of IgG, with very little IgM.

Antibody affinity – The affinity of antibodies in the secondary response is usually much higher. This is affinity maturation.

The characteristics of primary and secondary antibody responses are compared in *Figure 8.23*.

It is possible to detect antibody forming cells (AFCs) in the spleen following antigen challenge using plaque-forming cell assays (see Chapter 28). Studies show that the appearance of AFCs in the spleen precedes the rise in serum antibody titre by about one day.

Isotype switching depends on T cells

During a T-dependent immune response there is a progressive change in the predominant immunoglobulin class of the specific antibody produced, usually to IgG. This class switch is not seen in T-independent responses, where the predominant immunoglobulin usually remains IgM.

Isotype switching from IgM to IgG is not a random event. The IgG subclasses produced by the plasma cells vary depending on the stimulus. Thus in the mouse, complete Freund's Adjuvant yields predominantly IgG2 antibodies, whereas alum-precipitated protein antigens result in a predominantly IgG1 response. Switching to IgA or IgE also occurs, and cells producing these isotypes are concentrated in the mucosa-associated lymphoid tissues.

The molecular mechanisms of isotype switching are discussed in Chapter 6. Although there is universal agreement that T cells are important in controlling this phenomenon,

T cell proliferation

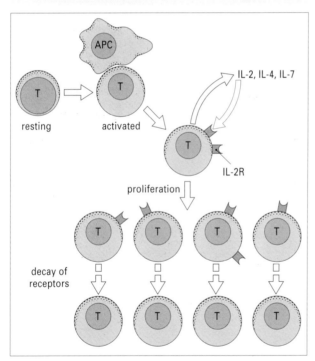

Fig. 8.21 Resting cells do not make T-cell growth-factor cytokines (IL-2, IL-4 or IL-7) and do not express large numbers of receptors for these molecules. Some receptors for IL-4 and IL-7 are present, but not for IL-2. Only the p75 chain of the IL-2 receptor is present, which has low affinity. Activation induces the p55 chain and this combines with p75 to give high affinity IL-2 receptor.

Activation induces production of mRNA and protein for IL-2 and IL-4. Secretion of IL-2 and IL-4 and interaction with receptors induces growth. This stimulation is autocrine (acting on the same cell) or paracrine (acting on the neighbouring cell). In the absence of antigen stimulation the IL-2 receptor population declines, leading to an end of the proliferative phase of the response.

The four phases of primary antibody response

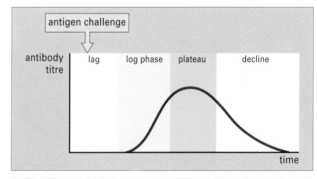

Fig. 8.22 Following antigen challenge the antibody response proceeds in four phases:

1. A lag phase, when no antibody is detected
2. A log phase, when the antibody titre rises logarithmically
3. A plateau phase, during which the antibody titre stabilizes
4. A decline phase, during which the antibody is cleared or catabolized.

The actual time course and titres reached will depend on the nature of the antigenic challenge and the nature of the host.

the signals that control the switch are not fully understood. IL-4, which is produced by TH2 cells, is important in the production of IgG1 and IgE. TGFβ is important in the switch to IgA production, and IFNγ, produced by TH1 cells, favours the production of IgG2a in mice.

Affinity maturation depends on cell selection

The antibodies produced in a secondary response to a T-dependent antigen have higher average affinity than those produced in the primary response. This is associated with the switch from IgM to IgG production, since there is no maturation in the affinity of the IgM response.

The degree of affinity maturation is inversely related to the antigen dose administered: high antigen doses produce poor maturation compared to low antigen doses (*Fig. 8.24*). It has been suggested that, in the presence of low antigen concentrations, only B cells with high affinity receptors bind sufficient antigen and are triggered to divide

and differentiate. However, in the presence of high antigen concentrations, there is sufficient antigen to bind and trigger both high and low affinity B cells (*Fig. 8.25*).

Although individual B cells do not usually change their overall specificity, the affinity of the antibody produced by a clone may be altered as a result of somatic hypermutation acting on the recombined antibody genes (see Chapter 6). It appears then, that two processes are involved in affinity maturation.

• Slight alterations in the antibody structure of daughter cells generate clones of higher affinity. Such changes occur late in the primary response to a T-dependent antigen.

• Antigen drives the selective expansion of high-affinity clones.

Somatic hypermutation is a common event in AFCs during T-dependent responses and is important in the generation of high-affinity antibodies. In this context it is a

Primary and secondary antibody responses

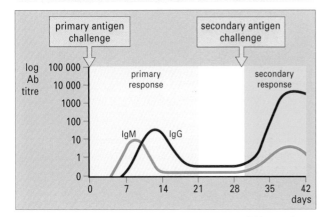

Fig. 8.23 In comparison with the antibody response following primary antigenic challenge, the antibody level following secondary antigenic challenge in a typical immune response appears more quickly, persists for longer, attains a higher titre, and consists predominantly of IgG. (In the primary response the appearance of IgG is preceded by IgM.)

Affinity maturation

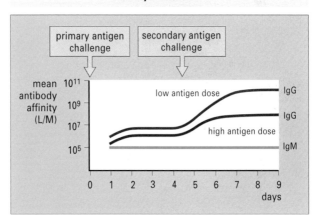

Fig. 8.24 The average affinity of the IgM and IgG antibody responses following primary and secondary challenge with a T-dependent antigen are shown. The affinity of the IgM response is constant throughout. The affinity maturation of the IgG response depends on the dose of the secondary antigen. Low antigen doses produce higher affinity immunoglobulin than high antigen doses.

Clonal selection by high and low antigen doses

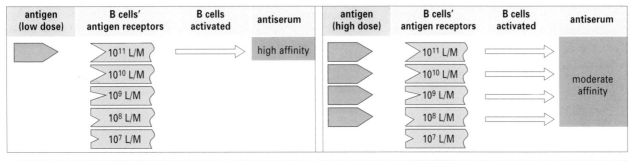

Fig. 8.25 Low antigen doses (left) bind to and trigger only those B cells with high affinity receptors, whereas high antigen doses (right) allow triggering of more B cell clones and therefore produce antibody responses with lower average affinity.

normal and beneficial event. However, the same process could yield high-affinity IgG autoantibodies, e.g. anti-DNA, which would be highly deleterious. This type of mutation has been demonstrated experimentally in long-term tissue culture. Its role in the development of common autoimmune diseases is not known.

Immunological memory

The capacity to mount a secondary response is based on immunological memory. (This memory is exploited by the process of vaccination.)

The cellular basis of memory lies in the expansion of antigen-specific lymphocyte populations during the primary response, so that there is an increased frequency of resting B and T cells capable of responding to that antigen in the future. Memory B cells differ qualitatively from unprimed B cells; they make IgG earlier and usually have higher affinity antigen receptors, due to selection during the primary response.

It is not likely that memory T cells have higher affinity receptors than unprimed T cells, as there is no hypermutation in T cells. However, memory T cells can respond to lower doses of antigen, implying that their overall set of receptors (including adhesion molecules) are more efficient. It is now known that immunological memory is not just due to increased numbers of the same cells. There are also changes in the properties of the cells themselves, indicated by changing patterns of expression of cell-surface molecules and cytokines. Memory CD4$^+$ T cells are capable of synthesizing cytokines more readily and rapidly.

Critical Thinking

■ What are the differences between interactions of T cells and APCs, and T cells and B cells?

■ Why is affinity maturation and immunoglobulin class regulation important in determining the type and effectiveness of an immune response? How can T cells control these processes

■ How is lymphocyte proliferation induced and regulated?

■ Can cytokines be harmful?

■ What is the difference between antigen recognition by T cells, and antigen recognition by B cells?.

FURTHER READING

Banchereau J et al. The CD40 antigen and its ligand. Ann Rev Immunol 1994;**12**:881.

Brodsky FM, Guagliardi L. The cell biology of antigen processing and presentation. Ann Rev Immunol 1994:**9**:707.

Chantry D, Feldmann M. The role of cytokines in autoimmunity. Biotechnol Ther 1991;**1**:361.

Clark EA and Ledbetter JA. How B and T cells talk to each other. Nature 1994;**367**:425.

Parker DC T cell-dependent B cell activation. Ann Rev Immunol 1993;**11**:331.

Romagnani S. Cytokine production by human T cells in disease states. Ann Rev Immunol 1994;**12**:227.

Ullman K, Northrop JP, Veirweij CL, Crabtree GR. Transmission of signals from T lymphocyte antigen receptor to the gene responsible for cell proliferation and immune function. Ann Rev Immunol 1989;**8**:421.

Non-adaptive immune defences allow leucocytes to detect and respond to the presence of pathogens, without involving the more recently evolved antigen-specific receptors of B cells and T cells.

Microbial structures are recognized early in a reaction, while specific immune responses are developing. Release of cytokines is a major determinant of the type of response that is subsequently activated.

The specific immune response is directed by helper T cells (TH) which respond to and release different cytokine profiles, and so drive distinct patterns of effector function.

Cell-mediated immune responses comprise numerous distinct effector functions. Activation of an inappropriate effector function can lead to failure to eliminate the pathogen and to chronic immunopathology.

There are two major types of cell-mediated effector mechanism. The first aims to destroy infected cells (with or without the help of antibody). The second involves pathways that activate phagocytes to kill organisms and tissue cells to resist infection.

Cytokine mediators play a central role in positive and negative regulation of immune reactions, and in integrating them with other physiological compartments such as the endocrine and haematopoietic systems.

Granuloma formation or chronic tissue-destructive inflammation occur when cell-mediated reactions are not resolved, due either to failure to eliminate an infection or an inability to clear an antigen which has become persistent. Immunopathology can result from microvascular damage secondary to excessive cytokine release, or from direct destruction of essential cells.

The term 'cell-mediated immunity' (CMI) was originally coined to describe localized reactions to organisms, usually intra-cellular pathogens, mediated by lymphocytes and phagocytes rather than by antibody (humoral immunity). It is now often used in a more general sense for any response against organisms or tumours in which antibody plays a subordinate role.

It is not possible, however, to consider cell-mediated and antibody-mediated responses entirely separately. Cells are involved in the initiation of antibody responses, and antibody acts as an essential link in some cell-mediated reactions. Moreover, no cell-mediated response is likely to occur in the total absence of antibody, which can modify cellular responses in numerous ways. For instance, formation of antigen–antibody complexes during an immune response leads to the release of chemotactic complement fragments which enhance accumulation of cells, and local inflammation. Antibody may also be involved in linking antigens to cells, via the cells' Fc receptors, thus modulating the cells' responses. In the case of phagocytic cells and killer cells, antibodies can link them to their targets.

Similarly, it should not be assumed that all cell-mediated immunity is dependent on T lymphocyte function – much of the initial defensive reaction to microorganisms depends on recognition of common microbial components by receptors that are not related to the antigen-specific receptors of T cells and B cells.

■ T-CELL-INDEPENDENT DEFENCE MECHANISMS

Phagocytosis must usually occur before cells can kill microorganisms
Chemotaxis allows the cells mediating protection to move towards target organisms

Numerous microbial components will cause chemotaxis of phagocytes towards the site of infection (*Fig. 9.1*). Some, such as bacterial endotoxin, do so by activating the alternative pathway of complement, so releasing C5a and C3a. Other microbial components are chemotactic in their own right. For

T-cell independent functions – I: phagocytosis

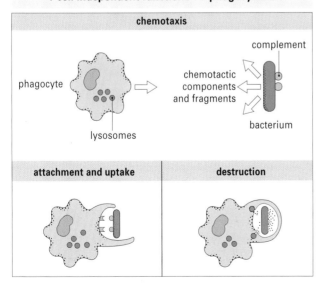

Fig. 9.1 Most of the effectors of T-cell-independent cell-mediated immunity are functional even in animals with no T cells, and in normal animals they play a protective role before the T-cell-mediated response gets under way. Subsequently these functions may be enhanced by T-cell-derived cytokines. Most microbial organisms release factors that are chemotactic for phagocytes. They are then taken up by phagocytosis, and killed without a requirement for further activation of the phagocyte. This process is assisted by the alternative complement pathway, which does not rely on antibodies.

instance, formyl peptides are chemotactic and are also directly stimulatory for phagocytes, which have receptors for these common bacterial products.

Binding of the organism to the phagocyte may induce uptake and trigger killing mechanisms

The next stage in the phagocytosis of an organism is its binding to the surface of the phagocytic cell. This binding is facilitated if complement has been activated leading to deposition of C3b, which can bind to the CR3 receptors on the phagocytes. Similarly, if antibody has bound to the pathogen then Fc receptors on the phagocyte may contribute to the uptake.

Some organisms prefer an intracellular habitat and have evolved ways of binding to surface structures so that although uptake is triggered normally, microbicidal pathways are not subsequently activated. These points, and the nature of the microbicidal pathways, are discussed in greater detail in Chapter 17.

Microbial components trigger cytokine release

Another mechanism that is independent of T-cell or antibody responses, and that plays a vital role in the initial stages of an infection, is the triggering of cytokine release from macrophages and other cells. All invading organisms appear to contain or release molecules that have this effect (see Chapter 17).

Cytokines are protein or glycoprotein mediators released from appropriately stimulated cells (see Chapter 8). The first cytokines to be identified came from lymphocytes and were termed lymphokines. The term cytokines now includes lymphokines (some of which are given interleukin [IL] designation), interferons (IFN), colony stimulating factors (CSF), and tumour necrosis factors (TNF).

Among the mediators released by macrophages in response to microbial components, TNFα and IL-12 are particularly important. In synergy with other mediators, these cytokines are known to have several rapid protective effects, rapidly enhancing non-specific antimicrobial activity:

* TNFα enhances the microbicidal capacity of macrophages and neutrophils.
* TNFα and IL-12 cause NK cells to release IFNγ. This further augments the microbicidal activity of macrophages.
* TNFα causes changes in endothelial cells and phagocytes which result in greater adhesion of the phagocytes to blood vessel walls, thus increasing the entry of the cells into sites of inflammation (Fig. 9.2).

These pathways may explain the paradoxical resistance of SCID (severe combined immunodeficient) mice, which lack functional T cells, to certain bacterial infections.

■ T-CELL-DEPENDENT CELL-MEDIATED RESPONSES

Cytokines released in the earliest stages of an infection help to determine the nature of the subsequent immune response. This is an important area, currently subject to intensive investigation. Before discussing it further we must outline the different types of cell-mediated response that can be activated, and how they are selected.

Figure 9.3 illustrates the most important functions of immunologically active cells (individual cells may perform more than one function) and emphasizes the central organizing role of CD4+ T helper (TH) cells. Different subsets of TH cells modulate the various types of cellular cooperation, and produce different blends of cytokines. Secondary effects of T cell activation include delayed hypersensitivity with granuloma formation (discussed below and in Chapter 17), or tissue-damaging immunopathology (see Chapter 25). Some T cells inhibit responses and are designated suppressor T cells (Fig.9.3). Some of these release the modulatory cytokine TGFβ and may well be true 'supressor' T cells; others may simply be regulatory cells that switch the response from the mechanism under study to one that the experimentalist is not measuring.

TH cells play a pivotal role in cell-mediated immunity

TH cells determine both specificity and mechanism in cell-mediated immunity:

* They direct the fine specificity of the response, i.e. they determine which antigens and which epitopes are recognized
* They are involved in the selection of the effector mechanisms to be directed against the selected target epitopes
* They aid proliferation of the appropriate effector cell types
* They enhance the functions of phagocytes and of other effector cells.

T-cell independent functions – II: cytokine release

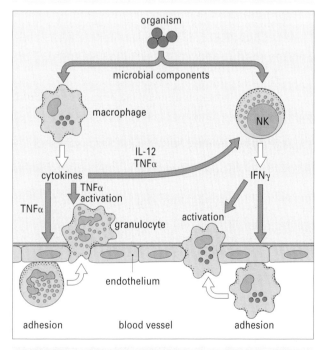

Fig. 9.2 A second early protective pathway is the triggering of cytokine release from macrophages and NK cells by microbial components alone, or in synergy with TNFα and IL-12. These rapidly increase the microbicidal potential of phagocytes, and increase their adherence to endothelial cells.

TH cells select the effector mechanisms to be used against target pathogens

TH cells, via their interaction with antigen-presenting cells bearing antigenic peptides associated with MHC Class II, play a major role in determining which epitopes become targets of the immune response (see Chapter 7). However, when confronted with an invading organism, the immune system must make a second, perhaps even more important 'decision'. It must select effector mechanisms appropriate for the infection in question. Not all the effector systems illustrated in *Figure 9.3* are activated equally in any one immune response. The three most easily recognizable patterns of effector mechanism that can be selected – and there may be many others – are as follows:

- CD8$^+$ cytotoxic T (Tc) cells
- Antibody plus mast cells and eosinophils
- Macrophage activation and delayed hypersensitivity.

This 'decision' is important because activation of inappropriate effector mechanisms can lead to enhanced susceptibility to the pathogen, rather than protection from it. For example, in a model of influenza virus infection, cytotoxic T cells protect, whereas macrophage activation increases susceptibility. In a similar way, macrophage activation protects mice from *Leishmania major*, whereas reactions that do not lead to macrophage activation can be detrimental, in spite of antibody production.

Differentiation into TH subsets is an important step in selecting effector mechanisms

Local patterns of cytokine and hormone expression help to select the effector mechanism to be activated. The initial pattern of cytokine triggering by the pathogen, and the local concentration of several steroid and vitamin D$_3$ metabolites in the lymphoid tissue, determine whether the TH cells that develop are of the TH1 or TH2 subset; these TH subsets in turn select the effector functions. For instance if an organism triggers release of IL-12 and IFNγ from macrophages and NK cells, the TH subset that develops will be biased towards TH1, whereas release of IL-4 and IL-10 will bias it towards TH2.

These subsets of TH cells probably represent different patterns of differentiation from the same precursors. In the mouse it is suggested that virgin (THP) cells, which have not previously been stimulated, release only IL-2. Short term stimulation leads to the development of TH0 cells which can release a wide range of cytokines (*Fig. 9.4*). After chronic stimulation, the specialized TH1 and TH2 subsets arise. Some cytokines are released by both types (IL-3, GM-CSF, and

The central role of TH cells in cell-mediated immunity

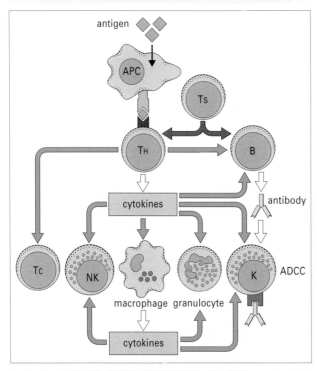

Fig. 9.3 Antigen-presenting cells (APCs) present processed antigen to helper T cells (TH), which are central to the development of immune responses. These cells recognize particular epitopes and thus select those as targets. They then select and activate the appropriate effector mechanisms. They can help B cells to make antibody and activate or suppress the actions of a variety of other effector cells. These are described in greater detail later, and include cytotoxic T cells (Tc), natural killer (NK) cells, macrophages, granulocytes and antibody-dependent cytotoxic (K) cells. Many of these effects are mediated by lymphokines, but cytokines from other cells, particularly macrophages, are also important. Both T and B cells may in turn be influenced by 'suppressor' (Ts) or regulatory cells.

Differentiation of murine TH cells

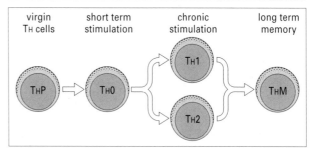

cytokines released				
THP	**TH0**	**TH1**	**TH2**	**THM**
	IFN$_γ$	IFN$_γ$		
IL-2	IL-2	IL-2		IL-2
	IL-4		IL-4	
	IL-5		IL-5	
			IL-6	
	IL-10		IL-10	

Fig. 9.4 The suggested differentiation of murine TH cells into subsets with distinctive patterns of lymphokine release. Similar subsets are found in man when cells are taken from sites of chronic inflammation rather than from the blood. These cytokine patterns influence the effector functions that are activated.

TNFα) while others are not. Thus TH1 cells release IL-2 and IFNγ, while TH2 cells release IL-4, IL-5, IL-6, and IL-10.

How these differing patterns of cytokine secretion may direct the response towards particular effector mechanisms is shown in *Figure 9.5*. For instance, TH1 cells tend to activate macrophages, and there is some evidence that they respond particularly well to antigen presented by these cells. TH2 cells tend to increase production of eosinophils and mast cells, and enhance production of antibody, including IgE; these cells respond well to antigens presented by B cells. Once established, each of these patterns of response is able to suppress the other, because the IFNγ from TH1 cells inhibits proliferation of TH2 cells, while IL-10 from TH2 cells reduces cytokine secretion from TH1 cells, and perhaps also from cytotoxic T cells and NK cells.

This specialization of TH cells was first recognized in the mouse, but is now clearly demonstrated in man. T-cell clones resembling TH2 cells have been isolated from the eyelids of patients with a severe pollen allergy who suffer from vernal conjunctivitis. On the other hand, T-cell clones taken from the cerebrospinal fluid of patients with multiple sclerosis, a primarily cellular response, are like murine TH1 cells. However, it seems likely that more types of TH cell will be discovered, since many patterns of inflammation fail to fit the TH1/TH2 classification.

CD8⁺ T cells can also be divided into subsets on the basis of cytokine expression

T cells expressing the CD8 membrane marker can also vary in their pattern of cytokine output. Many CD8⁺ cytotoxic T cells seem to make a spectrum of cytokines reminiscent of TH1 cells. CD8⁺ T cells that make a TH2-like pattern of cytokines may have regulatory or suppressor functions (Ts cells). The differentiation of CD8⁺ cells is also influenced by the CD4⁺ T cell subsets. CD8⁺ cytotoxic T cells tend to occur when TH1 activity is dominant, and to fade when TH2 is dominant.

■ CELL-MEDIATED CYTOTOXICITY

Cell-mediated cytotoxicity is a property not only of cytotoxic T cells, but also of certain other subpopulations of lymphoid cells and, under some circumstances, of myeloid cells. The effector cells at the bottom of *Figure 9.3* are all able to lyse target cells to which they are sufficiently closely bound. However, these cells do not necessarily operate in the same way, and confusion has arisen because the term 'cell-mediated cytotoxicity' covers several distinct phenomena. Thus, different receptors can be involved in the binding of the cytotoxic cell to the target, and in the triggering of the various killing mechanisms. There are three main types of receptor–ligand interaction involved (*Fig. 9.6*):

- Specific antigens (e.g. viral peptides on infected cells) are recognized by MHC-restricted T-cell receptors of cytotoxic T cells. These are mostly CD8+, but some CD4+ are also cytotoxic.
- Determinants, e.g. on tumour cells, are recognized by receptors on NK cells
- Antibody already bound to antigen (e.g. viral antigen on

Selection of effector mechanisms by TH1 and TH2 cells

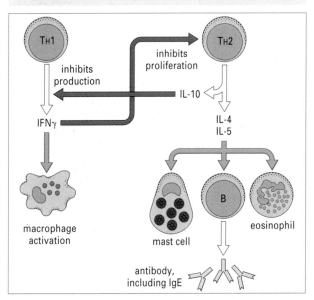

Fig. 9.5 Not only does their lymphokine output drive different effector pathways, but TH1 cells tend to switch off TH2 cells, and vice-versa.

Cell-mediated cytotoxicity

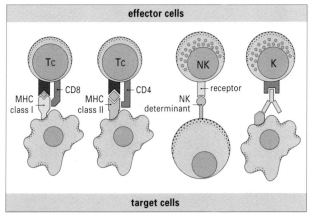

Fig. 9.6 Three different types of cell binding in cell-mediated cytotoxicity:
1. Cytotoxic T cells (mostly CD8⁺, some CD4⁺) bind their target while recognizing antigen and MHC determinants.
2. NK cells recognize an absence of autologous MHC Class I, and the presence of poorly defined ligands on tumour cells.
3. K cells recognize the Fc of IgG antibody bound to antigen on the target cell surface.

an infected cell) and recognized by Fc receptors of K cells; this is known as antibody-dependent cell-mediated cytotoxicity (ADCC).

This classification of receptor–ligand interactions into functional categories is, of course, a simplification. In reality, more than one type of interaction may be manifested by a particular cell type. Moreover, other receptor–ligand interactions can help to stabilize the bond between the cytotoxic cell and the target (*Fig. 9.7*), and can even help to trigger the killing event. For example, by adding antibodies against CD3, CD2 or CD16 (see Appendix) to cytotoxic T cells *in vitro*, it is possible to trigger the killing of cells that are bound to them. It is probable that binding of physiological ligands to these molecules can also trigger cytotoxic cells in this way.

Some types of cell-mediated cytotoxicity do not require antibody
One group of cytotoxic T cells recognizes peptides presented by MHC molecules on target cells
MHC-restricted cytotoxic T cells are a subpopulation of small lymphocytes (see Chapter 2). They are known to be derived from radiosensitive precursor cells. The majority are CD8$^+$ and therefore recognize antigens in association with class I MHC molecules. About 10% of MHC-restricted cytotoxic T cells are functionally distinct, being CD4$^+$ and class II restricted. The interaction of CD4 or CD8 with the appropriate MHC molecule probably helps to stabilize cell–cell recognition; antibodies to any of these cell surface molecules can inhibit killing (*Fig. 9.6*).

The most important role of cytotoxic T cells is probably the elimination of virus-infected cells (see Chapter 16). It therefore 'makes sense' that most Tc cells recognize antigen presented by Class I MHC molecules, since these are expressed on nearly all nucleated cells.

MHC-unrestricted cytotoxic cells include NK and LAK cell types
Several, partly overlapping cell populations have been shown to possess the property of non-specific, MHC-unrestricted killing. These include the following:
* Cells naturally present in spleen or peripheral blood populations, usually known as Natural Killer (NK) cells.
* Cells activated by culture in relatively high concentrations of IL-2, known as Lymphokine Activated Killer (LAK) cells.
* Mixed populations with non-specific killing activity developing in mixed lymphocyte cultures, or in cultures stimulated with the lectin phytohaemagglutinin (PHA).

NK cells – These cells are mostly derived from 'large granular lymphocytes' (LGLs), which comprise about 5% of human peripheral blood lymphoid cells (*Fig. 9.8*). The majority of NK cells are CD3$^-$CD16$^+$CD56$^+$ (see Appendix), and do not contain productive rearrangements of the T-cell receptor genes. Susceptibility to killing by NK cells is inversely correlated with expression of Class I MHC. So expression of correct autologous Class I MHC may function as a 'password' exempting the cell from NK-mediated lysis. Thus NK cells express receptors (Ly-49 family) for MHC and several related families of receptors, some having homology with lectins.

LAK cells – There is increasing evidence that the enhanced cytotoxic activity of peripheral blood or spleen cell populations that have been precultured with IL-2 is largely derived from precursor cells that are indistinguishable from NK cells. Thus LAK cells probably do not represent a separate lineage, but rather a consequence of activation. This type of cell is undergoing trials for the treatment of cancer in man: the patient's own T cells are stimulated *in vitro* with IL-2, and then returned to the patient.

Interactions between Tc and target cells

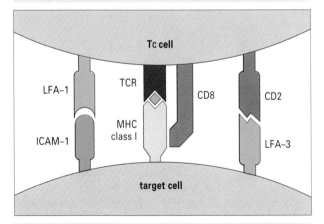

Fig. 9.7 Some of the ligands that may be involved in the interaction between cytotoxic cells and their targets.

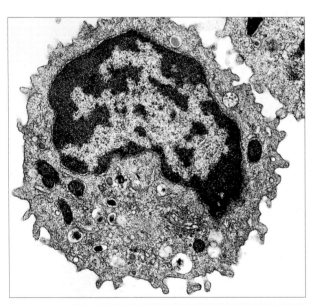

Fig. 9.8 A large granular lymphocyte. Large granular lymphocytes, which can be isolated by density gradient centrifugation, contain the majority of peripheral blood NK effector activity.

Mixed populations with non-specific killing activity – Stimulation of peripheral blood cells by autologous tumour cells, by mixed lymphocyte culture, or by phytohaemagglutinin, gives rise to many CD3$^+$CD8$^+$ cells which show typical class I-restricted cytotoxicity. However, clonal analysis of these complex cultures reveals some CD3$^+$ cells that express a T-cell receptor, but whose cytotoxic effects show little or no MHC restriction. These are particularly common when PHA has been used as a stimulus. Such cells may simply be recognizing determinants that are present on a wide range of target cells; alternatively, they may be recognizing unknown restriction elements. The situation is further complicated by the fact that such cultures also contain LAK cells, induced by IL-2 released by other lymphocytes in the culture.

Antibody-dependent cell-mediated cytotoxicity (ADCC) depends on binding of the cytotoxic cell to the target via antibody

Cells with cytotoxic potential that also possess Fc receptors for IgG may bind to and lyse target cells coated with IgG (*Fig. 9.9*). It is customary to refer to this as killer (K) cell activity

but it is now clear that this is a function that may be performed by several cell types with Fc receptors, including T cells and NK cells. Myeloid cells expressing Fc receptors can also show K cell activity, but probably use different killing mechanisms (discussed later).

Potential targets for K cell action include viral antigens on cell surfaces, MHC molecules and some epitopes present on tumours. Thus, monocytes and (according to some controversial reports) polymorphs may also be active against antibody-coated tumour targets. Some myeloid cells (monocytes and eosinophils) are certainly important effectors of damage to antibody-coated schistosomulae (see Chapter 18). In this reaction, which may also apply to other parasites, the important antibody classes appear to be the anaphylactic ones (IgE in all species, IgG in mice, and IgG2a in rats). This raises the intriguing possibility that IgE acts by first triggering mast cells to release eosinophil chemotactic factor, and then binding the arriving eosinophils onto the target (*Fig. 9.10*). This pattern of effector mechanisms is characteristically evoked when the helper T cell response is dominated by TH2 cells, since the IL-4 and IL-5 released by these cells enhances the generation of eosinophils, mast cells and IgE.

The mechanisms of ADCC are similar for cytotoxic T cells, NK cells and lymphoid K cells

Lymphoid cells use similar methods to kill targets, whatever receptor–target interaction is responsible (*Fig. 9.11*). One mode of killing by lymphoid cells involves three clear and distinct phases.
1. The cell binds to the target.
2. A Ca^{2+}-dependent phase, in which the vesicle contents of the cytotoxic cell are discharged – these modify the target so that it is programmed for death.
3. A late phase, when the target cell is killed.

This model is based on the observation that the vesicles of LGLs, NK cells and some cytotoxic T cells contain perforin, a monomeric pore-forming protein related to the lytic component (C9) of complement (see Chapter 13). The vesicles also contain a serine esterase that may be involved in the assembly of the lytic complex. In the presence of Ca^{2+}, the perforin monomers bind to the target cell membrane and polymerize to form transmembrane channels. Although in close contact with the perforin, the cytotoxic cell survives and can continue to kill further targets. It is believed to be

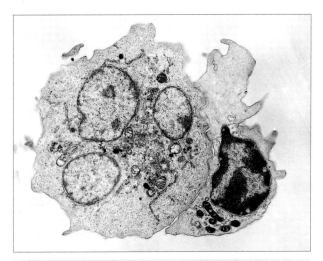

Fig. 9.9 K cell activity. Electron micrograph of a lymphocyte (right) engaging a target cell sensitized with antibody (left). ×2500. (Courtesy of Dr P. Penfold.)

Dual role for antibody in the immune reaction to schistosomes

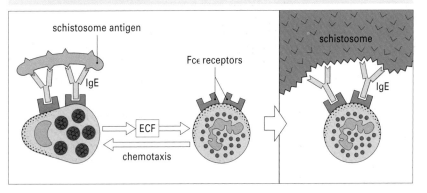

Fig. 9.10 Mast cells sensitized with anti-schistosome IgE release eosinophil chemotactic factor (ECF) following contact with schistosome antigen (left). The arriving eosinophils attach to the antibody-coated worm via their Fc receptors and are important effectors in damaging the parasites (right). This is therefore a form of ADCC mediated by cells of myeloid origin.

Cell-mediated cytotoxicity

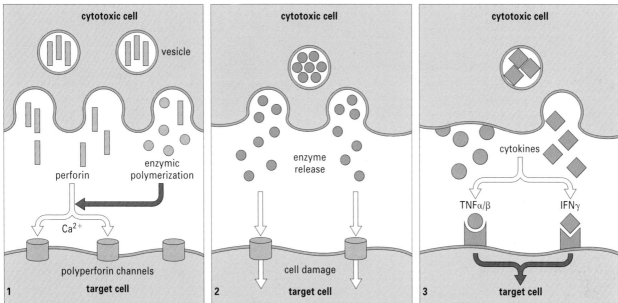

Fig. 9.11 Potential mechanisms for cytotoxic damage to target cells.
1. The cytotoxic lymphoid cell degranulates, releasing perforin and various enzymes into the immediate vicinity of the target cell membrane. In the presence of Ca^{2+} there is enzymic polymerization of the perforin to form polyperforin channels on the target cell.
2. Degradative enzymes or other toxic substances released from the cytotoxic cell may pass through the channels on the target to cause cell damage.
3. TNFα and LT (TNFβ) from the cytotoxic lymphoid cells or macrophages, and IFNγ either from the cytotoxic cell or from nearby lymphoid cells, trigger the target cell via its receptors. Susceptible cells die. This process takes longer than 1 and 2.

protected from autodestruction by a proteoglycan (chondroitin sulphate A) which is also present in the vesicles, and which may bind to and inactivate the perforin. The killing caused by perforin is in fact quite unlike the true lysis caused by complement. What is seen is apoptosis, with DNA fragmentation and disintegration of the cell into small, membrane-bound fragments known as apoptotic bodies. These are rapidly taken up and destroyed by other cells without provoking significant inflammation.

Some cytotoxic T cells do not seem to contain perforin, and can lyse targets in the absence of calcium. It has been suggested that these cells must use some other mechanism. This observation has been confirmed by recent studies using cytotoxic T cells derived from 'knockout' mice unable to express the perforin gene; cytotoxicity was reduced, but not eliminated. It appears, therefore, that other pathways exist for triggering apoptosis that do not involve the perforin-mediated pore-forming step.

Cytotoxic T cell vesicles may also contain TNFα, lymphotoxin (TNFβ) and NK cytotoxic factor (NKCF), which is partially neutralized by antibody to TNFα. The role of these cytokines is unclear because their known cytotoxic effects take much longer than the 3–4 hours required by cytotoxic T cells.

Myeloid cells use a range of mechanisms to kill their targets

TNFα alone is certainly responsible for many examples of tumour cell killing by macrophages, and in conjunction with IFNγ (released by T cells or NK cells) is powerfully synergistic in the killing of susceptible tumours (*Fig. 9.12*). It is not clear how these cytokines kill the target. There is increased activity of target cell cyclo-oxygenase and lipoxygenase, with some consequent intracellular free radical release, and this plays a role in some cases. There may also be release of free radicals from the mitochondrial electron transport pathways,

Mechanisms which may contribute to the cytotoxicity of myeloid cells

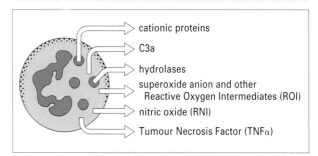

- cationic proteins
- C3a
- hydrolases
- superoxide anion and other Reactive Oxygen Intermediates (ROI)
- nitric oxide (RNI)
- Tumour Necrosis Factor (TNFα)

Fig. 9.12 Reactive oxygen intermediates (ROIs) and reactive nitrogen intermediates (RNIs), cationic proteins, hydrolytic enzymes and complement proteins released from myeloid cells may damage the target cell in addition to cytokine-mediated attack.

and there are changes in protein synthesis. Myeloid cells may also release toxic mediators that are used against phagocytosed pathogens, including reactive oxygen and nitrogen intermediates (ROIs and RNIs – see Chapter 17).

■ THE ROLE OF MACROPHAGES IN THE IMMUNE RESPONSE

Macrophages are involved at all stages of the immune response (*Fig. 9.13*). First, as already outlined, they act as a rapid protective mechanism that can respond before T-cell mediated amplification has taken place. Then they take part in the initiation of T cell activation by processing and presenting antigen (see Chapter 7). Finally, they are important in the effector phase of the cell-mediated response following T-cell mediated activation as inflammatory, tumoricidal and microbicidal cells (*Fig. 9.14*).

Some macrophage functions are enhanced following exposure to lymphokines
Circulating monocytes possess the ability to kill some organisms (see Chapter 17). Much of this ability is lost if they are cultured *in vitro*, but exposure to lymphokines, particularly

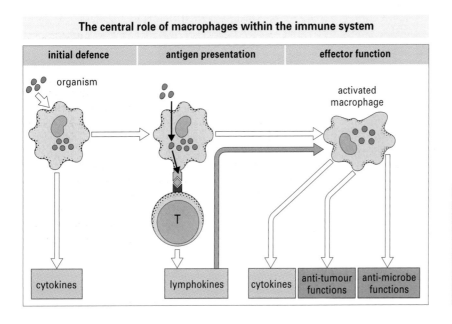

The central role of macrophages within the immune system

initial defence	antigen presentation	effector function

organism

activated macrophage

T

cytokines   lymphokines   cytokines   anti-tumour functions   anti-microbe functions

Fig. 9.13 Macrophages play a role in the initial response to infection before T- and B-cell enhanced immunity can act. They then act as antigen processing and presenting cells. Finally, when T cells respond to antigen they release lymphokines which activate macrophages.

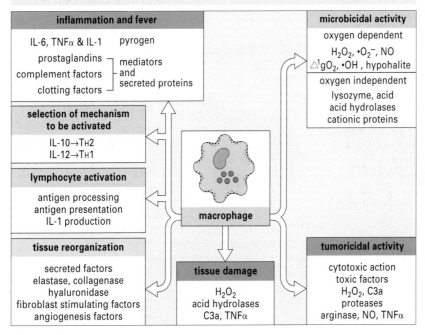

The central role of macrophages in immunity and inflammation

inflammation and fever

IL-6, TNFα & IL-1   pyrogen
prostaglandins ⎤
complement factors ⎬ mediators and secreted proteins
clotting factors ⎦

selection of mechanism to be activated

IL-10→TH2
IL-12→TH1

lymphocyte activation

antigen processing
antigen presentation
IL-1 production

tissue reorganization

secreted factors
elastase, collagenase
hyaluronidase
fibroblast stimulating factors
angiogenesis factors

macrophage

tissue damage

H_2O_2
acid hydrolases
C3a, TNFα

microbicidal activity

oxygen dependent
H_2O_2, •O_2^-, NO
$\triangle^1 gO_2$, •OH , hypohalite

oxygen independent
lysozyme, acid
acid hydrolases
cationic proteins

tumoricidal activity

cytotoxic action
toxic factors
H_2O_2, C3a
proteases
arginase, NO, TNFα

Fig. 9.14 Macrophages and their products are important in both the induction phases of inflammation and in tissue reorganization and repair (left). Macrophage effector functions are shown on the right. The effector functions may cause tissue damage, as in delayed hypersensitivity reactions.

IFNγ, restores it and also activates additional killing pathways which normal monocytes do not express.

The destruction of many intracellular parasites, and of some tumour cells *in vitro*, requires this lymphokine-mediated 'activation' of macrophages (*Fig. 9.15*). The classic experiment demonstrating this phenomenon involved animals immunized with BCG (Bacillus Calmette-Guérin, an avirulent variant of bovine tuberculosis). When subsequently challenged with PPD (a crude mixture of T-cell stimulating antigens from *Mycobacterium tuberculosis*) the animals were also protected against the unrelated bacterium, *Listeria monocytogenes*. It was concluded that the activation of macrophages involved an antigen-specific pathway, but that the enhanced microbicidal activity was not specific for the immunizing organism. Further experiments demonstrated that lymphocytes derived from a BCG-immunized mouse, when cultured *in vitro* with appropriate antigen (PPD for example), would release mediators that enhanced the ability of macrophages to kill or inhibit both the immunizing organism and unrelated organisms. The mediators in question were subsequently shown to be lymphokines.

Macrophages are heterogeneous

Macrophage activation is a complex phenomenon. Activated macrophages show enhanced ability to kill some microorganisms, but not others. For example, IFNγ used alone enables human monocytes to kill *Legionella*, but it leads to enhanced growth of *Mycobacterium tuberculosis*. There are several reasons for this complexity:

- Activated macrophages can express numerous different effector functions (*Fig. 9.14*). Antimicrobial functions are discussed in greater detail in Chapter 17.
- The monocyte/macrophage series is very heterogeneous; cells taken from different sites differ in such relevant characteristics as expression of class II MHC molecules and Fc receptors, lymphokine responsiveness and production of peroxidase. Most authors nevertheless believe that there is only one lineage of macrophages, and that these differences are due to environmental and maturational effects.
- The functions activated may depend not only on the macrophage, but also on the precise 'blend' of lymphokines and inflammatory stimuli to which it is exposed.

Several patterns of lymphokine-mediated effects can be recognized:

- Effects mediated by a single lymphokine working alone.
- Quantitative effects, increased or decreased according to the status of secondary signals.
- Cooperative (synergistic) effects, where one mediator has no effect unless a second mediator or bacterial product is present. For instance, the pathway that leads to formation of nitric oxide is activated by IFNγ, but subsequent exposure to TNFα greatly enhances the actual triggering of nitric oxide release (*Fig. 9.16*).

It is suggested that activation occurs in stages, and requires sequential stimuli; possible stimuli include lymphokines, endotoxin, various mediators and regulators of inflammation. Different effector functions may be expressed at each stage, and there are characteristic changes in macrophage appearance and physiology (*Fig. 9.17*).

Calcitriol is involved in the activation of human macrophages, and in regulation of TH1/TH2 balance

When human macrophages are exposed to IFNγ they express a 1-hydroxylase. This enzyme enables them to convert inactive circulating 25-hydroxycholecaliferol into the active

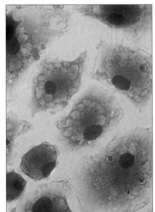
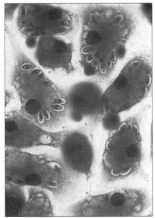

Fig. 9.15 Killing of *Leishmania* by activated macrophages.
The destruction of *Leishmania enriettii* by C57 strain mouse macrophages is enhanced by lymphokines. Parasites within the macrophages are destroyed during 48-hour culture with a lymphocyte supernatant containing lymphokines (left). Control cultures containing no lymphokine allow unrestrained growth (right). Giemsa stain, ×800. (Courtesy of Dr J Manuel.)

The activation of macrophages

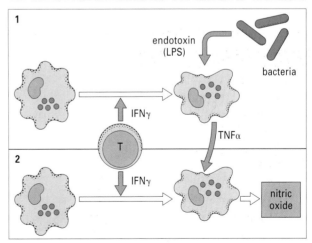

Fig. 9.16 The activation of macrophages may require interaction of several lymphokines and microbial factors.
1. Optimal release of TNFα from macrophages requires activation by IFNγ followed by exposure to microbial components with cytokine-triggering ability, such as endotoxin. This may then provide enough TNFα to trigger pathway 2.
2. IFNγ activates the pathway that leads to production of nitric oxide, but TNFα is required in order to trigger it.

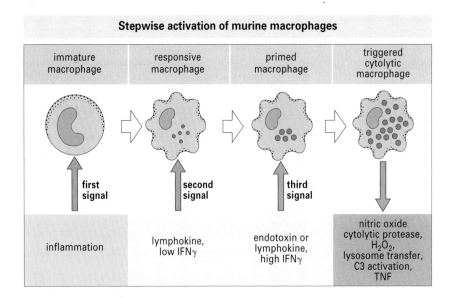

Stepwise activation of murine macrophages

immature macrophage	responsive macrophage	primed macrophage	triggered cytolytic macrophage
	first signal	second signal	third signal
inflammation	lymphokine, low IFNγ	endotoxin or lymphokine, high IFNγ	nitric oxide cytolytic protease, H₂O₂, lysosome transfer, C3 activation, TNF

Fig. 9.17 A hypothetical scheme for the stepwise activation of murine peritoneal macrophages to develop tumoricidal activity.

metabolite, 1,25-dihydroxycholecalciferol (also known as vitamin D₃, or calcitriol). Macrophages have receptors for this derivative, and it exerts additional activating effects on these cells (*Fig. 9.18*). It also exerts powerful negative feedback on Th1 lymphocytes, and may be one of the mechanisms that tends to shift the response from Th1 towards Th2 when elimination of the parasite fails, and the cell-mediated response becomes chronic. This pathway is of some importance in man,

since production of calcitriol can be so great in sarcoidosis or tuberculosis that it leaks from the site of macrophage activation into the peripheral circulation, where it can induce hypercalcaemia.

Macrophage effector functions are subject to both negative and positive regulation

There is also evidence that activated macrophages can be deactivated. Prostaglandin E may have this effect, and some effector mechanisms (but not all) are glucocorticoid sensitive. Recently a Macrophage Deactivating Factor (MDF) has been purified from a tumour cell supernatant. This factor blocks activation by IFNγ of increased capacity for production of ROIs and, to some extent, of nitric oxide (*Fig. 9.19*). IL-4, calcitonin gene related peptide (CGRP), and the TGFβ family of cytokines have similar effects.

■ GRANULOMA FORMATION

Sometimes the cell-mediated response fails to eliminate an infecting organism, or antigenic material cannot be eliminated because it is either resistant to degradation or derived from self components. If, in such cases, T cells continue to accumulate and release lymphokines, this leads to granuloma form-

The role of calcitriol (1,25-dihydroxycholecalciferol) in the activation of human macrophages

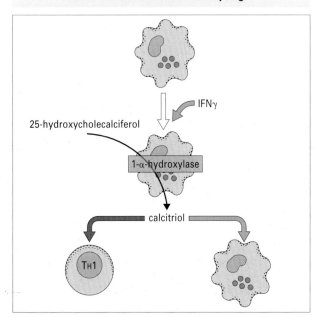

IFNγ

25-hydroxycholecalciferol

1-α-hydroxylase

calcitriol

Th1

Fig. 9.18 In man, exposure to IFNγ leads to increased expression of 1-α-hydroxylase, enabling macrophages to convert inactive circulating 25-hydroxycholecalciferol into calcitriol. This is an example of an autocrine feedback loop, which further activates the macrophage, while reducing Th1 activity.

Negative regulation of macrophages

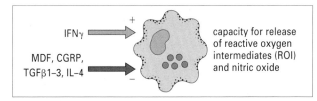

IFNγ +

MDF, CGRP, TGFβ1–3, IL-4 −

capacity for release of reactive oxygen intermediates (ROI) and nitric oxide

Fig. 9.19 Exposure of macrophages to IFNγ will increase their potential for release of both reactive oxygen intermediates, and nitric oxide. Several other factors oppose this activation.

ation. Granulomas are characteristic of infections with organisms which live at least partly intracellularly (e.g. *Mycobacterium tuberculosis, M. leprae, Leishmania spp.*, and *Listeria monocytogenes*), or organisms which are large and persistent (e.g. schistosome ova).

Granulomas characteristically contain macrophage-derived cell types of somewhat obscure function, including epithelioid cells and multinucleate giant cells (*Fig. 9.20*). Their morphology suggests secretory rather than phagocytic roles, and they are thought to result from chronic stimulation of macrophages by lymphokines.

Analysis of the T cells in granulomatous foci indicates that CD4$^+$ cells are located at the centre and CD8$^+$ cells around the periphery, suggesting that CD4$^+$ (TH) cells are of prime importance in inducing the accumulation and activation of other lymphocytes and macrophages (*Fig. 9.21*). If such granulomas are cultured *in vitro* they can be shown to release a variety of cytokines. For maximal granuloma development TH1 lymphokines and TNFα appear to be essential; in the murine schistosome model some TH2 cytokines are also required.

■ IMMUNOPATHOLOGY

There are a number of situations in which the cell-mediated response is itself responsible for part or all of the tissue damage resulting from infectious disease. It can also be involved in autoimmunity (*Fig. 9.22*). These mechanisms are described in detail in Chapters 17 and 22.

Cytotoxicity – Cytotoxic cells may kill virus-infected target cells that are essential to the host's survival, such as the cells of the central nervous system. If this occurs in response to a virus which does not itself cause cell death or dysfunction, the tissue damage is immunopathological.

Chronic inflammation – Cell-mediated mechanisms may be directed towards autoantigens (or towards unidentified cryptic infections or commensal organisms), and so cause chronic tissue-damaging inflammation (as in rheumatoid arthritis, Crohn's disease, sarcoidosis, psoriasis, and multiple sclerosis). The relative roles of putative infectious agents and of subsequent autoimmunity are often unknown as is the case with the destruction of the islets of Langerhans in the pancreas that leads to insulin-dependent diabetes.

Space-occupying lesions – The sheer size of a granuloma may compromise the function of the host tissue. Thus granulomas evoked by *M. leprae* can damage the nerves in which they form, and granulomas in the retina or brain can cause functional abnormalities.

Excessive cytokine release – Excessive release of cytokines (particularly TNFα) can lead to toxic shock syndrome, haemorrhagic necrosis and the Shwartzman reaction, and can also contribute to necrosis within sites of cell-mediated response (the Koch phenomenon). These mechanisms are discussed in Chapter 17.

■ THE CYTOKINE NETWORK

Cytokines form a complex communication network between cells

Cytokines (including lymphokines and interleukins) are hormone-like peptides or glycopeptides. They have been mentioned at intervals throughout this chapter because they work in parallel with other signals arising from direct cell-to-cell contact, providing a communication network involved in

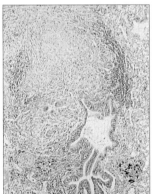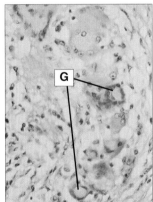

Fig. 9.20 A granulomatous reaction in pulmonary tuberculosis. The central area of caseous necrosis – in which much of the cellular structure is destroyed – is characteristic of tuberculosis in the lung (see Chapter 17). Apart from this necrosis, the histology is characteristic of chronic T-cell-dependent 'tuberculoid' granulomas. The lesion is surrounded by a ring of epithelioid cells and mononuclear cells. Multinucleate giant cells, thought to be derived from the fusion of epithelioid cells, are also present (left, ×170). Giant cells (G) are illustrated at a higher magnification (right, ×270). H&E stain. (Courtesy of Dr G. Boyd.)

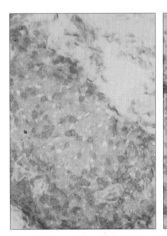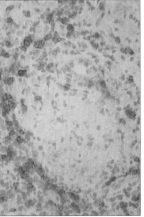

Fig. 9.21 CD4 and CD8 staining of a granuloma. Shown here is a dermal granuloma from a patient with borderline tuberculoid leprosy stained red with peroxidase-coupled antibodies to CD4 (left) and CD8 (right). CD4$^+$ TH cells are present in and around the lesion, while CD8$^+$ T cells occur mainly on the periphery. (Courtesy of Dr R. L. Modlin and Dr T. H. Rea.)

Pathways of cell-mediated immunopathology

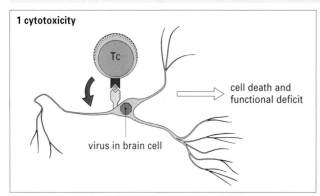

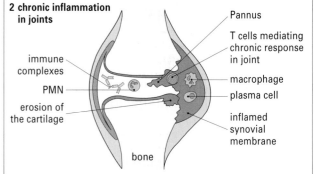

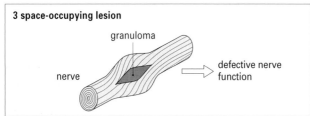

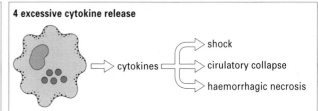

1 cytotoxicity

Tc

cell death and functional deficit

virus in brain cell

2 chronic inflammation in joints

Pannus

T cells mediating chronic response in joint

immune complexes

PMN

erosion of the cartilage

macrophage

plasma cell

inflamed synovial membrane

bone

3 space-occupying lesion

granuloma

nerve

defective nerve function

4 excessive cytokine release

cytokines

shock

cirulatory collapse

haemorrhagic necrosis

Fig. 9.22 Pathways of cell-mediated immunopathology.
1. Cytotoxic cells may kill virus-infected host cells that are essential to survival (e.g. nerve cells in the brain).
2. The response may be directed towards autoantigens (or perhaps to unidentified cryptic infections or commensal organisms), leading to chronic inflammation, as is seen in rheumatoid arthritis.
3. A granuloma may cause a bulky space-occupying lesion, impairing the function of sensitive tissues such as brain, retina and nerve.
4. Excessive release of cytokines can lead to several tissue-damaging syndromes, especially toxic shock syndromes with TNFα.

Effects of interleukin-6 (IL-6)

IL-2, IL-2R, proliferation, differentiation

T

B

plasma cells

mesangial cell proliferation

keratinocytes

growth

IL–6

platelets

hepatocytes

megakaryocytes

acute phase response

C–reactive protein etc.

monocytes

neutrophils

stem cells

Fig. 9.23 IL-6 is a typical cytokine, in that it has a range of effects on many organ systems.

every function of the immune response. The term 'lympho-kine' originally referred to mediators released from lymphocytes. The term 'interleukin' was coined in the hope that by numbering these mediators (interleukin-1, interleukin-2, and so on) a universal nomenclature could be created. It is misleading because it implies that these mediators only act as signals between white cells: although many of them do have this function, most also have functions that bypass leucocytes entirely. The best term is 'cytokine', which can be used to refer to any mediator that acts as a signal between cells, whatever the cell type.

Much of the confusion surrounding the nomenclature stems from the fact that cytokines are multifunctional. Thus many cytokines were discovered independently in several different laboratories, working with entirely different experimental systems. For example, TNFα was discovered almost simultaneously in two laboratories, one of which was studying weight loss in chronic infection and named the cytokine 'cachectin'. Similarly, IL-6 was originally identified as having different functions in unrelated assays (*Fig. 9.23*).

The advent of pure recombinant cytokines has greatly facilitated the identification of cytokine functions *in vitro*. However, such experiments can prove misleading when extrapolated to the situation *in vivo*. There are several reasons for this.

Firstly, cytokines do not operate individually *in vivo*. Perhaps each cytokine should be considered as a single 'word' in a 'sentence' of cytokines. Each cell responds to the whole 'sentence' and even the sequence of exposure to these mediators may be important. A mixture of cytokines can exert an effect which is not seen with any single one of the cytokines used alone, and there can be both synergistic and antagonistic effects (*Fig. 9.24*).

Secondly, there are inhibitors of cytokines *in vivo*. These can operate in three different ways (*Fig. 9.25*):
- Cytokine-like mediators bind to the cytokine receptor, but do not activate signal transduction. For example, there is an IL-1 inhibitor that is related to IL-1 itself, and that competes with IL-1 for IL-1 receptors.
- Extracellular domains of cytokine receptors that have been shed by the cell can bind the cytokine and so prevent its interaction with receptors on cell membranes. Soluble TNFα receptors do this.
- One cytokine can switch off the response to another, acting via a different receptor.

Cytokines can often exert autocrine effects (i.e. effects on the cell of origin). This is intelligible if one is able to bear in mind the presence of inhibitors *in vivo*, since the autocrine feedback can be 'intercepted' and modulated by inhibitory products of other cells.

Experiments *in vivo* partially resolve the problem of determining the true biological role of these multifunctional

Examples of interactions between cytokines

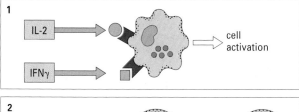

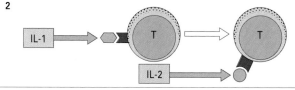

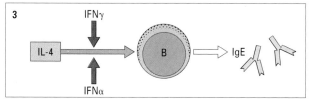

Fig. 9.24 Interactions between cytokines vary.
1. Synergy. Some cytokines, e.g. IL-2 and IFNγ, act synergistically to increase cell activation.
2. Receptor induction. Some cytokines act by inducing another receptor, a form of sequential synergy (a cascade effect).
3. Antagonism. Some cytokines are directly antagonistic, as shown by the contrasting effects of IL-4 and IFNγ on IgE production.

Three types of cytokine inhibitor

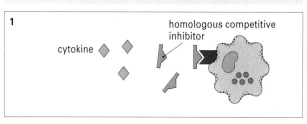

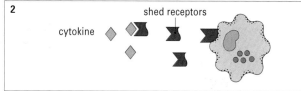

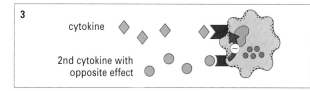

Fig. 9.25 Three types of cytokine inhibitor.
1. Molecules homologous to the cytokine and able to bind to its receptor without leading to signal transduction, act as competitive inhibitors. The gene for an IL-1 inhibitor of this type has been cloned. There may also be inhibitory glycosylation variants of some mediators.
2. The extracellular domains of TNF and IL-1 receptors can be shed. They bind their cytokine in the fluid phase, and so stop the cytokine from reaching receptors on cell membranes.
3. Other mediators, acting through quite separate receptors, can exert opposite effects on the cell (see also *Figs 9.5* and *9.24*).

cytokines. Cytokines can be injected, or released slowly from surgically implanted osmotic minipumps. Alternatively the animals can be treated with neutralizing antibodies to the cytokine. Finally, transgenic animals can be created which overexpress the chosen cytokine, or the gene for the cytokine can be selectively 'knocked out'.

Such experiments have led to quite unexpected results which had not emerged from experiments *in vitro*. For example, the development of transgenic mice that overexpressed the human IL-6 gene demonstrated for the first time the striking effects of IL-6 on the production of both megakaryocytes and platelets. Nevertheless, these experiments *in vivo* can be difficult to interpret. An effect can be secondary, due not to the injected or overexpressed cytokine but to another, possibly unidentified agent (the 'cascade effect').

The cytokine network has multiple physiological roles

It has often been pointed out that the evolution and function of the immune system parallels that of the nervous system in many ways. For instance, both systems have learning and memory functions based on cell-to-cell communication, and they share many mediators, receptors and antigens. Both systems need an internal communication network, and also a communication network that can control and interact with other organs. The nervous system is directly 'wired' to most other organs via nerves, but also uses the hypothalamus–pituitary–adrenal axis to send signals to the periphery. In contrast the immune system is composed mostly of free, mobile cells: cell-to-cell interactions are intermittent and mostly concerned with internal communication. Thus communication with other organs is largely cytokine mediated (*Fig. 9.26*). In addition to these direct effects, the immune system is integrated with the nervous and endocrine systems (see Chapter 11). For example, it shares with the nervous system an ability to signal via the hypothalamus–pituitary–adrenal axis, since several cytokines such as IL-1, IL-6 and TNF have direct effects on the hypothalamus or pituitary. In addition, lymphocytes can produce ACTH in response to CRF. Many cells of the immune system also express receptors for neurotransmitters, opioids and neuropeptides, and the role of these mediators in modulating immune responses is currently under investigation.

The known functions of the characterized cytokines are summarized elsewhere (see Appendix). The comments above should have made clear to the reader the need to interpret such data with caution. Not all the functions listed will turn out to be physiologically relevant, since many have been reported following experiments *in vitro* with single recombinant cytokines.

The physiological roles of the cytokine network

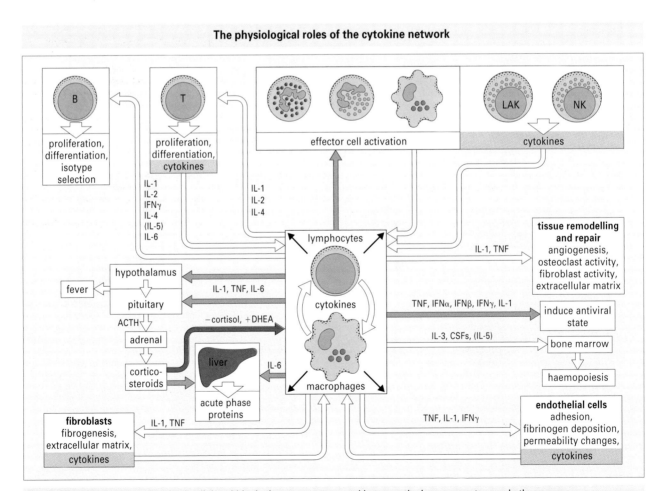

Fig. 9.26 Cytokines as communication links within the immune system, and between the immune system and other organs.

Critical Thinking

■ How does the initial recognition of a pathogen determine the type of immune effector function which will subsequently be mounted against it?

■ Why do most cytotoxic T cells recognize epitopes presented by Class I MHC, which is expressed on essentially all nucleated cells?

■ What happens if inappropriate cell-mediated effector functions are activated?

■ Does chronic tissue-damaging cell-mediated immunopathology result from TH1/TH2 imbalance?

■ To what extent do we misinterpret the roles of individual cytokines by working *in vitro* with pure recombinant cytokines?

■ Since several steroids affect T-cell function and cytokines act on the hypothalamo–pituitary–adrenal axis, should we talk about a 'cytokine network', or a 'cytokine/endocrine network'?

FURTHER READING

Akira S, Taga T, Kishimoto T. Interleukin-6 in biology and medicine. *Adv Immunol* 1993;**54**:1–78.

Bloom BR, Salgame P, Diamond B. Revisiting and revising suppressor T cells. *Immunol Today* 1992;**13(4):**131–36.

Bretscher PA, Wei G, Menon JN, Bielefeldt-Ohmann H. Establishment of stable, cell-mediated immunity that makes "susceptible" mice resistant to Leishmania major. *Science* 1992;**257**:539–42.

Cerami A, Beutler B. The role of cachectin/TNF in endotoxin shock and cachexia. *Immunol Today* 1988;**9**:29.

Cooper AM, Dalton DK, Stewart TA, Griffin JP, Russell DG, Orme IM. Disseminated tuberculosis in interferon gamma gene-disrupted mice. *J Exp Med* 1993;**178**:2243–47.

Grzych JM, Pearce E, Cheever A, *et al.* Egg deposition is the stimulus for the production of TH2 cytokines in murine schistosomiasis mansoni. *J Immunol* 1991;**146**:1322–40.

Janeway CA. The immune system evolved to discriminate infectious self from noninfectious self. *Immunol Today* 1992;**13(1)**:11–16.

Kabelitz D. Human gamma delta T lymphocytes. *Int Arch Allergy Immunol* 1993;**102**:1–9.

Kagi D, Ledermann B, Burki K, *et al.* Cytotoxicity mediated by T cells and natural killer cells is greatly impaired in perforin-deficient mice. *Nature* 1994;**369**:31–37.

Kaufmann SH. Immunity to intracellular bacteria. *Annu Rev Immunol* 1993;**11**:129.

Lukacs NW, Boros DL. Lymphokine regulation of granuloma formation in murine schistosomiasis mansoni. *Clin Immunol Immunopathol* 1993;**68**:57–63.

Moretta L, Ciccone E, Moretta A, Höglund P, Öhlén C, Kärre K. Allorecognition by NK cells: nonself or no self. *Immunol Today* 1992;**13(8):**300–306.

Mosmann TR, Coffman RL. Different patterns of lymphokine secretion lead to different functional properties. *Annu Rev Immunol* 1989;**7**:145–73.

Nathan CF, Murray HW, Wiebe ME, Rubin BY. Identification of interferon-γ as the lymphokine that activates human macrophage oxidative metabolism and antimicrobial activity. *J Exp Med* 1983;**158**:670.

Romagnani S. Human TH1 and TH2 subsets: doubt no more. *Immunol Today* 1991;**12**:256–57.

Rook GAW, Bloom BR. Mechanisms of pathogenesis in tuberculosis. In: B.R. Bloom, ed. *Tuberculosis; pathogenesis, protection and control.* Washington DC: ASM Press, 1994: 485–501.

Rook GAW, Hernandez-Pando R, Lightman S. Hormones, peripherally activated prohormones, and regulation of the TH1/TH2 balance. *Immunol Today* 1994;**15**:301–303.

Smith HR, Karlhofer FM, Yokoyama WM. Ly-49 multigene family expressed by IL-2-activated NK cells. *J Immunol* 1994;**153**:1068.

Trinchieri G. Interleukin-12 and its role in the generation of TH1 cells. *Immunol Today* 1993;**14**:335–38.

Unanue ER. Cellular studies on antigen presentation by class II MHC molecules. *Curr Opin Immunol* 1992;**4**:63–69.

Vassalli P. The pathophysiology of tumour necrosis factor. *Annu Rev Immunol* 1992;**10**:411–52.

Young JD, Liu C. Multiple mechanisms of lymphocyte mediated killing. *Immunol Today* 1988;**9**:140–44.

DEVELOPMENT OF THE IMMUNE SYSTEM

Most cells of the immune system derive from haemopoietic stem cells.

Development of different kinds of cells (cell lineages) is dependent on cell interactions and cytokines.

Lymphoid stem cells develop and mature within the primary lymphoid organs – this process is called lymphopoiesis.

T lymphocytes developing in the thymus are subject to positive and negative selection processes.

Mammalian B cells develop mainly in the fetal liver and bone marrow from birth onwards. This process continues throughout life. B cells also undergo a selection process at the site of B-cell generation.

The diverse antigen repertoires found in mature animals are generated during lymphopoiesis, by recombination of gene segments for the TCR and Ig

Germinal centres are sites of oligoclonal B-cell proliferation, antibody class switching, affinity maturation and development of immunological memory.

An efficient immune system depends on the interaction of many cellular and humoral components, which develop at different rates during fetal and early postnatal life. Many cells involved in the immune response are derived from undifferentiated haemopoietic stem cells (HSCs). These differentiate into various cell lineages under the influence of microenvironmental factors such as cell-to-cell interactions and the presence of soluble cytokines (*Fig. 10.1*).

In the chicken, HSCs originate from blood islands found within the embryonic yolk sac in the peri-aortic mesenchyme, and later in the bone marrow. In mammals, HSCs are found in the fetal liver, spleen and bone marrow;

Origin of the cells of the immune system

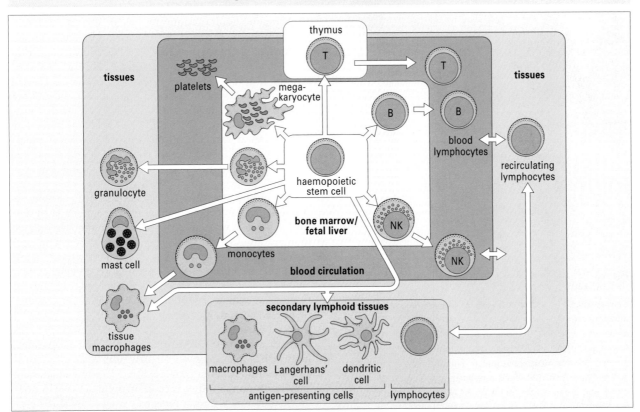

Fig. 10.1 All of the cells shown arise from the haemopoietic stem cell. Platelets produced by megakaryocytes are released into the circulation. Granulocytes pass from the circulation into the tissues. Mast cells are identifiable in all tissues. B cells mature in the fetal liver and bone marrow in mammals, while T cells mature in the thymus. The origin of the large granular lymphocytes with NK activity is uncertain, but is probably the bone marrow. Both lymphocytes and monocytes (which develop into macrophages) can recirculate through secondary lymphoid tissues. Langerhans' cells and dendritic cells act as antigen-presenting cells in secondary lymphoid tissues.

after birth and throughout adult life they are normally found only in the bone marrow. These 'self renewing' HSCs, under the influence of various growth and differentiation factors in sites of haemopoiesis, give rise to most or all the cells of the immune system.

Four major cell lineages arise from the HSCs:
- Erythroid (erythrocytes).
- Megakaryocytic (platelets).
- Myeloid (granulocytes and mononuclear phagocytes).
- Lymphoid (lymphocytes).

The myeloid and lymphoid lineages are critical to the functioning of the immune system.

Development of granulocytes and monocytes

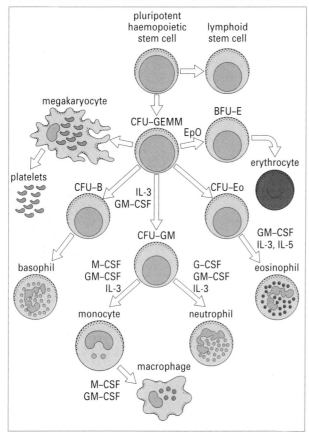

Fig. 10.2 Pluripotent haemopoietic stem cells generate CFU–GEMMs, which have the potential to give rise to all blood cells except lymphocytes. IL-3 and GM–CSF are required to induce this stem cell into one of five pathways (i.e. to give rise to megakaryocytes, erythrocytes via burst-forming units, basophils, neutrophils or eosinophils) and are also required during further differentiation of the granulocytes and monocytes. Eosinophil differentiation from CFU–Eo is promoted by IL-5. Neutrophils and monocytes are derived from the CFU–GM through the effects of G–CSF and M–CSF respectively. Both GM–CSF and M–CSF, and other cytokines (including IL-1, IL-4 and IL-6), promote the differentiation of monocytes into macrophages.
CFU = colony-forming unit (B = basophil, G = granulocyte, E = erythrocyte, M = monocyte); CSF = colony-stimulating factor; Ep0 = erythropoietin; Eo = eosinophil; BFU–E = erythrocytic burst-forming unit.

■ MYELOID CELLS

Myelopoiesis commences in the liver of the human fetus at about six weeks of gestation. Studies in which colonies have been grown *in vitro* from individual stem cells have shown that the first progenitor cell derived from the HSCs is the colony-forming unit (CFU), which can give rise to granulocytes, erythrocytes, monocytes and megakaryocytes (CFU–GEMM). Maturation of these cells occurs under the influence of colony-stimulating factors (CSFs) and several interleukins, including IL-1, IL-3, IL-4, IL-5 and IL-6 (*Fig. 10.2*). These factors, which are important in the positive regulation of haemopoiesis, are derived mainly from stromal cells in the bone marrow, but are also produced by mature forms of differentiated myeloid and lymphoid cells. Other cytokines (e.g. TGFβ) may downregulate haemopoiesis.

Neutrophils and monocytes develop from a common stem cell
Neutrophil development
The CFU–GM cell is the precursor of both neutrophils and mononuclear phagocytes. As the CFU–GM differentiates along the neutrophil pathway, several distinct morphological stages are seen. Myeloblasts develop into promyelocytes and myelocytes, which mature and are released into the circulation as neutrophils. The one-way differentiation of cells from the CFU–GM into mature neutrophils is probably the result of acquiring specific growth/differentiation factor receptors at different stages of development.

Surface differentiation markers disappear or appear on the cells as they develop into granulocytes (*Fig. 10.3*). For example, MHC class II molecules and CD38 are expressed on the CFU–GM, but not on mature neutrophils. Other surface molecules acquired during the differentiation process include CD13, CD14 at low density, CD15 (the Le^x hapten), the β$_1$ integrin, VLA-4 (CD49d, α chain), the β$_2$ integrins CD11a, b and c associated with CD18 β$_2$ chains, complement receptors and CD16 Fcγ receptors (see *Fig. 2.42*).

It is difficult to assess the functional activity of different developmental stages of granulocytes, but it seems likely that the full functional potential is realized only when the cells are mature. This conclusion is based on studies of fetal and neonatal immune systems, which are thought to contain few or no mature immune cells. There is some evidence that neutrophil activity, as measured by phagocytosis or chemotaxis, is lower in fetal than in adult life. However, this may be due, in part, to the lower levels of opsonins present in the fetal serum, rather than to a characteristic of the cells themselves. To become active in the presence of opsonins, neutrophils must interact directly with microorganisms and/or with cytokines generated by a response to antigen. This limitation could reduce neutrophil activity in early life. Activation of neutrophils by cytokines is also a prerequisite for their migration into tissues.

Monocyte development
CFU–GMs taking the monocyte pathway give rise initially to proliferating monoblasts. These differentiate into promonocytes and finally into mature circulating monocytes. Circulating monocytes are thought to be a replace-

Morphology and markers on developing granulocytes and monocytes

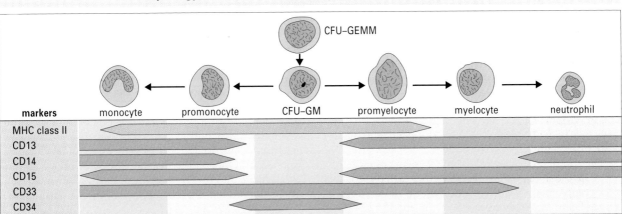

Fig. 10.3 Cells of the monocyte and neutrophil lineages develop from a common CFU–GM. Differentiation along either pathway results in loss of CD34. CD33 is maintained on monocytes but is lost from mature neutrophils, as are MHC class II molecules. CD14 is expressed on monocytes but only weakly on some granulocytes, possibly when they are activated.

ment pool for tissue-resident macrophages. The different forms of macrophages comprise the reticulo-endothelial system (see Chapter 2).

Like mature neutrophils, mature monocytes and macrophages lose CD34. However, unlike neutrophils, they continue to express significant levels of MHC class II molecules (*Fig. 10.3*). These molecules are clearly important for the presentation of antigen to T cells. Monocytes also acquire many of the same surface molecules as mature neutrophils (see *Fig. 2.29*).

As with granulocytes, it is difficult to assess the functional potential of different stages of monocyte development. However, studies of certain myeloid tumour cell lines *in vitro* (believed to represent distinct stages of monocyte differentiation) indicate that both phagocytic efficiency and Fc receptor-mediated cytotoxicity are optimal only in mature macrophages. Generation of the cytokine IL-1 by monocytes is equally good at birth and in adults, but enhanced function induced by IFNγ is lower in neonatal than adult monocytes.

Dendritic cells probably also develop from bone-marrow stem cells

In addition to macrophages, most of the classical antigen-presenting cells (APCs), which include the follicular dendritic cells, Langerhans' cells and interdigitating cells, are present at birth. Their origin is still unclear, but it is likely that most are derived from bone-marrow stem cells. One possibility is that they are derived from the same CD34⁺ precursor cell (CFU–GEMM). Morphological, cytochemical and functional differences would then be due to local microenvironmental influences such as cytokines. Alternatively, APCs could be derived from different stem cells and represent separate lineages of differentiation.

APCs are present in the thymus very early in development, and their function in MHC restriction and selection indicates that at least some APCs must be fully mature at this time. APC activity, however, is clearly suboptimal early in life. For example, neonatal rats fail to initiate a normal antibody response to sheep red blood cells unless they are also injected with APCs taken from adults (*Fig. 10.4*).

Development of APC function

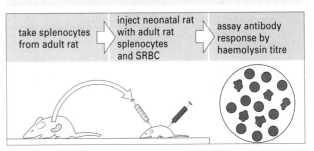

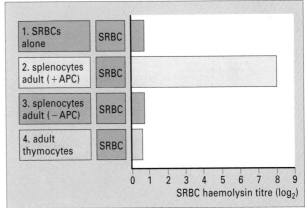

Fig. 10.4 Development of antigen-presenting cell function: antigen processing and presentation. In this experiment, groups of neonatal rats were injected with sheep red blood cells (SRBCs) alone (1), or SRBCs and spleen cells (including APCs) from adult rats (2), or SRBCs and adult, APC-depleted spleen cells (3), or SRBCs and adult thymocytes (4). In all cases the adult rat was of the same strain as the neonate. The antibody response was measured in each group. Neonatal rats injected with SRBCs alone do not make antibodies to this antigen. However, if they also receive adult splenocytes containing APCs with the antigen, they do make a response. Neither adult splenocytes (lacking APCs) nor thymocytes alone are sufficient for antibody production. Thus neonatal APCs are unable to process and present this antigen effectively.

■ THE COMPLEMENT SYSTEM

Lower levels of complement components are found early in life

The complement system is another important component of the innate immune system, and plays a major role in protection against microorganisms. At least 20 distinct plasma proteins have been identified as belonging to the system (see Chapter 13). These proteins appear during fetal development, and are detectable before circulating IgM (*Fig. 10.5*). They are present in the serum of neonates at 50–60% of adult levels.

The appearance in serum of complement components before IgM reflects the fact that, together with phagocytic cells, complement was the main immune protection for animals before the evolutionary development of antibodies. Thus, to some extent, ontogeny recapitulates phylogeny.

■ LYMPHOID CELLS

Lymphocytes develop in the primary lymphoid organs – T cells in the thymus, and B cells in the bursa of Fabricius (birds) or in the fetal liver and bone marrow (mammals). These cells then migrate to the secondary lymphoid tissues, where they can respond to antigen.

T cells develop in the thymus
Stem-cell immigration initiates development

The thymus develops from the third (and in some species also from the fourth) pharyngeal pouch, as an epithelial rudiment of endodermal origin which becomes seeded with blood-borne stem cells, possibly originating in the yolk sac. Relatively few stem cells appear to be needed to

give rise to the enormous repertoire of mature T cells with diverse antigen receptor specificities. At least in the mouse, two layers of embryonic tissue are involved in the formation of the thymic anlage: the ectoderm of the 3rd branchial cleft that forms the epithelium of the thymic cortex, and the endothelium of the 3rd pharyngeal pouch that differentiates into the epithelium of the thymic medulla.

Migration of stem cells into the thymus is not a random process but results from chemotactic signals periodically emitted from the thymic rudiment. In birds, stem cells enter the thymus in two or possibly three waves. This has been demonstrated using chicken and quail chimeras (*Fig. 10.6*). Once in the thymus, the stem cells begin to differentiate into thymic lymphocytes (called thymocytes), under the influence of the epithelial microenvironment.

Development of the complement system

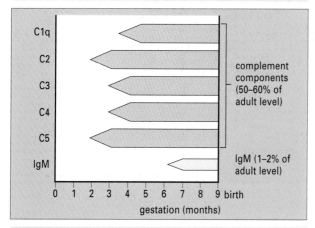

Fig. 10.5 This bar diagram shows the earliest times at which the components of the complement system can be detected in human fetal tissue. The levels of most complement components reach more than 50% of their adult value by birth. By comparison, immunoglobulins are not produced by the fetus until much later.

Stem cell colonization of the chick thymus

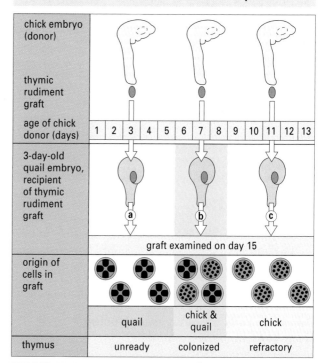

Fig. 10.6 Thymic rudiments from chick embryos of different ages were grafted onto 3-day-old quail embryos and later examined to determine the origin of cells in the thymus. Quail cells can be distinguished from chicken cells by the appearance of condensed chromatin in the resting cell. Grafts made at less than 6 days of age were later found to contain quail cells only (**a**), showing that they had not become colonized with chick stem cells before grafting. If the graft was made after 8 days it was later found to be colonized with chick lymphocytes (**c**). Grafts transferred between 6 and 8 days contained both chick and quail cells (**b**). The interpretation is that before 6 days the chick thymus is not ready to receive stem cells. There follows a window of colonization, after which (from day 8) the thymus is refractory to further colonization. Further studies indicate that there may be additional windows open later in embryogenesis.

Whether or not the stem cells are 'pre-T cells', i.e. are committed to becoming T cells before they arrive in the thymus, is controversial. Although the stem cells express CD7, substantial evidence exists that they are in fact multipotent.

T-cell development occurs as thymocytes move from cortex to medulla

The thymus is organized into lobules. Each thymic lobule has cortical and medullary areas (see Chapter 3) where epithelial cells, macrophages and bone marrow-derived interdigitating cells, rich in MHC class II antigens, are found. All three types of cell are important in the differentiation of the T lymphocytes (*Fig. 10.7*). For example, specialized epithelial cells in the peripheral areas of the cortex (thymic 'nurse' cells) contain intracytoplasmic thymocytes within vesicles in their cytoplasm and may be involved in the process of thymic education (see below). The subcapsular region of the thymus is the first to be colonized by stem cells arriving from the bone marrow. These cells develop into large, actively proliferating, self-renewing lymphoblasts which generate the thymocyte population.

There are many more developing lymphocytes (85–90%) in the thymic cortex than are in the medulla. Moreover, studies of function and cell surface markers have indicated that cortical thymocytes are less mature than medullary thymocytes. This reflects the fact that cortical cells migrate to, and mature in, the medulla. Most mature T cells leave the thymus via post-capillary venules located at the corticomedullary junction. However, other routes of exit may exist, including lymphatic vessels.

T cells alter their phenotype during maturation

As with the development of granulocytes and monocytes, 'differentiation' markers of functional significance appear or are lost during the progression from stem cell to mature T cell. Analyses of genes coding for αβ and γδ T-cell receptors, and other studies examining changes in surface membrane antigens, suggest that there are at least two pathways of T-cell differentiation in the thymus. It is not known whether these pathways are distinct, but it seems more likely that they diverge from a common pathway. Only a small proportion, less than 1%, of mature thymic lymphocytes express the γδ TCR. Most thymocytes differentiate into αβ TCR cells, which account for the majority (>99%) of T lymphocytes found in the secondary lymphoid tissues and in the circulation (see Chapter 2).

Phenotypic analyses have shown a succession of changes in surface membrane antigens during T-cell maturation (*Fig. 10.8*). The phenotypic variations can be simplified into a three-stage model.

Stage I (early) thymocytes – These thymocytes express CD7 together with CD2 and CD5. Proliferation markers such as the transferrin receptor (CD71) and CD38 (a marker common to all early haemopoietic precursors) are also expressed at this stage. Note that none of the proliferation markers are T lineage-specific. However, the commitment of early thymocytes to become T cells is shown by the TCR β-chain gene rearrangements, and by expression of the TCR-associated complex (CD3) in the cytoplasm but not on the membrane.

Position and structure of the thymus

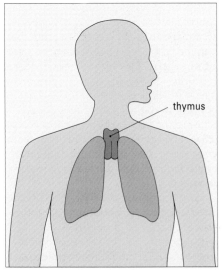
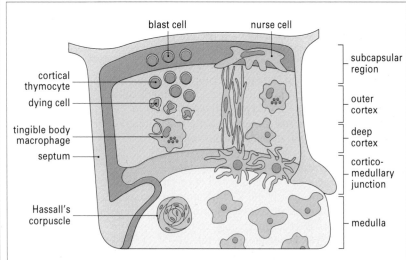

Fig. 10.7 The bilobed thymus is an encapsulated organ divided into lobules by septa. The cortex contains densely packed, dividing cortical thymocytes in a network of epithelial cells which extends into the medulla. The medulla contains fewer lymphocytes, but there are more bone-marrow derived antigen-presenting cells, both interdigitating cells and macrophages. There is a close association of the developing lymphocytes with epithelial cells and interdigitating cells, which are particularly numerous at the corticomedullary junction. The function of the whorled epithelial structures termed Hassall's corpuscles is unknown.

Fig. 10.8 Expression of human T-cell markers during development. Tdt (terminal deoxynucleotidyl transferase) is an enzyme which is present in thymic stem cells, decreases in stage II and is lost altogether in the medulla. Several surface glycoproteins appear during differentiation. CD1 is present on stage II cortical thymocytes and is lost in the medulla. CD2 and CD7 (the pan-T marker) appear very early in differentiation and are maintained through to the mature T-cell stage. CD5 appears at an early stage and persists on mature T cells. CD3 is expressed first in the cytoplasm in stage I cells (cyto), and then on the surface simultaneously with the TCR. In most stage II cells, both surface CD3 and the αβ TCR are expressed at low density,

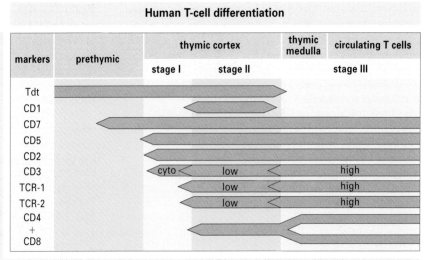

Human T-cell differentiation

markers	prethymic	thymic cortex		thymic medulla	circulating T cells
		stage I	stage II		stage III
Tdt					
CD1					
CD7					
CD5					
CD2					
CD3		cyto	low		high
TCR-1			low		high
TCR-2			low		high
CD4 + CD8					

but are present at high density on stage III cells. CD4 and CD8 are co-expressed on stage II cells (double positives). One of these molecules is lost during differentiation into mature stage III cells (single positives).

Stage II (intermediate or common) thymocytes – These account for around 85% of lymphoid cells in the thymus at any one time. They are characterized by the appearance of additional surface markers such as CD1, and by the co-expression of CD4 and CD8 on the same cell (such cells are called 'double positives'). Genes encoding the TCR α chain are rearranged in these intermediate thymocytes; both chains of the αβ receptor are expressed at low density on the cell surface in association with polypeptides of the CD3–antigen complex.

Stage III (mature) thymocytes – These show major phenotypic changes – namely loss of CD1, presence on the cell membrane of CD3 associated with the high density αβ TCR, and the distinction of two subsets of cells expressing either CD4 or CD8. The majority of thymocytes at this stage lack CD38 and the transferrin receptor, and are virtually indistinguishable from mature, circulating T cells. All these cells express the receptor CD44, thought to be involved in migration and homing to peripheral lymphoid tissues. L-selection also develops at this time.

T-cell receptor diversity is generated in the thymus

T cells have to recognize a wide variety of different antigens. The genes of the αβ and γδ TCR undergo somatic recombination during thymic development to produce functional genes for the different T-cell receptors (see chapter 6). The β and δ chains are encoded by V, D and J segments. The α and γ chains use only V and J segments. The first TCR genes to rearrange during T-cell development encode the γ chains and this is followed by rearrangement of the β and α chain genes. Through a random assortment of the different gene segments, a large number of productive rearrangements are made. These result in the expression of diverse variable-region peptide

sequences for both chains of the TCR. Thymocytes that make non-productive rearrangements are destroyed.

Initial surface expression of the TCR is at low density. This takes place within the subcapsular and outer cortex of the thymus, where there is active cell proliferation.

Positive and negative selection of developing T cells occurs in the thymus

Positive selection – T cells recognize antigenic peptides only when presented by self-MHC molecules on APCs (see Chapters 5 and 7). In effect, T cells show 'dual recognition' of both the antigenic peptides and the polymorphic part of the MHC molecules. (CD4, found on some subsets of T cells, also attaches to the class II molecule, but to the non-polymorphic portion.) Positive selection (also called thymic education) ensures that only those TCRs with a moderate affinity for self-MHC are allowed to develop further. There is evidence that positive selection is mediated through thymic epithelial cells, acting as APCs (*Fig. 10.9*). T cells displaying very high or very low receptor affinities for self-MHC undergo apoptosis and die in the cortex. Apoptosis is a pre-programmed 'suicide', achieved by activating endogenous nucleases that cause DNA fragmentation (*Fig. 10.10*).

T cells with receptors with intermediate affinities are rescued from apoptosis, survive, and continue along their pathway of maturation.

Negative selection – Some of the positively selected T cells may have receptors that recognize selfcomponents other than self-MHC. These cells are deleted by a 'negative selection' process, which occurs in the deeper cortex, at the corticomedullary junction and in the medulla. The thymocytes interact with antigen, interdigitating cells and macrophages. Only thymocytes that fail to recognize self-antigen are allowed to proceed. The rest undergo apoptosis and are destroyed. These, and all the other apoptotic cells generated in the thymus, are phagocytosed by tingible body macrophages in the deep cortex. The existence of negative selection (also called central tolerance) has recently received strong experimental support from murine studies in which specific Vβ families are eliminated by certain endogenous superantigens during thymic development (see Chapter 11).

T cells at this stage of maturation (CD4$^+$ CD8$^+$ TCR^{lo}) go on to express TCR at high density and lose either CD4 or CD8, becoming 'single positive' mature thymocytes. These separate subsets of CD4$^+$ and CD8$^+$ cells possess specialized homing receptors, and exit to the T-cell areas of the peripheral lymphoid tissues where they function primarily as mature 'helper' and 'cytotoxic' T cells respectively. Fewer than 5% of thymocytes leave the thymus. The rest die as the result of selection processes (*Fig. 10.11*) and failure to express antigen receptors.

The role of adhesion molecules and cytokines in thymic development

It has been shown that the adhesion of maturing thymocytes to epithelial and accessory cells is crucial for T-cell development. This adhesion is mediated by the interaction of complementary adhesion molecules, such as CD2 with LFA-3 (CD58), and LFA-1 (CD11a, CD18) with ICAM-1 (CD54).

Such interactions induce the production of the cytokines IL-1, IL-3, IL-6 and GM–CSF, which are required for T-cell maturation in the thymus. Thymocytes also express receptors for IL-2. This cytokine, together with other molecules, promotes cell proliferation which mainly occurs in the subcapsular and outer cortex.

Some T cells develop outside the thymus
Negative selection may occur in the periphery

Not all self-reactive T cells are eliminated during intrathymic development. This is probably because not all selfantigens are able to move through the thymic tissues. The thymic epithelial barrier may also limit access to some circulatory antigens. Given the survival of some self-reacting T cells, a separate mechanism is required to prevent

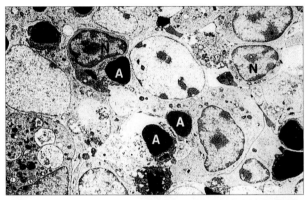

Fig. 10.10 Thymic cell apoptosis. Upper: Fetal thymic lobes in culture were treated with anti-CD3 antibodies – this simulates activation via the TCR and therefore triggers programmed cell death (apoptosis). This electron micrograph shows the heavy condensation of nuclear chromatin in apoptotic nuclei (A) as compared with the dispersed chromatin of normal cells (N). (Courtesy of Dr C. Smith.) **Lower:** Analysis of the DNA from apoptotic cells by agarose gel electrophoresis shows the characteristically ordered, ladder-like pattern created by bands of digested fragments.

T cell–MHC restriction occurs in the thymus

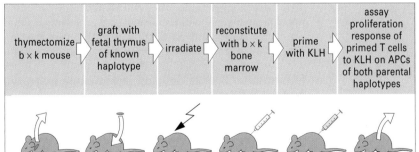

mouse type	engrafted fetal thymus type	proliferation response to APCs from each parental strain	
		H–2^b	H–2^k
b × k	b × k	++	++
b × k	b	++	−
b × k	b(dG-treated)	++	−
b × k	k	−	++
b × k	k(dG-treated)	−	++

Fig. 10.9 Host mice (F$_1$ [H–2^b × H–2^k]) were thymectomized, then grafted with 14-day fetal thymuses of various genotypes. They were subsequently irradiated to remove their resident T-cell populations, then reconstituted with F$_1$ bone marrow to provide stem cells. Following priming with antigen (keyhole limpet haemocyanin, KLH) the proliferative responses of lymph node T cells to KLH on APCs from each parental strain were evaluated. In some experiments,

thymus lobes were incubated before grafting with deoxyguanosine (dG), which destroys intrathymic cells of macrophage/dendritic cell lineage. The results show firstly that (1) the thymic environment is necessary for T cells to learn to recognize MHC, and (2) that bone-marrow-derived macrophages/dendritic cells (removed by dG treatment) are not required for this process to occur. (Adapted from Lo and Sprent, *Nature* 1986:**319**;672.)

T-cell differentiation and negative and positive selection in the thymus

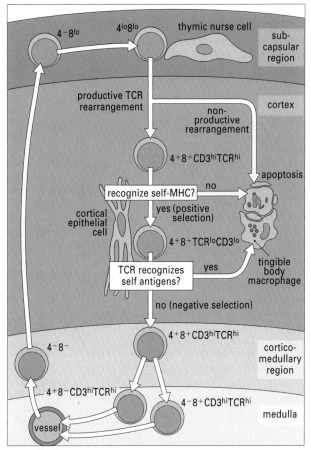

Fig. 10.11 In this model pre-thymic T cells are attracted to and enter the thymic rudiment. They proliferate below the sub-capsular region as large lymphoblasts, which replicate and give rise to a pool of cells entering the differentiation pathway. Many of these cells are associated with epithelial thymic nurse cells (TNCs), although the significance of this interaction is still debated. Cells in this region first acquire CD8 and then CD4 at low density. They also re-arrange their TCR genes and may express the products of these genes at low density on the cell surface. Maturing cells move deeper into the cortex and adhere to cortical epithelial cells. These epithelial cells are elongated and branched, and thus provide a large surface area for contact with thymocytes. The TCRs on the thymocytes are exposed to epithelial MHC molecules through these contacts. This leads to positive selection. Those cells which are not selected undergo apoptosis and are phagocytosed by macrophages. There is an increased expression of CD3, TCR, CD4 and CD8 during thymocyte migration from the subcapsular region to the deeper cortex. Those TCRs with self-reactivity are now deleted through contact with autoantigens presented by interdigitating cells and macrophages at the corticomedullary junction – a process called negative selection. Medullary epithelial cells might also contribute to this process. Following this stage, cells expressing either CD4 or CD8 appear and exit to the periphery via specialized vessels at the corticomedullary junction. (A process of negative selection may also occur in the cortex, leading to the elimination of cells whose TCRs have high affinity for self-MHC.)

their attacking the body. Recent experiments with transgenic mice have suggested that peripheral inactivation of self-reactive T cells (peripheral tolerance) could have two mechanisms:

- Downregulation of TCR and CD8 (in cytotoxic cells) so that the cells are unable to interact with target autoantigens.
- Anergy, due to the lack of crucial secondary activation signals provided by the target cells.

Peripheral tolerance is discussed in more detail in chapter 12.

Extrathymic T-cell development

Although the vast majority of T cells require a functioning thymus for their differentiation, small numbers of cells (often oligoclonal in nature) carrying T-cell markers have been found in athymic ('nude') mice. The possibility that these mice possess thymic remnants cannot be ruled out. However, there is accumulating experimental evidence to suggest that bone-marrow precursors can home to mucosal epithelia and mature to form functional T cells with $\gamma\delta$ TCRs, and probably also T cells with $\alpha\beta$ TCRs, without the need for a thymus. The importance of extrathymic development in animals that are euthymic (i.e. that have a normal thymus) is at present unclear.

T cells in the neonate are immature

Most T cells in neonatal blood are $CD45RA^+$, an observation that is consistent with the idea that they are mostly antigen-naïve. Furthermore, exposure of neonatal T cells to a variety of antigens results in the production of less interferon-γ (and probably other cytokines) than adult T cells.

Avian B cells develop in the bursa of Fabricius

Primary B-cell lymphopoiesis in birds occurs in a discrete lymphoepithelial organ, the bursa of Fabricius. The bursal rudiment develops as an outpushing of the hindgut endoderm and becomes seeded with blood-borne stem cells. Studies on chicken/quail chimeras have indicated that there is a window for the immigration of stem cells into the bursa between days 10 and 14 of embryonic life (see Chapter 15). Pyroninophylic cells – the putative stem cells – are seen in contact with epithelial cells. Bursal cell proliferation gives rise to the cortex and the medulla in each bursal follicle, which may be seeded by one or a few stem cells (*Fig. 10.12*).

Mammalian B cells develop in the bone marrow and fetal liver

Mammals do not have a specific discrete organ for B-cell lymphopoiesis. Instead, these cells develop directly from lymphoid stem cells in the haemopoietic tissue of the fetal liver (*Fig. 10.13*) from 8–9 weeks of gestation in humans, and by about 14 days in the mouse. Later the site of B-cell production moves from the liver to the bone marrow, where it continues into adult life. This is also true of the other haemopoietic lineages, giving rise to erythrocytes, granulocytes, monocytes and platelets. Recent data have indicated that B-cell progenitors are also present in the omental tissue of murine and human fetuses. Whether or not these B-cell progenitors precede those in the fetal liver remains to be established.

B-cell production in the bone marrow does not occur in distinct domains

B-cell progenitors in the bone marrow are seen adjacent to the endosteum of the bone lamellae. Each B-cell progenitor, at the stage of immunoglobulin gene rearrangement, may produce up to 64 progeny. These migrate towards the centre of each cavity of the spongy bone and reach the lumen of a venous sinusoid. In the bone marrow, B cells mature in close association with stromal reticular cells. The latter are found both adjacent to the endosteum and in close association with the central sinus, where they are termed adventitial reticular cells (*Fig. 10.14*). Reticular cells have mixed phenotypic features with some similarities to fibroblasts, endothelial cells and smooth muscle cells. They produce type IV collagen, laminin and the smooth-muscle form of actin. Experiments *in vitro* have

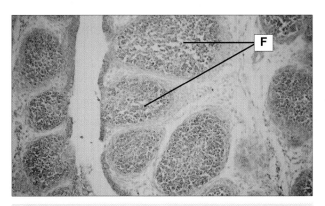

Fig. 10.12 Section of a bursa showing B cells developing in follicles (F). The bursa is also a site of some granulocytopoiesis for a short period of embryonic life. H&E stain, × 50.

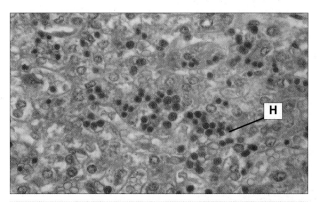

Fig. 10.13 Section of human fetal liver showing islands of haemopoiesis (H). Haemopoietic stem cells (HSCs) give rise to islands of differentiating lineage-specific cells, including B cells.

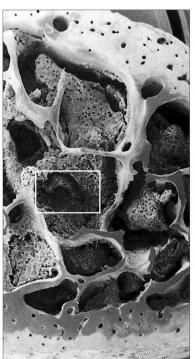

A model for B-cell differentiation in the bone marrow

progenitors | pre-B | immature/mature B

stromal reticular cell

phagocytosis

endosteum

central sinus

Fig. 10.14 Left: Low power scanning electron micrograph showing the architecture of bone and its relationship to bone marrow. A cavity has been picked out and is drawn schematically on the right. (Courtesy of Drs A. Stevens and J. Lowe). **Right:** Within the cavities of spongy bone, B-cell lymphopoiesis takes place with maturation occurring in a radial direction towards the centre (from the endosteum to the central venous sinus). Immature progenitor cells adjacent to the endosteal cell layer mature into pre-B cells, most of which die and are phagocytosed by bone-marrow macrophages containing tingible bodies (stained by haematoxylin). Cells which survive mature further and reach the central venous sinus. Association with reticular cells, and the presence of cytokines such as IL-7 is essential for all steps of B-cell maturation. (Adapted from Osmond D, Gallagher R. *Immunol Today* 1991:**12**;1–3).

shown that reticular cells sustain B-cell differentiation. Adventitial reticular cells may be important for the release of mature B cells into the central sinus.

B cells are also subject to selection processes

The majority of B cells (over 75%) maturing in the bone marrow do not reach the circulation but (like thymocytes) undergo a process of programmed cell death or apoptosis, and are phagocytosed by bone marrow macrophages. It has been suggested that B-cell–stromal interactions may mediate a form of positive selection that rescues a minority of B cells with productive rearrangements of their immunoglobulin genes from programmed cell death. Negative selection of autoreactive B cells may occur in the bone marrow or in the spleen, the site to which the majority of newly produced B cells are exported.

From kinetic data, it is estimated that about 5×10^7 murine B cells are produced each day. Since the mouse spleen contains approximately 7.5×10^7 B cells, a large proportion of B cells must die, probably at the pre-B cell stage due to non-productive rearrangements of receptor genes or if they acquire self-reactive antibody receptors.

Immunoglobulins are the characteristic markers of the B-cell lineage

Lymphoid stem cells, probably expressing terminal deoxynucleotidyl transferase, Tdt, proliferate, differentiate and undergo immunoglobulin gene rearrangements (see Chapter 6) to emerge as pre-B cells which express μ heavy chains in the cytoplasm. Some of these pre-B cells express small numbers of surface μ chains, associated with pseudo light chains. Allelic exclusion of either maternal or paternal immunoglobulin genes has already occurred by this time. The proliferating pre-B cells are thought to give rise to smaller pre-B cells. Once the B cell has synthesized light chains, which may be either κ- or λ-type, it is committed to the antigen-binding specificity of its sIgM antigen receptor. Thus, one B cell can make only one specific antibody, a central tenet of the clonal selection theory for antibody production. Surface immunoglobulin-associated molecules Igα and Igβ (CD79α and β) are present by the pro-B cell stage of development. A summary of B-cell differentiation, with expression of immunoglobulins and some other relevant molecules, is shown in *Figure 10.15*.

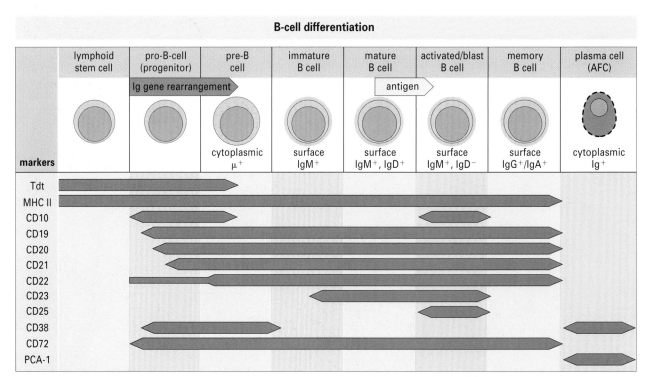

Fig. 10.15 B cells differentiate from lymphoid stem cells into virgin B cells and may then be driven by antigen to become memory cells or plasma cells. The cellular location of immunoglobulin is shown in yellow. The genes coding for antibody are rearranged in the course of progenitor cell development. Pre-B cells express cytoplasmic μ chains only. The immature B cell has surface IgM, and the mature B cell other immunoglobulin isotypes. On antigen stimulation the B cell proliferates and develops into a plasma cell or a memory cell following a phase of proliferation, activation and blast transformation. Memory cells and plasma cells are found at different sites in lymphoid tissue. Tdt is expressed very early in ontogeny. The diagram also shows the sequence of appearance of other relevant B cell surface markers. PCA-1 is found only on plasma cells. Note that CD38 is an example of a molecule found on early progenitors that is lost, only to reappear on the fully differentiated plasma cells.

Developing B cells develop characteristic surface markers

A sequence of immunoglobulin gene rearrangements and phenotypic changes takes place during B-cell ontogeny, similar to that described above for T cells. Heavy chain gene rearrangements occur in B-cell progenitors and represent the earliest indication of B-lineage commitment. This is followed by light chain gene rearrangements which occur at later pre-B cell stages. Certain B cell surface markers are expressed prior to immunoglobulin detection, namely class II MHC molecules, CD19, CD20, CD21 CD40 and the CD10 (CALLA) antigen. The last marker is a highly conserved neutral endopeptidase transiently expressed on early B progenitors before the appearance of heavy μ chains in the cytoplasm. CALLA is re-expressed later in the B-cell life history, following activation by antigen (*Fig. 10.15*). Other markers, e.g. CD23 and CD25 (IL-2 receptor α) are mostly found on activated B cells.

A number of growth and differentiation factors are required to drive the B cells through early stages of development. Receptors for these factors are expressed at various stages of B-cell differentiation. IL-7, IL-3 and low molecular weight B-cell growth factor (L–BCGF) are important in initiating the process of B-cell differentiation, whereas other factors are active in the later stages (*Fig. 10.16*).

B cells migrate and function in the secondary lymphoid tissue

Early B-cell immigrants into fetal lymph nodes (17 weeks in man) are sIgM⁺ and carry a T-cell marker (CD5). CD5⁺ B-cell precursors are found in the fetal omentum. Small numbers of CD5⁺ B cells are also found in the mantle zone of secondary follicles in adult lymph nodes.

Following antigenic stimulation, mature B cells can develop into memory cells or antibody-forming cells (AFCs). Surface immunoglobulin (sIg) is usually lost by the plasma cell (the terminally differentiated form of an AFC), since its function as a receptor is finished. Like any other terminally differentiated haemopoietic cell, the plasma cell has a limited lifespan, and eventually undergoes apoptosis (see *Fig 2.24*).

Immature and mature B cells respond in different ways to antigens. Treatment with anti-IgM antibodies or antigen results in loss of sIgM by capping and endocytosis in both mature and immature B cells. However, only mature B cells resynthesize sIgM in culture (*Fig. 10.17*). Since immature B cells can be induced to lose their antigen receptor, this could be one mechanism by which self-reactive B cells are rendered tolerant during development.

Resynthesis of sIgM on mature and immature B cells

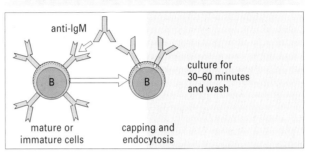

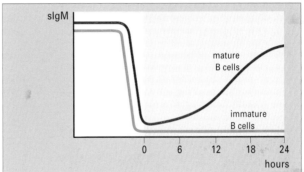

Fig. 10.17 Mature (adult) and immature (neonatal) B cells are incubated at 37°C together with antibody to their sIgM (anti-IgM) for 30–60 minutes; this causes capping of the sIgM and its internalization by endocytosis. The cells are then washed free of anti-immunoglobulin. As shown in the graph, mature B cells resynthesize their sIgM over the following 24 hours, but immature B cells do not.

Cytokine receptor expression during B-cell development

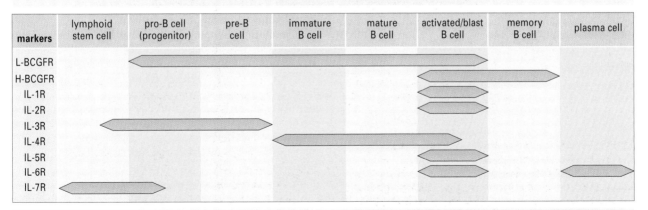

markers	lymphoid stem cell	pro-B cell (progenitor)	pre-B cell	immature B cell	mature B cell	activated/blast B cell	memory B cell	plasma cell
L-BCGFR		◁———————————————————————▷						
H-BCGFR						◁——————▷		
IL-1R						◁——▷		
IL-2R						◁——▷		
IL-3R		◁——————————▷						
IL-4R				◁——————————————▷				
IL-5R						◁——▷		
IL-6R						◁——▷		◁▷
IL-7R	◁——————▷							

Fig. 10.16 The whole life history of B cells from stem cell to mature plasma cell is regulated by cytokines present in their environment. Receptors for these cytokines are selectively expressed by B cells at different stages of development. IL-7 plays an important role in initiating events in B-cell differentiation. Some of these receptors now have CD markers (see Appendix).

DIVERSITY OF ANTIBODY SPECIFICITY

Antibody diversity is generated by genetic recombination

The variable region genes comprising V, D and J segments are present in every somatic cell in a germline configuration (see Chapter 6). During early B-cell development intervening sequences between D and J are deleted, bringing these genes closer together. Further rearrangements of the V, D and J segments of the variable region heavy chain genes (VH) occur during the progenitor stage of B-cell development (*Fig. 10.15*). The recombined heavy chain gene is expressed with a μ heavy chain gene in the cytoplasm of the large pre-B cell. These actively proliferating pre-B cells then rearrange their Vκ genes, and later their Vλ genes if the κ rearrangement has not been successful. When a light chain gene is productively rearranged the immature B cell expresses surface μ chains with the available light chain (κ or λ). Those cells not making productive rearrangements die by apoptosis. This is one explanation as to why so many pre-B cells die during development (see above). There is some evidence that pseudo-light-chain genes are expressed prior to κ and λ light chains, and that these may assemble small amounts of surface IgM on pre-B cells. This might be important in selection of early pre-B cells.

The generation of antibody diversity is not entirely random

Once the κ or λ light chains are being produced, the surface IgM on the immature B cell can act as a functional antigen receptor. The rearrangements of the V, D and J segments (heavy chains) and V and J segments (light chains) are thought to be randomly generated within the B cells. However, there is evidence in mice, rats and chickens for a programmed sequence of development of specific antibody specificities (*Fig. 10.18*). Antibody production, as distinct from antigen recognition by B cells is, however, dependent on both T cells and APCs. The reason for this programmed development of specificities at the molecular level within B cells is unclear, but it may reflect the biased utilization of V gene segments nearest to the D or J segments, with a 3' directional movement of the relevant recombinases and/or some negative selection of particular clones (possibly for self-reactivities).

CD5⁺ B lymphocytes are a distinctive cell population

Many of the first B cells to appear in ontogeny express CD5. These B cells express their immunoglobulins from unmutated or minimally mutated germline genes. $CD5^+$ B cells produce mostly IgM, but also some IgG and IgA. These so-called natural antibodies are of low avidity but, unusually, are polyreactive. They are found at high concentration in adult serum. $CD5^+$ cells may respond well to T_{ind} antigens. They may also be involved in antigen processing and antigen presentation to T cells, and probably play a role in both tolerance and antibody responses. Functions proposed for natural antibodies include the following: the first line of defence against microorganisms; clearance of damaged self components; and 'idiotype network' interactions within the immune system.

DIVERSITY OF ANTIBODY CLASS

B cells produce antibodies of five major classes: IgM, IgD, IgG, IgA and IgE. There are also 4 subclasses of IgG and 2 of IgA (see Chapter 4). Each terminally differentiated plasma cell is derived from a specific B cell and produces antibodies of just one class or subclass.

B cells switch immunoglobulin class by recombining heavy chain genes

The first B cells to appear during development carry surface IgM as their antigen receptor (see above). This is followed by expression of other classes of immunoglobulin. That the cells carrying non-IgM classes are the progeny of the IgM-bearing B cells was shown by experiments where chickens or mice treated with anti-μ antibodies failed to develop antibodies of any immunoglobulin class. The constant region genes encoding the different heavy chains (CH) are responsible for the antibody classes and subclasses. These are clustered at the 3' end of the immunoglobulin heavy chain (IgH) locus and appear in a particular sequence along the chromosome. B cells switch from IgM to the other classes or subclasses by a process of recombination between highly repetitive switch regions 3' to each CH gene, and by the deletion of intervening CH genes. The details of this pro-

Development of immune responsiveness

age (days)	Brucella	SRBC	DRBC	KLH	SSS$_{III}$
0	4.7	0	0	0	0
1	5.3	0	0	0	0
2		0	0		
3	7.3	2.9	0	0	0
4		5.4	0		
7			0.6	0	0
10–11			3.0	7.7	0
14–15			4.3	10.4	16%
20–22					70%
28					88%

Fig. 10.18 Five different antigens – *Brucella abortus*, sheep red blood cell (SRBC), donkey red blood cell (DRBC), keyhole limpet haemocyanin (KLH) and type III pneumococcal polysaccharide (SSS$_{III}$) – were injected into neonatal rats of different ages. The antibody responses were then measured. The responses to the first four antigens are expressed as log$_2$ antibody titres. The response to SSS$_{III}$ is expressed as a percentage of animals responding. Blank boxes indicate 'not tested'. Note how the ability to respond to different antigens appears at different times, indicating the programmed first appearance of antibodies of that specificity.

cess, which is known as isotype switching, are given in Chapter 6. Some B cells express IgM and IgD isotype on their surface. This is due to the differential splicing of long nuclear RNA transcripts of the CH genes.

Isotype switching happens during maturation and during proliferation

Most isotype switching probably occurs during proliferation. However, it can also take place prior to encounter with exogenous antigen during early clonal expansion and maturation of the B cells (*Fig. 10.19*). We know this because some of the progeny of immature B cells synthesize antibodies of other immunoglobulin classes, including IgG and IgA. Further B-cell differentiation results in synthesis of surface IgD – an antibody class that is found almost exclusively on B-cell membranes. Different classes of sIg on the same B cell have the same antigen specificity, that is to say they express the same V region genes, although later additional diversity within a single clone may be generated by somatic mutation following class switching. Evidence that some class switching can occur independently of antigen comes from experiments with vertebrates raised in gnotobiotic (virtually sterile) environments, which are severely restricted in their exposure to exogenous antigens. Such animals show a sequence of expression of different isotypes on B cells similar to that seen in control animals.

Isotype expression can be influenced by the type of antigen

It is well documented that certain antigens induce antibody responses dominated by different immunoglobulin isotypes. In mice for example, carbohydrates in bacterial cell walls give rise to T-cell independent immune responses which are dominated by IgG3 antibodies, whereas in responses to viral infections, IgG2a antibodies are more common. In man, the IgG2 subclass of antibodies dominates in anti-polysaccharide responses. This isotype bias could be mediated by two mechanisms:

- The B cell clones that are selected have already switched classes spontaneously (*Fig. 10.19*).
- Switching is induced *de novo* as the result of interaction with accessory cell-derived cytokines.

There is now considerable evidence for the role of T cells and their cytokines in *de novo* isotype switching. In the mouse, T cells in mucosal sites have been shown to preferentially stimulate IgA production. IL-4 preferentially switches B cells that have been polyclonally activated (by lipopolysaccharide, LPS) to the IgG1 isotype, with concomitant suppression of the other isotypes (*Fig. 10.20*). In a similar system, IL-5 induces a five-to-ten-fold increase in IgA production with no change in the other isotypes, while IFNγ enhances IgG2a responses but suppresses all the other isotypes. It is interesting that IL-4 and IFNγ, which act as reciprocal regulatory cytokines in expression of antibody isotypes, are derived from different TH subsets. TH1 cells produce IFNγ in the mouse; TH2 cells produce IL-4, IL-5 and IL-10 (see Chapter 8). More recently, similar subsets have been described in man, and T-cell derived IL-4 has been shown to be involved in the overproduction of IgE in atopic individuals.

B-cell differentiation: class diversity

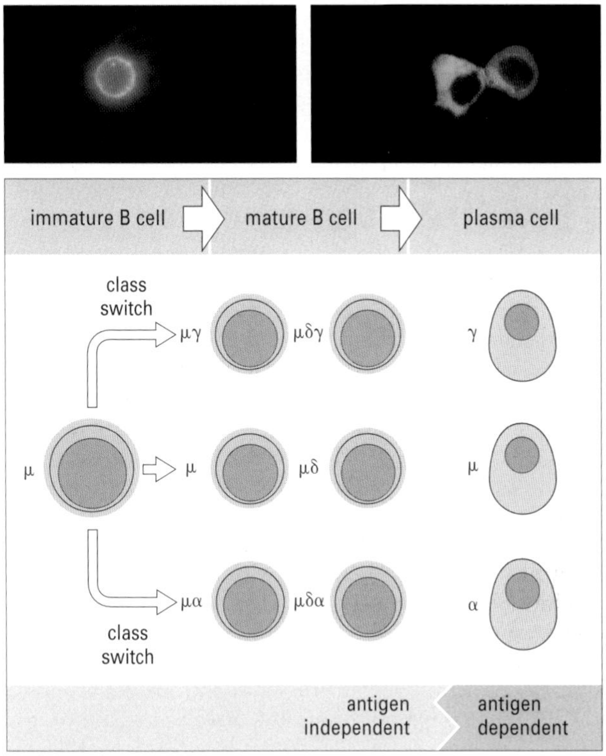

Fig. 10.19 Immature B cells produce IgM only, but mature B cells can express more than one cell surface antibody, since mRNA and cell surface immunoglobulin remain after a class switch. IgD is also expressed during clonal maturation. Maturation can occur in the absence of antigen, but the development into plasma cells (which have little surface immunoglobulin but much cytoplasmic immunoglobulin) requires antigen and (usually) T-cell help. The photographs show B cells stained for surface IgM (green, left) and plasma cells stained for cytoplasmic IgM and IgG (green and red, right). IgM is stained with fluorescent anti-μ chain, and IgG with rhodaminated anti-γ chain.

Isotype regulation by murine T-cell cytokines

TH	cytokines	immunoglobulin isotypes					
		IgG1	IgE	IgA	Ig3	IgG2b	IgG2a
TH2	IL-4	↑	↑	↓	↓	↓	↓
	IL-5	=	=	↑	=	=	=
TH1	IFNγ	↓	↓	↓	↓	↓	↑

Fig. 10.20 This figure shows the effects of IFNγ (product of TH1 cells) and IL-4 and IL-5 (products of TH2 cells) which result in an increase (↑), a decrease (↓) or no change (=) in the frequency of isotype-specific B cells following stimulation with the polyclonal activator – lipopolysaccharide (LPS) *in vitro*. Whereas IFNγ induces IgG2a isotype, IL-4 induces IgG1 and IgE antibodies. IL-5 enhances B cells secreting IgA.

The sequence of appearance of immunoglobulin classes by B cells during development is reflected in the serum immunoglobulins detected in the human fetus and neonate. IgM is synthesized before birth whilst IgG and IgA begin to appear around birth (*Fig. 10.21*). Serum IgG does not reach adult levels until 1–2 years after birth, and IgA takes even longer.

■ DEVELOPMENT OF MEMORY B CELLS

When B cells are activated by antigen (with T-cell help), they either mature into AFCs and then into end-stage plasma cells, or they develop into memory cells. There is now substantial evidence that germinal centres in the various lymphoid tissues (see Chapter 3) are important as sites of development of memory B cells. At these sites, the B cells undergo active hypermutation of their antibody variable-region genes, a process that can lead to death by apoptosis for some cells. As described below, cells with high-affinity receptors for foreign antigen are rescued from cell death by antigen presented within the germinal centres by follicular dendritic cells.

The process outlined above will now be described in more detail. Antigen-specific B cells colonizing the primary lymphoid follicles are primed by antigen and give rise to B-cell blasts. One or a very few B-cell blasts go on to form a germinal centre (*Fig. 10.22*). B-cell blasts prolifer-

ate at high rate and reach approximately 10^4 cells in 3–4 days. On the fourth day, the cells transform into centroblasts which have no surface immunoglobulin. These migrate to the interior-facing pole of the follicle where they form the dark zone. Centroblasts give rise to centrocytes which then re-express surface immunoglobulin and occupy the basal light zone of the germinal centre. During this period, following stimulation by antigen presented on follicular dendritic cells, hypermutation of the antibody variable-region genes in the B cell is thought to occur. Centrocytes are found in close association with follicular dendritic cells (FDCs), the interaction of which is mediated by LFA-1 (CD11a/CD18) and VLA-4 ($\alpha_4\beta_1$ integrin,

Schematic organization of the germinal centre

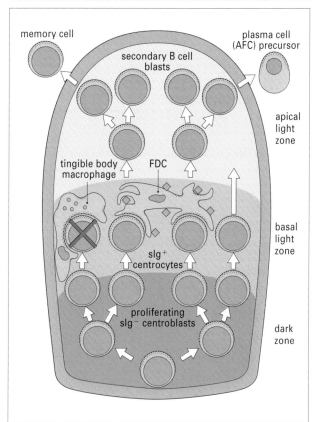

Fig. 10.22 Schematic organization of the germinal centre. In this model, the germinal centre is composed of three major zones, a dark zone, a basal light zone and an apical light zone. These zones are predominantly occupied by centroblasts, centrocytes and secondary blasts respectively. Primary B-cell blasts carrying surface immunoglobulin receptors (SIg^+) enter the follicle and leave as memory B cells or AFCs. Antigen-presenting follicular dendritic cells (FDCs) are mainly found in the two deeper zones, and cell death by apoptosis occurs primarily in the basal light zone where tingible body macrophages are also located. (Adapted from Roitt IM. *Essential Immunology* 7th ed. Oxford: Blackwell Scientific Press, 1991.)

Immunoglobulins in the serum of the fetus and newborn child

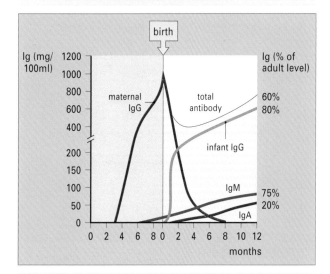

Fig. 10.21 IgG in the fetus and newborn infant is derived solely from the mother. This maternal IgG has disappeared by the age of 9 months, by which time the infant is synthesizing its own IgG. The neonate produces its own IgM and IgA: these classes cannot cross the placenta. By the age of 12 months, the infant produces 80% of its adult level of IgG, 75% of its adult IgM level and 20% of its adult IgA level.

CD49d/CD29) on the lymphocytes and ICAM-1 (CD54) and VCAM-1 (CD106) respectively on the FDC. Successful interactions of centrocytes bearing high-affinity receptors for antigen presented by the FDCs give rise to secondary blasts which leave the secondary follicles, either as memory cells or plasma cell precursors. Lack of centrocyte–FDC interaction leads to programmed cell death by apoptosis.

Critical Thinking

■ What factors are required for the development of granulocytes from haemopoietic stem cells?

■ How does development of myeloid cells differ from that of lymphoid cells? Why does it need to be different?

■ What are the main stages of T-cell development in the thymus?

■ What are the main similarities and differences between T and B cell development?

■ Why is cell death by apoptosis such a major feature of lymphocyte development?

■ What are the main functions of the germinal centres?

FURTHER READING

Boyd RL, *et al*. The thymic environment. *Immunol Today* 1993;**14**:445–59.

Gallagher RB, Osmond DG. To B, or not to B: that is the question. *Immunol Today* 1991;**12**:1.

Hamilton JA. Colony stimulating factors, cytokines and monocyte-macrophage – some controversies. *Immunol Today* 1993;**14**:18–24

Hannet II, Erkeller-Yuksel F, Lydyard PM, Denys V, DeBruyère M. Developmental and maturational changes in human blood lymphocyte subpopulations. *Immunol Today* 1992;**13**:215.

Rajewsky K, von Boehmer H, eds. Lymphocyte development. *Curr Opin Immunol* 1992;**4**:131–81.

Zouali M, MacLennan ICM. Molecular events in the development of the lymphocyte repertoire. *Immunol Today* 1992;**13**:41.

The immune response is subject to a variety of control mechanisms which serve to restore the immune system to a resting state when responsiveness to a given antigen is no longer required.

Many factors govern the outcome of any immune response. These include the antigen itself, its dose and route of administration and the genetic background of the individual responding to antigenic challenge.

Immunoglobulins can influence the immune response positively as anti-idiotype or through immune complex formation. They may also negatively influence immune responses by reducing antigenic challenge through masking of antigen determinants or clearance of antigen.

The antigen-presenting cell may affect the immune response through its ability to provide co-stimulation to T cells.

T cells can regulate the immune response. Transfer studies have shown that CD4[+] T cells can depress subsequent immune responses. CD8[+] T cells have also been implicated. Cytokine production by T cells has been shown to influence the type of immune response elicited by antigen.

Genetic factors which influence the immune system include both MHC-linked and non-MHC-linked genes. The neuroendocrine system influences immune responses. Genetic factors governing this system will also therefore affect the immune response.

The immune response, like all biological systems, is subject to a variety of control mechanisms. These mechanisms restore the immune system to a resting state when responsiveness to a given antigen is no longer required. An effective immune response is an outcome of the interplay between antigen and a network of immunologically competent cells. The nature of the immune response both qualitatively and quantitatively, is determined by many factors, including the form and route of administration of the antigen, the nature of the antigen-presenting cell, the genetic background of the individual and any history of previous exposure to the antigen in question or to a cross-reacting antigen. Specific antibodies may also modulate the immune response to an antigen. Some of these factors are discussed in detail elsewhere (see Chapters 8 and 9) and are dealt with only briefly here.

■ REGULATION BY ANTIGEN

T cells and B cells are triggered by antigen following effective engagement of their antigen-specific receptors. In the case of the T cell, this engagement is not with antigen itself but of processed antigenic peptide bound to MHC class I or class II molecules (see Chapter 7). The nature of an antigen, its dose and the route of administration have all been shown to profoundly influence the outcome of an immune response.

The nature of the antigen influences the type of immune response that occurs

Different antigens elicit different kinds of immune responses. Polysaccharide capsule antigens of bacteria generally induce IgM responses, whereas proteins can induce both cell-mediated and humoral immune responses. Intracellular organisms such as some bacteria, parasites or viruses induce a cell mediated immune response whereas soluble protein antigens induce a humoral response. A cell-mediated immune response is also induced by agents such as silica

An effective immune response removes antigen from the system. The lymphocytes then return to a quiescent state, since repeated antigen exposure is required to maintain T- and B-cell proliferation. However, some antigens (for example those of intracellular microorganisms) may not be cleared so effectively, leading to a sustained immune response which has pathological consequences (see Chapter 25).

Large doses of antigen can induce tolerance

Very large doses of antigen often result in specific T- and sometimes B-cell tolerance. T-independent polysaccharide antigens have been shown to generate tolerance in B cells following administration in high doses. Tolerance and its underlying mechanisms are discussed in Chapter 12.

The route of administration of an antigen can determine whether or not an immune response occurs

The route of administration of antigen has been shown to influence the immune response. Antigens administered subcutaneously or intradermally evoke an immune response whereas those given intravenously, orally or as an aerosol may cause tolerance or an immune deviation from one type of CD4[+] T cell response to another. For example, rodents that have been fed ovalbumin or myelin basic protein (MBP) do not respond effectively to a subsequent challenge with the corresponding antigen. Moreover, in the case of MBP, the animals are protected from the development of the autoimmune disease, experimental allergic encephalomyelitis (EAE). This phenomenon may have some therapeutic value in allergy; recent studies have shown that oral administration of a T cell epitope of the Der p1 allergen of house dust mite could tolerize to the whole antigen. With regard to mechanism(s) of such tolerance induction, both anergy and immune deviation have been implicated.

Similar observations have been made when antigen is given as an aerosol. Studies in mice have shown that aerosol administration of an encephalitogenic peptide inhibits the development of EAE that is normally induced by a conventional (subcutaneous) administration of the peptide (*Fig. 11.1*).

A clear example of how different routes of administration affect the outcome of the immune response is provided by studies of infection with lymphocytic choriomeningitis virus (LCMV). Mice primed subcutaneously with peptide in incomplete Freund's adjuvant develop immunity to LCMV. However, if the same peptide is repeatedly injected intraperitoneally, the animals become tolerized and cannot clear the virus (*Fig. 11.2*).

■ THE ANTIGEN-PRESENTING CELL

The nature of the APC initially presenting the antigen may determine whether responsiveness or tolerance ensues. Effective activation of T cells requires the expression of co-stimulatory molecules on the surface of the APC (see Chapter 8). Thus, presentation by dendritic cells or activated macrophages, which express high levels of MHC class II as well as costimulatory molecules, results in highly effective T cell activation (see *Fig. 8.4*). However, if antigen is presented to T cells by a 'non-professional' APC that is unable to provide co-stimulation, then unresponsiveness results. For example, when naive T cells are exposed to antigen by resting B cells they fail to respond and become tolerized. Adjuvants may facilitate immune responses by inducing expression of high levels of MHC and co-stimulatory molecules on APCs.

■ REGULATION BY ANTIBODY

Antibody has been shown to exert feedback control on the immune response. Passive administration of IgM antibody together with an antigen specifically enhances the immune response to that antigen, whereas IgG antibody suppresses the response. This was originally shown with polyclonal antibodies but has since been confirmed using monoclonal antibodies (*Fig. 11.3*).

The ability of passively administered antibody to enhance or suppress the immune response has certain clinical consequences and applications:

- **Certain vaccines** (e.g. mumps and measles) are not generally given to infants before one year of age. This is because levels of maternally-derived IgG remain high for at least six months after birth; the presence of such passively-acquired IgG at the time of vaccination would result in the development of an inadequate immune response in the baby.
- **In cases of Rhesus (Rh) incompatibility** the administration of anti-RhD antibody to Rh⁻ mothers prevents primary sensitization by fetally derived Rh⁺ blood cells, presumably by removing the foreign antigen (fetal erythrocytes) from the maternal circulation.

Peptide-induced inactivation of LCMV-specific T cells

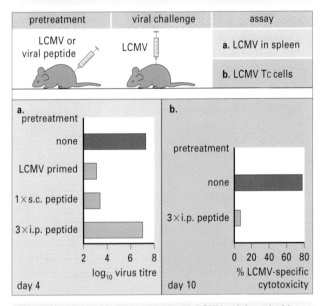

Fig. 11.2 Mice were either primed with LCMV or injected with 100 mg LCMV peptide. The peptide was given either subcutaneously (s.c.) or three times intraperitoneally (i.p.) with incomplete Freund's adjuvant. The animals were later infected with LCMV (day 0). The titre of virus in the spleen was measured on day 4. Animals that had been pretreated with subcutaneous peptide or with LCMV developed neutralizing antibody and protective immunity against the virus; animals pretreated with peptide i.p. did not develop immunity. Cytotoxic T cell activity was assessed in the mice on day 10. Mice that had received no pretreatment demonstrated Tc cells specific for the LCMV peptide. Mice pretreated with peptide i.p. failed to show such activity.

Aerosol administration of antigen modifies the immune response

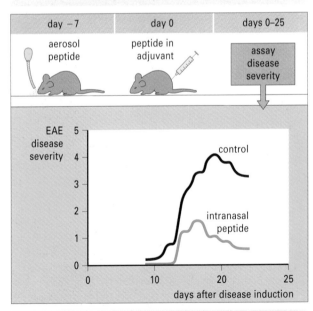

Fig. 11.1 Mice were treated with a single aerosol dose of either 100 mg peptide (residues 1–11 of myelin basic protein), or just the carrier. Seven days later the same peptide, this time in adjuvant, was administered subcutaneously. The subsequent development of EAE was significantly modified in pretreated animals.

Feedback control by antibody

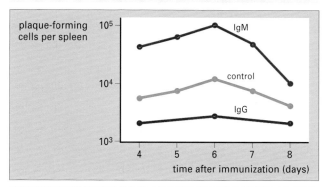

Fig. 11.3 Mice received either a monoclonal IgM anti-SRBC (sheep red blood cells), IgG anti-SRBC or medium alone (control). Two hours later, all groups were immunized with SRBC. The antibody response, measured over the following eight days, was enhanced by IgM and suppressed by IgG.

The mechanisms by which antibody modulates the immune response are not completely defined. In the case of IgM enhancing plaque forming cells, there are thought to be two possible interpretations:
- IgM-containing immune complexes are taken up by Fc receptors or C3 receptors on APCs and are processed more efficiently than antigen alone.
- IgM-containing immune complexes stimulate an anti-idiotypic response to the IgM, which amplifies the immune response. (Anti-idiotypes are discussed later in the chapter.)

IgG antibody can suppress specific IgG synthesis

For IgG-mediated suppression there are also various ways in which the antibody is known to act.

Antibody blocking – passively administered antibody binds antigen in competition with B cells (*Fig. 11.4*). The impact of the IgG in this case is highly dependent on the concentration of the antibody, and on its affinity for the antigen compared to the affinity of the B-cell receptors. Only high-affinity B cells compete successfully for the antigen. This mechanism is independent of the Fc portion of the antibody.

Receptor cross-linking – IgG antibody is also known to have an effect that is Fc dependent. Experiments have demonstrated that immunoglobulin can inhibit B cell differentiation by cross-linking the antigen receptor with the Fc receptor (FcγRII) on the same cell (see *Fig. 11.4*). In this case, the antibodies may recognize different epitopes.

Doses of IgG that are insufficient to inhibit completely the production of antibodies have the effect of increasing the average antibody affinity; this is because only those B cells with high-affinity receptors can successfully compete with the passively acquired antibody for antigen. For this reason, antibody feedback is thought to be an important factor driving the process of affinity maturation (*Fig. 11.5*).

Antibody-dependent B-cell suppression

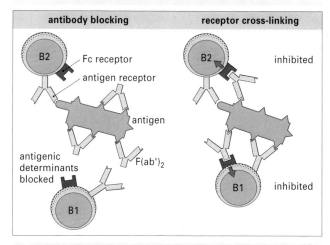

Fig. 11.4 Antibody blocking High doses of antibody (or its F(ab')₂ fragment) block the interaction between an antigenic determinant (epitope) and B-cell receptors for that determinant. The B cell is then effectively unable to recognize the antigen (B1). This receptor blocking mechanism also prevents B cell priming. B cells with receptors for different epitopes are unaffected (B2).

Receptor cross-linking Low doses of antibody (but not F(ab')₂) allow cross-linking by antigen of a B cell's Fc receptors and its antigen receptors. This allows B cell priming but inhibits antibody synthesis. The effect is not epitope-specific.

Antibody feedback affinity maturation

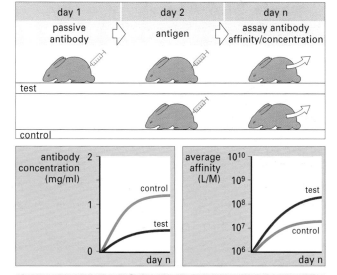

Fig. 11.5 The effect of passive antibody on the affinity and concentration of secreted antibody. One of two rabbits was injected with antibody (passive antibody) on day 1. Both rabbits were immunized with antigen on day 2 and the affinity and concentration of antibody raised to this antigen were assayed at a later time (day n). The antibody assay results show that passive antibody reduces the concentration, but increases the affinity, of antibody produced.

Regulatory effects of immune complexes

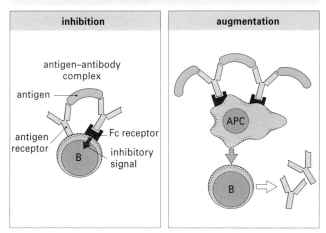

Fig. 11.6 Immune complexes can act either to inhibit or augment an immune response. **Inhibition** When the B cell's Fc receptor is cross-linked to its antigen receptor by an antigen–antibody complex, a signal is delivered to the B cell inhibiting it from entering the antibody production phase. Passive IgG may have this effect. **Augmentation** Antibody encourages presentation of antigen to B cells when it is present on an antigen-presenting cell (APC), bound via Fc receptors. (Complexes can also activate complement and then bind to APCs via their C3b receptors in an analogous way.) Passive IgM may have this effect.

Suppressor cells in immunological tolerance

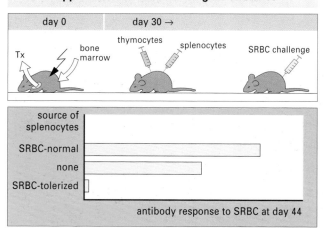

Fig. 11.7 Thymectomized and irradiated mice were reconstituted with bone marrow cells. After 30 days they were recolonized with thymocytes and splenocytes, and challenged with sheep red blood cells (SRBC). At day 44, recipients given splenocytes primed with an immunogenic dose of SRBC had made a strong response. Animals receiving no spleen cells had a moderate response. Animals receiving cells from mice tolerized to SRBC (with a high dose of antigen) did not respond, indicating that cells from tolerized animals had actively suppressed the response in the recipient.

Immune complexes may enhance or suppress immune responses

One of the ways in which antibody (either IgM or IgG) might act to modulate the immune response involves an Fc-dependent mechanism and immune-complex formation with antigen. Immune complexes can inhibit or augment the immune response (*Fig. 11.6*).

The immune response of patients with malignant tumours is often depressed, and it has been postulated that this is the result of the presence of circulating immune-complexes composed of antibody and tumour cell antigens.

■ REGULATION BY LYMPHOCYTES

T cells clearly modulate the immune response in a positive sense by providing T-cell help. Furthermore, the kind of help which is generated (TH1 versus TH2) affects the nature of the immune response, favouring either humoral or cell-mediated immunity. Additionally there is clear evidence that T cells are capable of downregulating immune responses (*Fig. 11.7*).

CD4⁺ T cells can prevent the induction of autoimmunity
The observation has been made, in many experimental models of autoimmune disease, that CD4⁺ T cells generated

Transfer of tolerance by CD4⁺ T cells

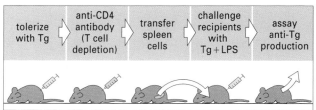

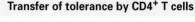

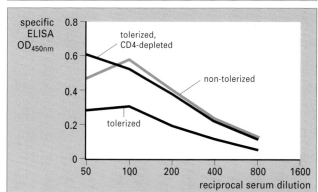

Fig. 11.8 Mice were injected with 200 μg of mouse thyroglobulin (Tg) to induce tolerance. (A control group was not tolerized.) Part of the tolerized group was further treated *in vivo* with depleting anti-CD4 antibodies, to remove CD4⁺ T cells. For each mouse in each of these three groups (non-tolerized; tolerized; tolerized and CD4-depleted), spleen cells were transferred into an irradiated syngeneic recipient. The recipients were then challenged with mouse thyroglobulin and LPS, and their anti-Tg antibody response was assayed using ELISA (see Chapter 28). Anti-CD4 treatment removed the ability to transfer tolerance.

following administration of high doses of autoantigen (often given in a soluble or deaggregated form) prevent further induction of autoimmunity. For example, CD4$^+$ T cells have been shown to prevent the development of autoantibodies to thyroglobulin (*Fig. 11.8*).

Furthermore, administration of an anti-CD4 antibody (blocking MHC class II-mediated antigen presentation) at the same time as an immunogenic dose of thyroglobulin not only prevents the development of autoimmunity, but also results in the development of a population of CD4$^+$ T cells that can transfer specific tolerance to naive recipients (*Fig.11.9*). The exact mechanism by which T cells exert such a negative influence is not entirely clear. However, recent experiments suggest that the production by TH cells of cytokines such as TGFβ, IL-4 and IL-10 can either partially or totally suppress an immune response.

TH cell subsets are involved in the regulation of immunoglobulin production

The production of different cytokines by different TH (CD4$^+$) lymphocyte subpopulations probably provides an explanation for certain observations regarding the regulation of IgE synthesis. Cross regulation of TH subsets has been demonstrated where cytokines such as IFNγ, secreted by TH1 cells, can inhibit the responsiveness of TH2 cells; IL-10 produced by TH2 cells down-regulates B7 and IL-12 expression by APCs, which in turn inhibits TH1 activation. Thus preferential activation of TH1 or TH2 cells may result in an immune deviation – the selection of a particular type of effector response. The selective biasing of responses may prove useful in the treatment of allergy.

CD8$^+$ T cells can transfer resistance and tolerance

CD8$^+$ T cells have also been shown to regulate immune responses. CD8$^+$ T cells have been found in the spleens of animals tolerized to MBP by oral dosing of the antigen (see above). These cells can adoptively transfer resistance to EAE *in vivo*. The T cells not only suppress T cell responses to MBP *in vitro*, but also perform bystander suppression to other unrelated antigens. This effect is thought to be mediated by TGFβ.

Regulation of the immune response by CD4$^+$ TH2 cells is a normal physiological process

The role of such CD4$^+$ or CD8$^+$ T cell-mediated regulatory effects in normal physiology has been questioned. However, the observation that CD4$^+$ T cells able to prevent autoimmunity can be found in unmanipulated normal animals supports their importance in normal homeostasis. Furthermore, the observation that dysregulated immune responses arise in rats and mice when CD4$^+$ TH2 cells, which normally make IL-4 and IL-10, are removed strongly suggests that regulation of the immune response by CD4$^+$ TH2 cells (rather than CD4$^+$ TH1 cells) is a normal physiological process and not an artefact (*Fig. 11.10*).

■ IDIOTYPIC MODULATION OF RESPONSES

Tolerance to self-antigens is established during ontogeny (see Chapter 10). However, during the neonatal period the unique binding regions of antigen-specific receptors on B and T cells are present at levels that are too low to generate tolerance.

Anti-CD4-induced suppression of experimental allergic thyroiditis (EAT)

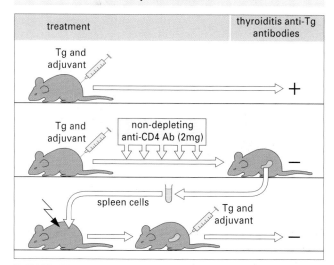

Fig. 11.9 Mice immunized with 50 µg of mouse thyroglobulin (Tg) develop thyroiditis and anti-Tg antibodies. If they are injected over a period of 11 days with a non depleting monoclonal anti-CD4 antibody to blockade CD4/ class II interaction, thyroiditis does not occur. Splenocytes transferred from these treated animals prevent irradiated recipients from developing thyroiditis following immunization with Tg. (Immunized mice that have received control T cells develop thyroiditis.)

Prevention by cytokines of colitis induced in *scid* mice

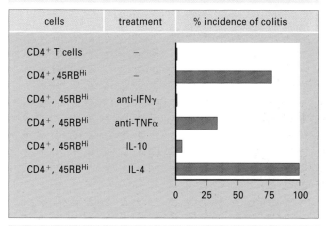

Fig. 11.10 The table shows the incidence of colitis in mice treated by transfer of different cell populations. Mice receiving unfractionated CD4$^+$ T cells are prevented from getting colitis. If they receive fractionated CD4 cells expressing high levels of CD45RB (CD45RB^{hi}), colitis develops. However, if the animals were also given either anti-IFNγ or anti-TNFα then the incidence of disease was reduced. IL-10 (but not IL-4) also modulates disease in these animals. These data suggest that IFNγ and TNFα are involved in the development of colitis, and that IL-10 can switch off the effector cells.

Similarly, although antibodies are present in the serum, tolerance only develops to their Fc portions because only these are present in sufficient concentration; tolerance does not develop to the unique determinants in the heavy and light chains that determine antigen binding specificity. Individual T-cell receptors and immunoglobulins are therefore immunogenic by virtue of these unique sequences, known as idiotypes. Antibodies formed against these antigen-binding sites are called anti-idiotypic antibodies, and are capable of influencing the outcome of an immune response.

Idiotypic determinants may be encoded in the germ line V region genes, or they may be generated by the process of recombination and mutation involved in producing functional V-region elements (see Chapter 6). Immunogenic epitopes in or around the binding site are termed idiotopes (*Fig. 11.11*). Jerne proposed that an immune network existed within the body which interacted by means of idiotype recognition. According to this proposition, when an antibody response is induced by antigen, this antibody will in turn invoke an anti-idiotypic response to itself. This hypothesis is conceptually very appealing, but the role of such an idiotype network in controlling a normal immune response is still hotly debated.

Idiotypic interactions may enhance or suppress antibody responses

There is good evidence that anti-idiotypes can affect the representation of recognized idiotypes in an immune response. For example, when C57Bl/6 strain mice are challenged with the hapten, NP, they produce antibodies that are largely restricted to a few defined idiotypes, for example the idiotype 146. Anti-idiotype to this antibody (idiotype 146) can enhance or suppress the production of idiotype 146 when the mice are subsequently challenged with NP on a carrier protein. The observed effect depends on the amount of anti-idiotype given (*Fig. 11.12*) and is idiotype-specific, as the overall level of anti-NP antibody is hardly affected. Most importantly, the amounts of anti-idiotype employed are within the normal physiological range for particular idiotype-bearing antibodies, which

suggests that idiotypic regulation may occur *in vivo*. This kind of observation has been made in other idiotypic systems.

Dramatic effects are observed when anti-idiotype is administered neonatally, where the effect may be lifelong. For example, the ability of neonatal mice to mount an anti-phosphoryl choline response is greatly reduced after being injected with anti-idiotype to T15 (T15 is a major idiotype in the response to phosphoryl choline). The reduction lasts many months. The response which these mice subsequently make is dominated by non-T15 immunoglobulins (*Fig. 11.13*).

■ NEUROENDOCRINE MODULATION OF IMMUNE RESPONSES

It has long been known that stressful conditions may lead to a suppression of immune functions, for example reducing the ability to recover from infection. (This effect is clearest in those cases where the stressful stimulus cannot be controlled.) However, it is much more difficult to make direct connections at the cellular or molecular level that explain these observations. Broadly, there are two main routes by which events occurring in the CNS could modulate immune function (*Fig. 11.14*):

- Most lymphoid tissues receive direct sympathetic innervation, both to the blood vessels passing through the tissues, and directly to the lymphocytes themselves.
- The nervous system directly or indirectly controls the output of various hormones, in particular, corticosteroids, growth hormone, thyroxine and adrenaline.

Modulation of idiotype by anti-idiotype

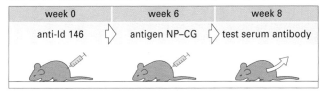

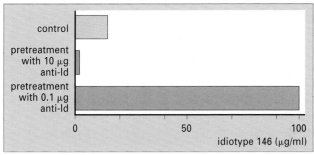

Fig. 11.12 Mice were injected at time 0 with either 10 μg or 0.1 μg of anti-idiotype (anti-Id) to the nitrophenyl (NP)-binding antibody 146. The animals were then challenged six weeks later with NP on the carrier, chicken globulin (CG). Two weeks later the serum titres of idiotype 146 (bar diagram), and total anti-NP (not shown) were assayed. Mice pretreated with 10 μg anti-Id showed suppression of idiotype 146, while mice treated with 0.1 μg showed enhanced production of idiotype 146, although the overall levels of anti-NP were similar in both groups.

Idiotopes associated with the antibody-combining site

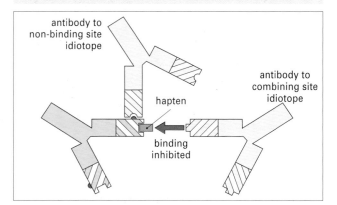

Fig. 11.11 An anti-idiotype serum may contain antibodies directed to various sites on the immunoglobulin molecule. Those associated with the combining site are site associated idiotopes. The binding to these can be inhibited by hapten. Antibodies to non-binding site idiotopes (non-site associated) are not inhibited by hapten.

Lymphocytes express receptors for many hormones, neuro-transmitters and neuropeptides, including ones for steroids, catecholamines (adrenaline and noradrenaline), enkephalins, endorphins, substance P and vasoactive intestinal peptide (VIP). Expression and responsiveness vary between different lymphocyte and monocyte populations, such that the effect of different transmitters may vary in different circumstances. However, one particularly important control is mediated by corticosteroids, endorphins and enkephalins, all of which may be released during stress, and all of which are immunosuppressive *in vivo*. The precise *in vitro* effects of endorphins vary greatly depending on the system and on the doses used; some levels are suppressive, and others enhance immune functions. It is certain, however, that the corticosteroids act as a major feedback control on immune responses. It has been found that lymphocytes themselves can respond to corticotrophin releasing factor to generate their own ACTH, which in turn induces corticosteroid release.

■ GENETIC CONTROL OF IMMUNE RESPONSES

The ability to make an immune response to a given antigen is inherited

It has long been recognized that the ability to make an immune response to any given antigen varies between individuals. Familial patterns of susceptibility to *Corynebacterium*

diphtheriae infection suggested that resistance or susceptibility might be an inherited characteristic. This proposal was supported by the finding that different strains of guinea pigs displayed different resistance patterns to diphtheria, and that this characteristic was inherited. In 1943 Fjord–Scheibel demonstrated, by selection of high-responder and low-responder guinea pig strains, that the production of diphtheria anti-toxin was controlled by a single gene, inherited as a Mendelian dominant trait. This study was also the first demonstration of the dominance of high responsiveness. Ninety per cent of offspring of the two high-responder animals were anti-toxin producers in the first generation, whilst it took five generations of inbreeding low-responders before ninety per cent of their offspring were low-responders.

B-cell suppression by anti-idiotype

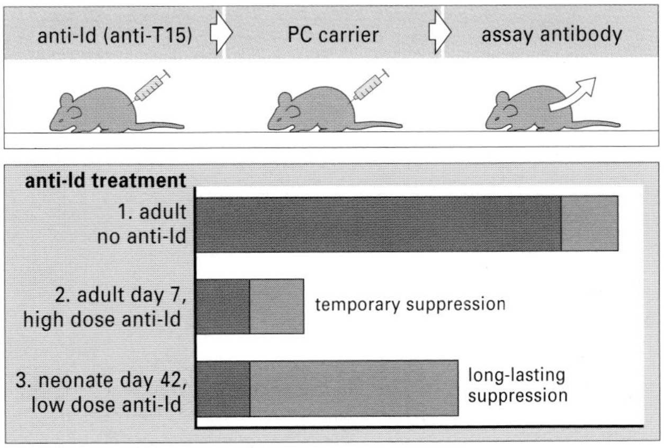

anti-Id (anti-T15) ⇨	PC carrier ⇨	assay antibody

anti-Id treatment

1. adult no anti-Id

2. adult day 7, high dose anti-Id — temporary suppression

3. neonate day 42, low dose anti-Id — long-lasting suppression

Fig. 11.13 Mice were pretreated with anti-idiotype to T15, either during the neonatal period or as adults. They were subsequently immunized with the hapten phosphoryl choline (PC) coupled to a carrier. The total antibody to PC was measured along with the T15 component of the response (darker area). Normal adult mice make a good response to PC that is dominated by T15 (1). Adult mice pretreated with anti-idiotype are temporarily suppressed with the loss of the T15 component, accounting for the reduction in the total anti-PC response (2). Mice treated with anti-idiotype in the neonatal period undergo long-term suppression of their T15+ B cells, but generate T15⁻ PC-specific cells to compensate (3).

Neuroendocrine interactions with the immune system

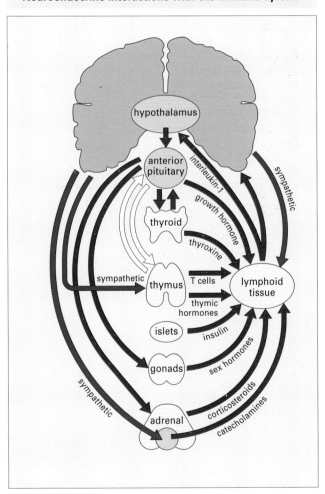

Fig. 11.14 The diagram indicates some of the potential connections between the endocrine, nervous and immune systems. Blue arrows indicate nervous connections, red arrows indicate hormonal interactions, and white arrows indicate postulated connections for which the effector molecules have not been established.

MHC haplotypes influence the ability to respond to an antigen

With the development of inbred mouse strains it became possible to analyze genetic influences more rigorously and it was conclusively demonstrated that genetic factors play a role in determining immune responsiveness. For example, strains of mice with different MHC haplotypes vary in their ability to mount an antibody response to specific antigens (*Fig. 11.15*). This function depends on MHC class II molecules, and is specific for each antigen – a high-responder strain for some antigens will be a low-responder strain for others. It was furthermore shown that genes within the MHC (see Chapters 5 and 7) play a fundamental role in influencing the response against infectious agents.

Non MHC-linked genes also influence the immune response

Considerable advances have been made in recent years: the elucidation of the structures of MHC class I and MHC class II; the analyses of polymorphic residues in the MHC and their influence on peptide binding; the ability to monitor the T cell repertoire following the generation of reagents and molecular methods for TCR detection; the development of transgenic mice; all these have contributed to an explosion of information about how genetic factors influence the immune response. However, genetic influences on the immune response are not always linked to the MHC. For example, severe combined immunodeficiency is due to the lack of a recombinase gene, and leucocyte adhesion deficiency is caused by mutations in the β_2-integrin subunit which lead to a failure of expression of LFA-1, CR3 and CR4.

MHC-linked immune response genes control all immune responses that involve antigen recognition by T cells

As discussed in previous chapters, the immune response depends upon the activation of clones of lymphocytes. In the case of T cells, these recognize antigen only when it is presented to them as peptide complexed to class I or class II major histocompatibility (MHC) antigens. For example, CD8[+] Tc cells specific for LCMV glycoprotein will only lyse virally infected target cells derived from an MHC class I matched mouse strain (*Fig. 11.16*); this recognition is learnt during ontogeny (*Fig. 11.17*).

The peripheral T-cell repertoire is influenced both by the range of self antigens, and by their ability to bind to the individual's MHC antigens. The ability of peptide to bind to MHC is determined by the amino acid sequences in the binding sites of the MHC molecules. We now know that most of the polymorphic residues in MHC molecules reside in the peptide-binding groove. Thus the extensive sequence polymorphism of MHC molecules has a deep impact on peptide

Strain differences in the antibody response

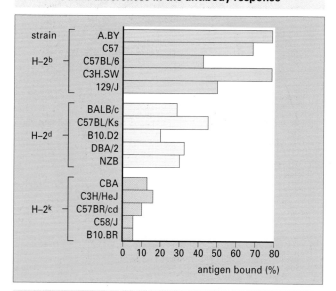

Fig. 11.15 Fifteen strains of mice were given a standard dose of the synthetic antigen (TG)-A-L. Antibody responses are expressed as the antigen-binding capacity of the sera. Animals of the H–2^b haplotype are high responders, H–2^d are intermediate and H–2^k are low responders. However there is some overlap between the levels of response in different haplotypes indicating that H–2-linked genes are not the only ones controlling the antibody response.

Genetic restriction of Tc cells

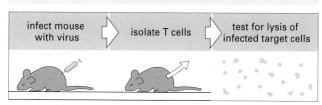

virus	mouse strain	H–2 region				percent lysis of infected targets of haplotype		
		K	I	S	D	H–2^s	H–2^k	H–2^d
LCMV	A.TL					25	1	64
Sendai	A.TL					63	4	24
LCMV	CBA					2	34	1
LCMV	A/J					0	30	64

Fig. 11.16 The Tc cells of virus-infected adult mice (strains A.TL, CBA and A/J) were tested for their ability to kill virus-infected target cells with haplotypes H–2^k, H–2^s and H–2^d. The strain A.TL is H–2K^s, H–2I^k and H–2D^d and its cells kill target cells infected with lymphocytic choriomeningitis virus (LCMV) only if the targets share the H–2K^s or the H–2D^d haplotypes. This shows that the antiviral cytotoxic T cells are class I restricted. Note that the cytotoxicity to LCM is determined mostly by the H–2D locus. By comparison, in A.TL mice infected with Sendai virus, the cytotoxicity is principally determined by the H–2K locus. Infection of CBA mice with LCMV confirms the importance of genetic restriction in these responses. The infection of A/J mice with LCM confirms the finding that cytotoxicity to LCMV is strongest to the H–2D-matched infected targets. Different viruses may associate preferentially with particular H–2K or H–2D MHC molecules to present a target for cytotoxic cells.

binding and, as a consequence, on T cell activation. It is now established that, during development, T cells are subjected to two selection processes in the thymus:

- Positive selection, based on an interaction of the TCR with MHC on thymic cortical epithelium.
- Negative selection, a result of a high-affinity interaction between the TCR and MHC–peptide presented on bone-marrow-derived cells in the thymus medulla.

T cells are positively selected in the thymus to recognize antigens presented on self MHC molecules

Early studies in this area used complex protocols involving thymectomy, irradiation, bone marrow reconstitution and thymus grafting. Using these techniques, it was shown that Tc cells were highly specific, and would only kill target cells which bore the same MHC antigens as those expressed on the thymus in which the T cell matured (*Fig. 11.18*). This, together with other data, suggested that the maturing T cell was educated to recognize antigen only in the context of MHC originally encountered in the thymus.

Experiments carried out on transgenic mice have helped to clarify this process, since it is possible to construct a trans-

genic animal whose T cells largely utilize a single TCR that recognizes a defined antigen. This antigen may also be expressed as a transgene. This simplifies the analysis, since the T cells under investigation represent the majority and can be recognized by means of clonotypic, or Vβ-specific antibodies. (Vβ is a variable domain of the TCR complex.) Thus a transgenic mouse, whose T cells largely express the TCR of a CD8$^+$ Tc cell clone that recognizes an LCMV glycoprotein presented by an H–2D^b class I molecule, can be generated and then used to show positive selection. In these transgenics the TCR can be identified using antibodies specific for Vβ8.

Different MHC molecules have different effects on the development of mature CD8$^+$ T cells expressing the transgenic TCR (*Fig. 11.19*). Only mice expressing the H–2^b molecule show a positive selection of CD8$^+$ T cells using the Vβ8 chain of the transgenic TCR. This shows that this receptor is only positively selected in mice expressing the appropriate MHC haplotype. Positive selection occurs on cortical thymic epithelial cells. It is thought that the peptides which mediate positive selection are naturally occurring thymic self peptides.

T cells that recognize self antigens are negatively selected in the thymus

Negative selection by clonal deletion has been demonstrated using monoclonal antibodies specific for murine TCR Vβ chains. Using this technique, it was possible to identify and count those T cells possessing TCRs with a given Vβ chain and to demonstrate that mice expressing I–E

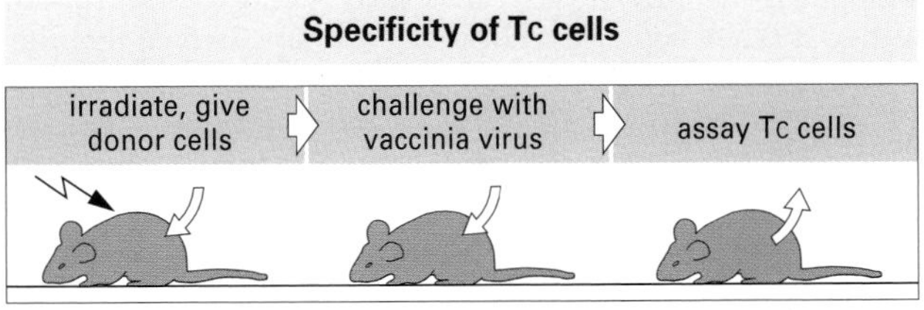

Specificity of Tc cells

experiment	source of donor (A×B) cells	recipient	cytotoxicity to: A-vaccinia	cytotoxicity to: B-vaccinia
1	bone marrow	A	+	–
2	bone marrow	B	–	+
3	spleen	A	+	+
4	spleen	B	+	+

Fig. 11.17 Recipient mice (type A and B) were irradiated and reconstituted with donor lymphocytes (bone marrow or spleen cells) from A×B mice. This produced chimeric animals, in which the lymphocytes were of the donor (A×B) type and other tissues were of the recipient type. The chimeras were then challenged with vaccinia virus; T cells from the spleen were removed and assayed for cytotoxicity against either type A or type B cells infected with vaccinia (denoted A-vaccinia and B-vaccinia). Mice reconstituted with (A×B) bone marrow cells can only kill infected targets of the same type as the recipient (1 and 2). Mature lymphocytes from the spleen of (A×B) mice can kill both A and B targets regardless of the recipient (3 and 4). The interpretation is that immature stem cells from the bone marrow undergo thymic 'education' in the recipient and can then only recognize antigen in association with the recipient's MHC haplotype. Mature cells from the donor's spleen, however, have already undergone thymic education. In most cases, for thymic education of donor cells to occur, the donor and recipient must share at least one class II region haplotype.

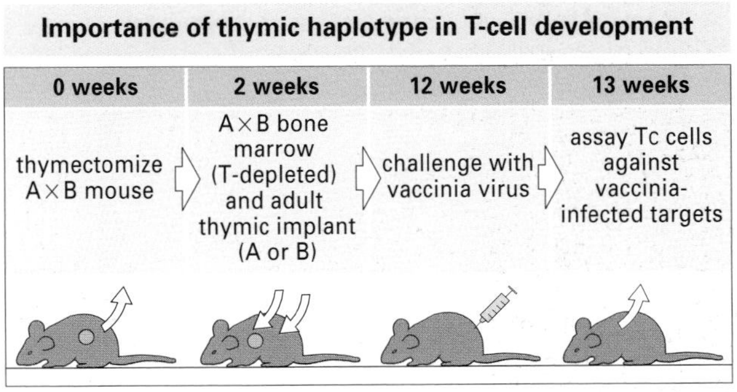

Importance of thymic haplotype in T-cell development

thymic donor	target cell haplotype A	target cell haplotype B
A	+	–
B	–	+

Fig. 11.18 Eight-week-old mice of MHC genotype (A×B) were thymectomized, irradiated and reconstituted with bone marrow that had been specifically depleted of T cells. Each mouse was then given a subcutaneous implant of adult thymus of either type A or type B haplotype. (The grafted tissue was first irradiated to destroy mature T cells. This leaves the thymic stromal cells intact.) Ten weeks after grafting, the mice were infected with vaccinia virus; their spleen cells were tested one week later for the ability to specifically kill virally infected target cells of haplotype A or B. Animals reconstituted with a type A thymus killed haplotype A targets, and those with a type B thymus killed haplotype B targets.

Positive selection in the thymus

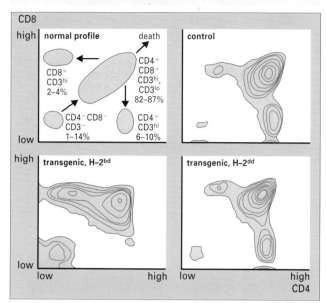

Fig. 11.19 Thymocytes were obtained from transgenic mice carrying the TCR of a CD8⁺ T cell that recognizes LCMV on H–2ᵇ. The thymocytes were analyzed for expression of CD4 and CD8 by fluorescence-activated cell sorting. In the normal developmental profile CD4⁻CD8⁻ cells become CD4⁺CD8⁺ and finally mature into CD4⁺CD8⁻, or CD4⁻CD8⁺, or die. In a control (non-transgenic mouse) the major population is CD4⁺CD8⁺, with smaller CD4⁺CD8⁻ and CD4⁻CD8⁺ populations. In a transgenic mouse expressing an H–2ᵇ allele, the T cells are positively selected in the thymus producing a much larger CD4⁻CD8⁺ population. No such selection occurs if the relevant H–2ᵇ allele is absent.

would delete Vβ17a⁺ T cells in the thymus. The presence of Vβ17a⁺CD4⁺CD8⁺ T cells but no mature Vβ17a⁺CD4⁺ T cells or Vβ17a⁺CD8⁺ T cells suggested that deletion occurred at the double positive (CD4⁺CD8⁺) stage of T-cell maturation. Deletion was shown to require expression of an endogenous ligand together with I–E, and not just I–E on its own.

Superantigens can cause the deletion of entire sets of T cell receptors

In some strains of mice, entire sets of T cell receptor-bearing T cells are deleted in the thymus. For example, Vβ6⁺ and Vβ8.1⁺ T cells are deleted in mice expressing the minor lymphocyte stimulating antigen Mls–1ᵃ and certain MHC class II molecules (*Fig. 11.20*). This ability of whole families of T cells to recognize Mls explains the intense proliferative response obtained when Mls mismatched cells are cultured together. It shows that responses to certain antigens involve all the T cells expressing certain Vβ chains (*Fig. 11.21*).

These antigens, some exogenous and some endogenous which elicit such a powerful response are called superantigens. Superantigens do not bind within the peptide binding groove of the MHC but directly bind MHC Class II and the β chain of the TCR (see Chapter 8). Staphylococcal enterotoxin B (SEB) is an example of an exogenous superantigen. T cells in the mouse which respond to this antigen have TCR with Vβ3 or Vβ8 chains. Mls antigens are a class of endogenous superantigens (see Chapter 8). However, it is now known that the Mls of any given mouse strain is in fact determined by the presence of endogenous mouse mammary tumour viruses (MMTVs) encoded in the genome of that strain. There are many different MMTVs, and each mouse strain has only some of them in its genome. These endogenous superantigens are expressed in the thymus and cause deletion (negative selection) of T cells expressing TCRs with Vβ3, Vβ6 or Vβ8.1.

T-cell deletion by superantigens

V region	antigen recognized	T cell population expressing V region	after tolerance by clonal deletion
Vβ17a	I–E, B cell peptide	5.6%	0.9%
Vβ6	Mlsᵃ	12.4%	0.3%
Vβ8.1	Mlsᵃ	7.5%	0.3%
Vβ3	Mls-2	4.1%	0.1%
Vβ3	SEB	5.7%	1.2%
Vβ8	SEB	18.9%	0.0%
Vβ11	I–E, peptide	5.0%	0.5%

Fig. 11.20 Superantigens can cause clonal deletion of T cells expressing certain Vβ chains. The absolute number of T cells utilizing particular Vβ chains varies between mouse strains. This table provides examples of deletion values obtained in certain strains; while the absolute levels may vary from strain to strain, the overall phenomenon holds true. (SEB = staphylococcal enterotoxin B.)

T-cell recognition of Mls-1ᵃ

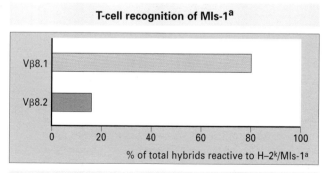

Fig. 11.21 A high frequency of T cells expressing Vβ8.1 recognize Mls–1ᵃ. T cell hybridomas were generated by fusing T cell blasts (expressing Vβ8.1 or Vβ8.2) from B10.Br (Mls–1ᵇ) lymph nodes with a variant of the T cell thymoma BW5147 (expressing neither Vα nor Vβ). These hybrids were separated by screening them with antibodies which recognized Vβ8.1 and (for comparison) Vβ8.2. They were then screened for reactivity against Mls–1ᵃ on H–2ᵏ stimulators. The great majority of the hybridomas reactive to this antigen were found to express Vβ8.1; a minority expressed Vβ8.2. This indicates the preference for use of Vβ8.1 in recognition of Mls–1ᵃ.

The transgenic mice described in the previous section (whose transgenes encode the α and β chains of a TCR specific for LCMV glycoprotein in the context of H–2D^b) have also been used to demonstrate how thymic selection can affect the ability of an animal to mount an immune response in later life. When neonatally infected with LCMV, these mice became tolerant to, and carriers of, the virus. When the maturing T-cell populations in these neonatally infected mice are examined, there is a marked reduction in CD4$^+$CD8$^+$ T cells, suggesting that clonal deletion of T cells has occurred at an early stage in ontogeny (*Fig. 11.22*). The expressed peripheral T-cell repertoire can therefore be shaped by both positive and negative selection (*Fig. 11.23*), thus affecting the immune response.

MHC-linked genes control the response to infections

MHC-linked genes have been shown to play a role in the immune response to infectious agents and also to self antigens. In some cases the gene involved is the MHC gene itself, but in others it is thought to be a gene that is simply linked to the MHC.

Susceptibility to infection by Trichinella spiralis *is affected by the I–E locus in mice*

The first observation that genes (*Ts-1* and *Ts-2*) within the MHC could influence the response to parasites involved the susceptibility to *Trichinella spiralis*. (It is interesting that such an effect should be noted with an antigenically complex organism, especially as these parasites express different antigens at different stages in their life cycle, with different APCs being involved in their presentation.) If different recombi-

nant mouse strains are infected with *T. spiralis* it can be seen that resistance or susceptibility is affected by the I–E locus. Mouse strains that express I–E appear to be susceptible (*Fig. 11.24*). An additional MHC-linked gene has been shown to influence the response to *T. spiralis*; in this case it is not an MHC-encoded gene but another gene in linkage disequilibrium. This gene, which has been designated *Ts-2*, maps between *S* and *D*, close to the TNF genes.

The I-E locus also influences susceptibility to **Leishmania donovani**

The I–E subregion has also been shown to influence susceptibility to *Leishmania donovani*. Using H–2 congenic mice it was shown that I–E-expressing mice were unable to combat visceral leishmaniasis. Direct involvement of the I–E product in this susceptibility was shown by the ability of anti-I–E antibody, but not the anti-I–A antibody, to enhance parasite clearance. Furthermore, insertion of an I–E transgene into a mouse strain lacking I–E makes them unable to clear parasites from the liver and spleen as effectively as the original strain.

Positive and negative selection on the thymus

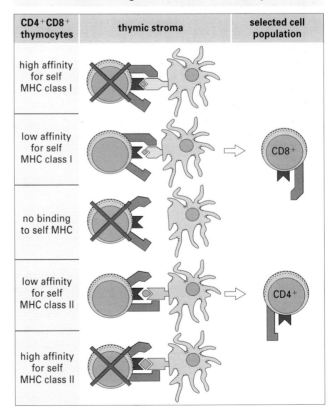

CD4$^+$CD8$^+$ thymocytes	thymic stroma	selected cell population
high affinity for self MHC class I		
low affinity for self MHC class I		CD8$^+$
no binding to self MHC		
low affinity for self MHC class II		CD4$^+$
high affinity for self MHC class II		

Fig. 11.23 CD4$^+$CD8$^+$ thymocytes interact with thymic stroma expressing MHC class I and MHC class II molecules complexed to self-peptides. Clones with high affinity for self-MHC class I or class II are deleted, as are clones that have no ability to recognize self-MHC. Clones with low affinity for self-MHC class I are positively selected and lose their CD4, to become CD8$^+$ T cells. Conversely, those that interact weakly with self-MHC class II molecules, mature into the CD4$^+$ population.

Tolerance to LCMV in transgenic mice

anti-LCMV (Vβ8.1) transgenic animal	neonatal LCMV infection	primary anti-LCMV response	thymocyte numbers	
			CD4$^+$CD8$^+$	CD8$^+$
Mls–1^b	–	+++	normal	normal
Mls–1^a	–	+	normal	low
Mls–1^b	+	–	low	low

Fig. 11.22 Tolerance induction in transgenic mice varies with the antigen. Transgenic mice expressing TCR specific for LCMV in the context of H–2D^b were examined for their ability to mount a proliferative and cytotoxic response to LCMV-infected cells. As this TCR also expresses Vβ8.1, it is possible to examine the influence of the presence of Mls–1^a on the ability to make such a primary response to LCMV. Mice can also be infected at birth with LCMV, and so the effect of neonatal exposure to the antigen recognized by the transgenic TCR can be assessed. A partial reduction in both proliferation and cytotoxicity is seen in mice expressing Mls–1^a and a total elimination of the response following neonatal exposure to the specific antigen. Analysis of the T-cell populations in these animals shows that LCMV-tolerant mice have markedly reduced numbers of CD4$^+$CD8$^+$ thymocytes and mature CD8$^+$ T cells. However, exposure to the self-superantigen (Mls–1^a) alone results in the deletion of only mature CD8$^+$ T cells. This suggests that different antigens may tolerize T cells at different times during their development.

Certain HLA haplotypes confer protection from Plasmodium falciparum

In humans, a comparison of the HLA haplotypes associated with severe malarial anaemia revealed that the HLA haplotype (DRB1*1302–DQB1*0501), which is common in West Africans and rare in other racial groups, provides protection from the lethal consequences of infection by *P. falciparum*. DRB1*1302 has been shown to bind different peptides from DRB1*1301 due to a single amino acid difference in the β chain. This would clearly influence the response to the malaria parasite.

MHC-linked genes have a major influence on susceptibility to autoimmune diseases
Associations with MHC genes

Insulin-dependent diabetes mellitus (IDDM), an autoimmune disease in which the beta cells of the pancreas are destroyed by cells of the immune system, is associated with HLA-DR3 and HLA-DR4. The highest risk is in fact seen in HLA-DR3/4 heterozygotes. Because of linkage disequilibrium, although the original associations were seen with DR, they are in reality with DQ. Molecular genetic analysis has permitted the association to be analysed in more detail, and it seems that the primary association in Caucasians is with DQB1*0302. In rheumatoid arthritis the predominant association is with HLA-DR4 or DR-1 in several ethnic groups; there is little association with HLA-DQ. The way in which these disease associations contribute to susceptibility remains unclear, but possible explanations include repertoire differences through positive and negative selection on different class II genes, or preferential binding of disease-inducing epitopes on bacteria or viruses to particular MHC molecules. Analysis of the amino acid sequences of peptide binding grooves of HLA-DR4 and DR-1 has supported this hypothesis by demonstrating the presence of differently charged residues in susceptible or resistant subtypes of HLA-DR.

Associations with MHC region

Another example of linkage disequilibrium is that provided by the association of autoimmunity in the (NZB x NZW) F₁ mouse with the H–2ᶻ of the NZW parent. It has been clearly demonstrated that this association was not with an MHC gene itself, but with the TNFα gene closely linked to the MHC genes. The NZW TNFα allele gives rise to the production of low amounts of TNFα. If the concentration of this cytokine is increased, the mice are protected from the development of lupus nephritis (*Fig. 11.25*).

Associations with genes involved in processing

Other MHC-linked genes have recently been identified which may influence immune responses. These genes are involved in the generation (by proteolysis) and transport of antigen peptide fragments. They are polymorphic, and such polymorphism has functional consequences. For example, in the rat, different allelic forms of the *cim* locus affect peptide loading into the class I MHC, which in turn affects the ability of the class I MHC molecule to be recognized as an alloantigen. It is therefore possible that some of the MHC-linked disease associations that have been identified are attributable to similar genes, involved in proteolysis and transport of antigen peptides to the MHC molecules for presentation to cells of the immune system.

Many non-MHC genes also modulate immune responses

The immune response is also governed by some genes outside the MHC region. However, these genes are generally less polymorphic than MHC genes and they make a lesser contribution to variations in disease susceptibility in a population than the MHC genes. Nevertheless, their effects have been clearly shown in autoimmune diseases, allergy and infection (*Fig. 11.26*). For example:

Susceptibility to *T. spiralis*

mouse strain	H–2 haplotype	I–E expression	resistance index	resistance phenotype
B10.BR	k	+	0	sus
B10.P	p	+	– 22	sus
B10.RIII	r	+	33	sus
B10	b	–	63	res/int
B10.S	s	–	100	res
B10.M	f	–	104	res
B10.Q	q	–	105	res

Fig. 11.24 Association of H–2 haplotype, expression of cell surface I–E molecules, and susceptibility to infection with Trichinella spiralis. The resistance index is measured as number of parasites present after a constant challenge, relative to strains B10.BR (susceptible = 0% resistance) and B10.S (resistant = 100% resistance). B10 shows intermediate resistance.

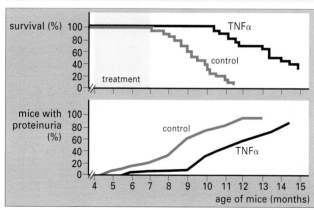

TNFα and lupus nephritis

Fig. 11.25 Upper: Twenty (NZB × NZW) F1 female mice were treated with recombinant murine TNFα. Their survival is compared with age- and sex-matched F1 controls.
Lower: Cumulative frequency of significant proteinuria (≥ 300 mg/dl) in (NZB × NZW) F₁ mice treated with TNFα, and in controls.

- Individuals with defects in the complement component C3 show an increased susceptibility to bacterial infections and a predisposition towards immune-complex disease.
- High IgE production in some allergy prone families has been shown to associate with the presence of an 'atopy gene' on human chromosome 11q.

Non-MHC-linked genes affect susceptibility to infection

Macrophages – play a key role in the immune system. Genes regulating their activity may therefore determine the outcome of many immune responses. A good example of such genetic control of macrophage function is provided by the *Lsh/Ity/Bcg* gene. This gene governs the early response to infection with *Leishmania donovani*, *Salmonella typhimurium*, *Mycobacterium bovis*, *M. lepraemurium* and *M. intracellulare*. Its influence is on the early phase of macrophage priming and activation, and it has wide-ranging effects, including

- Up-regulation of the oxidative burst.
- Enhanced tumoricidal activity.
- Enhanced antimicrobial activity.
- Up-regulation of MHC class II expression.

Recent studies have identified *Nramp* as a potential candidate for Bcg in the mouse. As *Nramp* encodes a membrane protein with homology to known transport proteins, the suggestion has been made that it may be implicated in the transport of NO_2^- into the phagolysosome and thus facilitate the killing of intracellular organisms. However, until *Nramp* has indeed been formally shown to encode the Bcg product either by transfection or by transgenesis, this is completely hypothetical.

Biozzi generated two lines of mice by selective inbreeding, based on their responsiveness to erythrocyte antigens. These high-responder and low-responder Biozzi mice make quantitatively different amounts of antibody in response to antigenic challenge. The basis for these differences has in part

been attributed to genetic differences in macrophage activity. These high- and low-responder strains also differ markedly in their ability to respond to parasitic infections, and this does not necessarily correlate with the amount of antibody they make (*Fig. 11.27*).

Eosinophils – play an important role in the host response to parasitic infection. It has been shown that the degree of eosinophilia following infection is genetically determined, with marked differences seen in different inbred strains of mice. Similar observations have been made in guinea pigs and sheep, where a consistent correlation has been found between resistance to nematode infection and the extent of eosinophilia.

Non-MHC linked genes also affect development of autoimmune disease

Major advances have recently been made in mapping the loci which govern susceptibility to the autoimmune disease, insulin-dependent diabetes mellitus (IDDM). This work has been largely carried out using the NOD mouse strain, which spontaneously develops an autoimmune disease similar to IDDM in man. At least 10 genetic loci have been identified in the NOD mouse (*Idd-1* to *10*). Only one locus (*Idd-1*) is linked to the mouse MHC on chromosome 17, and is thought to encode MHC class II antigens themselves. The other genes have been mapped to other chromosomes but their identity and functional roles in determining resistance or susceptibility are not yet known.

When the lymphoproliferative (*lpr*) gene is introduced into mouse strains it causes the development of a characteristic clinical syndrome. The mice develop anti-DNA antibodies, rheumatoid factor, circulating immune complexes and glomerulonephritis. There is also a lymphadenopathy in these mice involving an expansion of CD4⁻CD8⁻ T cells in the periphery. These T cells are not monoclonal, but have differently arranged TCRs. It was initially suggested that the syndrome was due to a defect in negative selection, but it was difficult to see how a gene such as *lpr* could mediate this effect. Recently it has been shown that mice with the *lpr* gene have a defect in the Fas antigen, which is encoded by a gene on chromosome 19 in the mouse. The Fas antigen is a cell surface protein which is a member of the tumour necrosis/nerve growth factor family, and which mediates apoptosis.

Role of non-MHC genes in resistance to infection

organism	resistant		susceptible	
	strain	haplotype	strain	haplotype
Mycobacterium lepraemurium	DBA/2J C3H/HeJ	d k	BALB/cJ C3H/A	d k
Salmonella typhimurium	DBA/2J	d	B10.D2, BALB/c	d d
M. tuberculosis	CBA, C3H	k	B10.BR	k
Listeria monocytogenes	B10.A B10.D2 B10.BR	a d k	A/J DBA/2, BALB/c CBA, C3H	a d k
Rickettsia tsutsugamushi	AKR SWR BALB/c	k q d	C3H, CBA DBA/1 DBA/2	k q d

Fig. 11.26 Different strains of mice vary in their resistance to the organisms listed. Different strains with the same MHC haplotype can be susceptible or resistant, showing that the MHC haplotype is not critical in determining resistance to infection.

Response of Biozzi mice to parasite infection

organism	Biozzi high	Biozzi low
T. cruzi	resistant	susceptible
P. berghei	resistant	susceptible
P. yoelii	resistant	susceptible
L. major	susceptible	resistant
S. mansoni	susceptible	resistant

Fig. 11.27 High- and low-responder Biozzi mice show a differential responsiveness to parasitic infections, which is not consistent within the high and low responder groups.

The defect in Fas antigen arising from the *lpr* mutation results in the failure of apoptosis. However, this defect does not appear to affect negative selection and the generation of a normal repertoire of mature single positive T cells in the thymus. Evidently Fas is only one of the ligands which mediate apoptosis. It is now proposed that the defect leads to the expansion of double negative T cells in the periphery and an acceleration of an autoimmune syndrome. The defect in apoptosis is also expressed in B cells and permits the accumulation of autoreactive B cells in the periphery.

Other studies further suggest that the *gld* gene, which has been shown to result in a similar autoimmune phenotype to that seen in lpr/lpr mice, may arise from a related defect. It is proposed that the *gld* encoded protein is the ligand for the Fas antigen. Thus mice which are gld/gld do not express the ligand, have a defect in apoptosis of peripheral B and T cells, and develop autoimmunity. The *gld* gene is located on chromosome 1 in the mouse and thus provides yet another example of a gene which affects immune function, but which is not MHC-linked.

Critical Thinking

■ Endogenous retroviral sequences modify the expressed T-cell repertoire of mice. What is the biological significance of such a modification?

■ Why would the immune system retain so many different ways of regulating the immune response?

■ The examples of regulation which are provided in this chapter are derived from contrived model systems. Is it possible to determine whether these mechanisms operate in a normal intact individual?

FURTHER READING

Aichele P, Kyburz D, Ohashi PS, *et al*. Peptide-induced T-cell tolerance to prevent autoimmune diabetes in a transgenic mouse model. *Proc Natl Acad Sci* USA 1994; **91**:444.

Blalock JE, Bost KL, eds. Neuroimmunoendocrinology. *Allergy;* vol 43. Basel: Karger.

Eisenberg RA, Sobel ES, Reap EA, Halpern MD, Cohen PL. The role of B cell abnormalities in the systemic autoimmune syndromes of *lpr* and *gld* mice. *Semin Immunol* 1994;**6**:49.

Gaulton GN, Greene MI. Idiotypic mimicry of biological receptors. *Annu Rev Immunol* 1986;**4**:253.

Gershon RK, Kondo K. Infectious immunological tolerance. *Immunology* 1972;**21**:903.

Goodnow CC, Adelstein S, Basten A. The need for central and peripheral tolerance in the B cell repertoire. *Science* 1990;**248**:1373.

Herman A, Kappler JW, Marrack P, Pullen A. Superantigens: mechanisms of T cell stimulation and role in immune responses. *Annu Rev Immunol* 1991;**9**:745.

Holt PG. Immunoprophylaxis of atopy: light at the end of the tunnel? *Immunol Today* 1994;**15**:484.

Jerne NJ. Towards a network theory of the immune system. *Ann Immunol (Paris)* 1974;**1235c**:373.

Mason D, MacPhee I, Antoni F. The role of the neuroendocrine system in determining genetic susceptibility to experimental allergic encephalomyelitis in the rat. *Immunology* 1990;**70**:1–5.

Metzler B, Wraith DC. Inhibition of experimental autoimmune encephalomyelitis by inhalation but not oral administration of the encephalitogenic peptide: influence of MHC binding affinity. *Internat Immunol* 1993;**5**:1159.

Nagata S, Suda T. Fas and Fas ligand: *lpr* and *gld* mutations. *Immunol Today* 1995;**16**:39.

Nossal GJV. Negative selection of lymphocytes. *Cell* 1994;**76**:229.

Powell D, Mason D. Evidence that the T cell repertoire of normal rats contains cells with the potential to cause diabetes. Characterization of the CD4+ T cell subset that inhibits this autoimmune potential. *J Exp Med* 1993;**177**:627.

Powrie F, Leach MW, Mauze S, Menon S, Caddle LB, Coffman RL. Inhibition of TH1 responses prevents inflammatory bowel disease in *scid* mice reconstituted with CD45RB^hi CD4+ T cells. *Immunity* 1994;**1**:553.

Rozzo SJ, Eisenberg RA, Cohen PL, Kotzin BL. Development of the T cell receptor repertoire in *lpr* mice. *Semin Immunol* 1994;**6**:19.

Stein KE, Soderstrom T. Neonatal administration of idiotype or anti-idiotype primes for protection against *Escherichia coli* K13 infection in mice. *J Exp Med* 1984;**160**:101.

Schwartz RH. A cell culture method for T cell clonal anergy. *Science* 1990;**248**:1349.

Vidal SM, Malo DM, Vogan K, Skamene, Gros P. Natural resistance to infection with intracellular parasites: isolation of a candidate for *Bcg*. *Cell* 1993;**73**:469.

Von Boehmer H. Positive selection of lymphocytes. *Cell* 1994;**76**:219.

Wakelin D, Blackwell JK. Genetic variations in immunity to parasite infection. In: *Immunology and Molecular Biology of Parasitic Infections*. Oxford: Blackwell Scientific Publications, 1991.

Zinkernagel RM, Pircher HP, Ohashi P, *et al*. T and B cell tolerance and responses to viral antigens in transgenic mice: implications for the pathogenesis of autoimmune versus immunopathological disease. *Immunol Rev* 1991;**122**:133.

Tolerance mechanisms are needed because the immune system randomly generates a vast diversity of antigen-specific receptors and some of these will be self-reactive; tolerance prevents reactivity against the body's own tissues.

Central thymic tolerance to self antigens (autoantigens) results from deletion of differentiating T cells that express antigen-specific receptors with high binding affinity for intrathymic self antigens. Low-affinity self-reactive T cells, and T cells with receptors specific for antigens that are not represented intrathymically, mature and join the peripheral T-cell pool.

Post-thymic tolerance to self antigens has three main mechanisms: self-reactive T cells in the circulation either ignore self antigens, for example when the antigens are in tissues sequestered from the circulation, or they may under certain conditions be deleted or rendered anergic and unable to respond.

B-cell deletion takes place in the bone marrow: differentiating B cells that express surface immunoglobulin receptors with high binding affinity for self membrane-bound antigens will be deleted after leaving their birth place.

B-cell anergy results when B cells with the potential to respond to soluble self proteins downregulate their surface IgM receptors.

Autoimmunity is a breakdown of tolerance. An example is when T cells that have previously ignored self antigens are stimulated by professional antigen-presenting cells that can deliver a powerful co-stimulator signal and can present an antigen, derived from an invading microorganism, which cross-reacts with a self antigen.

Artificial tolerance can be induced artificially by various regimes that may eventually be exploited clinically to prevent rejection of foreign transplants and to deal with autoimmune diseases.

■ INTRODUCTION

Immunological tolerance is a state of unresponsiveness which is specific for a particular antigen; it is induced by prior exposure to that antigen. The most important aspect of tolerance is self-tolerance, which prevents the body from mounting an immune attack against its own tissues. There is potential for such attack because the immune system randomly generates a vast diversity of antigen-specific receptors (see Chapter 6), some of which will be self-reactive. Cells bearing these receptors therefore must be eliminated, either functionally or physically.

Self-reactivity is prevented by processes that occur during development, rather than being genetically preprogrammed. Thus, while homozygous animals of histoincompatible strains A and B reject each other's skin, and their F_1 hybrid offspring (which express the antigens of both the A and B parents) reject neither A skin nor B skin, the ability to reject such skin reappears in homozygotes of the F_2 progeny. Thus it is clear that self–non-self discrimination is learned during development: immunological 'self' must encompass all epitopes (antigenic determinants) encoded by the individual's DNA, all other epitopes being considered as non-self.

Yet it is not the structure of a molecule *per se* that determines whether it will be distinguished as self or non-self. Factors other than the structural characteristics of an epitope are also important. Among these are:
- The time when lymphocytes are first confronted with epitopes.
- The site of the encounter.
- The nature of the cells presenting epitopes.
- The production of 'co-stimulatory' molecules by these cells.

History

Soon after antibody specificity was established, it was realized that there must be some mechanism to prevent autoantibody formation. As early as the turn of the century, Ehrlich coined the term 'horror autotoxicus', implying the need for a 'regulating contrivance' to stop production of autoantibodies. In 1938, Traub induced specific tolerance by inoculating mice *in utero* with lymphocytic choriomeningitis virus, producing an infection that was maintained throughout life. Unlike normal mice, these inoculated mice did not produce neutralizing antibodies when challenged with the virus in adult life. That cells carrying self and non-self antigens could develop within a single host, was reported in 1945 by Owen, who described an 'experiment of nature' in non-identical twin cattle. These exchanged haemopoietic (stem) cells via their shared placental blood vessels and each animal carried the erythrocyte markers of both calves. They exhibited life-long tolerance to the otherwise foreign cells, in being unable to mount antibody responses to the relevant erythrocyte antigens. Following this observation, Burnet and Fenner postulated that the time of encounter was the critical factor in determining responsiveness and hence recognition of non-self antigens. This hypothesis seemed logical, as the immune system is usually confronted with most self components before birth and only later with non-self antigens.

Experimental support came in 1953, when Medawar and his colleagues induced immunological tolerance to skin allografts (grafts that are genetically non-identical but are from the same species) in mice by neonatal injection of allogeneic cells (*Fig. 12.1*). This phenomenon was easily accommodated in Burnet's clonal selection theory (1957), which states that a particular immunocyte (a particular B cell or T cell) is selected by antigen and then divides to give rise to a clone of

Induction of specific tolerance in mice

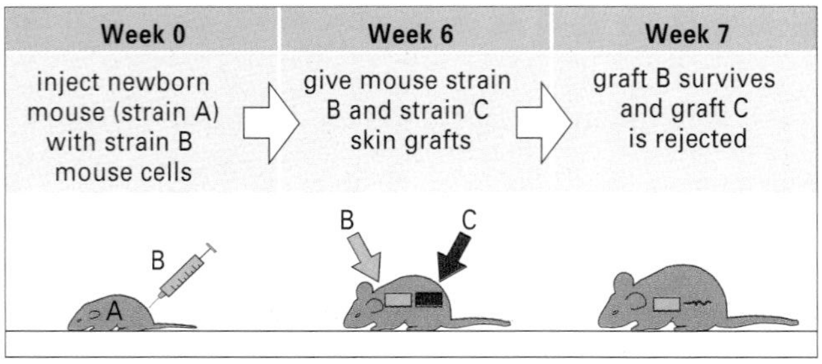

Week 0	Week 6	Week 7
inject newborn mouse (strain A) with strain B mouse cells	give mouse strain B and strain C skin grafts	graft B survives and graft C is rejected

Fig. 12.1 This demonstrates the induction of specific tolerance to grafted skin in mice by neonatal injection of spleen cells from a different strain. Mice of strain A normally reject grafts from strain B. However, if newborn mice of strain A receive cells from strain B mice, at 6 weeks of age they show tolerance towards skin grafts from the donor strain B, but reject grafts from other strains (C).

daughter cells, all with the same specificity. Antigens encountered after birth activate specific clones of lymphocytes, whereas when antigens are encountered before birth the result is the deletion of the clones specific for them, which Burnet termed 'forbidden clones'. Implicit in this theory is the need for the entire immune repertoire to be generated before birth, but in fact lymphocyte differentiation continues long after birth. The key factor in determining responsiveness is thus not the developmental stage of the individual, but rather the state of maturity of the lymphocyte at the time it encounters antigen. This was suggested by Lederberg in 1959, in his modification of the clonal selection theory: immature lymphocytes contacting antigen would be subject to 'clonal abortion', whereas mature cells would be activated. In the unborn and the neonate, most of the cells of the immune system have yet to reach maturity, so the individual is particularly susceptible to tolerance induction at this stage.

Key discoveries in the 1960s established the immunological competence of the lymphocyte, the crucial role of the thymus in the development of the immune system, and the existence of two interacting subsets of lymphocytes, T and B cells. This set the scene for a thorough investigation of the cellular mechanisms involved in 'tolerogenesis'.

In 1970, Bretscher and Cohn suggested that the distinction between immunity and tolerance depends on whether the lymphocyte receives a 'second' or co-stimulator signal in addition to the epitope presented to it: immunity requires both. Thirteen years later, Lafferty and his group provided much evidence from transplantation systems, supporting this view. For example, pancreatic islet tissue is not rejected by incompatible hosts if leucocyte antigen-presenting cells (APCs) capable of delivering the co-stimulator signal are removed by culturing the tissue under special conditions. If antigen in combination with the co-stimulator signal is later supplied by injecting leucocytes expressing the graft antigen, rejection occurs.

■ EXPERIMENTAL INDUCTION OF TOLERANCE

Transgenic technology has allowed the study of tolerance to authentic self antigens

Until recently, only artificially induced tolerance was amenable to experimental study: antigens or foreign cells were inoculated into an animal and the fate of responding T or B cells was investigated under a variety of circumstances. It was not clear, however, to what extent these experimental models resembled natural self tolerance.

Transgenic methods have now made possible the direct investigation of self tolerance. These methods allow one to introduce a specific gene into mice of defined genetic background and analyse its effects upon the development of the immune system. Furthermore, if the introduced gene is linked to a tissue-specific promoter, its expression can be confined to specific cell types (see Chapter 28). The protein product encoded by a 'transgene' is treated by the immune system essentially as an authentic self antigen (autoantigen), and its effects can be studied *in vivo* without the trauma and inflammation associated with grafting foreign cells or tissues. In addition, the parent strain and the transgenic strain are ideal for control experiments and lymphocyte transfer studies because they are congenic, i.e. they differ at only one locus.

There are four possible ways in which self-reactive lymphocytes may be prevented from responding to self antigens

- **Clonal deletion:** physically deleting cells from the repertoire at some stage during their maturation.
- **Clonal abortion:** preventing the further differentiation of the immature cell.
- **Clonal anergy:** downregulating the intrinsic mechanism of immune response.
- **Suppression:** inhibiting cellular activity through interaction with other cells, such as those producing inhibitory cytokines or idiotype-specific lymphocytes which recognize the antigen receptor itself.

Which of these fates awaits the self-reactive lymphocyte depends on numerous factors. Among these are (1) the stage of maturity of the cell being silenced, (2) the affinity of its receptor for the self antigen, (3) the nature of this antigen, (4) its concentration, (5) its tissue distribution, (6) its pattern of expression, and (7) the availability of co-stimulatory signals. As a general rule, if there is no co-stimulation, antigen is more likely to switch off the cell's ability to respond than it is to stimulate an immune response.

■ CENTRAL THYMIC TOLERANCE TO SELF ANTIGENS

Within the thymus, T cells develop from precursors that have not undergone rearrangement of their T-cell receptor (TCR) genes. The genes are rearranged during the development of thymic lymphocytes, so that T cells eventually express TCRs that enable them to recognize antigen degradation products or peptides when these are held in the groove of the MHC molecules encoded by the body's own major histocompatibility complex (MHC) (Chapters 5 and 7).

The thymus selects T cells with receptors that bind to antigen associated with MHC molecules but deletes cells with over-high avidity for self antigens

The high proliferative rate of thymocytes is paralleled by a massive rate of cell death: the vast majority of the double positive (CD4$^+$CD8$^+$) thymocytes die within the thymus. Among the factors which account for this are aberrant TCR gene rearrangement (so that no usable TCR is made), negative selection and failure to be positively selected. In positive selection, T cells that have some degree of binding avidity for polymorphic regions of MHC molecules are selected for survival (*Fig. 12.2*): the T cells encounter the MHC molecules on cortical epithelial cells, and binding is presumed to protect the cells from programmed cell death. This positive selection process ensures that the mature T cell recognizes peptides only in the binding cleft of self MHC molecules, and so will be self-MHC restricted. Positive selection does not, however, prevent the differentiation of T cells bearing TCR of high binding strength for both self peptides and MHC molecules. Some form of negative selection must therefore operate to silence these strongly self-reactive cells.

The avidity of interaction between TCR on thymocytes and epitopes on thymic stromal cells determines the type of selection

Since both positive and negative selection processes involve the recognition of self peptides associated with self MHC molecules, how can signals initiated through the same TCR lead to both processes? The difference between these two processes is related to the avidity of engagement, which is a function of both the affinity of the TCR for its epitope and the epitope concentration. A stronger engagement favours negative selection. The existence of qualitatively different signals for each selection process is probably the reason why the CD8's co-receptor function is essential for positive selection but is not required for negative selection unless the affinity of the TCR for the peptide is low.

Clonal deletion is the predominant mechanism of negative selection

This has been shown in a variety of experimental models. For example, in mice transgenic for a rearranged TCR directed to the male (H–Y) antigen, H–Y-autospecific T cells are deleted in male mice but not in female mice, which do not express H–Y.

The timing and localization of negative selection depend on a variety of factors

These include the accessibility of developing T cells to self-antigen, the combined avidity of the TCR and accessory molecules (CD8 or CD4) for the self-MHC–self-peptide complex, and the identity of the deleting cells. Negative selection does not require specialized antigen-presenting cells (APCs): it is normally a function of the thymic dendritic cells or macrophages, which are situated predominantly at the corticomedullary junction and are rich in class I and II MHCs and so can bind the T cells that have high avidity for self peptides

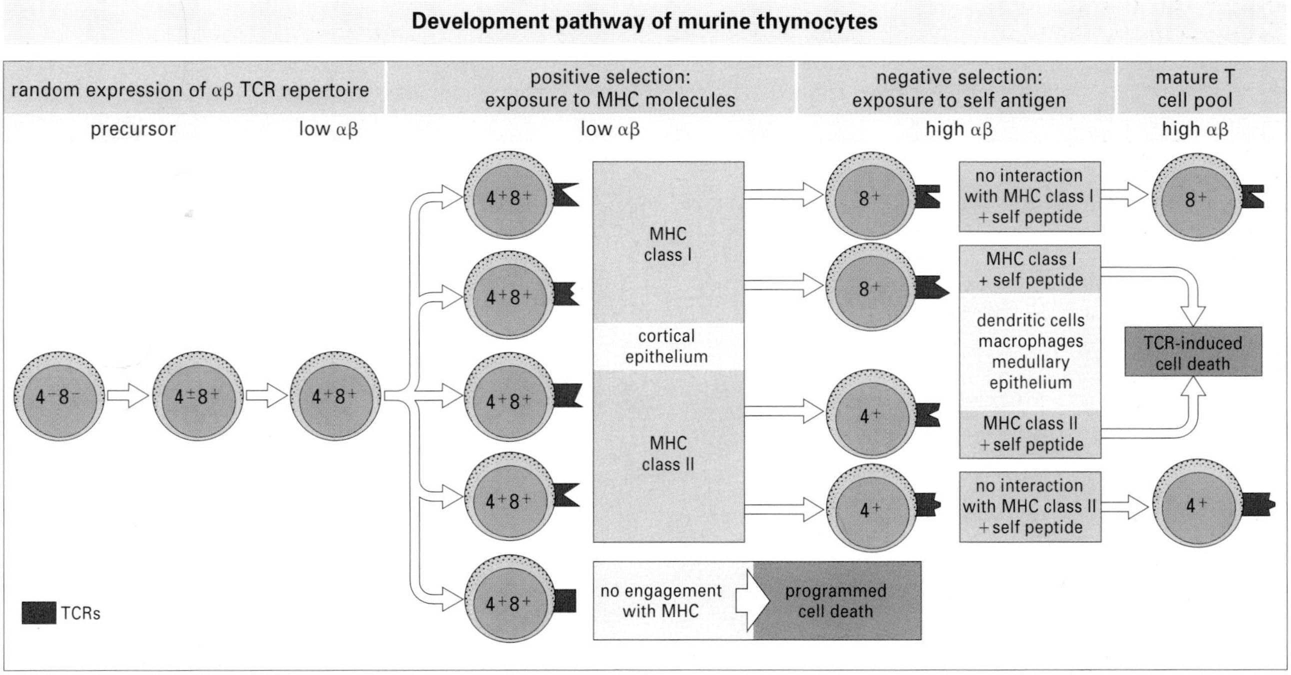

Development pathway of murine thymocytes

Fig. 12.2 Precursor thymocytes develop into cortical 'double positive' cells expressing low levels of the αβ TCR. These undergo positive selection for interaction with self MHC class I or class II molecules on cortical epithelium. Unselected cells (the majority) undergo programmed cell death (by apoptosis). Cells interacting with class I MHC lose CD4 and cells interacting with MHC class II lose CD8. Finally self-reactive cells are eliminated by their interaction with self peptides presented on cells at the corticomedullary junction and in the thymic medulla.

(*Fig. 12.3*). Some of the medullary and cortical epithelial cells can also be involved. Other cells participating in deletion may be the thymocytes themselves (*Fig. 12.3*).

Specialized 'veto' cells bearing self epitopes impart a negative signal, killing the self-reactive clone (*Fig. 12.4*). Under physiological conditions, veto signals occur when a T cell expressing a TCR for a self epitope binds to a veto cell that expresses the self epitopes. For the veto effect to occur, the TCR has to bind to the self epitope associated with MHC class I on the veto cell, while the CD8 of the veto cell binds to MHC class I on the T cell. Once binding has occurred, the T cell is killed.

■ POST-THYMIC TOLERANCE TO SELF ANTIGENS

Some self-reactive T cells escape thymic censorship

Potentially autoaggressive T cells, which have escaped negative selection in the thymus, are found in healthy individuals. These circulate either because the corresponding self antigen is not expressed in the thymus (in which case negative selection cannot occur); or because the T cells' TCRs have too low an affinity for the self-peptide–MHC complex displayed on thymic stromal cells; or because the concentration of surface MHC–peptide complex is too low. The question must therefore be asked: what mechanisms prevent autoimmunity?

Potentially self-reactive T cells can sometimes ignore their self antigen

Ignorance of self antigens (autoantigens) occurs:
- If self-reactive T cells are unable to penetrate an endothelial barrier that serves to sequester cells bearing self antigens.
- If they cannot be activated even after crossing these barriers because:
    (a) The self antigen is present in too low an amount to be detected.
    (b) The self antigen is present on tissue cells that express few or no MHC molecules.
    (c) The T cells perceive the self antigen requires help (e.g. in the form of cytokines delivered by TH cells) to be fully activated.

Such ignorance of self antigens is not a form of immunological tolerance, but it is an important factor in considering how some autoimmune states arise.

Potentially self-reactive T cells can be tolerized by self antigen on tissue cells or silenced by immunoregulatory cells

Peripheral deletion of mature T cells has been documented in several transgenic mouse models. For example, when mice transgenic for a TCR that recognizes lymphocytic choriomeningitis virus (LCMV) were infected with a form of virus known to cause persistent infection, this induced a cytotoxic

---

Thymic cells involved in negative selection

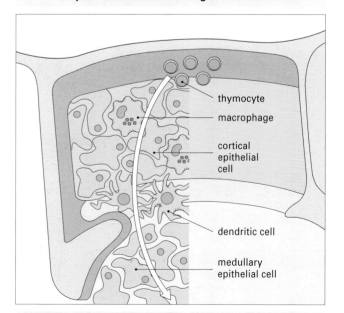

Fig. 12.3 The deleting population includes bone-marrow-derived macrophages, or dendritic cells, which are situated predominantly at the corticomedullary junction. Other cells involved in deletion may be the thymocytes themselves, through their veto function, and some types of thymic epithelial cells, possibly in the medulla.

The veto effect: three mechanisms

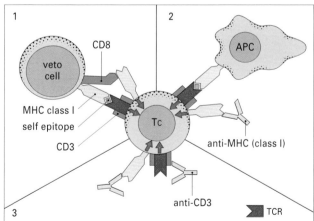

Fig. 12.4 1. Specialized veto cells bearing self epitopes can kill a self-reactive clone.
2. The veto effect can be mimicked using an APC to present self antigen to the T cell, combined with a monoclonal antibody which binds to the class I molecule of the T cell.
3. The veto effect can also be reproduced using a monoclonal antibody, as in (2), and another monoclonal antibody in place of the APC. This antibody binds to the CD3 molecule on the T cell, suggesting that the message coming from the TCR is passed to the cell via the CD3.

lymphocyte response followed by deletion of the LCMV-immune T cells. The phenomenon could be reproduced by injecting an LCMV peptide: after an initial clonal expansion, the transgenic CD8$^+$ T cells were deleted and tolerance was established. In the management of autoimmunity, therefore, administration of the relevant peptide should protect; indeed, this has recently been achieved in transgenic models of autoimmune diabetes and encephalomyelitis.

Anergy, a failure of the T-cell response, has been demonstrated *in vitro* when T cells are presented with antigen on 'non-professional' APCs: it occurs because these APCs cannot deliver a co-stimulatory signal, due to their lack of the molecules B7-1 and B7-2. These co-stimulator molecules are characteristically expressed by professional APCs, and their binding to the T cell's CD28 and CTLA-4 molecules produces a powerful co-stimulatory signal to the T cell (see Chapter 8). Anergy may also occur *in vivo* if self-reactive T cells gain access to tissue cells that do not express co-stimulator molecules; in such cases, the T cells may become anergic and escape deletion, at least initially.

There is evidence for some form of T-cell-dependent suppression of self-reactive cells. This probably occurs as a back-up mechanism to inhibit self-reactive T cells once they have been activated. One way in which T cells may suppress an immune response is by the inhibitory effects of cytokines such as TGF$_\beta$. Another way relates to the activities of two types of helper T cells, TH1 and TH2. Although these cells secrete a number of the same cytokines, they differ in their pattern of release of other cytokines. Thus TH1 and TH2 can antagonize each other and so play a role in immunoregulation (*Fig. 12.5*).

◼ B-CELL TOLERANCE TO SELF ANTIGENS

High-affinity IgG production is T-cell dependent (see Chapter 7). For this reason, and because the threshold of tolerance for T cells is lower than for B cells, the simplest explanation for non-self reactivity by B cells is a lack of T-cell help (*Fig. 12.6*).

In some circumstances B cells must be tolerized directly

For example, some microorganisms have cross-reactive antigens that have both foreign T-cell-reactive epitopes *and* other epitopes that resemble self epitopes and are capable of stimulating B cells. Such antigens could provoke a vigorous antibody response to self antigens (*Fig. 12.6*). Furthermore, in contrast to TCRs, the immunoglobulin receptors on mature, antigenically stimulated B cells can undergo hypermutation and may acquire anti-self reactivities at this late stage. Tolerance may thus be imposed on B cells both during their development and after antigenic stimulation in secondary lymphoid tissues.

Self-reactive B cells may be deleted or anergized depending on the affinity of the B-cell antigen receptor and the nature of the antigen

Tolerization by self antigens can lead to one of several results, such as deletion or anergy. The outcome depends on the affinity of the B-cell antigen receptor and on the nature of the antigen it encounters, whether this is an integral membrane

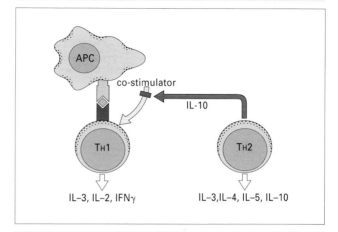

T-cell suppression of immune responsiveness

Fig. 12.5 Two subsets of TH cells, TH1 and TH2, exist. Each subset has a distinct pattern of cytokine production (white arrows). Through their production of IL-10, the TH2 cells may render TH1 cells anergic by interfering with the co-stimulator function of APCs.

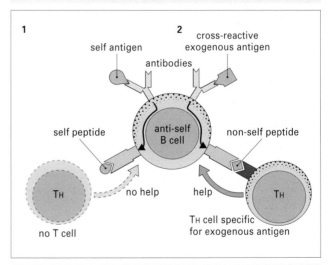

B-cell response to self or foreign antigens

Fig. 12.6 1. If TH cells are not available, either because of a hole in the T-cell repertoire (see Chapter 9), or because of deletion resulting from self-tolerance achieved intrathymically, any B cells that are self-reactive (anti-self) will nevertheless be unable to mount an anti-self antibody response.
2. Autoantibodies can be produced if an anti-self B cell collaborates with an anti-non-self TH cell in response to cross-reactive antigens containing both self and non-self determinants.
   This mechanism is discussed at greater length in Chapter 27 (cf. Fig 27.20).

protein or a soluble and largely monomeric protein in the circulation. The fate of self-reactive B cells has been determined using transgenic technology (*Figs 12.7* and *12.8*).

B cells that respond to membrane-bound self antigens are eventually deleted

The fate of self-reactive B cells encountering cell-membrane-associated self antigens that are capable of cross-linking the B cells' Ig receptors with high avidity may be summarized as follows. In the bone marrow, the number of immature self-reactive B cells is not reduced even though their IgM receptors are downregulated following exposure to the membrane-bound self antigens. Immature B cells are thus less readily deleted than are immature T cells during the early stages of differentiation. Nevertheless, these B cells have a very short lifespan and are destined to die (probably by apoptosis), generally prior to their arrival in the peripheral lymphoid tissues.

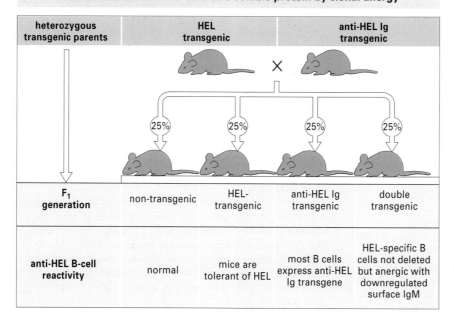

Tolerance induction in peripheral B cells by clonal deletion

heterozygous transgenic parents	MET-K^b transgenic		anti-K^b Ig transgenic
F$_1$ generation	non-transgenic	MET-K^b transgenic	anti-K^b Ig transgenic	double transgenic
anti-K^b B-cell reactivity	normal	no IgG anti-K^b reactivity	Ig anti-K^b antibody present	anti-K^b B cells deleted from lymph nodes and spleen

Fig. 12.7 Non-b haplotype mice were given the gene for H–2K^b, which is a foreign MHC class I and a membrane protein. The gene was controlled by the metallothionein promoter, specific for sites such as the liver (MET–K^b transgenic). These mice were crossed with other non-b mice which had been given the gene for anti-H–2K^b Ig antibodies (anti-K^b Ig transgenic). Double transgenic offspring expressed H–2K^b in the liver and exported B cells specific for H–2K^b from the marrow. However, these self-reactive B cells were partially deleted in the spleen and entirely deleted in the lymph nodes, and never had the chance to produce autoantibodies. No idiotype identical to the anti-K^b Ig in the transgenic parents was detected.

Tolerance induction in B cells to a soluble protein by clonal anergy

heterozygous transgenic parents	HEL transgenic		anti-HEL Ig transgenic
F$_1$ generation	non-transgenic	HEL-transgenic	anti-HEL Ig transgenic	double transgenic
anti-HEL B-cell reactivity	normal	mice are tolerant of HEL	most B cells express anti-HEL Ig transgene	HEL-specific B cells not deleted but anergic with downregulated surface IgM

Fig. 12.8 A mouse line was given the hen egg lysozyme (HEL) gene, linked to a tissue-specific promoter. The (largely soluble) HEL led to T- and B-cell tolerance. A second transgenic line (anti-HEL Ig) carried rearranged heavy and light chain genes encoding a high-affinity anti-HEL antibody. An allotype marker (IgH^a) distinguished this from endogenous immunoglobulin (IgH^b). The majority of B cells in these transgenics carried IgM and IgD of the 'a' allotype. Double transgenic offspring were highly HEL-tolerant, producing neither anti-HEL antibody nor plaque-forming cells. HEL-binding (self-reactive) B cells were not deleted; however, they had downregulated surface IgM, but not IgD, receptors. They behaved as anergic cells.

B cells that can bind soluble self antigens become anergic

When they are exposed to largely monomeric soluble antigens, self-reactive B cells are not deleted from the peripheral lymphoid tissues, where they can be found in large numbers, but are instead rendered anergic. This effect occurs only when the antigen is above a critical concentration threshold. Anergy is associated with downregulation of the membrane IgM, but not IgD, receptors. The anergic state is accompanied by an arrest in B-cell maturation in the follicular mantle zone of the spleen and by a striking reduction in marginal zone B cells with high levels of surface IgM. Thus, in contrast to B cells subjected to clonal deletion, anergic B cells do migrate to the periphery but, once there, they fail to interact with the corresponding TH cells, as an indirect result of the lack of IgM. Furthermore, their half life is 3–4 days compared with 4–5 weeks for normal peripheral B cells. The mechanism is probably not activity of suppressor T cells or of anti-idiotypic B cells, as no evidence for this has been found in transgenic models.

Anergy in B cells is reversible. Thus anergic B cells can respond to antigen-independent CD40-dependent signals from TH cells and then can take up physiological concentrations of antigen via IgD receptors to present to TH cells (see Chapter 8). On the other hand, upregulation of B7 molecules on the cell surface, after ligation of the antigen receptor, is impaired. This co-stimulatory defect of anergic B cells can be overcome if B cells are stimulated by inflammatory cytokines (such as IL-4) or various polyclonal activators (such as lipopolysaccharide). Furthermore, chronic T-cell activation by infectious agents can lead to 'bystander' B-cell activation via the CD40 pathway and cytokines.

■ ARTIFICIALLY INDUCED TOLERANCE *IN VIVO*

Tolerance can be induced artificially *in vivo* by a variety of means.

Chimerism is associated with tolerance

Tolerance can be induced by inoculation of allogeneic cells into hosts that lack immunocompetence, for example neonatal hosts, or adult hosts after immunosuppressive regimens such as total body irradiation, drugs (e.g. cyclosporin) or anti-lymphocytic antibodies (anti-lymphocyte globulin, anti-CD4 antibodies, etc.). For tolerance to be maintained, a certain degree of chimerism, the coexistence of cells from genetically different individuals, must be maintained. This is best achieved if the inoculum contains cells capable of self-renewal (e.g. bone marrow cells).

If mature T cells are present in the injected cell population, they may react against the histocompatibility antigens of their host and induce a severe and often fatal disease known as graft-versus-host disease.

Antibodies to T-cell co-receptors induce tolerance to transplants

Tolerance of transplanted tissues can be achieved in adult animals by monoclonal antibodies directed against the T-cell molecules, CD4 and CD8 (the antibodies can be either the T-cell-depleting or the non-depleting type). In this situation, tolerance of skin allografts is obtained even in the absence of cellular chimerism.

Soluble antigens readily induce tolerance

Tolerance is inducible in both neonatal and adult animals by administering soluble protein antigens in deaggregated form. T and B cells differ in their susceptibility to tolerization by these antigens. Thus, tolerance is achieved in T cells from spleen and thymus after very low antigen doses and within a few hours. Tolerance of spleen B cells requires much more time and higher antigen doses (*Fig. 12.9*). The antigen levels which will produce B-cell tolerance in neonates are about one-hundredth of those in adults.

Oral administration of antigens induces tolerance

Antigens administered orally induce tolerance through some (as yet unknown) mechanism that may involve an immuno-regulatory or a suppressor cell network generated in the gut wall.

Targeting antigen to naive B cells induces T-cell tolerance

In some experimental situations, antigen presented by naive B cells has induced antigen-specific T-cell tolerance. This may be because naive B cells, which do not express B7 and hence lack its T-cell co-stimulatory functions, can efficiently process antigen and present it to T cells. Accordingly, T-cell tolerance may be achieved by targeting the antigen to naive B cells, simply by attaching the antigen to a monoclonal antibody directed against the IgD molecule on the B cell surface.

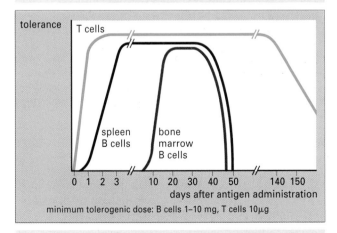

The relative susceptibilities of T cells and B cells to tolerization *in vivo*

tolerance

T cells

spleen B cells   bone marrow B cells

0 1 2 3   10 20 30 40 50   140 150
days after antigen administration

minimum tolerogenic dose: B cells 1–10 mg, T cells 10 μg

Fig. 12.9 A mouse was given antigen (human globulin – a T_{dep} antigen) at tolerance-inducing (tolerogenic) doses, and the duration of tolerance was measured. T-cell tolerance was more rapidly induced and more persistent than B-cell tolerance. Bone-marrow B cells may take considerably longer than splenic B cells to tolerize. Typically, considerably lower antigen doses are sufficient for T-cell tolerization: 10 μg as opposed to 1–10 mg, a 1000-fold difference.

Extensive clonal proliferation can lead to exhaustion and tolerance

Tolerance in T lymphocytes and to a lesser extent in B cells can be due to clonal exhaustion, the end result of a powerful immune response. Repeated antigenic challenge may stimulate all the antigen-responding cells to differentiate into short-lived end cells, leaving no cells that can respond to a subsequent challenge with antigen.

Antagonist peptides that signal inappropriately can induce tolerance

Some peptides, known as antagonist peptides, fit into the antigen-binding groove of MHC molecules but nevertheless do not activate specific T cells. This may be because they fail to transmit signals through the TCR, or because they transmit a negative signal or allow only partial signalling (*Fig. 12.10*). This might occur if the antagonists cannot induce the necessary conformational change in the TCR, or its dimerization, or recruitment into the peptide–MHC–TCR complex of co-receptor molecules. Whatever the case may be, antagonists block the response of T cells to the corresponding agonist peptide – i.e. the normal form, which can stimulate the cells. Specific T-cell tolerance is thus achieved by antagonists.

Slowly metabolized T-cell-independent antigens induce B-cell tolerance

T_{ind} antigens tend to be slowly metabolized *in vivo* and therefore tend to produce long-lasting B-cell tolerance, provided a large enough antigen dose is used. In very high concentration, T_{ind} antigens can actually blockade the surface receptors of fully differentiated antibody-forming cells (AFCs) and so prevent them from secreting antibody (*Fig. 12.11*).

Anti-idiotypic responses can be associated with tolerance

An antibody's combining site may act as an antigen and induce the formation of 'anti-idiotypic antibodies' (see Chapter 11). By cross-linking immunoglobulin on B cells, these antibodies can block B-cell responsiveness of the cell. Because in some animals most of the antibodies produced in response to particular antigens bear a particular idiotype, suppression of this idiotype by anti-idiotypic antibody can significantly alter the response. This type of tolerance will be partial, however, because it affects only those B cells carrying the idiotype.

Tolerance is induced by veto and suppressor cells

In some experimental systems, tolerance appears to have been induced and to have been transferable by veto cells (see *Fig. 12.4*), which can exist extrathymically, or by 'suppressor T cells', which may exert their effects through the release of certain inhibitory lymphokines.

Immune deviation may select an appropriate immune response

Although immune deviation is not strictly tolerance in terms of the antigen-specific functional or physical inactivation of cells, the use of certain cytokines may allow manipulation of selective immune responses. Since TH1-type cells are most active in cell-mediated immune responses such as delayed-type hypersensitivity and foreign graft destruction, interfer-

ence with their function by inducing TH2 cells may be beneficial in transplantation systems. For example, IL-10, a cytokine produced by TH2 cells, can suppress the activities of TH1 cells by an effect on APCs and may thereby diminish the damage caused by TH1 cells (see also *Fig. 12.5*).

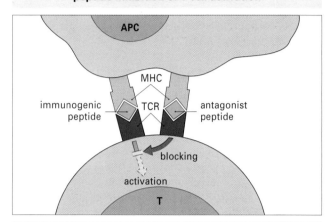

T-cell tolerance due to antagonist peptide inhibition of T-cell activation

Fig. 12.10 Antagonist peptides and immunogenic peptides both bind to the MHC molecules on professional antigen-presenting cells (APC). The interaction of the TCR with the MHC–antagonist peptide prevents stimulation by the immunogenic ligand through an inhibitory effect on the signalling pathways.

B-cell clonal deletion and AFC blockade

type of tolerance	minimum effective tolerogenic dose		isotype susceptibility	tolerance attainable
	dextran (500 kDa)	levan (6 kDa)		
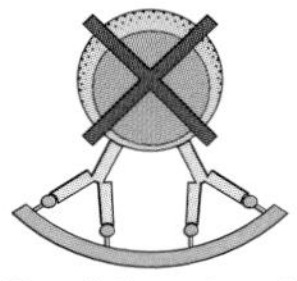 B-cell functional deletion	1 mg	10 mg	IgG>IgM	complete
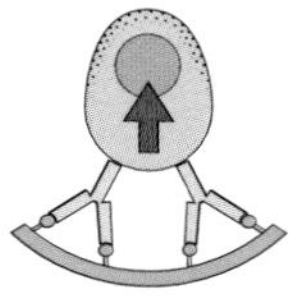 AFC blockade	0.01 mg	inactive	IgG<IgM	partial

Fig. 12.11 Binding of a T_{ind} antigen to the B cell's receptors may cause functional deletion of the B-cell clone, or reduce antibody production by interfering with processes involved in antibody secretion. These two tolerance mechanisms may be distinguished by the minimum effective dose of tolerogens and their molecular weight, the relative susceptibility of different classes of antibody affected and the level of tolerance attainable.

MAINTENANCE OF TOLERANCE *IN VIVO*

Persistence of antigen plays a major role in maintaining a state of tolerance to it *in vivo*: when the antigen concentration drops below a certain threshold, responsiveness is restored. If the tolerance results from clonal deletion or permanent anergy, recovery of responsiveness is related to the time required to generate new lymphocytes from their precursors. It can be prevented by measures such as thymectomy.

ARTIFICIALLY INDUCED TOLERANCE *IN VITRO*

B and T cells can be tolerized readily in vitro

Antigens that cross-link the immunoglobulin receptors on B cells but do not possess intrinsic mitogenic capacity can tolerize B cells. To tolerize mature B cells they must be at high concentration, but low concentrations work for immature B cells. A monoclonal anti-IgM antibody can be used to mimic this antigen cross-linking of the B-cell immunoglobulin receptors. High anti-IgM concentrations clonally abort pre-B cells, preventing their further differentiation to surface membrane IgM-bearing ($mIgM^+$) B cells. A lower concentration allows the pre-B cells to develop into morphologically normal B cells, with normal numbers of immunoglobulin receptors, but renders them profoundly anergic (Fig. *12.12*). Hence, both B-cell function and B-cell numbers can be modulated, via their surface immunoglobulin receptors, at the critical time of acquisition of these receptors (the pre-B to B cell transition).

Whether an antigen induces B-cell abortion, deletion or anergy depends on the degree of Ig-receptor occupancy and cross-linking

Factors contributing to the pathway a B cell will take include the antigen's valency (i.e. how many epitopes it has) and concentration, the receptor's affinity for the binding epitope of the antigen and the state of maturity of the B cell. At one end of the spectrum is clonal abortion, likely to occur in less mature cells, especially those possessing a higher affinity epitope-binding receptor or encountering antigens of higher valency and concentration (see *Fig. 12.13*). At the opposite end, no effect occurs at low concentrations and affinities. Clonal anergy is induced in circumstances that lie between these two extremes.

- **Clonal abortion:** multivalent antigen can, when given in appropriate concentrations, cause immature B cells to abort by preventing their further differentiation. 'Tolerizability' of pre-B cells is high.
- **Clonal deletion:** very strong negative signals can cause deletion of mature B cells.
- **Clonal anergy:** intermediate concentrations of multivalent antigen allows pre-B cells to develop into morphologically normal B cells, with normal numbers of immunoglobulin receptors, but renders them profoundly anergic.
- **Clonal ignorance:** antigen will not have any effect on B cells if its concentration is too low or if the affinity of the antigen receptors is too weak. Strictly speaking, this is not a form of tolerance.
- **Blockade of antibody-forming cells (AFCs):** excess of T_{ind} antigen interferes with antibody secretion by AFCs. Tolerizability of AFCs is low.

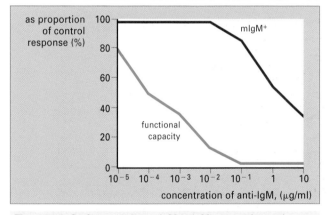

Sensitivity of B cells to anti-IgM

Fig. 12.12 Surface membrane IgM (mIgM) expression and functional capacity (responsiveness to lipopolysaccharide, LPS) are represented as a percentage of the normal response. Approximately 10 000 times more anti-IgM antibody is required to reduce mIgM expression as is needed to effect a similar reduction in functional capacity. As little as 10^{-3} μg/ml anti-IgM has a significant effect on LPS responsiveness without affecting mIgM expression.

Sensitivity of B cells

Stage of B-cell development	Strength of negative signal			
	very strong	strong	intermediate	weak
pre-B → B cell	abortion	abortion	anergy	no effect
B cell	deletion	anergy	no effect	no effect
AFC	blockade	no effect	no effect	no effect
memory B cell → secondary B cell	abortion	abortion	anergy	no effect

Fig. 12.13 As an immature B cell matures into an AFC, it becomes increasingly resistant to tolerization. The type of tolerance depends on the maturity of the cell and the strength of the signal received. This in turn depends on the affinity of the antigen receptor for the relevant epitopes, and the concentration and valency of the antigen which confronts the cell.

A second window of susceptibility to tolerization occurs transiently during the generation of B-cell memory

Secondary B cells (derived from memory B cells produced by T-cell-dependent stimulation – see Chapter 11) are highly susceptible to tolerization by epitopes presented multivalently in the absence of T-cell help (see Fig. *12.13*). Such a tolerance-susceptible stage probably ensures newly derived memory B cells that have acquired self-reactivity (as a result of accumulated somatic mutations) are purged from the repertoire.

T cells can be tolerized in vitro by antigen without APCs

If an influenza-specific T-cell clone is incubated for a few hours at 37°C with a high concentration of influenza peptide but no APCs (i.e. without co-stimulation), the T cells remain alive but become anergic. The outcome can be influenced by various lymphokines: some inhibit tolerance induction (e.g. IL-2 but not IFN$_\gamma$ or IL-1) and some reverse established tolerance (e.g. IL-2). These and other observations have suggested that altered regulation of the IL-2 pathway may be an intracellular lesion that characterizes the induction of tolerance in T cells.

■ TOLERANCE BREAKDOWN AND AUTOIMMUNITY

As there are many diverse tolerance-inducing mechanisms, it is probable that there are multiple ways in which tolerance can break down, leading to autoimmunity. Conditions predisposing to autoimmunity and the pathogenesis of autoimmune disease are discussed in more detail in Chapter 27.

Thymic selection may be flawed in individuals with certain MHC genotypes

Some MHC molecules may fail either to negatively select self-reactive T cells, or to positively select the immunoregulatory T cells required for the inhibition of activated self-reactive T cells. Other MHC molecules may negatively select T cells specific for epitopes of microorganisms, and the consequent failure to eliminate infections caused by these organisms may be associated with tissue damage and processing of self-antigen by professional APCs, leading to self-reactivity.

Antigen cross-reactivity may activate self-reactive T cells (molecular mimicry)

Self-reactive T cells that have ignored a given self antigen (for reasons given earlier) may be stimulated by professional APCs that can deliver a powerful co-stimulator signal *and* present an antigen (derived from an invading microorganism) that cross-reacts with the self antigen.

Sequestered self antigens may be released

Any factor causing release of self antigens previously inaccessible to T cells and to professional APCs may allow these to present the antigens to self-reactive T cells.

Cytokine production may be disturbed

The fact that clonal anergy is reversible in the presence of IL-2 (see earlier) suggests that disturbances in cytokine production may predispose to autoimmunity.

Immunoregulation may fail

Failure of suppression or defects in the regulation of T$_H$1 and T$_H$2 cells will cause immune deviation and may be associated with loss of tolerance.

■ POTENTIAL THERAPEUTIC APPLICATIONS OF TOLERANCE

A better understanding of tolerogenesis could be valuable in many ways. It could be used to promote tolerance of foreign tissue grafts or to control the damaging immune responses in hypersensitivity states and autoimmune diseases. The various ways of establishing artificial tolerance in adult animals are being investigated for their potential clinical applications. Some success has been obtained in the case of transplants associated with chimerism and performed under the umbrella of immunosuppressive agents. Treatment with monoclonal non-depleting anti-CD4 and anti-CD8 antibodies has also been used successfully for transplanting foreign tissues or organs in patients. The possibility that tolerance can be induced by orally feeding the target antigen and by using peptide antagonists may be used as a way to control some autoimmune diseases.

It is also important to learn how to activate T cells that ignore particular antigens, so as to enable the immune system to mount an appropriate active response. This could be exploited to limit the growth of tumours that may express their own unique tumour-specific genes as a membrane-bound antigen.

Critical Thinking

■ Why do self-reactive lymphocytes escape censorship?

■ Why do circulating self-reactive lymphocytes not normally cause autoimmunity?

■ What tips the balance towards autoaggression and how can this be prevented or curtailed?

FURTHER READING

Goodnow C. Transgenic mice and analysis of B-cell tolerance. *Annu Rev Immunol* 1992;**10**:489.

Miller JFAP, Flavell R. T cell tolerance and autoimmunity in transgenic models of central and peripheral tolerance. *Curr Opin Immunol* 1994;**6**:892–99.

Nossal GJV. Negative selection of lymphocytes. *Cell* 1994;**76**:229.

Waldmann H, Cobbald S. The use of monoclonal antibodies to achieve immunological tolerance. *Immunol Today* 1993;**14**:247.

The complement system is part of the innate immune system and has evolved mechanisms of self/non-self discrimination. The essence of this discrimination is the presence on host tissues of regulatory molecules that inhibit the activation of complement.

There are two main pathways for complement activation, the classical and alternative pathways. The classical pathway links the adaptive immune system, antibody, to the innate immune system, complement, by the binding to immune complexes of C1q.

There is continuous, 'tick-over', activation of C3 in plasma which leads to the deposition of small numbers of C3 molecules on host and foreign surfaces. On host surfaces, regulatory molecules promote the catabolism of such deposited C3 and inhibit further activation of complement. Alternative pathway activation is initiated when C3, activated by the 'tick-over' pathway, deposits on foreign surfaces, lacking regulatory molecules.

Complement proteins C3 and C4 possess an internal thioester bond which enables their covalent binding to amino and hydroxyl groups. This is a key step in the localization of complement activation to sites of inflammation.

The complement system contains two amplification mechanisms. The first is known as a 'triggered enzyme cascade'. The 'trigger' is the binding of a small number of C1q molecules, which then sequentially activate a series of zymogens (pro-enzymes) causing cleavage of a large number of C3 molecules.

The second amplification mechanism is a positive feedback loop, the 'amplification loop', which is initiated by the cleavage of a small amount of C3 to C3b. This participates in the formation of a C3 convertase enzyme, which cleaves yet more C3. Host cells contain molecules that inhibit this amplification loop by catabolizing C3b to inactive products. On foreign surfaces the amplification is unregulated.

The effector mechanisms of the complement system may be divided into five groups:
i) opsonization of microorganisms for phagocytosis; ii) direct killing of microorganisms by lysis; iii) chemotactic attraction to sites of inflammation and activation of leucocytes; iv) processing of immune complexes; and v) induction of specific antibody responses by augmentation of the localization of antigens to B lymphocytes and antigen-presenting cells.

Pathogenic microorganisms have evolved mechanisms to escape killing by the complement system and, in some cases, use the complement system to augment their pathogenicity.

The complement system may contribute to disease pathogenesis if activated systemically in vivo on a large scale, or if activation is focused on host tissues by autoantibodies.

■ INTRODUCTION

The term 'complement' was originally applied by Ehrlich to describe the activity in serum which could 'complement' the ability of specific antibody to cause lysis of bacteria. The discovery of this heat-labile activity in serum is usually attributed to Bordet (1895), although Nuttall had described a similar activity some years earlier. In 1907, Ferrata demonstrated that complement could be separated into two components by dialysis of serum against acidified water. This yielded a euglobulin precipitate and a water-soluble albumin fraction. Complement activity could only be demonstrated in the presence of both of these fractions, which he called mid-piece (C1) and end-piece (C2). Subsequently, Sachs and Omorokow showed that cobra venom inactivated another component (C'3), and Gordon found that a further component was destroyed by ammonia (C'4). The order of discovery of these components of complement does not correspond to their order of reaction, and this explains the apparent illogicality of the present-day nomenclature system.

The nomenclature of the complement system is complex

The proteins of the classical pathway and membrane attack system are each assigned a number and react in the order: C1q, C1r, C1s, C4, C2, C3, C5, C6, C7, C8, C9. Many of the proteins are zymogens, i.e. pro-enzymes requiring proteolytic cleavage to become active. The enzymatically-active form is distinguished from its precursor by a bar drawn above its notation, e.g. $\overline{C1r}$. The cleavage products of complement proteins are distinguished from the parent molecules by suffix letters; conventionally the small initial cleavage fragment is designated the 'a' fragment and the larger portion, the 'b' fragment, e.g. C3a and C3b. (An exception to this rule is seen for C2, so that the small fragment is designated C2b and the large fragment, C2a.)

The proteins of the alternative pathway are known by the term 'Factors', and are identified by single letters. Conventionally, 'Factor' can be abbreviated to 'F' or even omitted altogether, so that 'Factor B' may be represented as 'FB', or quite simply as 'B'.

Regulatory proteins are symbolized by abbreviations that are usually derived from a name related to a functional activity of the molecule: for example, decay accelerating factor (DAF) accelerates the breakdown of the classical pathway C3 convertase.

Complement receptors are named either according to their ligand (e.g. C5a receptor) or using the Cluster of Differentiation (CD) system. There is also a numbering system for receptors of the major fragments of C3, complement receptor types 1 to 4 (CR1 to CR4). This has the unfortunate consequence that some receptors have three names in current usage: the receptor for C3b is variously referred to as C3b receptor, CR1 and CD35.

Complement proteins can be grouped into superfamilies

Proteins in a superfamily – for example, the immunoglobulin supergene family (see Chapter 4) – share numerous structural and functional features. Within the complement system many proteins may be assigned to such families.

Classification of complement proteins into superfamilies provides a useful framework for understanding their structural and functional relationships

This idea is illustrated by the complement control proteins (CCPs), also known as regulators of complement activation (RCA). The members of this family of proteins are:

- Factor H: a plasma globulin with an elongated configuration
- C4-binding protein (C4-bp): a heptameric plasma protein with a 'spider-like' configuration
- Decay accelerating factor (DAF, CD55): a membrane protein attached by an unusual glycophospholipid 'foot'
- Membrane cofactor protein (MCP, CD46): a transmembrane protein that acts as a cofactor for cleavage of C3b
- Complement receptors type 1 (CR1, CD35) and type 2 (CR2, CD21): cellular receptors with transmembrane domains.

The CCPs are all encoded in a closely linked gene cluster on chromosome 1. Despite apparently dissimilar structures, they all contain a domain of approximately 60 amino acids, called the short consensus repeat (SCR). SCRs may appear many times in each molecule, and are encoded by tandemly-arranged homologous exons. They provide the structural scaffold of each molecule, and may also provide the binding specificity of the protein.

These six proteins also share a number of functions in the complement cascade: Factor H, C4-bp, DAF, MCP and CR1 all inhibit stable formation of the classical and alternative pathway of C3 convertase enzymes, respectively $\overline{\text{C4b2a}}$ and $\overline{\text{C3bBb}}$. Some also share other functions that are overlapping, though not identical. These functions include: inhibiting the binding of C2 to C4b, and Factor B to C3b; promoting the dissociation of C2a from C4b, and Bb from C3b; and acting as cofactors to Factor I, the enzyme responsible for the catabolism of C3b and C4b.

Note that there are other molecules that contain the SCR, yet do not interact with proteins of the complement system; they include IL-2 receptor, β_2-glycoprotein I and Factor XIII of the blood clotting system.

Most complement proteins have a 'mosaic' structure

The molecular basis of relationships within these families has become apparent following cloning of their genes. It is now believed that during evolution, exons have been duplicated and 'shuffled' between different genes. These duplicated segments of DNA have evolved in parallel and have often maintained closely related structures and functions, although in some cases activities have been lost, or new ones acquired.

Many complement proteins consist of a 'mosaic' of exons derived from different families. For example, C1s, an enzyme of the classical pathway, contains exons from the serine esterase and low density lipoprotein (LDL) receptor (LDL-B) families, as well as the short consensus repeat domain from the complement control protein superfamily. Similarly, C6, 7, 8 and 9, components of the pore-forming membrane attack complex, share features with perforin and with eosinophil cationic protein.

Complement is one of the major effector pathways of inflammation

The complement system is part of the innate immune system and consists of many proteins that act as a cascade, where each enzyme acts as a catalyst for the next. The most important component is C3, which is present in the circulation in amounts similar to some immunoglobulins (1–2 mg/ml).

The two main pathways for complement activation reflect the innate and adaptive immune response. The classical pathway links to the adaptive immune system through the binding of immune complexes to C1q. The alternative pathway (innate) is activated by the chance binding of C3b to the surface of a microorganism.

The activities of complement *in vivo* can be illustrated by the diseases associated with deficiencies of individual complement proteins. Individuals with such deficiencies (see Chapter 21) have increased susceptibility to two types of disease: recurrent infections by pyogenic (abscess forming) bacteria; and illnesses characterized by the production of autoantibodies and immune complexes. These observations suggest that complement has a role both in defence against bacteria, and also in the disposal of immune complexes, which would otherwise lead to autoimmunity and immune-complex disease (see Chapter 24).

The consequences of complement activation are:
- Opsonization
- Activation of leucocytes
- Lysis of target cells (*Fig. 13.1*).

Opsonization – involves complement proteins coating the surface of the target. Phagocytic cells carrying receptors for these complement components are then able to bind the target, leading to cell activation and endocytosis of the target.

Activation of leucocytes – Polymorphs and macrophages have specific receptors for small complement fragments that are generated on the target by the complement cascade. These fragments diffuse away from the target, and stimulate directed cellular movement (chemotaxis) and activation when bound by effector cells.

Lysis of target cells – The end point of the complement cascade is the insertion of a hydrophobic 'plug' into the target cell lipid membrane bilayer. This causes osmotic disruption and lysis of the target.

Complement can distinguish self from non-self

Although part of the innate immune system, complement has evolved mechanisms for self/non-self discrimination. The key step in the distinction of self from non-self by complement is the rapid and widespread binding of C3b to non-self, such as microorganisms or immune complexes, while the individual's own cell surfaces are protected by surface molecules that very effectively limit C3b deposition.

■ ACTIVATION OF COMPLEMENT

The complement cascade can be activated in two ways, known as the classical and alternative pathways. Both pathways lead to the formation of a convertase that cleaves C3 to C3a and C3b. This is the pivotal step in the process of complement activation (*Fig. 13.2*).

The classical pathway convertase is a combination of C4 with C2, $\overline{C4b2a}$ and the alternative pathway convertase is a combination of C3 with FB, $\overline{C3bBb}$. The C3b generated by these two enzymes binds to the target membrane and becomes a focus for further C3b production – this part of the cascade is called the amplification loop.

Both kinds of C3 convertase can be turned into a C5 convertase by the addition of a further molecule of C3b; C5 convertase catalyses the first step in a cascade that leads to the production of membrane attack complexes.

The classical pathway is activated mainly by immune complexes

The classical pathway is the main antibody-directed mechanism for the activation of complement (*Fig. 13.3*); C1 is the first enzyme complex in the cascade.

Activation is initiated by the binding of C1 to complexed antibody

C1 is a pentamolecular Ca^{2+}-dependent complex consisting of a single C1q molecule, two C1r and two C1s molecules (*Fig. 13.4*). The first step in the classical pathway is the binding of antibody to two or more of the 6 globular domains of C1q. C1q binds with high avidity to the CH2 domains (part of the Fc region) of aggregated IgG molecules in an immune complex. It can also bind to the CH3 domains of a single IgM molecule whose conformation has been modified from a 'planar' to a 'staple' configuration by binding to antigen.

Multiple binding of the globular domains of C1q to complexed IgG or IgM is believed to lead to a conformational change in the C1 complex. This causes one of the C1r molecules to activate itself (by autocatalysis), and then the other C1r, to yield two active $\overline{C1r}$ enzymes. These two enzymes then cleave the two C1s molecules to give active $\overline{C1s}$ serine esterases.

**Three major biological activities
of the complement system**

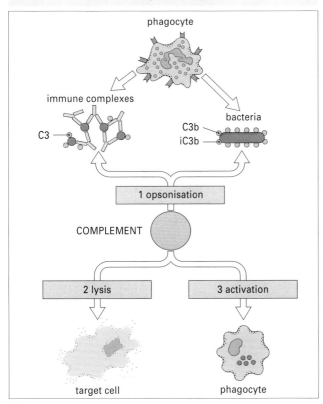

Fig. 13.1 (3) Activation of phagocytes, including macrophages and neutrophils, (2) lysis of target cells, and (1) opsonization (coating) of microorganisms and immune complexes, so that they can be recognized by cells expressing complement receptors.

**Comparison of the classical and
alternative complement pathways**

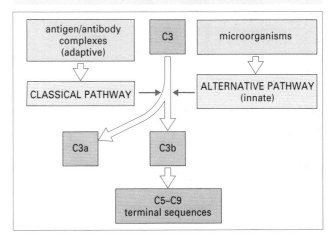

Fig. 13.2 Both pathways generate a C3 convertase, which converts C3 to C3b, the central event of the complement pathway. C3b in turn activates the terminal lytic complement sequence, C5–C9. The first stage leading to C3 fixation by the classical sequence is the binding of an antigen to its antibody. The alternative pathway does not require antibody, and is initiated by the covalent binding of C3b to hydroxyl groups on the microorganism's cell membrane. The alternative pathway provides non-specific 'innate' immunity, whereas the classical pathway probably represents a more recently evolved link with adaptive immunity.

Activators of complement

	immunoglobulins	microorganisms			other
		viruses	bacteria	other	
classical pathway	complexes containing IgM, IgG1, IgG2 or IgG3	murine retroviruses, vesicular stomatitis virus	–	*Mycoplasma*	polyanions, esp. when bound to cations, PO_4^{3-}(DNA, lipid A, cardiolipin), SO_4^{2-}(dextran sulphate, heparin, chrondroitin sulphate) arrays of terminal mannose groups (via mannan-binding protein)
alternative pathway	complexes containing IgG, IgA or IgE (less efficient than the classical pathway)	some virus-infected cells (e.g. EBV)	many strains of Gram-positive and Gram-negative organisms	trypanosomes, *Leishmania*, many fungi	dextran sulphate, heterologous erythrocytes, carbohydrates (e.g. agarose)

Fig. 13.3 This table summarizes the activators of the classical and alternative pathways.

Structure of C1

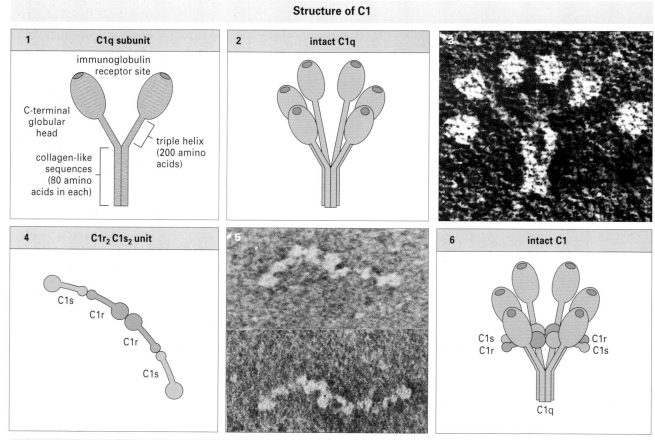

Fig. 13.4 Each subunit of C1q is Y-shaped with each branch of the Y ending in a globular head (**1**). C1q consists of 3 of these subunits joined together (**2**, **3**). There are six polypeptide chains in each subunit, giving 18 in the whole C1q molecule. The receptors for the Fc regions of IgG are in the globular heads, which form a ring in the C1q molecule. A unit consisting of two C1r molecules and two C1s molecules (**4**, **5**) lies across the C1q molecule (**6**). The catalytic sites of C1r are close together at the centre of the ring. The cohesion of the C1 complex is dependent on Ca^{2+}.(**3** and **5** from Ross *op. cit.*, reproduced courtesy of Dr. N. Hughes-Jones.)

The classical pathway can also be activated in an antibody-independent fashion

C1q belongs to a family of calcium-dependent lectins, known as the collectins (collagenous lectins). This protein family includes mannan-binding protein (MBP), conglutinin and lung surfactant proteins A and D. MBP in serum can bind to terminal mannose groups on the surface of bacteria, and is then able to interact with a serine proteinase known as MASP (mannan-binding protein-associated serine proteinase). MASP is homologous in structure to C1r and C1s: the interaction of MBP and MASP is analogous to the interaction of C1q with C1r and C1s, and leads to antibody-independent activation of the classical pathway.

C1q is also able to bind directly to certain microorganisms, including mycoplasmas and some retroviruses (though not HIV), in an antibody-independent process.

C1 cleaves C4 and generates activated C4b

The complement protein C4 contains an internal thioester bond in a sequence that is closely homologous to a thioester-containing sequence in C3 (see below). When $\overline{\text{C1s}}$ cleaves C4, two fragments are generated: C4a (which has weak anaphylatoxic activity) and a larger, unstable intermediate, C4b*. (The * denotes the unstable state of the molecule in which the nascent binding site is activated.) Within a few milliseconds this is attacked by nucleophilic groups in its immediate vicinity. The majority of C4b* is hydrolysed by water to form inactivated iC4b. However, C4b* can also form covalent bonds with amine or hydroxyl groups on cell surface molecules, to form surface bound C4b.

Two isotypes of C4 exist, C4A and C4B, encoded by tandem genes within the major histocompatibility complex.

When activated, C4A preferentially binds to amine groups, forming an amide bond, whereas C4B mainly binds to hydroxyl groups via an ester linkage. Thus C4A binds mainly to amino groups in proteins, and C4B to hydroxyl groups in carbohydrates.

Surface-bound C4b acts as a binding site for C2, leading to the formation of classical C3 convertase

Surface-bound C4b now acts as a binding site for the zymogen C2. The bound C2 is a substrate for $\overline{\text{C1s}}$, and is cleaved to release C2b. The large C2a segment remains bound to C4b to form $\text{C4}\overline{\text{b2a}}$, the classical pathway C3 convertase enzyme.

C3b generated by C3 convertase can bind covalently to cell surface molecules

C3 belongs to a family of proteins containing an unusual post-translational modification to their structure. An internal thioester bond is formed from closely positioned glutamine and cysteine residues by the elimination of ammonia. This bond is metastable and the electrophilic (electron-accepting) carbonyl group $(-C^+{=}O)$ of the thioester is susceptible to attack by nucleophilic groups (electron donors), such as hydroxyl and amine groups in adjacent proteins and carbohydrates. This reaction allows C3 to bind covalently to their molecules (*Fig. 13.5*).

Proteolytic cleavage of C3a from the N-terminus of the C3 α chain by C3 convertase, results in a conformational change that makes the internal thioester bond very unstable. This now becomes a nascent binding site within C3b*, which is extremely susceptible to interaction with adjacent nucleophiles. As is the case with C4*, the majority of C3b* will interact with water, but some will also bind to proteins and sugars in the immediate vicinity of the activation site. Since C3 convertases are usually generated on non-self surfaces or on immune complexes, this means that C3b deposition will also be confined mostly to these places. The bound C3b then acts as a focus for further complement activation via the alternative pathway amplification loop (see below) (*Fig. 13.6*).

Classical pathway activation is regulated very efficiently

Classical pathway activation is regulated in the fluid phase by two mechanisms. The first is C1 inhibitor, a serine proteinase inhibitor (serpin) that binds and inactivates $\overline{\text{C1r}}$ and $\overline{\text{C1s}}$.

The second mechanism blocks the formation of the classical pathway C3 convertase enzyme, $\text{C4}\overline{\text{b2a}}$. The formation of $\text{C4}\overline{\text{b2a}}$ is inefficient in the fluid phase, due to the presence of Factor I and C4 binding protein (C4-bp), which together catabolize C4b. C4-bp also promotes the dissociation of C2a from $\text{C4}\overline{\text{b2a}}$.

Classical pathway activation is also regulated by inhibiting complement binding to host cell surfaces. This is achieved by the complement control proteins (CCPs), including decay accelerating factor (DAF, CD55), CR1 (CD35) and membrane cofactor protein (MCP, CD46). These molecules operate in the following ways (*Fig. 13.7*):

- They inhibit the binding of C2 to C4b (DAF or CR1)
- They promote 'decay acceleration', the dissociation of C2a from C4b (DAF or CR1)
- They act as cofactors to promote the catabolism of C4b by Factor I (MCP or CR1).

Activation of the C3 thioester bond

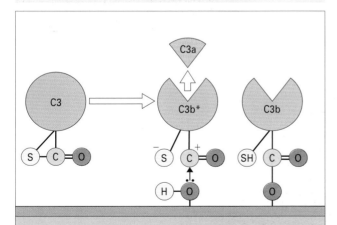

Fig. 13.5 The α chain of C3 contains a thioester bond formed between a cysteine and a glutamine residue. Following cleavage of C3 into C3a and C3b*, the bond becomes unstable and susceptible to nucleophilic attack by electrons on –OH and –NH$_2$ groups, allowing the C3b to form covalent bonds with proteins and carbohydrates.

The classical pathway

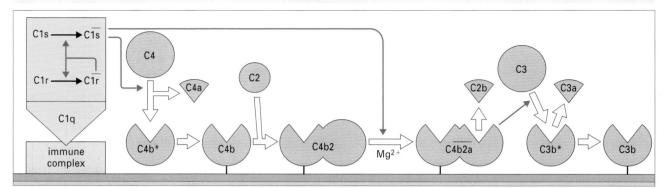

Fig. 13.6 Following the binding of C1q to immune complexes, C1r catalyses its own activation and that of C1s. C̄1s̄ then cleaves C4a from C4, leaving C4b*, which immediately binds to adjacent proteins or carbohydrates. Surface-bound C4b now binds C2 in the presence of Mg²⁺. C̄1s̄ cleaves C2b from this complex to leave C2a. (Note that the usual nomenclature is reversed with C2, and C2a refers to the larger segment. There have been proposals to change this nomenclature and implement a clearer system, but in this book the original designations are used.) The C̄4b2a̅ complex is the classical pathway C3 convertase. Here and in subsequent diagrams in this Chapter on complement, enzymatic reactions are shown using a red arrow

The alternative pathway of complement activates spontaneously

Tick-over activation continuously generates low levels of C3b* in serum

The internal thioester bond in native C3 is susceptible to spontaneous hydrolysis by water, generating an activated form of C3 known as C3i. This steady, low level, spontaneous C3 activation in plasma is known as tick-over activation. C3i then acts as a binding site for Factor B (see *Fig. 13.8*) to produce C3iB. (This is analogous to the binding of C2 to C4b.) The Factor B bound to C3i is cleaved by Factor D to release Ba. The remaining complex, C̄3̅iBb̅, is a fluid phase, alternative pathway C3 convertase (*Fig. 13.8*).

Because the convertase is operating in the fluid phase, most of the C3b* generated by C̄3̅iBb̅ is hydrolysed and inac-

tivated by water. However, if it should happen to come into contact with a non-self surface, such as a bacterial cell membrane, it will covalently bind and initiate the amplification loop of the alternative pathway. C3b that binds to autologous cell surfaces is prevented from initiating the amplification loop by the complement control proteins.

Microorganisms offer 'protected' surfaces for C3b

Surfaces that are good activators of complement are known as 'protected' surfaces (*Fig. 13.12*). Protected in this sense means that bound C3b is protected from proteolytic degradation. Non-self surfaces such as bacterial cell membranes are 'protected' for C3b because C3b has a higher affinity for Factor B than Factor H at these sites, and is therefore more likely to form a stable convertase. Non-self surfaces also lack the host regulatory proteins that inhibit complement activation.

Although the precise structural requirements for a protected surface are not understood, the carbohydrate composition seems to be important. The presence of acidic sugars, such as sialic acid, seem to help in protecting self membranes from amplified C3b deposition.

Initial binding of a molecule of C3b to a protected surface is followed by an amplification step that results in the binding of many more molecules of C3b to the same surface. The key to this rapid amplification of C3b is the formation of a surface-bound C3 convertase enzyme.

The alternative pathway amplification loop uses a positive feedback mechanism

Surface-bound C3b binds Factor B to give C3bB. This becomes a substrate for Factor D, a serine esterase that cleaves Factor B to release a small fragment, Ba, leaving C̄3̅bBb̅ bound to the surface. The C̄3̅bBb̅ dissociates fairly rapidly unless it is stabilized by the binding of properdin (P), forming the complex, C̄3̅bBbP̅. This constitutes the surface-bound C3 convertase enzyme of the alternative pathway.

Regulation of C3 convertases

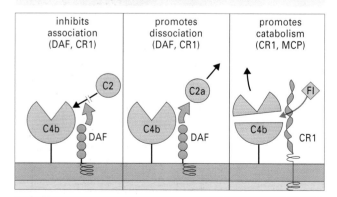

Fig. 13.7 Decay accelerating factor (DAF) and CR1 inhibit the association between C4b and C2, and promote dissociation of the C̄4b2a̅ complex. CR1 and membrane cofactor protein (MCP) promote Factor I (FI) mediated cleavage of C4b. These molecules control the interactions between C3b and Factor B in a similar way.

C3 tick-over

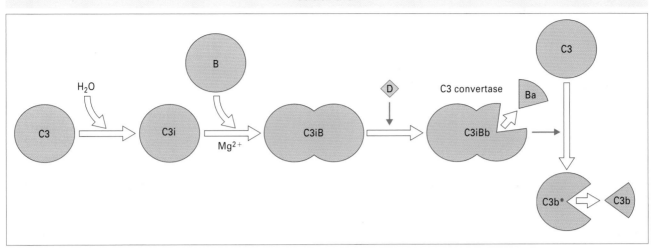

Fig. 13.8 The thioester bond of native C3 becomes hydrolysed by water forming C3i (C3(H₂O)), which binds to Factor B in the presence of Mg²⁺. Following cleavage of B by Factor D, this complex forms a fluid phase C3 convertase which can directly cleave C3 into C3a and C3b.

Analogous action of the classical and alternative pathways

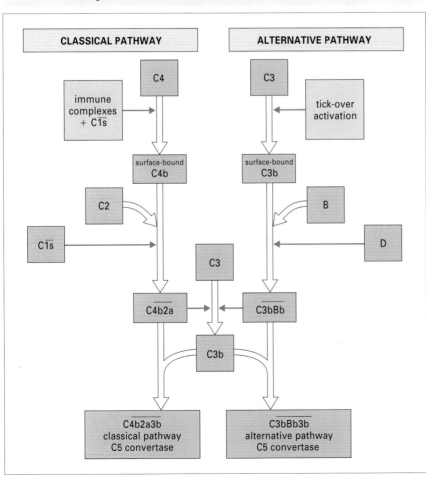

Fig. 13.9 Both pathways generate a C3 convertase: $\overline{C4b2a}$ (classical pathway) and $\overline{C3bBb}$ (alternative pathway). In the classical sequence, C1s is activated by complexed antibody and splits both C4 and C2. The small fragments, C4a and C2b, are lost and the major components form $\overline{C4b2a}$. In the alternative pathway, surface-bound C3b (generated by tick-over activation) binds Factor B, which is split releasing a small fragment, Ba. The major fragment, Bb, remains bound to form $\overline{C3bBb}$. This converts more C3, so creating positive feedback. Activator surfaces, on microorganisms for example, stabilize C3b by facilitating its combination with Factor B. This activity promotes alternative pathway activation. The C3 convertases of both pathways may bind further C3b to yield C5 convertase enzymes. These activate the next component of the complement system, C5. The classical pathway C5 convertase is $\overline{C4b2a3b}$, and the alternative pathway C5 convertase is $\overline{C3bBb3b}$.

The amplification loop of C3 activation

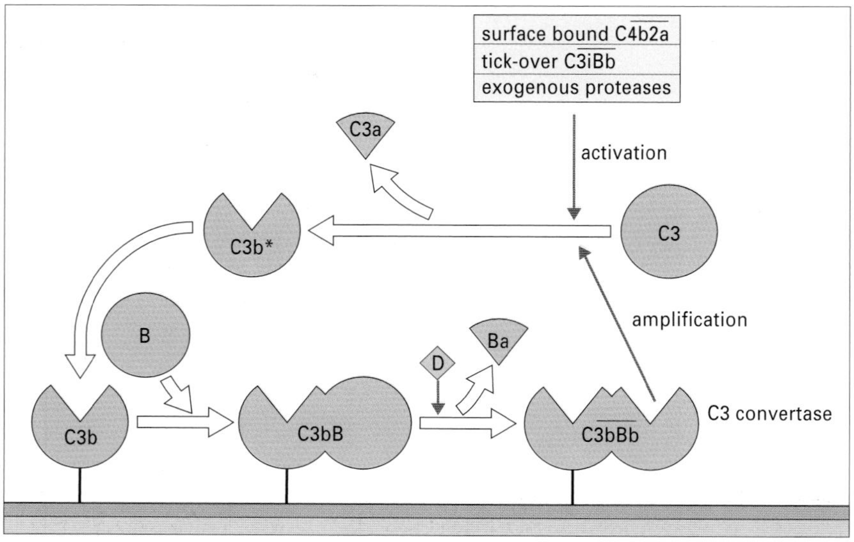

surface bound C4b2a
tick-over C3iBb
exogenous proteases

activation

amplification

C3 convertase

Fig. 13.10 C3b may be generated either by a classical pathway C3 convertase C4b2a or by an alternative pathway C3 convertase. C3b then binds to Factor B in a Mg^{2+}-dependent complex and is acted on by Factor D. This releases Ba and generates the alternative pathway, C3 convertase C3bBb. This in turn can act on more C3 to generate further C3b. Thus there is a positive feedback loop, which amplifies the initial complement activation.

C3bBbP cleaves many more C3 molecules; the location of the convertase means that C3b* thus generated will tend to bind to the nearby protected surface, rather than elsewhere (*Fig. 13.10*).

Note that the amplification loop also works for C3b deposited as a result of (antibody-dependent) classical pathway activation.

Alternative pathway and amplification loop activation are regulated

Activation of the alternative pathway in the fluid phase, where C3b does not bind to surfaces, is tightly regulated by proteins similar or identical to the complement control proteins that inhibit classical pathway activation. Factor H, encoded by a member of the RCA gene cluster and homologous to C4-bp, promotes the dissociation of Bb from both C3i and C3b. Factor H also functions as a cofactor to Factor I for the catabolism of C3i and C3b (*Fig. 13.11*).

Breakdown of C3b

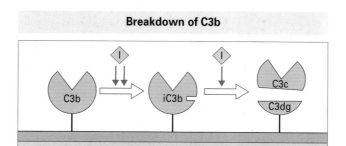

Fig. 13.11 Factor I cleaves C3b in three places to release C3c, leaving C3dg, a fragment of the α chain still bound to the substrate. The first two cleavages are promoted by Factor H (MCP or CR1) and produce an intermediate, iC3b. The third cleavage is promoted by CR1.

Regulation of the amplification mechanism is important for the host: this is a positive feedback system, and it will cycle until all C3 is completely cleaved unless it is regulated. (It was originally discovered in a patient with an hereditary deficiency of the regulatory enzyme, Factor I. Lacking Factor I, his amplification loop had cycled to exhaustion, so that all the C3 in his serum was converted to C3b.)

On autologous cell membranes, both DAF and CR1 accelerate the dissociation of C3bBb, promoting the release of C3b from the complex. CR1 and MCP both act as co-factors for the cleavage of C3b by Factor I (see *Fig. 13.7*). These reactions are exactly analogous to the activities of DAF, MCP and CR1 in controlling the activity of classical pathway C4b2a when it is bound to cell membranes.

To summarize, regulation of the fate of C3b bound to surfaces is the critical step enabling the non-specific distinction of self from non-self by the complement system. There are two possible outcomes for bound C3b:

- Amplification – C3b acts as a binding site for Factor B, forms a convertase enzyme, and focuses the deposition of more C3b to the same surface
- Inhibition – C3b is catabolized by Factor I using one of three cofactors, Factor H (from plasma), and CR1 or MCP (surface-bound).

The nature of the surface to which the C3b is bound regulates which of these two outcomes is most likely (*Fig. 13.12*). It is the presence of intrinsic molecules such as DAF, CR1, and MCP, on self surfaces, particularly the cell membranes, that effectively limits the formation of C3 convertase enzymes. On the other hand, non-self surfaces, for example bacterial cell membranes, act as a protected site for C3b since factor B has a higher affinity for C3b than does Factor H at these sites. Thus the deposition of a few molecules of C3b on to a non-self surface is followed by the formation of the relatively stable alternative pathway C3 convertase enzyme, C3bBbP, which focuses more C3b deposition in the near vicinity.

Formation of the membrane attack complex constitutes the final phase of complement activation

The final phase of activation of the complement cascade is the formation of the membrane attack complex (MAC) by the enzymatic cleavage of C5, a protein homologous to C3 and C4 but lacking the internal thioester bond.

C5 must be bound to C3b before it can be cleaved by the C5 convertase enzyme. The classical pathway C5 convertase enzyme is a trimolecular complex, $C\overline{4b2a3b}$ in which the C3b is covalently bound to the C4b. C5 binds selectively to the convertase because it has a higher binding constant to C3b when it is bound to C4b, than for C3b which is bound to other cell surface molecules. The alternative pathway C5 convertase enzyme is also a trimolecular complex, $C\overline{3bBb3b}$, in which one C3b is covalently bound to the other. Cleavage of C5 releases the small peptide fragment C5a, which is a potent anaphylatoxin.

The membrane attack complex is formed by non-enzymatic assembly of C5b-9

The remainder of the formation of the MAC is non-enzymatic. C5b binds C6, forming C5b6, and this then binds C7 to form a C5b67 complex (*Fig. 13.13*). The binding to C7 marks the transition of the complex from a hydrophilic to a hydrophobic state that preferentially inserts into lipid bilayers. C8 then binds to this complex, followed by a stepwise addition of up to 14 C9 monomers, resulting in the formation of a lytic 'plug' or pore-forming molecule, first observed in electron micrographs by Humphrey and Dourmashkin (*Fig. 13.13*). Although a small amount of lysis occurs when C8 binds to C5b67, it is the polymerized C9 that causes the majority of lysis. (Note that C5b6789 is usually abbreviated to C5b–9, and the earlier stages may be shortened in a similar way, e.g. C5b–8.)

Hydrophobic molecules that polymerize to form pores are a common mechanism for cellular cytotoxicity. T lymphocytes kill target cells by inserting a pore-forming molecule known as perforin into their membranes (see Chapter 9). Perforin has structural homology to C9, and similar molecules are found in the granules of eosinophils (the eosinophil cationic proteins). Certain bacterial toxins, such as streptolysin O, are also pore-forming molecules.

Formation of the membrane attack complex is regulated to reduce 'reactive lysis'

Once the hydrophobic C5b67 complex has formed it can insert itself into other cell membranes close to the primary surface on which complement activation is focused. This process of 'reactive lysis' could, if unregulated, have damaging consequences to self/host tissues.

C5b67 can be inactivated in the fluid phase

A number of proteins can inhibit reactive lysis by binding to fluid phase C5b67 before it attaches to self membranes. The most abundant of these is S protein, also known as vitronectin, which is present in plasma. It forms the SC5b67 complex, which is unable to insert into lipid bilayers. If C8 binds to C5b67 in the fluid phase this also forms a complex incapable of membrane insertion, as does the binding of low density lipoprotein (LDL).

Host cells bear membrane proteins that protect against lysis by the MAC

It has been known for some time that erythrocytes are poorly lysed by homologous complement, but readily lysed by complement derived from other species. This observation is explained by findings that host cells bear membrane proteins that protect against lysis by the MAC. Two proteins have been characterized that mediate this species restriction.

Regulation of the amplification loop

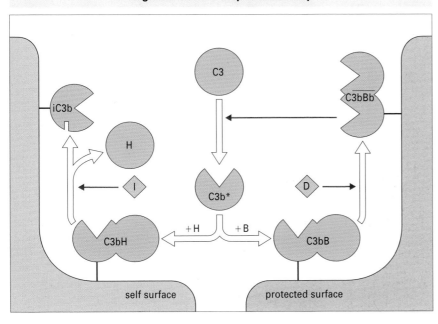

Fig. 13.12 Alternative pathway activation depends on the presence of protected surfaces. 'Protected' means that bound C3b is protected from proteolytic degradation. C3b which has bound to an activator surface binds factor B. This generates the alternative pathway C3 convertase, C3bBb, which drives the amplification loop. However, on self surfaces the binding of Factor H is favoured and C3b becomes inactivated by Factor I. Thus the binding of Factor B or Factor H controls the development of alternative pathway reactions. In addition to this mechanism, self cell membranes also bear a series of regulatory proteins which inhibit complement activation (see **Figs. 13.7** and **13.14**).

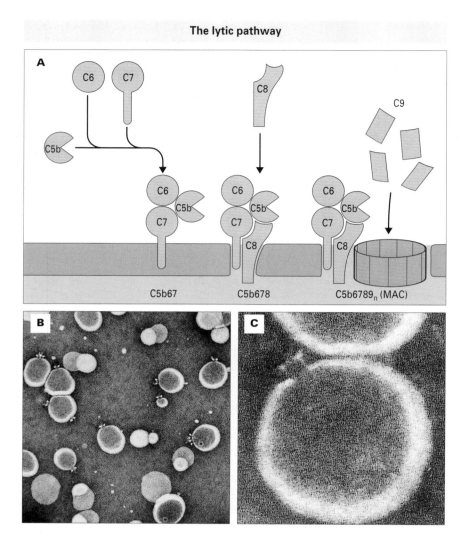

Fig. 13.13 A C5b binds C6 and C7 to give C5b67, which is hydrophobic and has a membrane binding site allowing the complex to attach to plasma membranes close to the reaction site. C8 binds to this complex on C5b and penetrates the membrane, where it can polymerize a number of molecules of C9 to generate the membrane attack complex (MAC).
B and **C** Electron micrographs of the membrane attack complex. The funnel-shaped lesion (**C**) is due to a human C5b–9 complex reincorporated into lecithin liposomal membranes ×234 000. (Courtesy of Professor J. Tranum-Jensen and Dr S. Bhakdi).

CD59 is a protein anchored by a glycophospholipid foot. It is widely distributed in cell membranes, binds to C8 in C5b–8 complexes, and inhibits the insertion and unfolding of C9 into cell membranes (*Fig. 13.14*).

A second protein, homologous restriction factor (HRF), has similar activity to CD59 but is probably a weaker inhibitor of C9 insertion. HRF is a 65 kDa glycophospholipid-linked membrane protein, whose sequence is not yet known.

Note that nucleated cells (such as cells of the host's immune system) are much more resistant than erythrocytes to lysis by complement, because they can actively remove MAC by endocytosis and exocytosis of fragments of membrane containing MAC.

■ COMPLEMENT RECEPTORS

Many of the fragments of complement proteins produced during activation bind to specific receptors on the surface of immune cells. This is an important mechanism for the mediation of the physiological effects of complement, including uptake of particles opsonized by complement, and activation of the cell bearing the receptor.

CD59 inhibits C9 binding to C5b-8

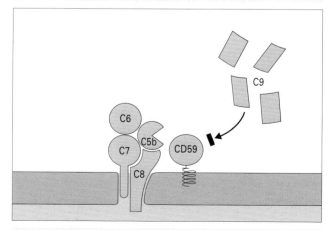

Fig. 13.14 CD59 binds to C8 in the C5b–8 complex and blocks the attachment of C9 and thus the formation of the MAC.

There are four receptors for the covalently fixed fragments of C3

Three products of C3 (sometimes called opsonic fragments) bind to the membranes of target cells: C3b, iC3b and C3dg. Four different receptors for these opsonic fragments are known, and are named complement receptor types 1 to 4 (CR1, CR2, CR3 and CR4); their ligands and their cellular distribution are shown in *Fig 13.15*.

CR1 has multiple physiological activities as a receptor for C3b and iC3b

The first complement-dependent cellular binding reaction to be recognized was a phenomenon that was later named 'immune adherence'. In this reaction, trypanosomes or other microbes opsonized with antibody and complement adhere to the platelets of rodents and to the erythrocytes of primates.

The receptor mediating these binding reactions is CR1, (also called the immune adherence receptor, or the C3b/C4b receptor, or CD35). CR1 is thought to have four physiological activities.

- It is an opsonic receptor on neutrophils, monocytes and macrophages, mediating endocytosis or phagocytosis by appropriately primed cells (*Fig. 13.16*).
- It acts as a cofactor to Factor I for the cleavage of C3b to iC3b, and for the subsequent cleavage of iC3b to C3c and C3dg. Factor H is probably more important than CR1 as a cofactor for the cleavage of C3b to iC3b, but CR1 is probably the sole cofactor for the cleavage of iC3b. In this role, CR1 protects self cells from attack by complement.

- On erythrocytes or platelets (depending on the species), CR1 may serve to pick up opsonized immune complexes or bacteria and transport them to the cells of the fixed mononuclear phagocytic system (*Fig. 13.17*).
- On B lymphocytes, CR1 may serve with CR2 as a receptor mediating lymphocyte activation.

CR2 is a receptor involved in the activation of B lymphocytes and is also the Epstein–Barr virus receptor

CR2 (CD21) – is located on B lymphocytes, follicular dendritic cells and certain epithelial cells; its ligands are iC3b, C3dg, IFNα, and the Epstein Barr virus (EBV). CR2 on B cells appears to function as an accessory receptor to antibody in activating specific immune responses. Ligation of CR2 by iC3b or C3dg lowers the threshold for triggering B-cell activation by ligation of the antigen-specific B-cell receptor, membrane-bound antibody. Thus immune complexes, containing cross-linked antigen and complement are more effective at activating B cells than antigen alone.

Opsonization and phagocytosis

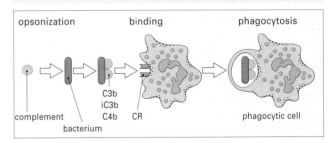

opsonization   binding   phagocytosis

complement   bacterium   C3b iC3b C4b   CR   phagocytic cell

Fig. 13.16 Steps in the uptake of a particle such as a bacterium opsonized by either C3b or C4b.

Complement receptors for fragments of C3

receptor	ligands	cellular distribution
CR1 (CD35)	C3b>iC3b C4b	B cells, neutrophils, monocytes, macrophages, erythrocytes, follicular dendritic cells, glomerular epithelial cells
CR2 (CD21)	iC3b, C3dg Epstein–Barr virus interferon-α	B cells, follicular dendritic cells, epithelial cells of cervix and nasopharynx
CR3 (CD18/CD11b)	iC3b zymosan certain bacteria fibrinogen factor X ICAM-1	monocytes, macrophages, neutrophils, NK cells, follicular dendritic cells
CR4 (p150-95) (CD18/CD11c)	iC3b fibrinogen	neutrophils, monocytes, tissue macrophages

Fig. 13.15 Complement receptors for fragments of C3. CR1 binds C3b more strongly than iC3b. These receptors allow cells to take up particles or immune complexes bearing that particular fragment.

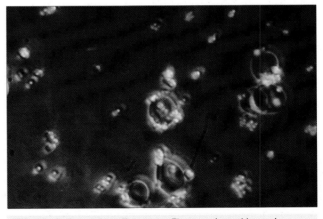

Fig. 13.17 Immune adherence. Fluoresceinated bacteria opsonized with antibody and complement are seen adhering to human erythrocytes. This reaction is mediated by C3b, iC3b and C4b on the bacteria binding to CR1. (Courtesy of Professor G. D. Ross.)

The main pathophysiological activity of CR2 follows from its role as the receptor for EBV. The *in vivo* tissue distribution of this virus corresponds to the locations of CR2, and it seems likely that EBV enters cells by binding directly to CR2 without the involvement of complement.

CR3 and CR4 are members of the leucocyte (β_2-) integrin family of adhesion molecules

The leucocyte integrins are heterodimers containing a common β-chain (CD18) and one of three different α-chains (CD11a,11b or 11c). Leucocyte integrin CD18/11a is known as LFA-1 (lymphocyte function-associated antigen type 1); CD18/11b is CR3; and CD18/11c is CR4 (also known as p150, 95).

These three molecules belong in turn to a superfamily of structurally related cell surface receptors and adhesion molecules, the integrins, which includes the fibronectin and vitronectin (S protein) receptors, and the fibrinogen receptor on platelets. The binding of these receptors to their ligands is calcium-dependent.

CR3 (CD18/11b) – occurs on cells of myeloid lineage and is an important receptor and adhesion molecule. It mediates phagocytosis of particles opsonized with iC3b, and is also a lectin, able to bind certain carbohydrates. Some yeasts, including *Saccharomyces cerevisiae*, bind directly to CR3 without the mediation of complement, as do other microorganisms such as *Staphylococcus epidermidis* and *Histoplasma capsulatum*. Other ligands for CR3 include fibrinogen, Factor X and ICAM-1.

CR4 (p150-95, CD18/11c) – is the least well characterized of this group of receptors, but has been shown to bind to iC3b in a calcium-dependent manner. It also binds to fibrinogen and is involved in the adhesion of monocytes and neutrophils to endothelium. It is distributed on cells of both myeloid and lymphoid lineages, and is strongly expressed on tissue macrophages, where it may be an important receptor for particles opsonized with iC3b.

The C5a receptor belongs to the rhodopsin superfamily of G-protein coupled receptors

Two small fragments of complement proteins, C3a and C5a, can trigger the degranulation of mast cells, and are known as anaphylatoxins. The effects of the anaphylatoxins C3a and C5a are mediated by binding to specific receptors. These have been well characterized for C5a and are present on all cells derived from the myeloid lineage (neutrophils, eosinophils, basophils and mast cells, monocytes and macrophages).

The C5a receptor belongs to the rhodopsin superfamily of G-protein coupled receptors, characterized by a serpentine structure with seven hydrophobic, transmembrane domains. The C5a receptor is homologous in structure to several receptors mediating chemotactic signals, including the f-met-leu-phe receptor (binding bacterial peptides) and receptors for the chemokines, IL-8 and Rantes.

Following receptor-binding, C5a is internalized and degraded to inactive peptide fragments; this is an important mechanism for regulating and limiting C5a activity.

Other complement receptors bind to the collectins

A 70 kDa molecule has been identified which binds to the collagen-like tail (see *Fig. 13.4*) of C1q, and to other members of the collectin family such as MBP. This receptor is located on polymorphs, monocytes, macrophages, B cells, platelets and endothelial cells. Its physiological function is uncertain, but it may augment the uptake of immune complexes opsonized with C1q or bacteria coated with MBP.

■ BIOLOGICAL EFFECTS OF COMPLEMENT

The biological activities of the complement system may be divided into those that are beneficial to the host and those that are harmful.

The major beneficial activities are:
- Promotion of the killing of microorganisms
- The efficient clearing of immune complexes
- The induction and enhancement of antibody responses.

Complement may cause harm to the host under several circumstances:
- If activated systemically on a large scale; e.g. in Gram-negative septicaemia
- If activated by tissue necrosis, e.g. during myocardial infarction
- If activated by an autoimmune response to host tissues.

Complement promotes the killing of microorganisms

Enhancing the killing of microorganisms is achieved in several ways:
- By generation of anaphylatoxins, which increase vascular permeability and therefore recruit other components of the inflammatory response to the site of the infection
- By opsonizing the microorganisms to enhance phagocytosis
- By insertion of the membrane attack complex into the cell membranes of microorganisms.

Anaphylatoxins are potent inducers of inflammation

Activation of the complement system results in the generation of the anaphylatoxins C5a and C3a. Their physiological role is to recruit inflammatory cells to sites of inflammation and activate their effector mechanisms.

Systemic administration of C5a, or profound intravascular activation of complement such as may be associated with Gram-negative bacterial sepsis, may be associated with the development of cardiovascular collapse and bronchospasm; this state resembles anaphylaxis and is the origin of the term anaphylatoxin.

Actions of C5a – C5a is a potent activator of all types of cells of the myeloid lineage (*Fig. 13.18*). Neutrophils respond to C5a by chemokinesis and chemotaxis. They degranulate and the respiratory burst is activated, leading to the production of oxygen free radicals. Membrane arachidonic acid is mobilized with production of prostaglandins and eicosanoids. Surface expression of adhesion molecules also increases, which promotes adhesion to vascular endothelium (*Fig. 13.18*). Monocytes and macrophages show similar responses, and also secrete IL-1 and IL-6. Basophils and mast cells degranulate and release histamine and other vasoactive mediators.

As a consequence of this cellular activation, there are indirect effects on blood vessels, increasing vascular permeability, and on smooth muscle, causing contraction. C5a may also synergise with other inflammatory mediators; for example, the generation of IL-1 by monocytes is synergistically stimulated by combinations of C5a with IFNγ or endotoxin.

Half-life of C5a – This is extremely short in the circulation, as might be predicted for such a potent mediator of inflammation. The circulating enzyme, carboxypeptidase N, cleaves the C-terminal arginine from C5a, producing C5a-des-arg, which is much less active in all of its biological activities than C5a, though retaining significant chemotactic activity. Ligation of the C5a receptor is followed by rapid internalization of ligand and intracellular C5a is rapidly proteolysed to inactive fragments.

Actions of C3a – C3a is much less active than C5a, and its receptor is not yet characterized. It induces weak neutrophil aggregation and activation of the respiratory burst. In contrast to C5a, it is not significantly chemotactic.

Note that the production of anaphylatoxins results not only from complement activation, but also from activation of other enzyme systems that directly cleave C3, C4 and C5. Such enzymes include plasmin, kallikrein, tissue and leucocyte lysosomal enzymes (especially neutrophil elastase), and bacterial proteases such as gingipain-1 (derived from *P. gingivalis* and associated with periodontal disease).

Fixed C3b and C4b act as opsonins enhancing phagocytosis

The covalent fixation of C3b and C4b to bacteria and immune complexes generates ligands for complement receptors on phagocytic cells. This promotes the clearance and destruction of bacteria and immune complexes. In addition to inducing phagocytosis, ligation of complement receptors on neutrophils, monocytes and macrophages may also stimulate exocytosis of granules containing proteolytic enzymes and free radical production through a respiratory burst (*Fig. 13.19*).

Complement deficiency is associated with an increase in the number of infections

The physiological role of complement as an opsonin and a bacteriolysin is elegantly illustrated by two different hereditary deficiency states in humans. Deficiency of either the classical pathway components and C3, or of the CR3/CR4/LFA-1 receptor family, produces a similar spectrum of infections by pyogenic bacteria. The fact that deficiency of either the opsonin or the receptor has similar consequences, demonstrates convincingly that complement plays an important role in the destruction of these bacteria through phagocytosis and intracellular destruction.

In contrast, deficiencies of MAC components are associated almost exclusively with increased susceptibility to infections by *Neisseria meningitidis*. This suggests that host defence against these bacteria, which are characterized by their ability to survive in the intracellular milieu, depends on their lysis in plasma by complement.

Complement seems to be of less importance in host defence against viral infections, where T cells play a more important role. Complement deficiency is not associated with undue susceptibility to viral infections.

The membrane attack complex also plays a part in the inflammatory response

The traditional view of the MAC was that it killed cells by channel formation and lysis. In recent years, however, it has become apparent that nucleated cells, such as those of the

Biological effects of C5a and C5a-des-Arg

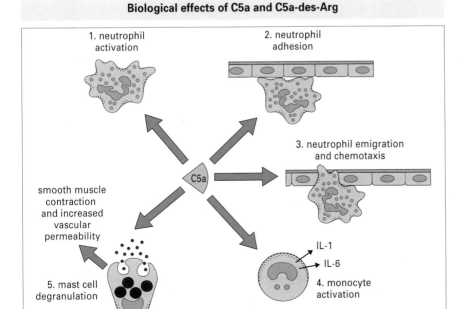

Fig. 13.18 C5a causes (1) neutrophil activation, (2) increased expression of adhesion molecules, (3) emigration of neutrophils and chemotaxis, (4) monocyte activation and (5) mast cell degranulation, which in turn causes smooth muscle contraction and increased vascular permeability.

Role of C3 in bacterial clearance and killing

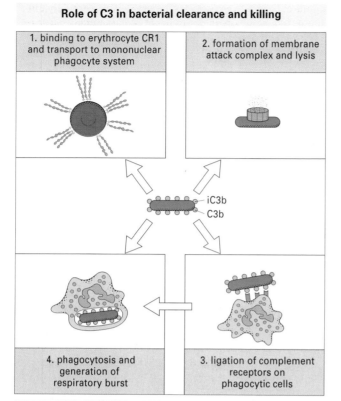

Fig. 13.19 C3 bound to bacteria as C3b or iC3b (1) binds to CR1 on erythrocytes, which transport bacteria through the circulation, (2) acts as a focus for the deposition of lytic membrane attack complex on the bacterial cell membrane, (3) ligates complement receptors on phagocytic cells, which in turn (4) activates the phagocytic cell leading to bacterial phagocytosis, respiratory burst generation and bacterial killing.

host's immune system, are relatively resistant to lysis by the MAC; this is partially due to the presence of regulatory molecules such as CD59, but also because the cells can endocytose and exocytose portions of membrane containing MAC. Even so, the perturbation of the membrane bilayer by sublethal MAC incorporation can stimulate cells of the immune system (depending on their innate capabilities) to release and metabolize arachidonic acid, to undertake oxidative metabolism, or to release granules or cytokines. These responses may play an important role in amplifying inflammation at sites of complement activation.

Pathogenic microorganisms resist complement-mediated attack

The interplay between the complement system and microorganisms may be viewed as the product of a continuing evolutionary battle. As the complement system has evolved, probably driven in large part by selective pressure from infectious diseases, so microorganisms have in turn evolved mechanisms of evasion, and in some cases have even taken advantage of the complement system to promote their own pathogenesis. Indeed, pathogenic organisms are only

pathogenic by virtue of their ability to evade host defence mechanisms to some extent.

Some bacteria direct deposition of C3b and MAC to sites where they cannot be effective

Certain Gram-negative bacteria possess long, O-linked, lipopolysaccharide coatings which, although they efficiently activate complement, direct the covalent binding of C3 and the attachment of the MAC away from the bacterial cell membrane, so that opsonization and lysis is impossible. In such a case, the adaptive immune response in the form of bactericidal antibody might function by directing complement activation to sites on the bacteria which would result in effective opsonization or lysis.

Other bacteria have surface coats that resist opsonization

A number of microorganisms resist complement using surface molecules that do not allow alternative-pathway activation and amplification of C3 deposition. For example, the possession of a capsule rich in sialic acids distinguishes certain pathogenic Gram-positive bacterial strains from their nonpathogenic counterparts. On such a capsule, C3b binds Factor H rather than Factor B, leading to catabolism of C3b.

Some microorganisms express molecules that inhibit complement activation

Another strategy used by microbes to evade the complement response is to express regulatory inhibitory molecules similar to those used by their hosts. Molecules on microorganisms with Fc-receptor activities have been known for some time, e.g. staphylococcal protein A, and the Fc receptor present on many herpes viruses. A recent finding is that Herpes simplex also expresses a molecule with complement-receptor activity, glycoprotein-C. *Candida albicans* also expresses CR2 and CR3-like molecules; the latter has antigenic homology with human CR3. These molecules may protect microorganisms from the normal consequences of antibody and complement binding. For example, such IgG or C3 may be blocked from recognition by opsonic receptors on host phagocytic cells. Another strategy is to express regulatory molecules that inhibit complement activation. For example, trypanosomes express a DAF-like and a CD59-like molecule, while schistosomes achieve similar ends by absorbing host DAF.

Certain microorganisms use the complement system to enhance their pathogenesis

Penetration of host cells is an essential step in the pathogenesis of viral infections. Several viruses have been found to use membrane-bound molecules of the complement system as receptors to gain entry to cells; these include Epstein–Barr virus using CR2, measles virus using membrane cofactor protein (MCP, CD46), and certain echoviruses using decay accelerating factor (DAF, CD55).

Other viruses may gain access to cells indirectly via antibody and C3b fixed to the virus. Examples of this include antibody-enhanced uptake of flaviviruses (including Dengue virus) via macrophage Fc receptors, and CR3-mediated uptake of West Nile virus (also a flavivirus) by C3 fixed to viral particles.

Complement plays an important accessory role in the induction of immune responses

The complement system helps to present antigen to antigen-presenting cells and to B cells (*Fig. 13.20*). For example, the localization of immune complexes to the germinal centres of lymph nodes, essential for the formation of memory B cells, is a complement-dependent process.

B cells and APCs carry a range of complement receptors:
- B cells carry CR1, which binds C3b and iC3b, and CR2, which binds iC3b and C3dg
- Monocytes and macrophages bear CR1 and CR3
- Follicular dendritic cells are the only cells that have been shown to bear all three receptors (CR1, CR2 and CR3).

Humans with hereditary deficiency of C3 have only mild impairment of antibody production. However, C2-, C3- or C4-deficiency in guinea pigs markedly impairs the primary and secondary antibody responses to low immunizing doses of T-cell dependent antigens. This evidence suggests that complement plays an accessory, but not crucial role in the efficient induction of antibody responses.

Complement is important in the processing of immune complexes

In the 1940s, Heidelberger observed that complement inhibited the formation of precipitating antigen–antibody lattices. Immune complex lattice size is influenced by many factors, including:
- The concentration of the reactants (antibody and antigen)
- The affinity of the antibody for its antigen
- The valency of both antibody and antigen, with high valency favouring large lattice formation.

The classical pathway of complement inhibits the formation of precipitating immune complexes in plasma. In the same way, activation of the alternative pathway can solubilize immune complexes that have already been precipitated, including those in tissues. This is achieved by the covalent incorporation of C3 into immune-complex lattices. C3 binding may disrupt immune-complex lattices by reducing the capacity of the antibody to bind to epitopes on the antigen, thus limiting the possibilities for forming large lattices (see Chapter 24).

The activation of complement by immune complexes is normally beneficial. Immune complexes bearing C3 are efficiently removed from tissues and from the circulation by monocytes and other phagocytes (*Fig. 13.20*). However, there are circumstances in which complex production continues at a high level. Complement activation by immune complexes may then prove deleterious, as is the case in subacute bacterial endocarditis and SLE.

Complement is important in the pathogenesis of some diseases

Systemic complement activation generates large amounts of anaphylatoxins

Under some circumstances the consequences of complement activation *in vivo* are deleterious rather than beneficial (*Fig. 13.21*). The state of shock that can follow Gram-negative bacteraemia is partially mediated by complement, which is systemically activated by endotoxin. Large quantities of C3a and C5a are generated, causing activation and degranulation of

neutrophils, basophils and mast cells. Intravascular neutrophil aggregation leads to clotting and deposition of emboli in the pulmonary microvasculature. In these vessels, neutrophil products (including elastase and free radicals) may cause the condition of shock lung. This is characterized by interstitial pulmonary oedema due to damage to small blood vessels, exudation of neutrophils into alveoli, and arterial hypoxaemia.

Circulation of blood through heart-lung bypass machines, or over cuprophane dialysis membranes, may lead to extra-corporeal activation of complement, accompanied by transient leucopenia, thought to be caused by aggregation of neutrophils in the lungs.

Tissue necrosis activates complement

Tissue injury following ischaemic necrosis can also cause complement activation and abundant deposition of MAC. A possible pathophysiological role for complement activation following

Role of C3 in processing of immune complexes

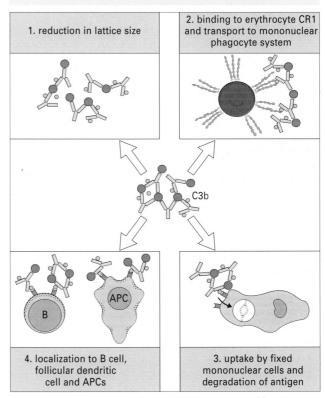

1. reduction in lattice size	2. binding to erythrocyte CR1 and transport to mononuclear phagocyte system

C3b

| 4. localization to B cell, follicular dendritic cell and APCs | 3. uptake by fixed mononuclear cells and degradation of antigen |

Fig. 13.20 C3 binds to immune complexes and (1) reduces the lattice size of the complex; (2) promotes the binding of immune complexes in the circulation to CR1 on erythrocytes which transport immune complexes through the circulation; (3) promotes the uptake of immune complexes by fixed mononuclear phagocytic cells leading to the degradation of antigen; and (4) promotes the localization of antigen in the form of immune complexes to B lymphocytes and to antigen presenting cells, including the specialized follicular dendritic cells of lymph nodes.

tissue ischaemia has been demonstrated in experimental models of myocardial infarction, in which complement depletion reduced the size of tissue injury. Infusion of soluble recombinant CR1 has recently been shown to have a similar effect.

Complement activation may cause tissue injury following the formation of immune complexes in vivo

Complement activation is an important cause of tissue injury in diseases mediated by immune complexes. Such complexes may form in tissues, for example, in glomeruli of patients with autoantibodies to glomerular basement membrane so that immune complexes form in the glomeruli; in myasthenia gravis the complexes form at motor end-plates, due to the presence of autoantibodies to acetylcholine receptors (see Chapter 23). Alternatively, circulating immune complexes may become trapped in blood vessel walls (see Chapter 24). In bacterial endocarditis, for example, an infected heart valve is the source of immune complexes that deposit in the kidney and other microvascular beds.

Complement mediates inflammation in these diseases in two major ways:

*   Activated leucocytes are attracted to sites of immune-complex deposition by locally produced anaphylatoxins, and then bind to C3b and C4b fixed to the immune complexes. This is the mechanism of damage in Goodpasture's syndrome; the inflammation which can be inhibited by either complement depletion or by neutrophil depletion.
*   The membrane attack complex (MAC) causes cell membrane injury, and thus stimulates prostaglandin synthesis from arachidonic acid.

This is the mechanism of damage in membranous nephritis, which may be induced experimentally by antibodies to subepithelial antigens. Inflammation is unaffected by neutrophil depletion, but is almost totally inhibited in animals deficient in C5. (The basement membrane is presumed to act as a physical barrier to neutrophil exudation, so that the heavy proteinuria is caused by deposition of membrane attack complex.)

Complement in the pathogenesis of disease

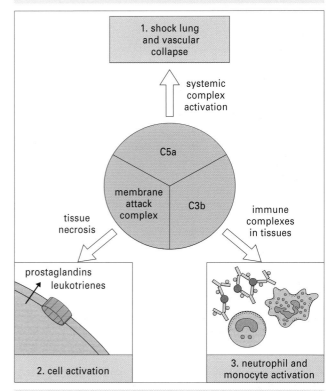

Fig. 13.21 Complement may cause disease pathogenesis by (1) systemic production of anaphylatoxins, e.g. following Gram-negative sepsis; (3) fixation of C3 to immune complexes localized in tissues causing recruitment and activation of tissue and circulating leucocytes; and (2) insertion of membrane attack complex into host cells leading to cellular activation and stimulation of membrane arachidonic acid metabolism.

Critical Thinking

■ How is the complement system inhibited from damaging host tissue?

■ How is complement activation initiated?

■ What are the amplification steps in complement activation?

■ What are the effector mechanisms of complement?

■ What is the internal thioester bond in C3 and C4 and what is its importance in the complement system?

■ What are the mechanisms for localization of complement activation to foreign surfaces?

■ What are the interactions between the complement system and microorganisms?

FURTHER READING

Ahearn JM, Fearon DT. Structure and function of the complement receptors, CR1 (CD35) and CR2 (CD21). *Adv Immunol* 1989;**46**:183–219.

Atkinson JP, Farries T. Separation of self from non-self in the complement system. *Immunol Today* 1987;**8**:212–15.

Bhakdi S, Tranum Jensen J. Complement lysis: a hole is a hole. *Immunol Today* 1991;**12**:318–20.

Campbell RD, Law SKA, Reid KBM, Sim RB. Structure, organisation, and regulation of the complement genes. *Annu Rev Immunol* 1988;**6**:161–95.

Carrell RW, Boswell DR. Serpins: the superfamily of plasma serine proteinase inhibitors. In: Barrett A, Salveson G, eds. *Proteinase Inhibitors*. Amsterdam: Elsevier, 1986:403–20.

Cooper NR. The classical complement pathway: activation and regulation of the first complement component. *Adv Immunol* 1985;**37**:151–216.

Cooper NR. Complement evasion strategies of microorganisms. *Immunol Today* 1991;**12**:327–31.

Couser WG. Pathogenesis of glomerulonephritis. *Kidney Int Suppl* 1993;**42**:S19–S26.

Esser AF. Big MAC attack: complement proteins cause leaky patches. *Immunol Today* 1991;**12**:316–18.

Farries TC, Atkinson JP. Evolution of the complement system. *Immunol Today* 1991;**12**:295–300.

Frank MM, Fries LF. The role of complement in inflammation and phagocytosis. *Immunol Today* 1991;**12**:322–26.

Gerard C, Gerard NP. C5a anaphylatoxin and its seven transmembrane-segment receptor. *Annu Rev Immunol* 1994;**12**:775–808.

Holmskov U, Malhotra R, Sim RB, Jensenius JC. Collectins: collagenous C-type lectins of the innate immune defense system. *Immunol Today* 1994;**15**:67–74.

Hourcade D, Holers VM, Atkinson JP. The regulators of complement activation (RCA) gene cluster. *Adv Immunol* 1989;**45**:381–416.

Kishimoto TK, Larson RS, Corbi AL, Dustin ML, Staunton DE, Springer TA. The leukocyte integrins. *Adv Immunol* 1989;**46**:149–82.

Klaus GGB, Humphrey JH. A re-evaluation of the role of C3 in B-cell activation. *Immunol Today* 1986;**7**:163–65.

Lachmann PJ, Walport MJ. Deficiency of the effector mechanisms of the immune response and autoimmunity. In: Whelan J, ed. *Ciba Foundation Symposium 129: Autoimmunity and Autoimmune Diseases*. Chichester:Wiley, 1987:149–71.

Law SK, Dodds AW. C3, C4 and C5: the thioester site. *Biochem Soc Trans* 1990;**18**:1155–59.

Loos M, Reid KBM, Colomb M. C1, the first component of complement: structure function relationship of C1q and collectins, C1-esterases, and C1-inhibitor in health and disease. *Behring Institute Mitteilungen*, 1993;**93**:1–328.

Morgan BP. *Complement: clinical aspects and relevance to disease*. London and New York: Academic Press, 1990.

Muller–Eberhard HJ. The membrane attack complex of complement. *Annu Rev Immunol* 1984;**2**:503–28.

Muller–Eberhard HJ, Schreiber RD. Molecular biology and chemistry of the alternative pathway of complement. *Adv Immunol* 1980;**29**:1–53.

Porter RR, Reid KBM. The biochemistry of complement. *Nature* 1978;**275**:699–704.

Reid KBM, Porter RR. The proteolytic activation systems of complement. *Annu Rev Biochem* 1981;**50**:433–64.

Reid KBM, Day AJ. Structure–function relationships of the complement components. *Immunol Today*, 1989;**10**:177–80.

Ross GD, ed. *Immunobiology of the Complement System*. New York: Academic Press, 1986.

Schifferli JA, Ng YC, Peters DK. The role of complement and its receptor in the elimination of immune complexes. *N Engl J Med* 1986;**315**:488–95.

Smith GL, Virus strategies for evasion of the host response to infection. *Trends Microbiol* 1994;**2**:81–88.

Walport MJ, Lachmann PJ. Complement. In (eds) Lachmann PJ, Peters DK, Rosen FS, Walport MJ. *Clinical Aspects of Immunology*, 5edn. Oxford: Blackwell Scientific Press, 1993:347–75.

CELL MIGRATION AND INFLAMMATION

Inflammation is a response that brings leucocytes and plasma molecules to sites of infection or tissue damage. The principal effects are an increase in blood supply, an increase in vascular permeability to large serum molecules, and enhanced migration of leucocytes across the local vascular endothelium and in the direction of the site of inflammation.

The migration of cells is a complex process that depends on which populations of cells are involved, their state of activation and how they interact with endothelium in different vascular beds throughout the body.

The activation state of cells partly determines their pattern of migration: resting or naive lymphocytes tend to migrate across high endothelial venules into lymphatic tissues, whereas activated lymphocytes tend to migrate to inflammatory sites.

Adhesion molecules that control leucocyte migration fall into families that are structurally related: the cell adhesion molecules (CAMs) of the immunoglobulin supergene family, the selectins and their carbohydrate ligands, and the integrins. Endothelial adhesion molecules are induced by cytokines. The expression of leucocyte adhesion molecules is determined by the cell population involved and by the cell's state of differentiation.

Chemotactic molecules are important both in directing cell migration and in triggering leucocytes at the endothelial surface to initiate their migration.

Inflammatory mediators released by mast cells, platelets and leucocytes in immune reactions, or following tissue damage act in concert with molecules released by the plasma enzyme systems to control vascular permeability and blood supply.

Under normal conditions, leucocytes migrate through all the tissues of the body – the cells present in the blood are the ones that are in transit between different tissues. Each population of cells has a particular pattern of migration. The pattern also depends on the cells' state of differentiation and activation:

- **Phagocytes**, including neutrophils and monocytes, leave the bone marrow and migrate to peripheral tissues, particularly at sites of infection or inflammation. Neutrophils make a one-way trip, but monocytes differentiate into macrophages and may recirculate back to the secondary lymphoid tissues to act as antigen-presenting cells (APCs).
- **Virgin lymphocytes** migrate from the thymus and bone marrow to the secondary lymphoid tissues. After activation by antigen, activated T cells tend to move to sites of inflammation (*Fig. 14.1*), while B cells and memory T cells seed other lymphoid tissues.
- **Dendritic cells**, such as the Langerhans cells of skin, are originally derived from bone-marrow stem cells which colonize various organs. After taking up antigen, they may migrate to local lymph nodes to present antigen to CD4$^+$ T cells.

One purpose of this migration is to give the small numbers of lymphocytes which are specific for any particular antigen the chance to encounter that antigen. Lymphatic drainage pathways and the migration of cells ensure that lymphocytes, APCs and antigen from infected or inflamed tissue converge on the lymph nodes, while blood-borne antigens are handled by the spleen. The initial clonal expansion of antigen-specific lymphocytes takes place in the secondary lymphoid tissues before cells are released into the efferent lymphatics and thence into the circulation (*Fig. 14.2*). Migration of these cells from the blood stream then depends on the expression of adhesion molecules on the endothelium: in inflammatory sites, the endothelium expresses adhesion molecules which are recognized by receptors on activated lymphocytes, or phagocytes that direct cell traffic to these areas. The reactions that develop in tissues in response to damage or infection are termed inflammatory reactions. They have three major components:

- **Blood supply** to the area increases, bringing leucocytes and serum molecules to the affected site.
- **Capillary permeability** increases, allowing exudation of the serum proteins (antibody, complement, kininogens, etc.) required to control the infection.
- **Leucocyte migration** into the tissue increases.

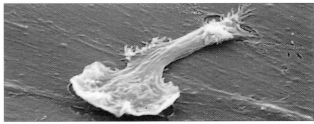
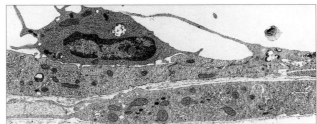

Fig. 14.1 Lymphocyte interactions with endothelium. The scanning electron micrograph (upper) shows an antigen-activated T cell binding to retinal endothelium *in vitro*. The migrating cell attaches to the endothelium and then extends pseudopodia, to probe the endothelial cell for a suitable migration point. (Courtesy of Dr J. Greenwood.) The electron micrograph (lower) shows a lymphocyte adhering to brain endothelium close to the interendothelial cell junction, in an animal with experimental allergic encephalomyelitis. Adhesion precedes transendothelial migration into inflammatory sites. (Courtesy of Dr C. Hawkins.)

When immune reactions occur in tissues, in response to antigen challenge, there is usually a phased appearance of different cell populations. The types of cells seen, their preponderance and their time of arrival, depend primarily on the nature of the antigenic challenge and on the site where the reactions

occur. In general, neutrophils are the first cells to arrive at sites of acute inflammation caused by infection. They represent the major cell type for several days. From the first day onwards mononuclear phagocytes and lymphocytes start to arrive. CD8$^+$ T cells and small numbers of B cells usually arrive later. The outcome of an acute reaction depends on whether antigen or the infectious agent is cleared. If it is not, a chronic inflammatory reaction develops. In this case, few neutrophils are seen, but large numbers of CD4$^+$ T cells and mononuclear phagocytes accumulate. Reactions to parasite infections (e.g. schistosomiasis) often lead to an accumulation of eosinophils. Eosinophils, together with basophils and macrophages, are also prevalent in the wall of the bronchus following asthmatic attacks.

Recirculation of lymphocytes and antigen-presenting cells

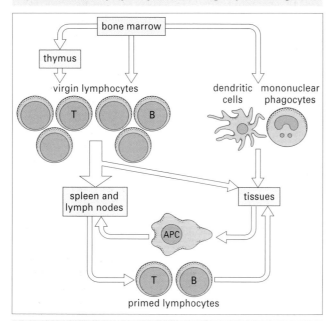

Fig. 14.2 Virgin lymphocytes from the primary lymphoid tissues such as bone marrow migrate to secondary lymphoid tissues, i.e. the spleen and lymph nodes. Antigen-presenting cells (APCs), including dendritic cells and mononuclear phagocytes, also derive from bone-marrow stem cells. These APCs enter tissues, take up antigen and transport it to the lymphoid tissues to be presented to T cells and B cells. Primed lymphocytes then migrate from the lymphoid tissues and accumulate preferentially at sites of infection or inflammation.

■ PATTERNS OF CELL MIGRATION

There are two main stages in leucocyte migration. The first is the attachment of circulating cells to the vascular endothelium, and this is followed by movement between or through the endothelial cells (*Fig. 14.3*). In the second stage, after traversing the endothelium, cells migrate towards the site of infection or inflammation, under the guidance of chemotactic stimuli. These processes are controlled partly by cell-surface molecules on the migrating cells, which allow them to interact with endothelium, tissue cells or extracellular matrix, and partly by a variety of soluble signalling molecules (chemokines and other chemotactic molecules).

The patterns of cell migration are complex, and depend not only on the type of cell, but also on its state of differentiation or activation. Moreover, vascular endothelium varies throughout the body, and this influences cell migration. In particular, the high endothelial venules (HEVs) found in secondary lymphoid tissues are quite different from those found in non-lymphoid tissues (see Chapter 3). Among non-lymphoid tissues the small-vessel endothelium varies considerably between different tissue types, and in all cases the molecules present on endothelium are modulated locally when inflammatory responses develop. All these factors affect

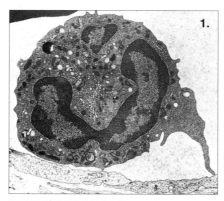
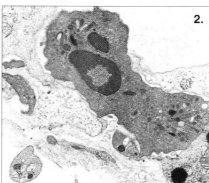
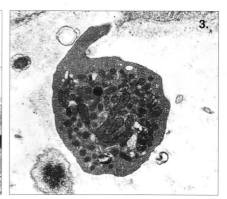

Fig. 14.3 Three phases of neutrophil migration. 1. A polymorphonuclear leucocyte adheres to the capillary endothelium. **2.** The leucocyte penetrates between the endothelial cells. **3.** A neutrophil which has traversed the endothelium. The entire process is sometimes referred to as 'diapedesis'. × 4000. (Courtesy of Dr I. Jovis.)

which types of cells migrate across different endothelial beds. In general, leucocyte migration across endothelium depends on the surface charge of the interacting cells, the haemodynamic shear force in the vascular bed, and the expression of complementary sets of adhesion molecules on both the leucocytes and the endothelium. For these reasons, leucocyte migration takes place across venules where surface charge is lowest, haemodynamic shear is low and adhesion molecules are selectively expressed (*Fig. 14.4*).

Lymphocyte migration into lymphoid tissue and sites of inflammation differs

Different patterns of movement occur at different stages of a lymphocyte's life span. For example, resting T cells tend to migrate across HEVs into secondary lymphoid tissues, while activated cells tend to migrate into sites of inflammation. Moreover, there is selective migration to particular regions. For example, lymphocytes isolated from Peyer's patches tend to relocalize to the gut on reinfusion, while splenic lymphocytes preferentially return to the spleen.

Migration into lymph nodes, Peyer's patches and mucosal lymphoid tissues occurs across HEVs (see Chapter 3). Up to 25% of the lymphocytes that enter a lymph node via the blood may be diverted across HEVs. In contrast, only a tiny proportion of those circulating through other tissues will migrate across the regular endothelium of venules at each transit. Nevertheless, this low-level migration is very important. It allows lymphocytes to patrol throughout the body, and is much enhanced if an inflammatory response develops.

HEVs are therefore particularly important in controlling lymphocyte recirculation. Normally they are present only in the secondary lymphoid tissues, but they are induced at sites of chronic inflammation. In addition to having a peculiar

shape, lymphoid HEVs' cells express distinct sets of heavily glycosylated, sulphated adhesion molecules, which bind to circulating T cells and direct them to the lymphoid tissue. These differ from the adhesion molecules that control migration to acute inflammatory sites. Moreover, the HEVs in different lymphoid tissues have different sets of adhesion molecules. In particular, there are separate molecules controlling migration to Peyer's patches, mucosal lymph nodes and other lymph nodes. These molecules were previously called vascular addressins (see p. 14.5), and their expression on different HEVs accounts for the way in which lymphocytes relocalize to their own lymphoid tissue.

Migration is controlled by both leucocytes and endothelium

Leucocyte migration is controlled by the adhesion molecules on both the endothelium and leucocytes, by the migratory capacity of the leucocytes, and by the presence of chemotactic agents. To explain the complex and varied patterns of cell migration, the large numbers of factors that modulate these must be considered. They include:

- **The state of activation of the lymphocytes or phagocytes:** the expression of adhesion molecules and their functional affinity vary depending on the type of cell and whether it has been activated by antigen, cytokines or cellular interactions.
- **The types of adhesion molecules expressed by the vascular endothelium:** this is related to its anatomical site and to whether it has been activated by cytokines.
- **The particular chemotactic molecules and cytokines present in the tissue:** receptors vary between leucocyte populations, so that particular chemotactic agents act selectively on some cells only.

We will look at the different types and distribution of adhesion molecules before considering their role in the mechanisms of cell migration.

■ INTERCELLULAR ADHESION MOLECULES

Intercellular adhesion molecules are membrane-bound proteins that allow one cell to interact with another. Often these molecules traverse the membrane and are linked to the cell's cytoskeleton, so that as the cell moves it can use them to gain traction on other cells, or on the extracellular matrix, as it moves. In many cases, a particular adhesion molecule can bind to more than one ligand, employing different binding sites. Although the binding affinity of individual adhesion molecules to their ligands is usually low, the avidity of the interaction can be high because of clustering of the molecules in patches on the cell surface.

Cells can modulate their interactions with other cell types, either by increasing the numbers of adhesion molecules on the surface or by altering their affinity/avidity (*Fig. 14.5*). There are two ways in which cells can alter the level of expression of adhesion molecules: many cells retain large intracellular stores of these molecules in vesicles, which can be directed to the cell surface within minutes following cellular activation. Alternatively, new molecules can be synthesized and transported to the cell surface, which usually takes several hours.

Leucocyte migration across endothelium

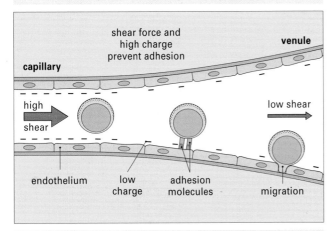

Fig. 14.4 Leucocytes circulating through a vascular bed may interact with venular endothelium via sets of surface adhesion molecules. In the venules, haemodynamic shear is low, surface charge on the endothelium is lower and adhesion molecules are selectively expressed. If leucocytes are correctly stimulated, adhesion can precede migration.

Modulation of leucocyte adhesion

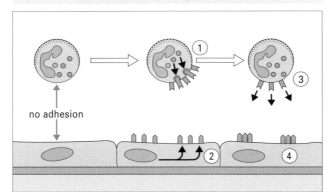

Fig. 14.5 There are four ways in which leucocyte binding to endothelium may become enhanced. 1. Many cells hold stores of adhesion molecules, which can be rapidly moved to the cell surface. 2. Endothelial cells at sites of inflammation may synthesize new adhesion molecules. 3. Molecules such as LFA-1 can increase their affinity following cell activation. 4. Reorganization of adhesion molecules on the cell surface may result in the formation of high avidity patches. In practice, cells may use several mechanisms and affinity changes may follow the initial interaction between the cells.

Endothelial cell adhesion molecules

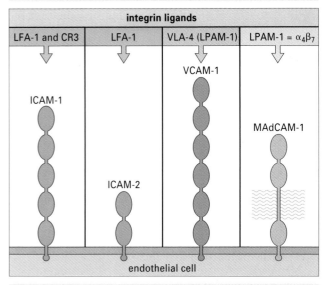

Fig. 14.6 The molecules ICAM-1, ICAM-2, VCAM-1 and MAdCAM-1 are illustrated diagrammatically with their immunoglobulin-like domains. Their integrin ligands are listed above. MAdCAM-1 also has a heavily glycosylated segment which binds L-selectin.

A bewilderingly large number of adhesion molecules have been identified that have a role in leucocyte migration. Nevertheless, they fall into four families which are structurally related. Migration is a complex process, and several sets of adhesion molecules are involved during the complete event.

Several endothelial adhesion molecules belong to the immunoglobulin supergene family

The immunoglobulin supergene family includes the cellular adhesion molecules (CAMs) ICAM-1 (intercellular CAM-1), ICAM-2, VCAM-1 (vascular CAM-1) and MAdCAM-1 (mucosal adhesion CAM-1). All members of this family are expressed, or inducible, on vascular endothelium. ICAM-1 has five extracellular domains; the two N-terminal domains are structurally homologous to the two extracellular domains of ICAM-2. VCAM-1 has six extracellular domains and MAdCAM-1 is a composite molecule which includes Ig-like domains (*Fig. 14.6*).

Integrins on leucocytes are involved in adhesion to endothelium and to extracellular matrix

The integrins are a major group of adhesion molecules, present on many cells, including leucocytes. Each member of this large family of molecules consists of two non-covalently bound polypeptides (α and β), both of which traverse the membrane. They fall into three main subfamilies, depending on whether they have a β_1, a β_2 or a β_3 chain. Recent discoveries suggest that the assortment of α chains with β chains is not quite as precise as originally thought. Broadly speaking, the β_1-integrins are involved in binding of cells to extracellular matrix, the β_2-integrins are involved in leucocyte adhesion to endothelium or to other immune cells, and the

Integrins

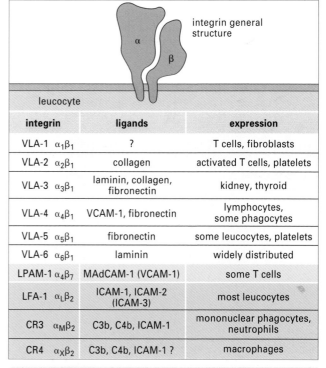

integrin		ligands	expression
VLA-1	$\alpha_1\beta_1$	?	T cells, fibroblasts
VLA-2	$\alpha_2\beta_1$	collagen	activated T cells, platelets
VLA-3	$\alpha_3\beta_1$	laminin, collagen, fibronectin	kidney, thyroid
VLA-4	$\alpha_4\beta_1$	VCAM-1, fibronectin	lymphocytes, some phagocytes
VLA-5	$\alpha_5\beta_1$	fibronectin	some leucocytes, platelets
VLA-6	$\alpha_6\beta_1$	laminin	widely distributed
LPAM-1	$\alpha_4\beta_7$	MAdCAM-1 (VCAM-1)	some T cells
LFA-1	$\alpha_L\beta_2$	ICAM-1, ICAM-2 (ICAM-3)	most leucocytes
CR3	$\alpha_M\beta_2$	C3b, C4b, ICAM-1	mononuclear phagocytes, neutrophils
CR4	$\alpha_X\beta_2$	C3b, C4b, ICAM-1 ?	macrophages

Fig. 14.7 The general structure of an integrin consisting of two non-covalently linked chains is shown at the top. The table gives the properties of some of the integrins involved in leucocyte binding to endothelium or extracellular matrix.

β_3-integrins (cytoadhesins) are involved in the interactions of platelets and neutrophils at inflammatory sites or sites of vascular damage. There are, however, several exceptions to this simple scheme, and additional β chains have been described (e.g. β_7). Each β chain may associate with one of a number of different α chains to make different adhesion molecules. *Figure 14.7* illustrates some of the integrins used by leucocytes during cell movement.

Selectins are a group of adhesion molecules on leucocytes and endothelium which bind to carbohydrate

The selectins include the molecules E-selectin and P-selectin, expressed on endothelium and platelets, and L-selectin which is expressed on some leucocytes (*Fig. 14.8*). They are transmembrane molecules, with a number of extracellular domains homologous to those seen in complement control proteins (e.g. factor H). The extracellular region also has a domain related to the epidermal growth factor (EGF) receptor and an N-terminal domain that has lectin-like properties (i.e. it binds to carbohydrate residues), hence the name selectins. Unsurprisingly, the ligands that selectins bind to carry carbohydrate moieties.

Carbohydrate ligands for selectins are associated with various glycoproteins on lymphocytes and endothelium

The carbohydrate ligands for the selectins may be associated with several different proteins. For example, glycam-1 expressed on HEVs has numerous *O*-linked carbohydrates which bind to L-selectin on lymphocytes and directs these cells to peripheral lymph nodes. However, L-selectin may also bind to carbohydrate on MAdCAM-1, expressed on mucosal HEVs. These carbohydrate molecules, descriptively called vascular addressins, are primarily present on HEVs of lymphoid tissues but may be induced at other sites during chronic inflammation (*Fig. 14.9*).

E-selectin and P-selectin expressed on activated endothelium bind to the sialyl Lewis-X carbohydrate associated with CD15, present on many leucocytes. They serve to slow leucocytes in the first phase of migration (*Fig. 14.10*).

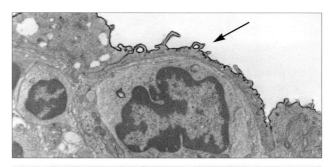

Fig. 14.9 Mucosal addressin on endothelium.
The immunoelectron micrograph has been stained to show MAdCAM-1 as a dark border (arrow), on the luminal surface. In this instance the molecule is expressed on brain endothelium in chronic relapsing experimental allergic encephalomyelitis, induced by immunization of Biozzi AB/H mice with myelin basic protein. (Courtesy of of Drs J. K. O'Neill and C. Butter, with permission from *Immunology*.)

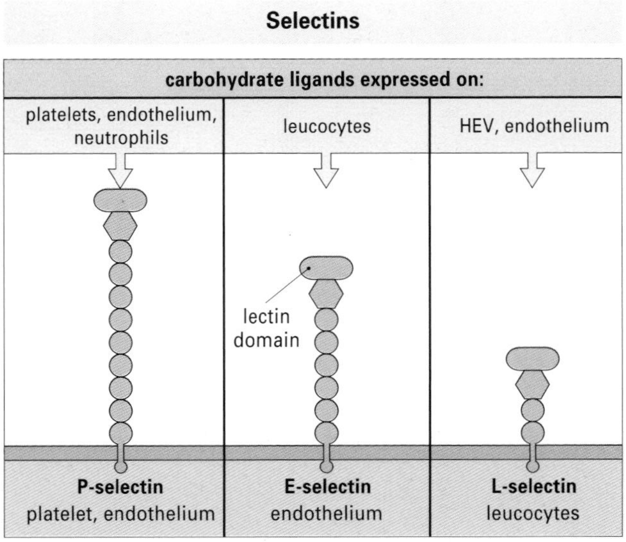

Three-step model of leucocyte adhesion

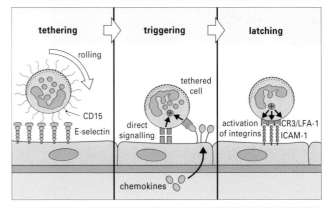

Fig. 14.10 The three steps of leucocyte adhesion are illustrated by a neutrophil, although different sets of adhesion molecules would be used by other leucocytes in different situations. *Tethering*: the neutrophil is slowed as it rolls down the endothelium, by interaction of E-selectin with CD15 on the leucocyte. *Triggering*: the tethered cell is triggered either by direct interaction with surface molecules on the endothelium or by chemokines and other chemotactic molecules held on the endothelium. *Latching*: the triggering upregulates integrins (CR3 and LFA-1) so that they bind to ICAM-1 induced on the endothelium.

Selectins

carbohydrate ligands expressed on:		
platelets, endothelium, neutrophils	leucocytes	HEV, endothelium
	lectin domain	
P-selectin platelet, endothelium	**E-selectin** endothelium	**L-selectin** leucocytes

Fig. 14.8 The structures of three selectins are shown. They have terminal lectin domains which bind carbohydrates on the cells listed, and also share other structural features.

■ MECHANISMS OF CELL MIGRATION

The process of leucocyte migration across endothelium requires several consecutive steps to occur. The first three are shown in *Figure 14.10*.

- **Tethering:** leucocytes are slowed as they pass through a venule and roll on the surface of the endothelium before being halted. This is mediated primarily by selectins interacting with carbohydrate.
- **Triggering:** the arrested leucocytes now have the opportunity to respond to cytokines, chemotactic agents and surface molecules on the endothelium and extracellular matrix. These may activate the cell and induce a programme of migration.
- **Latching and activation:** this upregulates the affinity of the leucocytes' integrins, which engage the cellular adhesion molecules on the endothelium and start to migrate.
- **Migration:** cells contact the basement membrane using new sets of adhesion molecules, and migrate beneath the endothelium.
- **Digestion:** enzymes are released which digest the collagen and other components of the basement membrane, allowing cells to migrate into the tissue.

Adhesion molecules control cell attachment and transendothelial migration

Different sets of adhesion molecules and chemotactic agents are used for each type of cell movement.

Leucocyte migration in inflammation – Neutrophils appear early at sites of acute inflammation and this is in part controlled by the cytokine induction of E-selectin on the surface of endothelium in these areas. Stimulation *in vitro* of endothelium with cytokines such as tumour necrosis factor-α (TNFα) or interleukin-1 (IL-1) induces expression of E-selectin over a period of 4–12 hours, but expression wanes by 24 hours (*Fig. 14.11*), and this molecule appears early during inflammatory reactions *in vivo*. Cells transfected with the gene for E-selectin express high levels of this adhesion molecule and bind neutrophils strongly. These facts suggest that the slowing of neutrophils by E-selectin is a critical first step in their migration.

Also important in migration of neutrophils, lymphocytes and monocytes are the β_2-integrins LFA-1 and CR3, which are expressed on leucocytes and bind to the endothelial CAMs belonging to the immunoglobulin supergene family. LFA-1 binds to ICAM-1 and ICAM-2 expressed on vascular endothelium. *In vitro*, the endothelial expression of ICAM-2 is constitutive, and it has been suggested that ICAM-2 determines the basal level of binding of lymphocytes to different types of endothelium. For example, ICAM-2 expression is relatively low on brain endothelium, and cell migration across normal cerebral endothelium is also relatively low. In contrast ICAM-1 is normally present at low levels on endothelium, but can be induced by cytokines (TNFα, IL-1 and IFNγ, depending on the species). ICAM-1 is induced over 8–96 hours *in vitro*, which corresponds to the later arrival of monocytes and lymphocytes (*Fig. 14.11*). The function of CR3 in phagocyte accumulation has been pinpointed by studies *in vivo* using antibodies to CR3, which inhibit phagocyte migration. Notably, a group of patients who suffer from leucocyte adhesion deficiency (LAD) syndrome, and who suffer from severe infections due to poor phagocyte accumulation, are deficient in all the β_2-integrins (LFA-1, CR3, CR4). CR3 recognizes a site on ICAM-1, as distinct from that recognized by LFA-1.

VCAM-1 is also induced in inflammatory sites and *in vitro* with a similar time course to ICAM-1 (*Fig. 14.11*). This molecule binds to the integrin VLA-4, present on some lymphocyte populations. There are, however, subtle differences in which cytokines induce E-selectin, ICAM-1 and VCAM-1 in different species and different vascular beds. This allows for cell migration across endothelium in inflammation to be fine-tuned, contributing to the phased arrival of the different leucocyte populations. Lymphocyte binding to endothelium can be modulated using antibodies to adhesion molecules on lymphocytes or endothelium, or by using soluble adhesion molecules, and this holds out prospects for therapy of diseases in which immunopathological events occur.

Normal leucocyte migration – A distinction must be drawn between the molecules described above, which control cell movement into inflammatory sites, and those which control normal lymphocyte traffic. Naive lymphocytes express L-selectin, which contributes to their attachment to carbohydrate ligands on HEVs in mucosal and peripheral lymph nodes. Once they have stopped on the HEV, migrating lymphocytes may use the integrin $\alpha_4\beta_7$ (LPAM-1) to bind to MadCAM-1 on the HEVs of mucosal lymph nodes or Peyer's patch. Since the expression of $\alpha_4\beta_7$ allows migration to mucosal lymphoid tissue, while $\alpha_4\beta_1$ (VLA-4) allows attachment to VCAM-1 on activated endothelium, or fibronectin in tissues, expression of one or the other of these molecules can alternately direct naive lymphocytes to lymphoid tissue or activated T cells to inflammatory sites.

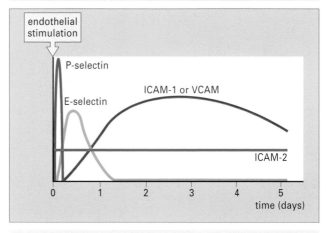

Expression and induction of endothelial adhesion molecules

Fig. 14.11 The graph shows the time course of induction of different endothelial molecules on human umbilical vein endothelium *in vitro*, following stimulation by TNFα.

Interaction of leucocytes with the extracellular matrix – Once they have crossed the endothelium and entered the tissues, the cells must interact with the proteins of the extracellular matrix (collagen, laminin, fibronectin, etc.), as well as the tissue cells. As lymphocytes leave the blood vessel, they lose some of their surface molecules (e.g. L-selectin) which are no longer required. The functional phenotype changes from that of a circulating cell to one adapted to move through tissues.

Many of the leucocyte molecules which allow interaction with extracellular matrix belong to the β_1-integrin group, and are known as very late antigens (VLAs), so called because they were first identified on the T-cell surface at a late stage after T-cell activation. The whole group of β_1-integrins are now referred to as VLA molecules, even though most of them are not expressed only on lymphocytes. This group includes receptors for collagen (VLA-2 and VLA-3), laminin (VLA-3 and VLA-6) and fibronectin (VLA-3, VLA-4 and VLA-5). The fact that some of these molecules appear late after lymphocyte activation suggests that cells go through a programme of differentiation, and that the ability to interact with extracellular matrix is one of the last functions to develop.

Chemotactic molecules trigger migration and control directional movement of leucocytes

The integrins used by leucocytes to migrate across endothelium are present on the surface of the cell or are stored in granules to be released to the surface, but they are mostly non-functional and require an activation signal from the endothelium to become active. This signal can be supplied directly by the endothelial cell or it may come from signalling molecules released from the tissue and retained on the endothelium. Many of these signalling molecules are also chemotactic. They include C5a, leukotriene-B_4 (LTB$_4$), and various low-molecular weight cytokines, referred to as chemokines (*Fig. 14.12*).

Chemotactic and chemokinetic functions differ: chemotaxis is the directional migration of cells up a concentration gradient of a chemotactic molecule, while chemokinesis is non-directional migration. For directional migration to occur, the cell must be responsive to gradients of the chemotactic mediator, a concentration difference of possibly as little as 0.1% between the leading and trailing edges of a migrating cell. In chemokinesis, mediators such as histamine enhance the overall motility of cells.

Chemokines The chemokines are a group of at least 18 heparin-binding molecules, including IL-8, and are released at inflammatory sites. They act via a group of three receptors (so far identified) that are expressed on different leucocyte populations. Some of the chemokines act selectively on particular populations of leucocytes: for example, macrophage inflammatory protein-1β (MIP-1β) selectively stimulates CD8$^+$ T cells. By binding to endothelium they can trigger a cell which has been tethered by selectins, activating its integrins and initiating migration – provided of course that the leucocytes express the correct integrins and the endothelium is expressing the corresponding ligand. Some of the chemokines can activate cells, some are primarily chemotactic, some have both functions. Why there should be so many chemokines is not known, but they presumably contribute to the selective control of leucocyte migration. Several other inflammatory mediators are either chemotactic or chemokinetic.

Other chemotactic molecules Several molecules are chemotactic for neutrophils and macrophages (*Fig. 14.12*). Both of these cells have an f.Met-Leu-Phe (f.MLP) receptor. This receptor binds to peptides blocked at the N terminus by formylated methionine. Since prokaryotes (e.g. bacteria) initiate all protein translation with this amino acid whereas eukaryotes do not, this provides a simple specific signal for the presence of bacteria, towards which phagocytes should move. Neutrophils and macrophages also have receptors for C5a and LTB$_4$, both of which are generated at sites of inflammation – C5a following complement activation and LTB$_4$ following activation of a variety of cells, particularly macrophages and mast cells. In addition, molecules generated by the blood clotting system, notably fibrin peptide B and thrombin, attract phagocytes.

The first cells to arrive at a site of inflammation, if activated, are able to attract others. For example, IL-8 released by activated monocytes can induce neutrophil and basophil chemotaxis. Similarly, macrophage activation leads to metabolism of arachidonic acid, with release of LTB$_4$.

▪ INFLAMMATION

Inflammation is the body's reaction to invasion by an infectious agent, antigen challenge or even just physical damage. In addition to the enhanced cell migration, detailed above, serum molecules also leak into inflammatory sites. In contrast with cell migration, which occurs across venules, serum exudation occurs primarily across capillaries, where blood pressure is higher. This event is controlled in two ways:

Chemotactic molecules

factor	characteristic	source	action on
C5a	77 amino acid peptide	N terminus of C5 α chain	
f.Met-Leu-Phe	tripeptide with blocked N terminus	prokaryotes	neutrophils, eosinophils, macrophages
LTB$_4$	arachidonic acid metabolite via lipoxygenase pathway	mast cells, basophils, macrophages	
Chemokines (IL-8, MIP-α, MIP-1β, RANTES, etc.)	10kDa proteins	different leucocyte populations	selective actions on different leucocyte populations

Fig. 14.12 The table lists molecules which are chemotactic for different leucocyte populations, depending on the expression of specific receptors. Some of the chemokines are chemotactic while others trigger cells.

- Blood supply to the area increases.
- Capillary permeability increases.

The increase in capillary permeability is caused by retraction of the endothelial cells and possibly also by increased vesicular transport across the endothelium. This permits larger molecules to traverse the endothelium than would ordinarily be capable of doing so and thus allows antibody, complement and molecules of other plasma enzyme systems to reach the inflammatory site.

Inflammation is controlled by chemokines, plasma enzyme systems, cytokines, and the products of mast cells, platelets and leucocytes

The development of inflammatory reactions is controlled by chemokines, by products of the plasma enzyme systems, and by vasoactive mediators released from leucocytes (*Fig. 14.13*). The mediators controlling different types of inflammatory reaction differ. Fast-acting mediators, such as vasoactive amines and the products of the kinin system (see below), modulate the immediate response. Later, newly synthesized mediators such as leukotrienes are involved in the accumulation and activation of other cells.

Once leucocytes have arrived at a site of infection or inflammation, they release mediators which control the later accumulation and activation of other cells. However, in inflammatory reactions initiated by the immune system, the ultimate control is exerted by the antigen itself, in the same way as it controls the immune response itself. For this reason, the cellular accumulation at the site of chronic infection, or in autoimmune reactions (where the antigen cannot ultimately be eradicated), is quite different from that at sites where the antigenic stimulus is rapidly cleared.

Plasma enzyme systems – There are four major plasma enzyme systems that have an important role in haemostasis and control of inflammation. These are the clotting system, the fibrinolytic (plasmin) system, the kinin system and the complement system. In many ways the complement system acts as a link between immunological events and inflammatory systems (see Chapter 13). The kinin system generates the mediators bradykinin and lysyl-bradykinin (kallidin). Bradykinin is a very powerful vasoactive nonapeptide, which causes venular dilation, increased vascular permeability and smooth muscle contraction. Bradykinin is generated following the activation of Hageman factor (XII) of the blood clotting system, whereas kallidin is generated following activation of the plasmin system or by enzymes released from damaged tissues.

Auxiliary cells – These cells, including mast cells, basophils and platelets, are important sources of the vasoactive mediators histamine and 5-hydroxytryptamine (serotonin), which produce vasodilation and increased vascular permeability. Many of the proinflammatory effects of C3a and C5a result from their ability to trigger mast-cell granule release, demonstrated by the fact that they can be blocked by antihistamines. Mast cells and basophils are also a route by which the adaptive immune system can trigger inflammation – IgE sensitizes these cells for antigen-specific triggering of granule release. The interactions of these systems are shown in *Fig. 14.14*.

Mast cells are also an important source of slow-reacting inflammatory mediators, including the leukotrienes, prostaglandins and thromboxanes (see Chapter 22). Platelets may also be activated by the immune system – by immune complexes or by platelet activating factor (PAF) from neutrophils, basophils and macrophages. This is thought to be important in Type II and Type III hypersensitivity reactions.

Inflammatory mediators

mediator	origin	actions
histamine	mast cells, basophils	increased vascular permeability, smooth muscle contraction, chemokinesis
5-hydroxy-tryptamine (5HT – serotonin)	platelets, mast cells (rodent)	increased vascular permeability, smooth muscle contraction
platelet activating factor (PAF)	basophils, neutrophils, macrophages	mediator release from platelets, increased vascular permeability, smooth muscle contraction, neutrophil activation
neutrophil chemotactic factor (NCF)	mast cells	neutrophil chemotaxis
IL-8	monocytes and lymphocytes	polymorph and monocyte localization
C3a	complement C3	mast-cell degranulation, smooth muscle contraction
C5a	complement C5	mast-cell degranulation, neutrophil and macrophage chemotaxis, neutrophil activation, smooth muscle contraction, increased capillary permeability
bradykinin	kinin system (kininogen)	vasodilation, smooth muscle contraction, increased capillary permeability, pain
fibrinopeptides and fibrin breakdown products	clotting system	increased vascular permeability, neutrophil and macrophage chemotaxis
prostaglandin E_2 (PGE$_2$)	cyclo-oxygenase pathway	vasodilation, potentiates increased vascular permeability produced by histamine and bradykinin
leukotriene B$_4$ (LTB$_4$)	lipoxygenase pathway	neutrophil chemotaxis, synergizes with PGE$_2$ in increasing vascular permeability
leukotriene D$_4$ (LTD$_4$)	lipoxygenase pathway	smooth muscle contraction, increasing vascular permeability

Fig. 14.13 The table lists major inflammatory mediators, which control blood supply and vascular permeability or modulate the movement of cells.

Cytokines – These are also important in signalling between cells as inflammatory reactions develop. In the initial stages, cytokines such as IL-1 and IL-6 may be released from cells of the tissue where the inflammatory reaction is occurring. Once lymphocytes and mononuclear cells have started to enter the inflammatory site, they may become activated by antigen and release cytokines of their own (IL-1, TNF, IL-4, IFNγ) which further enhance cellular migration by their actions on the local endothelium. Other cytokines, such as IL-8, are chemotactic or can activate incoming cells.

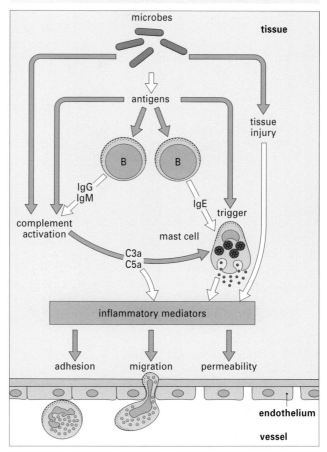

The immune system in acute inflammation

Fig. 14.14 The adaptive immune system modulates inflammatory processes via the complement system. Antigens (e.g. from microorganisms) stimulate B cells to produce antibodies including IgE, which binds to mast cells, while IgG and IgM activate complement. Complement can also be activated directly via the alternative pathway. When triggered by antigen, the sensitized mast cells release their granule-associated mediators and eicosanoids (products of arachidonic metabolism, including prostaglandins and leukotrienes). In association with complement (which can also trigger mast cells via C3a and C5a), the mediators induce local inflammation, facilitating the arrival of leucocytes and more plasma enzyme system molecules.

Critical Thinking

■ If you could make a 'knockout' mouse that lacked a functional gene for VCAM-1, what effect do you think this would have on the migration of lymphocytes, or the migration of neutrophils?

■ If you place some purified C5a on the base of a blister, what effect would you expect this to have on local leucocyte traffic, blood flow and vascular permeability? How would these effects be mediated?

■ Indomethacin is a drug which inhibits the production of prostaglandins and leukotrienes. What effect would you expect it to have on an inflammatory reaction, and why?

■ You are investigating the processes which occur during chronic rejection of kidney allografts. Which of these adhesion molecules might be worth looking for on the endothelium: P-selectin, E-selectin, VLA-4, ICAM-1, ICAM-2, LFA-1, MAdCAM-1? Why?

FURTHER READING

Davies P, Bailey PJ, Goldenberg MM, Ford-Hutchinson AW. The role of arachidonic acid oxygenation products in pain and inflammations. *Annu Rev Immunol* 1984;**2**:335–58.

Dustin ML, Springer TA. Role of lymphocyte adhesion receptors in transient interactions and cell locomotion. *Annu Rev Immunol* 1991;**9**:27–66.

Hemler ME. VLA proteins in the integrin family: structures, functions and their role on leucocytes. *Annu Rev Immunol* 1990;**8**:365–400.

Hynes RO. Integrins: versatility, modulation and signalling in cell adhesion. *Cell* 1992;**69**:11–25.

Male DK. Cell traffic and inflammation. In: Male DK, Champion B, Cooke A, Owen M., Trowsdale J. *Advanced Immunology*. 3rd ed. London: Mosby, 1995: Chapter 14.

Proud D, Kaplan AP. Kinin formation: mechanism and role in inflammatory disorders. *Annu Rev Immunol* 1988;**6**:49–83.

Shimizu Y, Newman W, Gopal TV, *et al*. Four molecular pathways of T cell adhesion to endothelial cells. Roles of LFA-1, VCAM-1 and ELAM-1 and changes of pathway hierarchy under different activation conditions. *J Cell Biol* 1991;**113**:1203–12.

Springer TA. Adhesion receptors in the immune system. *Nature* 1990;**346**:425–34.

Springer TA. Traffic signals for lymphocyte recirculation and leucocyte emigration: the multistep paradigm. *Cell* 1994;**76**:301–14.

Phagocytosis and encapsulation are important in eliminating non-self material in invertebrates, with circulating white blood cells mediating these processes in many species.

Recognition of foreign transplants is evident early in evolution, but there is little evidence for specificity and clonal expansion in invertebrates.

Lectins and prophenoloxidase are involved in recognition of self/non-self.

Cytokine-like molecules effect immunoregulation in many invertebrates.

Immunoglobulins are absent from all invertebrates, although Ig-like domains are found in many invertebrate phyla. An inducible, broad spectrum, humoral immunity is found in some coelomate invertebrates.

Clonally-restricted antigen receptor molecules are central to the vertebrate anticipatory immune response which generates effector and memory cells.

B cells and IgM are universally found in jawed vertebrates. Although additional non-μ heavy chains are found in ectotherms, antibody affinity remains low. Recombinant DNA technology reveals several patterns of Ig gene organization during vertebrate phylogeny.

The major histocompatibility complex (MHC) has been identified in cartilaginous fish. Co-evolving T cells have been described from bony fish upwards and their T cell receptor molecules are currently being investigated.

Natural killer (NK) cells, phagocytes, complement components and immunoregulatory cytokines constitute non-adaptive elements of the immune systems of vertebrates.

An evolutionary progression towards the sophisticated mammalian immune system is apparent from detailed studies of a range of vertebrates. However, the phylogenetic origins of the vertebrate adaptive immune system, particularly at the molecular level, remain uncertain despite extensive research into invertebrate immunity. Nevertheless, much can be learned about the origins of vertebrate non-adaptive (innate) immunity (e.g. phagocytosis) from the examination of invertebrates. Since invertebrates comprise over 95% of all animal species – they occur as solitary or colonial animals, with or without body cavities (coelomate/acoelomate), with or without blood systems – there are many suitable experimental subjects.

Figure 15.1 shows a simplified evolutionary tree of the animal kingdom with the coelomate invertebrates divided into two main evolutionary lines, based principally upon embryological differences. One line, leading to the molluscs, annelids and arthropods (the protostomes) diverged early in evolution from the pathway forming the echinoderms, tunicates and vertebrates (the deuterostomes). Research on invertebrate immunity has concentrated on arthropods and molluscs because many of these are pests transmitting diseases or competing for agricultural products. Consequently, work with groups that are phylogenetically relevant to the vertebrates (e.g. tunicates and echinoderms) has been neglected. In addition, since the ancestors of vertebrates are now extinct, attempts to trace the origin of vertebrate immunity within the invertebrates, in groups such as the tunicates (*Fig. 15.2*), are speculative and assume that some living animals are close relatives of the vertebrate ancestor. *Figure 15.1* also shows cellular and humoral immune phenomena discovered in the invertebrates.

Figure 15.3 presents possible steps in the evolution of vertebrate blood cells and immunity. Despite the success of the invertebrates, only vertebrates possess lymphocytes with a highly specific long-term memory component. What environmental pressures might have led to the increased sophistication of the vertebrate immune system? Perhaps the enhanced threat of cancer and of viral infections in these complex, long-lived animals was important, favouring the development of a finely tuned immune system, with circulating effector cells recognizing foreign peptides presented by major histocompatibility complex (MHC) glycoproteins on the surface of infected or mutated cells.

■ INVERTEBRATE IMMUNITY

Classification of blood cells in invertebrates

Most invertebrates possess white blood cells (leucocytes), but usually lack red blood cells (erythrocytes). The leucocytes can be fixed, free within blood vessels, or occupy fluid-filled body cavities called the coelom (coelomocytes) or haemocoel (haemocytes).

The first blood cells probably evolved from a free-living, protozoan-like ancestor. In primitive metazoans such as sponges, coelenterates and flatworms, wandering phagocytic amoebocytes not only function in host defence but are also involved in nutrition and excretion. In coelomates (both protostomes and deuterostomes), whose bodies are larger and more complex, a circulatory system is required to transport food and waste substances around the body. The amoebocyte-like cells, no longer required to gather food, probably migrated from the surrounding connective tissue into the circulatory system. Here, an array of cell types evolved, some of which took on specific roles in immune reactivity (*Fig. 15.4*).

Due to the huge diversity of invertebrates, and in contrast to the vertebrates, it is impossible to categorize free leucocytes into well defined classes by staining and morphology alone. However, a functional scheme can be devised with five main groups of cells (see *Fig. 15.4*):

Immunopotentialities of vertebrates and invertebrates

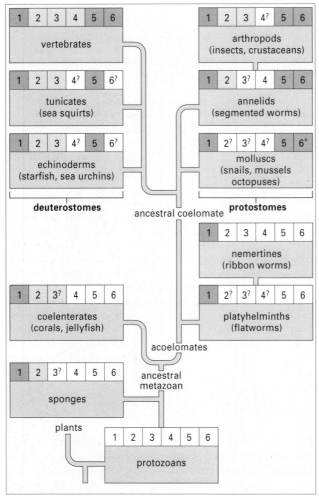

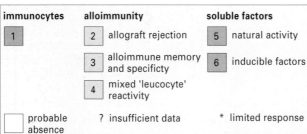

Fig. 15.1 Partial evidence for certain cellular and humoral immune phenomena in diverse invertebrate and vertebrate phyla is shown.

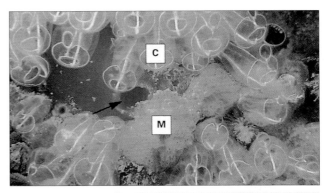

Fig. 15.2 Two colonial sea squirts (tunicates), *Clavelina lepadiformis* (C) and *Morchellium argus* (M), competing for space. An underlying solitary tunicate can be seen towards the centre (arrowed). The diameter of an individual *Clavelina* is approximately 4 mm. (Courtesy of Dr P. Dyrynda).

Evolution of the immune system

evolutionary step or selection pressure	immunological implications
single-celled animals	recognition and discrimination
multicellularity (including colonial forms)	histocompatibility system, allogeneic recognition and short-term memory
mesoderm and circulatory system, nutrition and defence as separate functions	freely circulating and more diverse blood cell types, cellular immunity and erythrocytes
cancer and viral infections associated with increasing complexity and longevity	immunosurveillance of own cells for those that are infected or cancerous
ancestral protovertebrates	increased recognition and discriminatory powers?
lower vertebrates: increased size, longer life span and reduced reproductive potential compared with invertebrates	true lymphocytes, lymphoid tissue and antibody production (IgM), longer-term memory
emergence onto land, exposure to irradiation and development of high pressure blood vascular systems	bone marrow, additional antibody classes, T- and B-lymphocytes, lymphoid organs with increased complexity, GALT
amniotes (reptiles, birds, mammals) with loss of free-living larval form	advanced differentiation of immunocompetent cells allowing increased diversity and efficiency of immune system
homoiothermy provides a more favourable environment for pathogens	increased efficiency of immune system, integrated cellular and humoral responses, germinal centres in secondary lymphoid organs, lymph nodes
viviparity with maternal–foetal interactions	additional fine-tuning of immune system to avoid rejection by mother

Fig. 15.3 Evolutionary steps of possible significance in the phylogeny of blood cells and the immune system. (Adapted from Rowley AF, Ratcliffe NA, eds. *Vertebrate Blood Cells.* Cambridge: Cambridge University Press, 1988; with permission.)

- **Progenitor cells**, together with a variable array of haemopoietic tissue, may act as stem cells for the other cell types. Superficially, they resemble vertebrate lymphocytes (*Fig. 15.5*) although evidence for true homology is strictly limited.
- **Phagocytic cells** (*Fig. 15.6*) are probably the only blood cell type present throughout the animal kingdom. They correspond to the mammalian granulocyte or macrophage but have different surface markers.
- **Haemostatic (granular) cells** are involved in coagulation and wound healing, and are important effectors of non-self recognition.
- **Nutritive cells** are present in only a few species.
- **Pigmented cells** are present in many species but may contain respiratory pigment, thus resembling vertebrate erythrocytes in a few species.

Invertebrates lack lymphocytes and antibodies but have very efficient host defence mechanisms

Invertebrate immune systems apparently lack immunoglobulins, interactive lymphocyte sub-populations and lymphoid organs. Nevertheless, the huge numbers and diversity of invertebrates attests to the efficiency of their host defences.

Like vertebrates, invertebrates have extremely effective physicochemical barriers as a first line of defence (*Fig. 15.4*). The mucus that surrounds the body of many coelenterates, annelids, molluscs, and some tunicates entraps and kills potential pathogens (*Fig. 15.7*). Tough external skeletons such as tests or shells form barriers to invasion in some coelenterates and molluscs, echinoderms and arthropods.

Once these barriers are breached, would-be invaders are then exposed to a range of interacting cellular and humoral defence reactions.

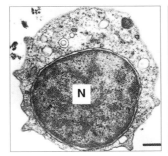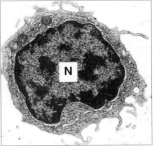

Fig. 15.5 **Electron micrographs of a lymphocyte-like cell from the tunicate, *Ciona intestinalis* (left), and a lymphocyte from a fish, the blenny, *Blennius pholis* (right).** Note the similarity in morphology; both cells have a large nucleus and a thin rim of undifferentiated cytoplasm. Scale bar = 0.5 μm (Courtesy of Dr A.F. Rowley, from *Endeavour (New Series)* **13**;72–77, with permission. © Maxwell Pergamon Macmillan plc, 1989.)

Cells and tissues of invertebrate immune systems

cells/tissues	role(s) in immunity/physiology
mucus, cuticle, shells, tests and/or gut barrier	physicochemical barriers to invasion
five groups of free and sessile white blood cells	mediate cellular and many of the humoral defence reactions
I progenitor cells	may act as stem cells for other cell types
II phagocytic cells	phagocytosis, encapsulation, clotting, wound healing and killing
III haemostatic cells	plasma gelation and clotting by cell aggregation; non-self recognition, lysozyme and agglutinin production
IV nutritive cells	encapsulation reactions and wound healing? nutritive role?
V pigmented cells	role in defence (if any) unknown; respiratory function
fixed cells such as pericardial cells, nephrocytes or pore cells etc.	pinocytose colloids and small particulates; synthesize lysozyme (pericardial cells) and other antimicrobial factors?
haemopoietic organs – well organized in some invertebrates	haemopoiesis and phagocytosis; synthesize antimicrobial factors in a few animals
fat body (insects), mid gut and sinus lining cells (molluscs, crustaceans)	synthesize immune proteins and agglutinins (fat body), phagocytosis (mid-gut cells), clearance of foreign particles (sinus lining cells)

Fig. 15.4 Invertebrate immune systems. (Adapted from Ratcliffe NA. *Immunol Lett* 1985:**10**;253–70; Elsevier Science Publications, with permission.)

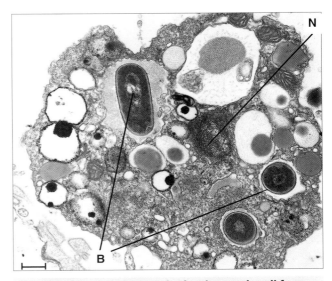

Fig. 15.6 **Electron micrograph of a phagocytic cell from the tunicate, *Ciona intestinalis*.** Note the ingestion of three bacteria (B) by this cell. Nucleus (N). Scale bar = 0.5 μm. (Courtesy of Dr A.F. Rowley.)

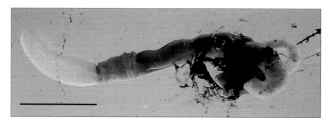

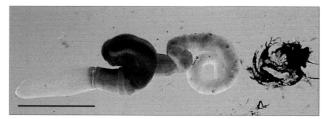

Fig. 15.7 Foreign particle entrapment and removal by the mucus layer surrounding the acorn worm, _Saccoglossus ruber_. A specimen was placed in a suspension of carbon in sea water for 2–3 minutes, then transferred to clean sea water. After 12 minutes large amounts of carbon were still enmeshed in the mucus layer surrounding the animal (**left**). By 15 minutes the carbon was completely removed, wrapped in a ball of mucus (**right**). Trapped microorganisms are probably dealt with in a similar fashion. Acorn worms are in a group of 'higher invertebrates' related to the tunicates. Scale bar = 5 mm. (Courtesy of Dr D.A. Millar.)

- Blood clotting/coagulation and wound healing.
- Phagocytosis.
- Encapsulation responses.
- Natural and inducible antimicrobial factors.

These reactions depend on non-self recognition and receptor molecules present in the blood and on the surfaces of the blood cells.

Activation of prophenoloxidase to phenoloxidase in arthropods

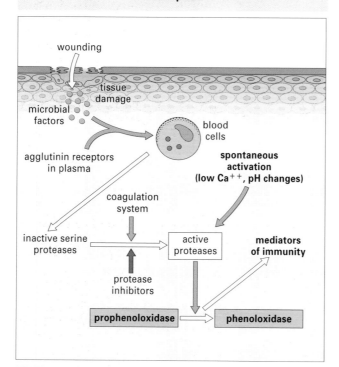

Fig. 15.8 Possible scheme for activation of prophenoloxidase (PpO) to phenoloxidase (PO) in arthropods. Activation is stimulated at the wound site by tissue damage, microorganisms and changes in Ca^{2+} and pH, which may lead to plasma coagulation and the generation of factors mediating later events in immunity. (Based largely on data from Drs K. Söderhäll, M. Ashida and N.A. Ratcliffe.)

Wounds are rapidly closed by coagulation of body fluids induced both by haemostatic cells and plasma components

Invertebrates rapidly seal wounds caused by injury or parasitic invasion, and so prevent the fatal loss of body fluids. The wound is closed by the extrusion of the fat body or gut, by muscular contraction, by coagulation of body fluids, by blood cell aggregation and clotting, and/or by melanin deposition. Leucocyte migration to the wound is probably stimulated by cytokine-like factors (see below).

Plasma gelation or coagulation at wound sites occurs mainly in arthropods, although it has also been reported in annelids and echinoderms. Coagulation involves haemostatic cells, which aggregate at the injury and discharge their contents, causing the plasma to gelate and strengthen the cell clot. There is also a contribution from plasma components in many species. The coagulation process, as in mammals, involves a complex enzyme cascade which is activated at the wound site by damaged tissue, microbial components, and changes in Ca^{2+} or pH. It has been likened to the alternative pathway in complement activation. The system is so sensitive that in horseshoe crabs it is elicited by as little as 4 ng/ml of _Escherichia coli_ endotoxin. The coagulation process is extremely important, as it forms a highly sensitive method of recognizing foreign invaders through the degranulation of haemostatic cells. Gelation may involve the enzyme prophenoloxidase (PpO) which, upon conversion to phenoloxidase (PO) by a cascade of serine proteases, may generate factors mediating later events in immunity (_Fig. 15.8_). The PpO cascade has recently been shown to be present in other invertebrates, such as annelids and tunicates.

Phagocytic cells ingest microbial invaders whilst larger invaders are enclosed in multicellular capsules

Phagocytic cells occur throughout the invertebrates and, with natural humoral factors (see below), form the first line of defence against microorganisms (see _Fig. 15.6_). Chemotaxis, attachment, ingestion and killing phases have all been described, and are similar to those seen in vertebrates. However, recognition of the target is not mediated by Fc receptors, and C3b-like receptors have only been reported on the phagocyte surface in one species. Phagocytosis can occur, as in vertebrates, without opsonic factors. However, it is enhanced in molluscs, arthropods and tunicates by plasma lectins and by components of the prophenoloxidase cascade.

If invading pathogens are too large or too numerous then they are enclosed in multicellular aggregates, termed nodules or capsules, resembling mammalian granulomas (*Fig. 15.9*). Sequestered organisms are thought to be killed by lysosomal enzymes and lysozyme present in leucocytes, and by peroxidase and reactive oxygen species (recorded in a few annelids, molluscs and arthropods).

Both phagocytosis and encapsulation are dependent on cell cooperation between the haemostatic and phagocytic cells (see below).

The body fluids of invertebrates contain a range of naturally occurring and inducible humoral defence factors

Naturally occurring defence factors – Invertebrates probably lack immunoglobulins but their body fluids contain a range of humoral defence factors. These include agglutinins, lysozyme and other lysins, non-lysozyme bactericidins, lysosomal enzymes and immobilization factors. There is also some evidence for the presence of components of the complement system. For example, sea urchin phagocytes may bear C3b-like receptors, and a humoral lytic system similar to complement has been reported. Furthermore, blood from a caterpillar has been found to react with bound cobra venom factor (cobra C3b) to produce a C3-convertase activity that cleaves bovine C3, generating a molecule similar to C3b. The prophenoloxidase cascade of arthropods has also been compared with the alternative pathway of the complement system, since both are activated directly by microbial components and involve a series of sequentially activated proteases (*Fig. 15.8*). Confirmation that the forerunners of the alternative complement pathways arose in invertebrates awaits detailed molecular analysis.

Inducible humoral defence factors – Although it is known that agglutinin and haemolysin levels can sometimes be enhanced in invertebrates, inducible antimicrobial factors from insects are the only molecules to have been studied in great detail. There is now evidence for their presence in a few other invertebrates but their more widespread detection and characterization may await the correct immunogens and/or immunization schedule. In insects such as moths, flies and bees, up to 15 antibacterial proteins can be induced within a few hours of injection of an antigen (*Fig. 15.10*). Many of these peptides have been purified and sequenced; they have a broad spectrum activity which only lasts a few days, and are therefore very different from vertebrate immunoglobulins. Recently, similar antibacterial proteins have been found in certain vertebrates (see p 15.14) and these molecules probably represen ancient, but still important, immune factors. One such factor, a cecropin called P4 or haemolin (*Fig. 15.10*), has homology (38%) with certain immunoglobulin domains. It could represent a primitive form of immunoglobulin, but may have evolved independently in invertebrates. In the American cockroach, a different sort of inducible protein has been detected which is much more like vertebrate immunoglobulin. It has a molecular mass of 700 kDa, is highly specific and lasts weeks rather than days. Again, detailed comparison with vertebrate immunoglobulin awaits molecular characterization.

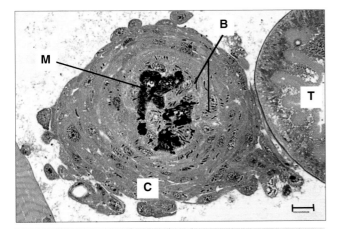

Fig. 15.9 Encapsulation of bacteria by the blood cells of a caterpillar. Final-stage larvae of the butterfly *Pieris brassicae* were injected with bacteria (heat-killed *Bacillus cereus*). After 24 hours, the capsules that had formed around the bacteria were excised and sectioned. Note the dark pigmented core of melanin (M), the multilayered sheath of blood cells (C), rod-shaped bacteria (B), and the attachment of the capsule to the Malpighian tubule (T). Scale bar = 10 μm.

Inducible immune proteins of *Hyalophora cecropia*

immune protein	molecular mass	function and properties
P4 (haemolin)	48 000	main immune protein, non-self recognition?
P5 attacins A–F	21–23 000	narrow spectrum antibacterial activity against some Gram-negative bacteria
P7 (lysozyme)	15 000	kills some Gram-positive bacteria
cecropins A–F (6 proteins)	~ 4 000	some have broad spectrum antibacterial activity against both Gram-positive and Gram-negative bacteria

Fig. 15.10 Inducible immune proteins of the moth, *Hyalophora cecropia*, isolated from the blood 10 hours after immunization with bacteria (*Enterobacter cloacae*). (Based on the work of H Boman, Hultmark and colleagues.)

Non-self recognition and cell–cell cooperation are mediated by various factors

Invertebrates can discriminate, often quite specifically, between various foreign substances. Factors present in invertebrate body fluids acting as recognition molecules include agglutinins, components of the prophenoloxidase cascade and an insect cecropin called haemolin.

Purified agglutinins – From the blood of molluscs, insects and tunicates, these enhance the recognition of test particles *in vitro*, as well as their clearance from the circulation *in vivo*. Such agglutinins also occur on the surface of blood cells to form bridging molecules between the leucocyte and the foreign particle, as in the mammalian immune system.

The prophenoloxidase (PpO) system – In arthropods, this is also a likely source of recognition factors. During conversion of PpO to phenoloxidase (PO) (see *Fig. 15.8*) recognition factors are released from haemostatic cells which enhance phagocytosis and encapsulation. An agglutinin, purified from cockroach blood and termed BDL1, has recently been shown to activate the PpO cascade, so that

a unifying concept is now available for these two recognition systems. BDL1 also has many structural and functional similarities to the mannose-binding proteins (MBPs) of vertebrates. (The MBPs are lectins; they are essential components of vertebrate non-specific immunity because they can bind to the surface of invading microorganisms, and activate complement-mediated attack.) Like MBPs, BDL1 activates complement and has collagenous and carbohydrate-recognition domains.

Haemolin – In addition to agglutinins and PpO, the blood of insects also contains an immune protein called haemolin. It has four immunoglobulin-like domains that bind to bacterial surfaces, and may be involved in the recognition of non-self molecules.

The process of non-self recognition and subsequent phagocytosis involves cell–cell cooperation between haemostatic cells and phagocytic cells (*Fig. 15.11*). Thus, although invertebrates lack interacting antigen-presenting cells and lymphocyte subpopulations, the various immunocytes cooperate during cell-mediated immunity.

Two hypothetical models for cell–cell cooperation in arthropod immunity

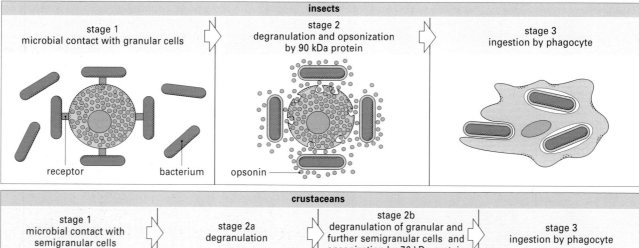

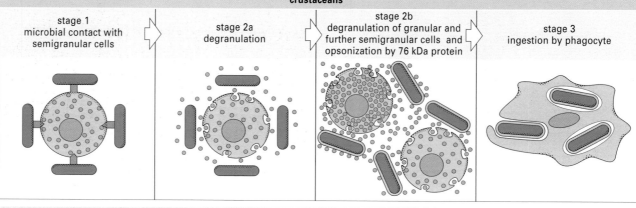

Fig. 15.11 Schemes derived from experiments which observed the reactions of purified blood cell populations to test particles. In insects, non-self recognition (stages 1 and 2) is carried out by the granular (haemostatic) cells, and ingestion (stage 3) by the phagocytes. The crustacean model has an extra amplification step at stage 2b, in which semigranular and granular cells interact to enhance the response. The 90 kDa and 76 kDa proteins detected in insects and crustaceans, respectively, are opsonic (recognition) molecules generated by activation of the prophenoloxidase cascade. (Adapted from Ratcliffe NA. In: Warr GW, Cohen N, eds. *Phylogenesis of Immune Functions*. Oxford: CRC Press, 1991:62. Data on crustaceans from the work of Professor K. Söderhäll and associates.)

The cellular and humoral defence reactions of vector species also act as determinants of infection by parasites

Evidence is accumulating to suggest that the immune capability of certain invertebrate disease vectors (e.g. mosquitoes, tsetse flies, sandflies, blackflies, kissing bugs and pulmonate snails) is an important determinant of their ability to transmit disease (malaria, sleeping sickness, tropical sores, river blindness, Chagas' disease and blood flukes). For example, in mosquitoes and pulmonate snails encapsulation responses have been reported to effectively sequester and possibly kill the enclosed parasites. In addition, recent research has identified gut-associated agglutinins in mosquitoes, tsetse flies, sandflies and kissing bugs as possibly playing major roles in growth and survival of invading protozoan parasites taken in with a blood meal. In some *Glossina* tsetse flies, for example, the inhibition of the midgut agglutinin with D-glucosamine significantly increases midgut infection rates with *Trypanosoma brucei rhodesiense*. Prophenoloxidase may also be important; female *Glossina morsitans morsitans* tsetse flies show low levels of mature salivary gland infections with *T.b. rhodesiense* compared with male flies, and have much higher levels of PpO than the male flies. The inducible antibacterial peptides present in the blood of *Simulium* blackflies have also been shown to kill immature stages of nematode worm parasites. Much has yet to be learned in this exciting new research field, including the methods adopted by the parasites to evade the vectors' immune defences.

Host defences are regulated by a network of cytokines, some of which resemble vertebrate interleukins

Cytokine-like molecules found in invertebrates may regulate the host defences by a network resembling that seen in vertebrates. The fact that molecules related to cytokines are present in protozoans suggests they are to be found throughout the animal kingdom. For example, a protozoan pheromone, Er-1, has structural and functional similarities to interleukin-2 (IL-2). In addition, molecules with activities resembling those of IL-1α, IL-1β and tumour necrosis factor (TNF) have recently been isolated and characterized from annelids, echinoderms and tunicates. IL-1α and IL-1β were detected using a vertebrate assay system (the murine thymocyte proliferation assay) and were shown to be inhibited by polyclonal antisera to vertebrate IL-1. Invertebrate IL-1 stimulates the 'blood' cells of these primitive animals to aggregate, phagocytose and proliferate. TNF-like activity from invertebrates has been detected with the L929 cytotoxicity assay, normally used for vertebrate TNF.

A range of other molecules with cytokine-like activity has been reported from invertebrates. In insects, these include a plasmatocyte (leucocyte-type) depletion factor, a leucocyte activator (termed haemokinin), and various stimulants for encapsulation and phagocytosis. A factor produced by the leucocytes of echinoderms (the sea-star factor) is mitogenic for mammalian lymphocytes and also induces the accumulation of starfish white blood cells. Finally, an inflammatory cytokine from tunicates has been shown to affect antibody production, phagocytosis and

cell-mediated cytotoxicity in vertebrates, and leucocyte phagocytic activity in prawns. Additional molecular characterization of these molecules is awaited.

Many invertebrates can reject allogeneic and xenogeneic grafts

Vertebrate immunity is characterized by a high degree of specificity and enhanced reactivity (memory, or anamnesis) following a second exposure to antigen. These processes are governed by the lymphocytes and the major histocompatibility complex (MHC). To determine levels of specificity and memory in invertebrates, transplantation, implantation and cytotoxicity studies have been undertaken. Such transplantation studies are difficult to perform in invertebrates, due to their tough exoskeletons or delicate outer layers. It can also be difficult to judge whether rejection has occurred. Despite these difficulties, it is now known that most invertebrates destroy xenografts, and allogeneic recognition has been observed in the sponges, coelenterates, annelids, insects, echinoderms and tunicates (*Figs 15.1, 15.12 and 15.13*). The apparent lack of allogeneic recognition in the molluscs probably reflects the technical problems in grafting these animals. Not all the groups exhibiting allograft rejection produce reactions characterized by specificity and memory; the reactions are usually strictly limited and short term (see *Fig. 15.1*). The great variability in results of grafting may stem from the temperature-dependence of the rejection process and the lack of appreciation of this by some workers.

It is not surprising that allogeneic recognition occurs in colonial invertebrates such as the sponges, coelenterates and tunicates, as the integrity of the colony is constantly threatened by overgrowth from adjacent colonies (*Fig.*

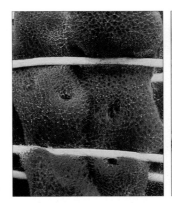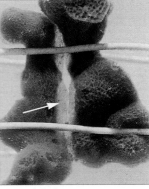

Fig. 15.12 Demonstration of cell-mediated immunity in sponges: allogeneic incompatibility and isogeneic compatibility. Two intact fingers of sponge (*Callyspongia* spp) from the same colony and two from different colonies are parabiosed (their circulations are fused) by being held together with vinyl-covered wire. **Left:** The interfacial fusion between isogeneic parabionts (intracolony) persists indefinitely. × 0.5. **Right:** Incompatibility between allogeneic parabionts (intercolony) results in a cytotoxic interaction and necrosis (arrow) after 7–9 days (24–27°C). × 0.25. (Courtesy of Dr W.H. Hildemann.)

15.2). Work with the larvae of tunicate colonies has shown that both allorecognition and fertilization are controlled by a single gene locus with multiple alleles. Thus, there are similarities between this tunicate system and the mammalian histocompatibility genes.

Once again, note that the limited specificity and memory of invertebrate allorecognition and xenorecognition does not seem to hamper their immune system or success. After all, invertebrates rapidly respond to pathogens and parasites and are hugely abundant.

The ancestors of MHC and molecules with immunoglobulin-like domains occur in invertebrates

The presence of allogeneic recognition in many invertebrates indicates that the ancestors of the major histocompatibility complex (MHC) could be present in these animals. Since invertebrates do not possess immunoglobulins, it is possible that the MHC may be ancestral to and separate from the immunoglobulin system of vertebrates. On this argument, primitive vertebrates retained MHC and evolved the immunoglobulin system separately, to provide a more precise recognition potential in the form of circulating antibodies and cell surface receptors. With further vertebrate evolution, the MHC and immunoglobulin systems would have become more closely integrated to provide the high level of control necessary for interacting antigen-presenting cells (APCs) and lymphocytes. The above proposal is, however, hypothetical; there is no evidence, structural or functional, that invertebrate cells express either MHC glycoproteins or dimeric cell receptors for alloantigens. In addition, invertebrates may lack mixed leucocyte reactivity (see *Fig. 15.1*) which is a functional marker of the MHC in vertebrates. This lack of supporting data has led to some counter-hypotheses; some argue that the MHC evolved in vertebrates from heat shock proteins (see later).

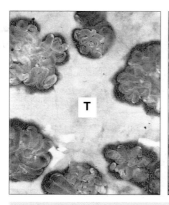
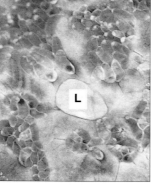

Fig. 15.13 Transplantation immunity in echinoderms: allograft rejection in starfish (*Dermasterias*). Left: In spite of the technical difficulties involved, this autograft (T) remains in perfect condition 300 days after transplantation. **Right:** An allograft (L) rejected at 287 days (14–16°C) is blanched and contracted. Rejection involves lymphocyte–like cells and larger phagocytic cells. × 4. (Courtesy of Dr W.H. Hildemann.)

The discovery of β_2-microglobulin-like molecules in earthworms, crustaceans and insects, however, does support the idea that MHC precursors may have arisen in the invertebrates. Although β_2-microglobulin in vertebrates is encoded by a gene not linked to the MHC, it associates with class I MHC molecules and belongs to the immunoglobulin supergene family. Thus MHC molecules may be the descendants of a single domain molecule like β_2-microglobulin that has been expanded by gene rearrangement, gene duplication and natural selection.

Finally, there is a group of molecules including Thy-1 (present in squid brain), and amalgam, fasciclin II, neuroglian and haemolin (all from insects), which also belong to the immunoglobulin superfamily; it has been suggested that these evolved to mediate interactions between cells, and could potentially produce an immune system recognizing 'non-self'. Such a step may have already been made in insects with haemolin (see above).

■ VERTEBRATE IMMUNITY

Compared with the immense variety of forms seen within the invertebrate phyla, vertebrates possess a fairly uniform basic plan of organization and are members of just one phylum – the Chordata. Although there is considerable evolutionary divergence within vertebrate stock, which includes jawless fish, cartilaginous and bony jawed fish, amphibians, reptiles, birds and mammals, the basic cellular and molecular components of anticipatory immunity are strikingly conserved throughout extant gnathostome (jawed) species. However, increased specialization of lymphoid tissues and lymphocyte functions, together with greater variety of immunoglobulin classes, appear to be associated with more complex grades of organization. The most complex structural and functional immune systems are seen in mammals.

T Cells and evolution of the MHC

Mammalian T-cytotoxic (Tc) and T-helper (TH) lymphocyte subsets, possessing $\alpha\beta$ T-cell receptors (TCRs), recognize most foreign antigens only when presented in suitable form by self-encoded, polymorphic MHC molecules. The phylogeny of certain T-cell populations (e.g. cytotoxic T lymphocytes [CTLs] and those involved in mixed leucocyte reactivity [MLR]) and the evolution of MHC are therefore dealt with together (*Fig. 15.14*).

Jawed vertebrates from cartilaginous fish upwards have all been shown to possess an MHC, by functional criteria and/or through molecular and genetic characterization. (Functional criteria require that MLR and acute allograft rejection are shown to be controlled by a single polymorphic genetic region, and that phenomena such as T–B cell collaboration, the generation of antigen-specific cytotoxic responses (e.g. to allogeneic cells) and thymic education of T-lineage cells are all under MHC control.)

The MHC has been well characterized in the ectothermic vertebrate Xenopus

Recent evidence indicates that MHC genes evolved in

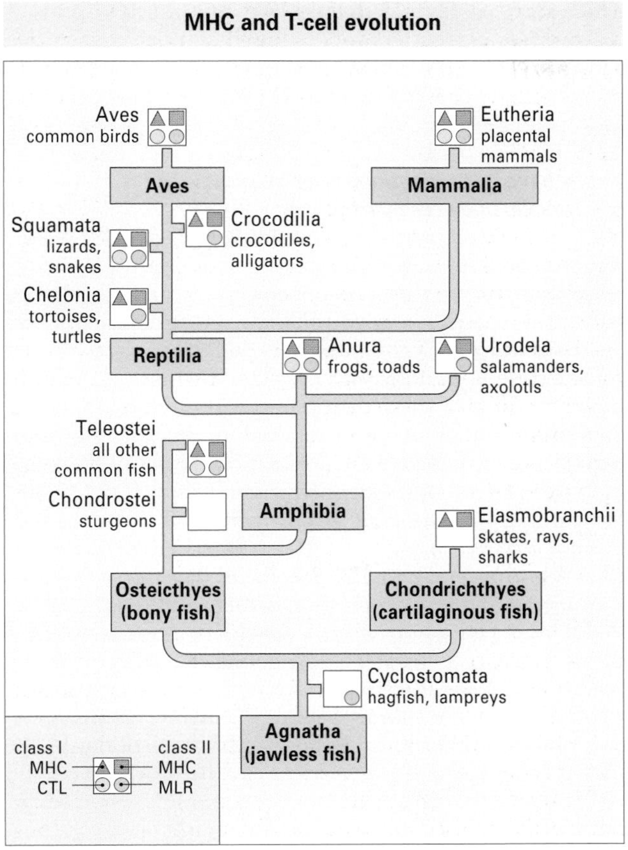

MHC and T-cell evolution

Fig. 15.14 This vertebrate phylogenetic tree illustrates aspects of MHC and T-cell evolution. Evidence for two functional indications of an MHC (cytotoxic T lymphocytes, CTL, and mixed leucocyte reaction, MLR) is shown, together with current biochemical and molecular evidence for the expression of class I and II MHC proteins and genes. A blank box indicates insufficient evidence for that characteristic.

cartilaginous fish whose ancestors diverged from other vertebrates > 400 million years ago. However, the best studied ectothermic (cold-blooded) vertebrate with respect to MHC genes and proteins is the clawed frog, *Xenopus*. Its MHC (the XLA) is compared with the avian MHC (B locus) and murine MHC (H–2) in *Figure 15.15*.

Classical MHC (Ia) in Xenopus – *Xenopus* class Ia proteins are polymorphic, with approximately 20 alleles. These proteins are expressed on the surfaces of all adult cells, highest expression being on haemopoietic cells. The class Iα-chains of *Xenopus* are 40–44 kDa, with three domains, and are non-covalently bound to β_2-microglobulin. *Xenopus* class I MHC proteins are unusual in that they are encoded by just one gene locus (contrast 3 in humans and 2 in mice).

Non-classical MHC (Ib) in Xenopus – The first *Xenopus* class I gene to be identified was one of a large family of mono-morphic, non-classical (class I) MHC-like molecules. It occurs on a different chromosome from the 'classical' (MHC Ia) genes. This class Ib gene apparently encodes a molecule with homologies to protein-binding regions of the heat shock protein 70 (Hsp 70) family. It has recently been suggested that the peptide-binding region of class I MHC molecules evolved from pre-existing Hsps. (Hsps are evolutionarily conserved molecules found in all organisms, which act as 'chaperones' and are involved in protein folding and intracellular transport.) Non-classical MHC-like proteins have been found associated with the epithelial surfaces of every vertebrate studied, and may have varying functions; some are thought to recognize the Hsps of pathogens or infected/stressed self cells, and subsequently present these conserved peptides to T cells with restricted TCR repertoires.

MHC class II in Xenopus – *Xenopus* class II MHC molecules are polymorphic (about 30 alleles) and are expressed constitutively on only a limited range of adult

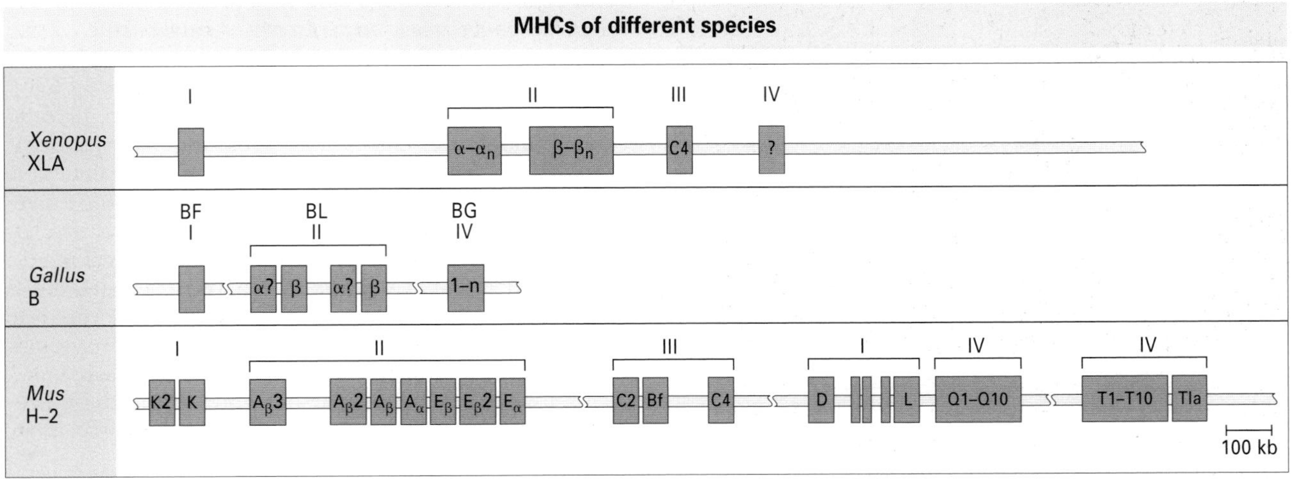

MHCs of different species

Fig. 15.15 The MHC can be identified in all jawed vertebrates. Speculative organization of MHC loci is here shown for the clawed frog (*Xenopus*) and the chicken (*Gallus*). The architecture of the mouse (*Mus*) H–2 complex is well known. Distances for *Xenopus* and *Gallus* are arbitrary. (Courtesy of Dr L. Du Pasquier.)

cells, including thymocytes, B and T cells, and various APCs such as putative Langerhans-like cells of the skin epidermis (see *Fig. 15.16*). Class II proteins are composed of MHC-encoded α and β chains, both of which are 30–35 kDa transmembrane glycoproteins. The genes for *Xenopus* MHC class II β chains encode polypeptides with nearly 50% homology to mammalian class II β chains. An invariant chain is transiently associated with class II during biosynthesis. *Xenopus* has three MHC class II β gene loci (as in humans).

MHC expression in Xenopus *varies with each stage of the life cycle*

One particularly interesting feature of MHC expression in *Xenopus* is that classical class I MHC molecules are not expressed on any cell surface prior to metamorphosis. In contrast, class II molecules appear early in the tadpole on B cells and on several epithelial cells that are in direct contact with the external environment. This shows that classical class I expression is not essential for early development or for functioning of the larval immune system. However, there remains the possibility that non-classical class I proteins play a role in larval immunity. Class II-restricted cellular immunity may well play a crucial role during this ontogenetic period. The widespread distribution of class II MHC in tadpoles compared with adults suggests that this pattern might represent the way in which antigen was presented in a more primitive immune system.

MHC in other vertebrates

MHC class I and II proteins and polymorphic class II genes have recently been identified in cartilaginous fish. Amongst teleosts, genes have been characterized for MHC class I and β$_2$-microglobulin in rainbow trout, and for MHC class II in carp.

Axolotls, which display relatively poor T-cell reactivity to alloantigens, possess α and β chains of MHC class II molecules, which are not very polymorphic. These amphibians also express MHC-encoded erythrocyte antigens,

which show similarities to class Ia chains (44 kDa) and to polymorphic class IV molecules found on nucleated chicken erythrocytes. These may also exist in *Xenopus*. Class Iα chains and heterodimeric class II molecules also occur in various reptiles.

T cells have been identified phenotypically and functionally in diverse vertebrates

αβ and γδ TCRs, together with CD3, CD4 and CD8 co-receptor molecules, have been identified in birds. Some of these receptors, or their component chains, are now beginning to be identified in amphibians. For example, genes from Mexican axolotl thymocytes and splenocytes reveal considerable homology with avian and mammalian TCR β chains. A 55 kDa surface protein is expressed on *Xenopus* thymocytes and on thymus lymphoid tumour cell lines, and sequencing indicates a TCR-δ-like molecule. Anti-*Xenopus* monoclonal antibodies identifying candidate CD5 (71–88 kDa, and expressed on all T cells) and CD8 (35 kDa, and expressed on cytotoxic T cells) are now available. Although gene segments encoding TCR β chains have recently been identified in rainbow trout, monoclonal antibodies specific to fish T cells have not yet been produced. There is no conclusive evidence at present for functional T cells in cartilaginous fish, although lack of T cells would seem surprising in view of the evidence for a polymorphic MHC by this stage of evolution. The cellular and molecular basis of the MLR shown by hagfish leucocytes awaits further clarification.

Temperature plays a crucial role in immune responses in ectotherms. In catfish, low temperatures inhibit T-cell (but not B-cell) proliferation. These effects are due to the lower level in fish T cells of certain saturated fatty acids (e.g. oleic acid) which can fluidify membranes. Diets high in appropriate fatty acids may therefore allow fish to adapt better to low temperatures. Oleic acid can also reverse the suppression of *in vitro* responses of mammalian T cells that occurs at low temperatures, although the precise temperature-sensitive signalling events have not yet been elucidated.

B cells and immunoglobulin evolution

Immunoglobulin heavy and light chains have been characterized in diverse vertebrates

Proteins from hagfish initially described as antibodies have now been identified as complement proteins C3–C5. Indeed, no immunoglobulin superfamily molecules have yet been found in the agnathan (jawless) hagfish and lamprey.

All jawed vertebrates make antibodies to a wide range of antigens. However, ectotherm antibodies are of relatively low affinity and display poor immunological memory compared with antibodies from endothermic (warm-blooded) vertebrates. The structure of antibodies is evolutionarily conserved, with multi-domain, heavy and light immunoglobulin polypeptide chains (see Chapter 4). These immunoglobulins may be expressed on the B cell surface as antigen receptor or secreted into the circulation by activated B cells.

Polymeric IgM is universally found in jawed vertebrates (*Fig. 15.17*) and is the major serum antibody of fish. Each heavy μ chain comprises four constant domains and one variable domain; disulphide bonds link heavy and light

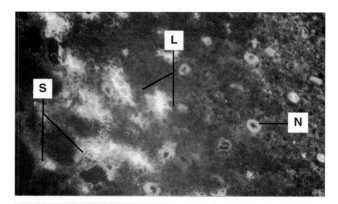

Fig. 15.16 Immunofluorescence showing class II MHC-positive dendritic cells in *Xenopus*. 'Langerhans-like' cells (L) frequent the basal epidermal layer of the skin. Also visible are class II⁺ neck cells of the skin gland opening through the epidermis (N), and skin glands below the epidermis (S). × 100.

chains. The μ-chain family displays considerable phylogenetic diversity; for example, only 24% amino acid sequence homology exists between catfish and mouse μ chains.

Non-μ low molecular weight antibodies are found in some cartilaginous fish, such as skates, rays and sharks (see *Fig. 15.17*), although the evolutionary relationship of IgR to other H-chain isotypes is uncertain. Amphibians, reptiles and birds possess a heavy chain isotype called IgY, with four constant domains, believed to be the precursor of mammalian IgG and IgE, with which IgY shares common structural and functional properties. The IgY of axolotls may also be a secretory immunoglobulin, as in the gut this immunoglobulin isotype becomes associated with 'secretory-component-like' molecules. It is interesting that fish lack IgE, yet teleosts display Type I hypersensitivity reactions which may reflect tissue-bound homocytotropic antibody. *Xenopus* IgX which, unlike IgY, is thymus-independent, is possibly the equivalent of mammalian secretory IgA, since this isotype is mainly found in the gut. IgA first appears in advanced birds.

Distribution of immunoglobulins in vertebrates

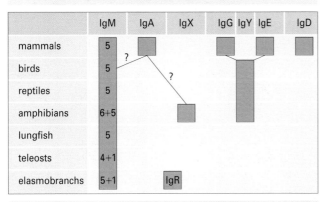

	IgM	IgA	IgX	IgG	IgY	IgE	IgD
mammals	5						
birds	5						
reptiles	5						
amphibians	6+5						
lungfish	5						
teleosts	4+1						
elasmobranchs	5+1		IgR				

Fig. 15.17 Distribution and possible relationships of immunoglobulins in the vertebrates. Polymeric IgM is found in all jawed vertebrates, but with varying numbers of basic units (2H + 2L chains), as shown. Monomeric IgM is also found in blood of cartilaginous (elasmobranch) and teleost fish. Non-μ heavy chain isotypes are found in diverse groups, but the roles of many remain uncertain. (Courtesy of Dr G.W. Warr.)

Light chain diversity also occurs in many ectotherms. Two antigenically-distinct types of light chains, one of which is κ-like, have been demonstrated in *Xenopus*, and two exist in catfish, trout and alligators. Both κ- and λ-like light chains are known to exist in sharks, indicating that divergence of the ancestral light chain into isotypes occurred prior to the emergence of cartilaginous fish.

Immunoglobulin genes in lower vertebrates are organized in one of four ways

Analysis of the immunoglobulin gene loci in ectotherms using recombinant DNA technology has advanced rapidly in recent years, revealing four patterns of organization.

Amphibians, teleosts and holostean fish – These have a mammalian type ('translocon') form of IgH organization. For example, in *Xenopus* there are approximately 80–100 VH, 15D and 9JH segments (*Fig. 15.18*). Both framework and complementarity-determining regions are found. Each *Xenopus* heavy chain constant region (IgM, IgX, IgY) is coded for by four CH exons. Two separate chromosomes, each with VL, JL and CL segments code for *Xenopus* light chains. Teleost immunoglobulin light chain genes show the 'multicluster' organization typifying shark immunoglobulin genes (see below).

Multiple rearrangements of *Xenopus* immunoglobulin genes, similar to those occurring in mammals, proceed during B-cell development and allelic exclusion exists, resulting in monospecific B lymphocytes. Recombinase-activating genes (involved in immunoglobulin gene rearrangements) are found in *Xenopus*, but antibody (V region) diversity is quite low, there being only some 5×10^5 different antibody molecules in adults. The restricted affinity maturation seen following B-cell activation in *Xenopus* (and in other ectotherms) apparently does not relate to absence of somatic mutations of immunoglobulin genes. Rather it is believed to relate to lack of efficient selection of mutants due to absence of appropriate germinal centres in ectotherm lymphoid organs. Lymph nodes with germinal centres are only found in birds/mammals. Although *Xenopus* larvae possess all three Ig isotypes found in adults, larval and adult antibody repertoires are different. The adult repertoire is effected by gene rearrangments occurring in a new wave of B-cell development after metamorphosis. The third hypervariable region in the adult is diversified by random addition of N residues, but this does not occur in larvae.

Fig. 15.18 The IgH locus in *Xenopus* is of similar architecture to that seen in teleost fish and resembles that in mammals. Recombination signal sequences adjoin all the gene segments. D segments rearrange first to JH; later, VH genes arrange to D–J. The rearranged V–D–J genes are finally joined to a constant region gene, producing IgM, IgX or IgY. (Based on data from Dr L. Du Pasquier.)

Xenopus IgH locus

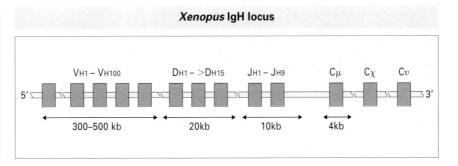

The generation of antibody diversity in birds – This involves a second pattern of immunoglobulin gene organization and takes place in a unique site, the cloacal bursa of Fabricius (*Fig. 15.19*). The chicken Ig light chain locus has a single V gene which is initially rearranged and joined to a single J–C unit (*Fig. 15.20*). Multiple D region genes also exist in the chicken IgH locus. Rearrangement takes place only for a limited period during early development when stem cells colonize the bursa, whereas in mice and humans immunoglobulin gene rearrangements occur in the B-cell precursors throughout life. Subsequently, in the chicken, stretches of nucleotide sequences from pseudogenes (adjacent to the single V gene), replace 10–120 base-pair segments within the rearranged immunoglobulin gene sequences. This high frequency gene conversion mechanism (which is also seen in rabbits) operates throughout the time B cells proliferate in the bursa.

A third pattern of Ig gene loci is seen in cartilaginous fish – Here both heavy (μ) and light (λ- and κ-like) immunoglobulin chains are coded for by many small discrete gene clusters (cassettes) (*Fig. 15.21*), within which V, (D), J and C genes are all found. Each immunoglobulin gene cluster differs in DNA sequence from other clusters. These sequences are in germline configuration. Shark antibodies apparently possess a diverse array (many millions) of binding specificities, but lack inter-individual immunoglobulin variation, since diversity is encoded in the germline, rather than by somatic mechanisms. The use of somatic gene rearrangements to accomplish immunoglobulin diversity (as in teleosts, amphibians, birds and mammals) is therefore not universal to vertebrates. These cartilaginous fish have a high level of natural antibodies to a diverse set of antigens, similar to the polyspecific (frequently auto-reactive) IgM antibodies of mammals, which are secreted by CD5+ B cells early in ontogeny. Whether the cluster arrangement of immunoglobulin gene subunits seen in sharks can achieve B-cell clonal restriction is not certain, although increase in specific antibodies without a general increase in serum Ig is found in sharks, implying that clonal selection is operating.

A new immunoglobulin superfamily molecule, possibly the evolutionary forerunner of immunoglobulin and TCR, has very recently been identified in the nurse shark. The molecule has one variable and five constant domains and is found as a dimer in the serum; it is coded for by a gene locus that undergoes rearrangements and somatic diversification.

Preliminary studies reveal that a novel IgH locus (clusters of V–D genes distributed along the chromosome) may be present in coelocanths, the evolutionary 'relics' recently found to be alive in the Indian Ocean.

The bursa of Fabricius

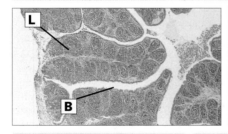
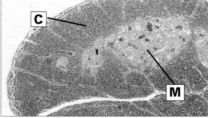
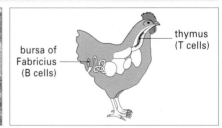

Fig. 15.19 The two central organs in the avian immune system are the thymus (**centre**) and the bursa of Fabricius (**left**). Lymphocytes developing in the thymus are termed T cells and those in the bursa, B cells. Lymphoid follicles (L) and bursal lumen (B) are marked, as are the cortex (C) and medulla (M) of the thymus. H&E stain, × 20.

Genetic basis of antibody diversity in chickens

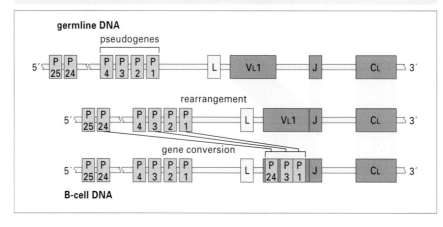

Fig. 15.20 The chicken germline immunoglobulin light chain locus has less than 30 kb of DNA. A single functional V gene (VL) lies 2 kb upstream from a single J–C unit, with an adjacent cluster of 25 pseudogenes (P) in a 19 kb region. Rearrangement occurs briefly during early B-cell development. Antibody diversity is achieved by gene conversion between P and the rearranged sequence. The arrangement shown (P1, P3 and P24) is illustrative; converted segments do not necessarily lie in order in the V gene segment.

Shark immunoglobulin VH loci

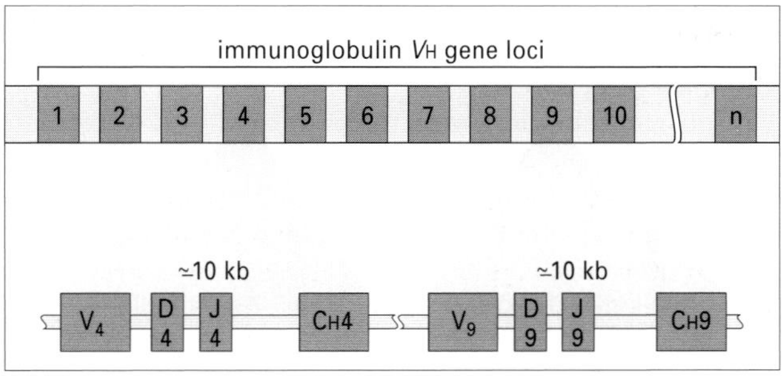

Fig. 15.21 In the shark there is a series of about 200 heavy chain gene clusters, each with a single V, D, J, and C gene segment. The fourth and ninth clusters are shown expanded. V_H, D_H and J_H segments are closely linked and occur within approximately 1.3 kb. Together with the C_H segment, they occupy only about 10–15 kb. The arrangements of genes within a cluster appears to be encoded in the germ line, rather than by somatic rearrangement mechanisms, which may account for the lack of inter-individual variation associated with the immune response of this species. (Based on data of Dr J.J. Marchalonis and Dr G.W. Litman.)

Cells of the non-adaptive immune system
Natural killer (NK) cells occur in most vertebrates

Mammalian NK cells are a large granular lymphocyte population distinct from T and B cells which, unlike Tc cells, can spontaneously lyse transformed cell lines that do not express MHC antigens. NK-like lymphoid cells have been demonstrated in several lower vertebrate groups including birds, reptiles, amphibians and teleost fish. Indeed, non-specific cytotoxic cells have recently been demonstrated in protochordates; these can kill mammalian tumour cell lines. In both cartilaginous and bony fish, macrophages have been shown to display spontaneous cytotoxicity, and antibody-dependent cellular cytotoxic (ADCC) reactions are found in sharks.

Monoclonal antibodies raised against catfish NK-like cells are able to modulate killing of human transformed lines by both fish and human NK cells, suggesting an evolutionary conservation of antigen-receptor molecules involved. Candidate NK cells, which mediate MHC-unrestricted cytotoxicity, have been identified in the chicken. They resemble mammalian NK cells in being cytoplasmic $CD3^+$ but surface TCR^-CD3^-, and often express CD8. These features indicate the close relationship of NK cells to T cells. Both avian and mammalian NK cells are, however, extra-thymically derived.

Phagocyte activity in fish

There is special interest in promoting disease resistance in fish in aquaculture. In this respect, parameters for enhancing fish phagocyte activity are being considered in some detail. The considerable progress in establishing long-term *in vitro* cultures of fish leucocytes (e.g. from catfish and carp) will undoubtedly foster work in this area. Enhanced activity of fish phagocytes to bacterial antigens, possibly due to release of macrophage-activating factors, can read-

ily be achieved by injecting killed pathogens and their products. β-glucans (polysaccharides from cell walls of yeasts and fungi) are also being used as enhancers of phagocyte-mediated immunity in fish, and are proving to be good adjuvants for vaccines although their mechanism of action awaits clarification. Cytokines such as fish T-cell-derived 'gamma interferon' and human TNFα, synergize in elevating the respiratory burst pathways of trout macrophages, which leads to production of bactericidal oxygen free-radicals (superoxide anion and hydrogen peroxide). Mammalian TGFβ can inhibit fish macrophage activation. Chemokine-like factors are found in fish and these can influence fish phagocyte locomotion. Since stress-induced immunosuppression may well be a problem in fish aquaculture, the recently reported ability of the immunoactive peptide FK-565 to block such immunosuppression is of interest.

Leukotrienes and other lipid mediators (collectively known as eicosanoids) are known to be involved in a variety of inflammatory processes in mammals. There is now evidence that eicosanoids are produced in fish (and amphibians) and play an important role in inflammatory responses in fish. For example leukotriene B_4 enhances the migration of rainbow trout leucocytes, and eicosanoids can modulate trout T-cell proliferation. Since dietary lipids can modulate fish eicosanoid production, dietary considerations are crucial in developing fish vaccination, and this is currently an active research area.

Non-antigen-specific molecules
Complement classical, alternative and lytic pathways are well developed in vertebrates

Agnathans possess antibody-independent, complement-like proteins. In hagfish these have homology with mammalian C3, C4 and C5, and act as opsonins, for which a 105 kDa receptor has been found on phagocytic leucocytes. Both the classical (antibody-mediated) and alternative pathways of complement activation have been demonstrated in all other vertebrate classes, although it remains uncertain whether the alternative complement pathway exists in cartilaginous fish.

Complement components C1–C9, together with factors B and D, have all been isolated in carp. Considerable homology exists between the gene for C3 in *Xenopus* and the gene for mammalian C3. Characterization of other complement components in anurans includes C1q, C4, C5, the membrane attack complex, and factor B. Basic properties of mammalian complement (such as thermolability, and requirements for Ca^{2+} and Mg^{2+}) are shared by fish and amphibian complement. Understandably, however, the temperature range over which ectotherm complement remains active is greater, with activity remaining at 4°C. Despite this, heat-inactivation can be achieved at a lower temperature; *Xenopus* serum, for example, is entirely stripped of complement activity by treatment at 45°C for 40 minutes. Guinea-pig complement may be used successfully in haemolytic antibody assays *in vitro* using antibody from adult amphibians. For most fish species and larval *Xenopus*, the complement used must be from the same species or a closely-related species.

Cytokines functionally similar to those in mammals are found in lower vertebrates

In comparison with the constantly increasing availability of data at the molecular level concerning the evolution of immunoglobulins, TCR and the MHC, research on cytokines, and especially cytokine receptors, of lower vertebrates rather lags behind. Bioassays have, however, revealed that several groups of cytokines do exist in many vertebrate classes. These include interleukins, interferons, tumour necrosis factor, colony stimulating factors and chemokines.

For example, T-cell growth factors (TCGF), able to promote the proliferation of T-cell lymphoblasts *in vitro*, have now been identified from culture supernatants of stimulated T lymphocytes taken from bony fish, urodele and anuran amphibians, snakes and chickens (*Fig. 15.22*). The purification of *Xenopus* TCGF indicates a protein of molecular mass 16 kDa, with biochemical and functional similarity to mammalian IL-2. The 'IL-2' gene and receptors for *Xenopus* 'IL-2' have not yet been identified.

'IL-1-like' activity has been detected in the macrophages of bony fish, amphibians and birds. 'Interferon-like' factors, with macrophage-activating and anti-viral function, have also been discovered in ectotherms (e.g. in farmed fish where viral diseases can decimate fish stocks). Interferon from flatfish has recently been sequenced, but bears little resemblance to any other interferon. This lack of homology may be the reason why oligonucleotide probes based on conserved sequences of mammalian cytokines have not been very successful in identifying ectotherm cytokine genes. Successes include fibroblast growth factor in amphibians, TGFβ (TGFβ5 in *Xenopus*, where it can inhibit T-cell proliferation and TGFβ4 in chickens), and flatfish IL-2. Evolutionary conservation of TNF receptors is indicated, since the activat-ing effects of human TNFβ on rainbow trout macrophages can be blocked by pre-incubating these phagocytes with anti-human TNF (p55) receptor antibodies.

Anti-microbial peptides

Anti-microbial peptides structurally related to invertebrate antibacterial proteins (described earlier) are also important immune factors of the vertebrate immune system. Thus, cecropins have been discovered in pig intestine, and defensins are found in mammalian phagocytes and certain intestinal cells, where they control microbial growth. Another family of peptides, called magainins, are secreted by granular glands in the skin and gut of *Xenopus*. Magainins have broad-range biocidal activity against Gram-negative and Gram-positive bacteria, fungi and protozoa. Moreover, they have also been shown to be cytotoxic for various human malignant cells. Several magainins have now been synthesized in the laboratory and are being considered as potential therapeutic agents in humans. Squalamine, a steroid that acts as a systemic antibiotic in sharks, has similarly become a candidate for human drug development.

■ LYMPHOMYELOID TISSUES IN LOWER VERTEBRATES

The lymphomyeloid system produces and stores lymphocytes, granulocytes and other blood cells, and provides the anatomical framework to allow appropriate immunocyte/antigen interaction.

Fish lymphomyeloid tissues

The agnathan hagfish possesses neither thymus nor spleen, its lymphocytes developing in head kidney or in the gut.

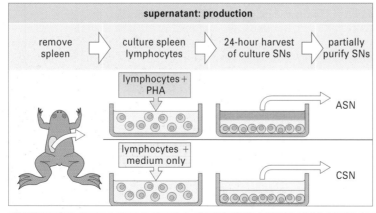

T-cell growth factor in *Xenopus*

supernatant: production				supernatant: assays		
				induces ³H-thymidine incorporation in:		supports growth of T cell lines
remove spleen	culture spleen lymphocytes	24-hour harvest of culture SNs	partially purify SNs	resting splenocytes	T lymphoblasts	
lymphocytes + PHA → ASN				+	+ + +	+ + +
lymphocytes + medium only → CSN				–	–	–

Fig. 15.22 Active culture supernatants (ASNs) are harvested from PHA-stimulated *Xenopus* splenocytes and compared with supernatants from control cultures (CSNs). The supernatants are initially partially purified. The ASNs appear to contain cytokines since they induce considerable proliferation of T lymphoblasts (but are less stimulatory for resting splenocytes) and support the growth of alloreactive T-cell lines; CSNs have no comparable effects. A similar but reduced level of activity can be generated in supernatants from mixed leucocyte culture. T-cell growth factor activity in *Xenopus* resides in a 16 kDa protein which, in view of biochemical and functional properties, may well represent amphibian IL-2. (Courtesy of Dr N. Cohen.)

A primitive spleen and bone marrow-like tissue are found in the lamprey.

Jawed fish lack lymphoid bone marrow, lymph nodes and nodular gut-associated lymphoid tissue (GALT) (*Fig. 15.23*). However, they have a well-developed thymus and spleen, diffuse GALT and lymphomyeloid tissue associated with kidney and liver (*Fig. 15.24*). One notable feature of fish lymphomyeloid tissue is the abundance of melano-macrophage centres within the liver of 'primitive' forms and also within the spleen and kidney of teleost fish (*Fig. 15.25*). These centres are heavily laden with pigments, for example haemosiderin, ceroid, melanin and, in particular, lipofuscin. Pigment accumulation in the fish 'macrophage aggregates' may be partly related to the animals' high levels of unsaturated fats, which maintain membrane fluidity at low temperatures; these fats are particularly prone to peroxidation and formation of lipofuscin.

Amphibian lymphomyeloid tissues
The thymus
The adult *Xenopus* thymus lies just under the skin, behind the middle ear. Detachment of the thymus from the pha-

Evolution of lymphomyeloid tissues in vertebrates

vertebrate group	lymphomyeloid tissue					
	thymus	spleen	bone marrow	lymph nodes	GALT-associated	kidney/liver
mammals	■	■	■	■	■	■
birds	■	■	■	■	■	■
reptiles	■	■	■	◨	■	■
frogs/toads	■	■	■	◨	■	■
salamanders/newts	◨	■	□	□	◨	■
lungfish	■	■	■	□	■	■
teleost fish	■	■	□	□	■	■
sharks/rays	■	■	□	□	■	■
jawless fish	□	◨	□	□	◨	■

■ presence/homology	□ probable absence
◨ partial evidence	

Fig. 15.23 Lymphoid and myeloid compartments are intermingled in fishes and amphibians.

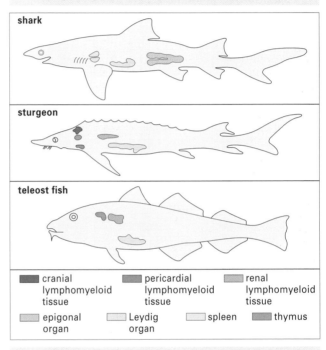

Lymphomyeloid tissues in different types of fish

shark

sturgeon

teleost fish

■ cranial lymphomyeloid tissue   ■ pericardial lymphomyeloid tissue   ■ renal lymphomyeloid tissue

■ epigonal organ   □ Leydig organ   □ spleen   ■ thymus

Fig. 15.24 Note that the intestines of sharks and sturgeons are also rich in lymphomyeloid tissue (in the spiral valve). (Courtesy of Dr R. Fänge.)

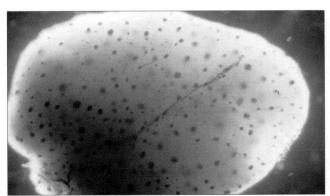

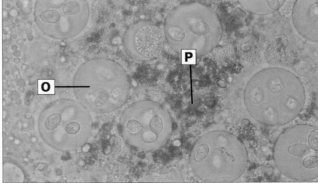

Fig. 15.25 Melano-macrophage centres (MMCs) in fish liver. Gross and microscopic views of liver of a cyptinodontid fish (*Rivulus marmoratus*) experimentally infected with the coccidian parasite *Calyptospora funduli*. At 60 days post-infection, distinct MMCs have appeared (left, × 60). The squash preparation (right, × 600) shows that these MMCs consist of degenerating oocysts (O) of the parasite and associated host pigment (P). The mononuclear phagocytes play a dominant role in MMC formation. (Courtesy of Dr W. K. Vogelbein.)

ryngeal epithelium occurs early in development, as it does in most other vertebrates except teleost fish. The thymus is differentiated into an outer cortex and a central (paler-staining) medulla. The rapidly-proliferating cortical lymphocytes are particularly sensitive to irradiation (*Fig. 15.26*). Apoptosis in the *Xenopus* thymus is enhanced by *in vitro* glucocorticoid treatment. Elevated *in vivo* levels of corticosteroids can induce thymic atrophy in *Rana*.

There is considerable evidence that the ectotherm thymus, like its counterpart in endotherms, produces lymphocytes with T-cell functions. The ultrastructure of thymic lymphocytes and neighbouring epithelial cells is shown in *Figure 15.27*. Several other stromal cell types are found within the amphibian thymus, including large dendritic (interdigitating) cells, macrophages, cysts and granular cells. Myoid cells are also found, as they are in the reptilian and mammalian thymus (see *Fig. 15.27*). Myoid cells may be involved in promoting circulation of tissue fluids within the thymus and may also act as a source of macrophage-stimulating factors. Thymic epithelial cells, which express MHC class II antigens early in development, appear to be involved in 'educating' T-lineage cells (see below). Nurse cell-like complexes of stromal cells and enclosed thymocytes have been found in the frog thymus and may represent sites of T cell education. B cells have also been found in the thymus of diverse vertebrate species, including amphibians, though this organ is not involved with their production. High endothelial venules have been described in the *Rana* thymus, which may promote cell immigration.

The spleen

The spleen is a major peripheral lymphoid organ in all jawed vertebrates. Together with the 'lymph nodes' and kidneys, it traps antigen, houses proliferating lymphocytes after their stimulation by antigen, and provides for the appropriate release of these cells and their products. Thymus-dependent and -independent lymphoid zones within the spleen have been demonstrated in *Xenopus* (*Fig. 15.28*). The white pulp follicles are rich in B cells (*Fig. 15.29*), shown by selective staining of this region with anti-immunoglobulin monoclonal antibodies. Splenic T cells, found especially in the perifollicular (marginal zone) regions, lack surface immunoglobulin, but a population will bind with anti-T cell monoclonal antibodies (see *Fig.*

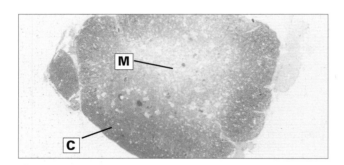

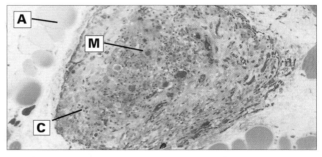

Fig. 15.26 Thymus of young adult *Xenopus*: effect of irradiation. Normal thymus (left, × 35) has an extremely lymphoid cortex (C) and a paler-staining, less cellular medulla (M). Gamma-irradiated thymus (9 days after 3000 rad irradiation) is shown on the right (× 90). Note the dramatic loss of lymphocytes from the cortex (C) following irradiation, but retention of some lymphocytes in the medulla (M). The irradiated thymus is reduced in size. Adipose tissue (A) surrounds the thymus. Toluidine blue stain.

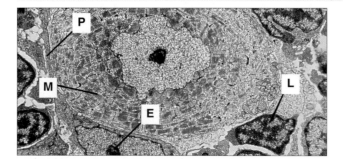

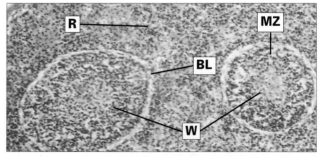

Fig. 15.27 Electron micrograph of thymus medulla of larval *Xenopus*. The myoid cell nucleus is surrounded by concentric rings of striated myofibrils (M) resembling those of skeletal muscle. The nuclear chromatin of the small lymphocytes (L) is organized into a series of electron-dense zones; the cytoplasm is scant with few organelles. The epithelial cell nuclei (E) have evenly-dispersed chromatin and prominent nucleoli; the cytoplasm is extensive and projections (P) extend in an interdigitating fashion between lymphocytes and other cell types to form a supportive network. × 700. (Courtesy of Dr J. J. Rimmer.)

Fig. 15.28 Spleen section of adult *Xenopus*. Thymus-dependent (perifollicular red pulp or marginal zone [MZ]) and thymus-independent (white pulp) areas are shown. In *Xenopus* (unlike many other ectotherms) the white pulp (W) is clearly separated from the surrounding red pulp (R) by lightly-staining boundary layer cells (BL). Concentrations of lymphocytes are also seen in the red pulp. H&E stain, × 80.

15.29). Blood vessels enter the spleen through the white pulp central arteriole, which is in close association with noradrenergic sympathetic nerve fibres. This nerve innervates the spleen and plays an immunomodulatory role. Capillaries leave the central arteriole and empty into the surrounding red pulp marginal zone; capillary walls contribute to the boundary layer. Experimental studies with India ink-stained and fluoresceinated antigens reveal that it is the red pulp that initially receives material circulating in the blood. Circulating antigens are later trapped within the white pulp follicles, that is they are closely associated with potential antibody-producing cells (*Fig. 15.30*). Antigen is held on the surfaces of large dendritic cells, whose cytoplasmic processes extend pseudopods through the boundary layer and into the marginal zone, which is rich in T cells. The overall arrangement of the amphibian spleen is similar to that of the mammalian spleen, although germinal centres have not been identified in the former. The spleen of amphibians plays an important role in B-cell development in both the larva (along with the liver) and in the adult, where it constitutes the main site of B-cell differentiation. Surprisingly, B lymphocytes of *Xenopus* do not constitutively express CD5, the marker found on 'primitive' natural antibody-producing B1 cells of mammals.

The lymphomyeloid nodes

Lymphomyeloid nodes, bearing a superficial functional resemblance to the lymph nodes of endothermic vertebrates, are seen for the first time in vertebrate evolution in 'advanced' amphibians such as the ranid and bufid frogs and toads, but not in urodeles or in *Xenopus*. The lymphomyeloid nodes of anurans are different from their mammalian counterparts in being mainly blood-filtering organs, although they can also trap material from surrounding lymph. Although a major site of antibody-producing cells, the anuran lymphomyeloid nodes do not have the clearly defined architecture of mammalian lymph nodes and germinal centres are not seen. In the adult frog, 'lymph nodes' are found in the neck and axillary regions; the lymph gland of the larva is structurally similar (*Fig. 15.31*).

Gut-associated lymphoid tissue

Nodular gut-associated lymphoid tissue (GALT), analogous to the mammalian GALT system, occurs throughout

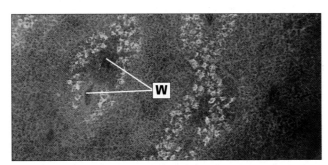

Fig. 15.29 Adult *Xenopus* spleen, showing B and T cell-rich zones. Left: B cells frequent the white pulp follicle (W); they are also seen in the marginal zone (MZ) and red pulp (R), mainly as densely-staining plasma cells. Anti-B-cell (anti-IgM) mAb stain, ×100.

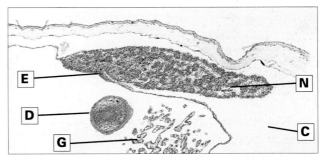

Right: T cells are seen concentrated in the marginal zone, just outside the white pulp follicle (W). They are seen especially in the perifollicular (marginal) zone (MZ) and lack surface immunoglobulin. Anti-T-cell stain, ×200.

Fig. 15.30 Immunofluorescence of adult *Xenopus* spleen showing antigen trapping. The frog was injected with human IgG. Three weeks later frozen sections were prepared and incubated with fluorescein-labelled anti-human IgG. The bright apple-green fluorescence shows the presence of antigen within white pulp follicles (W). The antigen is trapped in a dendritic pattern, similar to that seen in mammals and birds, where it appears to be held on reticular cell surfaces. × 35.

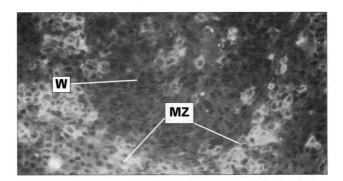

Fig. 15.31 Lymph gland section of larval *Rana*. The elongated (paired) lymphomyeloid node (N) is seen attached ventrally to the epithelium (E) of the gill chamber and projects into a large lymphatic channel (C). Gills (G), and a digit (D) of the anterior limb lying in the gill chamber are seen medially; the larval skin lies laterally. The lymph gland consists of an extensive lymphoid parenchyma with phagocytes and intervening sinusoids (pale-staining). The lymph gland is mainly a blood-filtering organ. H&E stain, ×25

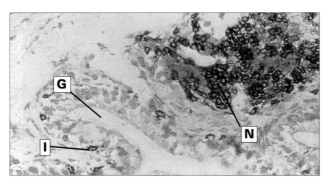

Fig. 15.32 Cryostat section of *Xenopus* small intestine stained with anti-CD5 (a pan T cell) monoclonal antibody and visualized by immunoperoxidase staining. Intraepithelial T cells (I) and nodular collections of T cells (N) in lamina propria can be seen, as can the gut lumen (G). T cells from both locations are lost after early thymectomy. × 300.

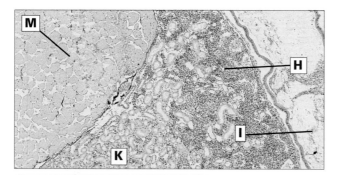

Fig. 15.33 Kidney section in larval *Rana* showing haemopoietic tissue. Haemopoietic tissue (H) is extensive in the intertubular regions where lymphocytes, granulocytes and other developing blood cell types are found. Myotomal muscles (M) and a loop of the intestine (I) lie adjacent to the mesonephros. H&E stain, × 25. (K = kidney tubules.)

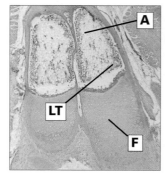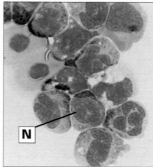

Fig. 15.34 Bone marrow. Left: Lymphomyeloid tissue (LT), an important source of antibody-producing cells, in bone marrow from Rana. Femur (F) and adipose tissue (A) are also marked. H&E stain, × 20. **Right:** A bone marrow cytocentrifuge preparation from *Xenopus*, showing peroxidase-positive neutrophilic granulocytes (N). × 700. (Cytocentrifuge preparation, courtesy of Dr I. Hadji-Azimi.)

the small intestine in amphibians. In *Xenopus*, GALT contains both IgM and IgX-secreting plasma cells. Immunohistochemistry with anti-T cell monoclonal antibodies reveals both nodular (lamina propria) and intra-epithelial T cells in *Xenopus* intestine (*Fig. 15.32*).

Kidney and liver
The kidney is a major lymphomyeloid organ in amphibians (*Fig. 15.33*), as it is in fish, but this function wanes in the kidneys of reptiles, birds and mammals. In anurans, B-cell development in ontogeny begins in the kidney and/or liver. These organs are, in fact, intimately involved with the early differentiation of erythroid, lymphoid and myeloid cells in diverse vertebrates.

Bone marrow
Bone marrow is found in amphibians, but its immunological role awaits clarification. In adult *Rana pipiens*, bone-marrow lymphomyeloid tissue is readily evident (*Fig. 15.34*) and is an important source of antibody-producing cells. In *Xenopus*, on the other hand, bone marrow appears to be more rudimentary and is mainly a site for the differentiation of neutrophilic granulocytes (*Fig. 15.34*).

■ AMPHIBIAN MODELS FOR STUDYING ONTOGENY OF IMMUNITY

In recent years, several isogeneic and inbred families of *Xenopus* have become available for immunological research. Different *Xenopus* families, that are either MHC compatible or possess one or two MHC haplotype differences, are proving invaluable for investigating the ontogeny of the immune system.

The development of the thymus
Thymus development and thymectomy experiments
Xenopus is ideally suited for investigating the role of the thymus in immune system development, since the free-living larva can be thymectomized very early in life when the thymus is still immature (*Figs 15.35 and 15.36*). In *Xenopus* the paired thymus develops from the dorsal epithelium of the second pharyngeal pouches. Experimental studies reveal that lymphoid precursor cells first enter the thymic epithelial rudiments at 3–4 days of age. A T-cell differentiation antigen, the XTLA-1 marker (120 kDa), recognized by anti-thymocyte mouse monoclonal antibody XT-1, begins to appear on the thymic lymphoid cell population at seven days. A majority of thymocytes express T cell surface antigens by 10 days of age, when candidate T cells are first identified in the periphery. The thymus involutes at metamorphosis when a new wave of colonization by stem cells occurs. Following metamorphosis, thymocyte numbers increase, reaching maximal levels at 15–16 months. Early thymectomy of *Xenopus* (at 4–8 days of age) has clearly demonstrated the existence of T-dependent (T_{dep}) and T-independent (T_{ind}) components of immunity (*Fig. 15.37*). Following this early thymectomy, XT-1$^+$ T cells (and also CD5$^+$ and CD8$^+$ T cells) are no longer found in larval and adult lymphoid organs, whereas surface-IgM$^+$ B cells are plentiful (*Fig. 15.38*). The thymus therefore

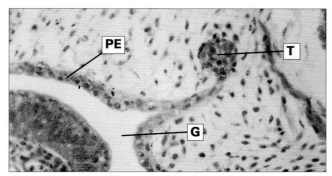

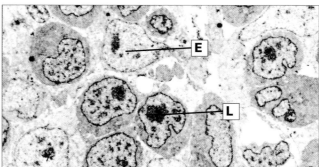

Fig. 15.35 *Xenopus* thymus at 3 days and 7 days. Left: At 3 days, developing thymus (T) is still attached to the pharyngeal epithelium (PE) and composed mostly of epithelial cells. A gill pouch (G) is also shown. H&E stain, × 100. **Right:** At 7 days, the thymus consists of less than 1000 cells of two major types. The epithelial cells (E) have a prominent nucleolus, dispersed chromatin and pale-staining cytoplasm. Lymphoid cells (L) possess large amounts of densely-staining cytoplasm with an abundance of free ribosomes and mitochondria. At 7 days, the XT-1 marker begins to appear on the thymic lymphoid cell population, and MHC class II proteins are first expressed on epithelial cells. Electron micrograph × 500.

appears to be critical for T-cell maturation at this level of evolution. However, it should be noted that early-thymectomized *Xenopus* sometimes chronically reject MHC-disparate skin grafts. Following rejection, their splenocytes become positive when tested in mixed lymphocyte culture, even to stimulators with an MHC distinct from the original donors, but not when stimulated with the T-cell mitogen, PHA. The nature of these alloreactive cells remains uncertain.

Thymectomy of larvae at various time points during development suggests that different T-cell functions require the presence of the thymus for varying periods in order to become established in the periphery (*Fig. 15.39*). Studies in intact animals reveal that alloimmune reactivity (*in vivo* and *in vitro*), together with the ability of splenocytes to respond to T-cell mitogens, develops early in the tadpole's larval life, whereas good IgY antibody responses are only seen in the froglet, which expresses appropriate T-cell helper function.

Thymic education in Xenopus *involves positive selection and limited negative selection*

Foreign thymus, grafted into early-thymectomized *Xenopus*, can promote the differentiation of host precursor cells along a T-cell pathway (*Fig. 15.40*). The *in vivo* development of thymuses, with epithelial and lymphoid compartments expressing different MHC markers, can readily be achieved by a different surgical approach. This involves joining the anterior part of one 24-hour embryo, containing the thymic epithelial buds, to the posterior portion of an MHC-incompatible embryo, from which the haemopoietic stem cells, including lymphocytes, arise (*Fig. 15.41*).

These two experimental systems have been used to explore the role played by thymic stromal cells in thymic education. This involves negative selection (establishing tolerance of T cells to self antigens) and positive selection (restricting the MHC-antigen specificities with which helper and effector T-cell populations preferentially interact). These experiments on *Xenopus* have indicated involvement of the foreign thymus epithelium in positive selection and

in inducing tolerance towards skin grafts of thymus MHC type, although interestingly this tolerance does not appear to prevent a mixed lymphocyte reaction towards thymus donor cells. Recently, similar findings have been made with bird and mammal embryos. However, in mammals the view

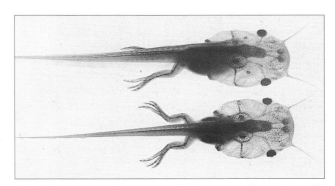

Fig. 15.36 *Xenopus* thymus at 38 days. The pigmented paired thymus lies behind the eyes (**upper**); its absence is readily apparent in the sibling thymectomized at 7 days (**lower**).

Effect of thymectomy in *Xenopus*

	antibody response to:		allograft rejection	mitogen response to:	
	LPS (T_{ind})	SRBC (T_{dep})		LPS (B cells)	PHA (T cells)
normal	+	+	fast	+	+
thymectomized	+	−	slow	+	−

Fig. 15.37 *Xenopus*, thymectomized at 4–8 days, are assessed for antibody response, cell-mediated response to skin allografts and mitogen response *in vitro*. (LPS = lipopolysaccharide; SRBC = sheep red blood cells; PHA = phytohaemagglutinin.)

T- and B-cell population in *Xenopus*

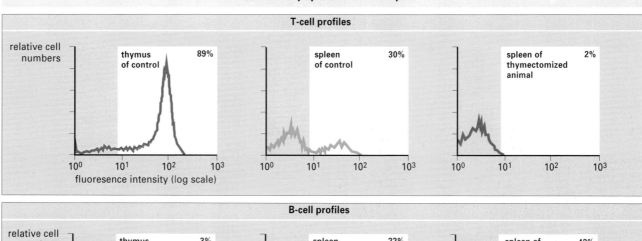

T-cell profiles

relative cell numbers

thymus of control — 89%

spleen of control — 30%

spleen of thymectomized animal — 2%

fluoresence intensity (log scale)

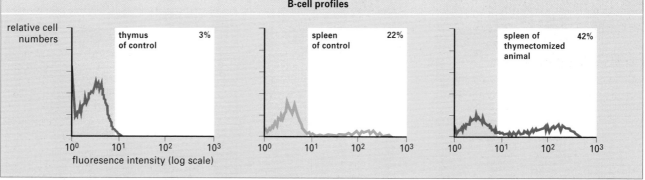

B-cell profiles

relative cell numbers

thymus of control — 3%

spleen of control — 22%

spleen of thymectomized animal — 42%

fluoresence intensity (log scale)

Fig. 15.38 Cells from the thymus and spleen of a control (4-month-old) *Xenopus*, and from the spleen of a 7-day thymectomized sibling, were stained first with either mouse anti-T cell (XT–1) monoclonal antibody (mAb) or with mouse anti-B cell (anti-IgM) mAb. FITC-labelled anti-mouse-immunoglobulin was used as secondary antibody. T and B cells were then identified using a fluorescence-activated cell sorter. Early larval thymectomy deletes the XT-1⁺ T cell population from the spleen, which now shows a proportional increase in B-cell numbers. The percentage shown on each graph represents the proportion of positive cells, i.e. those to the right of the marker (grey) set to exclude 98% background fluorescence.

Sequential emergence of T-cell subsets

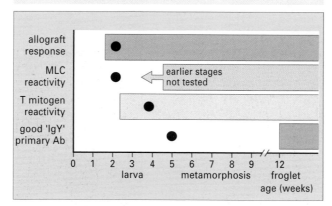

allograft response

MLC reactivity — earlier stages not tested

T mitogen reactivity

good 'IgY' primary Ab

0 1 2 3 4 5 6 7 8 9 12

larva | metamorphosis | froglet

age (weeks)

Fig. 15.39 Ontogeny of immune reactivity, and the effect of thymectomy at different ages in *Xenopus*. The allograft response, mixed lymphocyte reactivity and T mitogen reactivity all appear early. They are followed much later by TH cells, particularly those TH cells which permit the 'IgY' primary antibody response. (• Indicates the age after which thymectomy will no longer impair this particular function.)

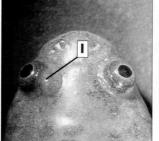
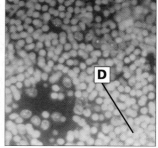

Fig. 15.40 Thymus implantation to thymectomized *Xenopus*. Left: The clawed frog (*X. laevis*) was thymectomized at 7 days of age. A thymus from a larval *X. borealis* donor was then implanted subcutaneously in late larval life. This thymus implant (I) grew well, lying adjacent to the left eye following metamorphosis. **Right:** A section of the implanted thymus was examined by fluorescence microscopy. Donor-derived cells (D) can be distinguished from host cells, because *X. borealis* nuclei display brightly fluorescent spots, whereas *X. laevis* cells stain homogeneously dull green. The thymus is now repopulated with host lymphocytes whereas many stromal cell types remain 'spotted' (i.e. they are of donor origin). Quinacrine stain, × 300.

persists that thymic interdigitating (dendritic) cells, which are a stromal population of extrinsic origin, rather than thymic epithelial cells, play a crucial role in negative selection by deleting T cells with high affinity for self MHC.

Ontogeny of alloimmunity, allotolerance and antibody production

Onset of alloimmunity (to MHC antigens) and specific antibody responses in tadpoles correlates with the appear-

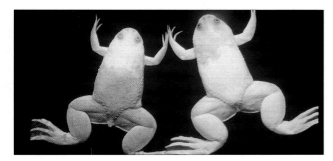

Fig. 15.41 Chimeric toads. Chimeric *Xenopus* were made by exchanging the anterior and posterior regions of two embryos 24 hours after fertilization. At this stage, the thymic anlage (e.g. thymic epithelium) is in the anterior region; all the lymphocyte precursors are in the posterior. One embryo was from an albino variant with white skin and red eyes, the other embryo was from a normal *Xenopus*. These chimeras are useful for studying thymic education. (Courtesy of Dr M. Flajnik and Dr L. DuPasquier.)

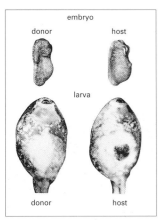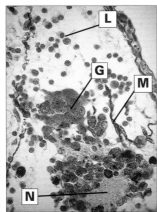

Fig. 15.42 Transplantation of embryonic tissue in *Rana* – ontogeny of alloimmunity. Left: A piece of neural fold removed from one embryo (tail-bud stage) is transplanted to the mid-ventral surface of another embryo (host). Intimately associated with the neural folds are the neural crest elements which are precursors of diverse cell types, including pigment cells. The pigment cells that differentiate are an externally visible means of following the progress of the embryonic transplant. The host larva has developed a distinctive mass of graft-derived pigment cells. **Right:** The section shows differentiated graft elements, large ganglion cells (G) with prominent nucleoli, other nervous tissue (N) and melanin (M), 15 days after transplantation. Despite the earliness of the transplantation, lymphocytes and granulocytes are invading the graft (L = leucocyte invading). H&E stain, ×100. (Courtesy of Dr E.P. Volpe.)

ance of the necessary T and B cell populations in the periphery (*Fig. 15.42*) and can occur when the lymphoid system contains less than a million lymphocytes. Immunological memory can be transferred over metamorphosis, but whether this reflects transfer of memory cells or is due to antigen persistence is unknown. Immunocompetent larvae (but not adults) can, nevertheless, readily be rendered tolerant to allogeneic skin; such allotolerance induction is particularly easy at metamorphosis (*Fig. 15.43*). The size of grafts applied and the degree of histoincompatibility appear to be critical. Those that are only slightly incompatible are always tolerated by larval and peri-metamorphic *Xenopus*. Tolerance induced by grafting foreign skin and lymphoid tissues in larval life is seldom 'complete' since signs of anti-donor reactivity (such as an MLR) can still be demonstrated before or after metamorphosis. Presumably tolerance is mediated by suppression or anergy.

Models for the study of lymphoid cell origins

Embryonic transplantation of cytogenetically-distinct gill buds in *Rana pipiens*, *Xenopus laevis* and the newt *Pleurodeles waltlii* confirmed that, as in endotherms, thymic lymphocytes develop from extrinsic precursor cells which colonize the thymus. In *Xenopus*, lymphoid precursor cells destined for the thymus have been shown to arise from both ventro-lateral plate mesoderm (ventral blood islands) and dorso-lateral plate mesoderm of the embryo. Two waves of stem cell entry into the thymus occur in young *Xenopus*, one during early larval life, the other during metamorphosis, which presumably allows the adult T cells to be educated in an environment where adult-specific antigens are expressed.

Several *Xenopus* haemopoietic lineages have recently been shown to express the leucocyte common antigen CD45, with tyrosine phosphatase activity.

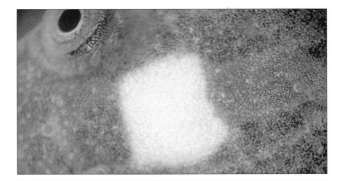

Fig. 15.43 Skin graft tolerance in *Xenopus*. Allogeneic skin, even from an MHC-disparate donor, may be tolerated by a larval or metamorphosing recipient. Subsequent skin grafts (here a piece of white belly skin) from the same donor are similarly retained by the adult frog. However, skin from a different donor is rejected within 3 weeks at 25°C.

Metamorphosis presents a problem for the immune system

Immunologists are intrigued to know how amphibians escape the risk of dying from an autoimmune disease at metamorphosis, since adult-specific cell markers are first expressed at this time. The significance of MHC class I first being expressed at metamorphosis remains to be elucidated. The involvement of suppressor functions seems likely. On the other hand, high plasma corticosteroid levels and increased expression of corticosteroid receptors on lymphocytes are found during the metamorphic climax. Such hormonal alterations may directly impair cell-mediated immunity, possibly by inhibiting IL-2 production. Amphibian metamorphosis is a fascinating period for probing the interplay between neuroendocrine and immune systems, which will undoubtedly have significance outside purely phylogenetic considerations.

Critical Thinking

■ Which cellular and humoral immune mechanisms are found in invertebrate phyla?

■ Discuss the fundamental differences that exist between the immune systems of invertebrate and vertebrate organisms. What evolutionary pressures may have lead to the developments in vertebrates?

■ What solutions have evolved in different vertebrates to the problem of generating antibody diversity?

■ What is known about the evolution of the major histocompatibility complex and associated T-cell phylogeny?

■ To what extent is the amphibian, *Xenopus laevis*, a useful model for exploring the ontogeny of the immune system?

■ What major gaps exist in our knowledge of the evolution of immunity? Outline what approaches you would adopt to address these shortcomings.

FURTHER READING

Clem LW, Warr G, eds. *Developmental and Comparative Immunology.* Oxford: Pergamon Press 1984, vol. 18 supp.1:1–164. Proceedings of the 6th Congress of Developmental & Comparative Immunology.

Cooper EL, ed. *Developmental and Comparative Immunology.* New York: Pergamon Press, 1992.

Cohen N, Sigel MM, eds. *The Reticuloendothelial System. Ontogeny and Phylogeny.* New York: Plenum, 1982.

Du Pasquier L. Evolution of the immune system. In: Paul WE, ed. *Fundamental Immunology.* 2nd ed. New York: Raven Press, 1989; 139–65.

Du Pasquier L, Schwager J, Flajnik MF. The immune system of *Xenopus. Annu Rev Immunol* 1989;**7**:251–75.

Du Pasquier L. Phylogeny of B cell development. *Curr Opin Immunol* 1993;**5**:185–93.

Flajnik MF. Primitive vertebrate immunity: what is the evolutionary derivation of molecules that define the adaptive immune system? In: *Antimicrobial Peptides.* Wiley, Chichester. CIBA Foundation Symposium 1994; **186**:224–32.

Flajnik MF, Hsu E, Kaufman JF, DuPasquier L. Changes in the immune system during metamorphosis of *Xenopus. Immunol Today* 1987;**8**:58–64.

Greenberg AS, Avila D, Hughes M *et al.* A novel antigen receptor gene family that undergoes rearrangement and extensive somatic diversification in sharks. *Nature* 1995 (in press).

Horton JD. Amphibians. In: Turner RJ, ed. *Immunology: A Comparative Approach.* Chichester: Wiley, 1994; 101–36.

Humphreys T, Reinherz EL. Invertebrate immune recognition, natural immunity and the evolution of positive selection. *Immunol Today* 1994;**15**:316–20.

Lackie AM, ed. Immune mechanisms in invertebrate vectors. *Zoological Society of London Symposia*, **56**. Oxford: Oxford University Press, 1986.

Iwanaga S, Söderhäll K, Vasta G, eds. *Invertebrate Immunology.* New Jersey: SOS Publications, 1995.

Marchalonis J, Schluter SF. Development of an immune system. In: Primordial Immunity: Foundations for the Vertebrate Immune System. *Ann NY Acad Sci* 1994;**712**:1–12.

Miller NW, McKinney EC. In vitro culture of fish leukocytes. In: *Biochemistry and Molecular Biology of Fishes*, vol 3. Elsevier, 1994:341–53.

Raison RL, Coverley J, Hook JW, et al. A cell surface opsonic receptor on leucocytes from the phylogenetically primitive vertebrate, *Eptatretus stouti. Immunol Cell Biol* 1994;**72**:326–32.

Ratcliffe NA, Rowley AF, eds. *Invertebrate Blood Cells.* Vols 1 & 2. London: Academic Press, 1981.

Ratcliffe NA, Rowley AF, Fitzgerald SW, Rhodes CP. Invertebrate immunity: basic concepts and recent advances. *Int Rev Cytol* 1985;**97**;183–350.

Robert J, Guiet C, Du Pasquier L. Lymphoid tumors of *Xenopus laevis* with different capacities for growth in larvae and adults. *Devel Immunol* 1994;**3**:297–307.

Rowley AF, Ratcliffe NA, eds. *Vertebrate Blood Cells.* Cambridge: Cambridge University Press, 1988.

Secombes CJ. The phylogeny of cytokines. In: Thomson AW, ed. *The Cytokine Handbook.* London: Academic Press, 1991;387–412.

Secombes CJ. Enhancement of fish phagocyte activity. *Fish Shellfish Immunol* 1994;**4**:421–36.

Smith LC, Davidson EH. The echinoid immune system and the phylogenetic occurrence of immune mechanisms in deuterostomes. *Immunol Today* 1992;**13**:356–62.

Stewart J. Immunoglobulins did not arise in evolution to fight infection. *Immunol Today* 1992;**13**:396–99.

Turner RJ, ed. *Immunology A Comparative Approach.* Chichester: Wiley, 1994.

Warr G. The immunoglobulin genes of fish. *Devel Comp Immunol* 1995;**19**:1–12.

Warr G, Cohen N, eds. *Phylogenesis of Immune Functions.* Oxford: CRC Press, 1991.

Viruses are obligate intracellular parasites. They vary in their complexity and replication strategies. Some produce acute infection and are eliminated from the host, whereas others persist indefinitely producing late disease.

Innate immune mechanisms restrict the early stages of infection and delay spread of virus. These defences include interferon and NK cells.

Antibody restricts the spread of virus to neighbouring cells and tissues by neutralizing virus infectivity. This is an important defence mechanism in preventing re-infection.

Cytotoxic T cells recognize virus infected cells. They are able to destroy infected cells early in the virus replication cycle before new viral progeny appear.

Viruses have evolved strategies to avoid recognition by the host. These include latency, antigenic variation and the production of decoy proteins that interfere with the host's antiviral defences.

Viruses may directly disrupt the function of the immune system by initiating immunosuppression and immunodeficiency disorders, and by triggering autoimmune disease.

■ MODES OF VIRUS INFECTION

Viruses are obligate intracellular parasites, and require the host cell's biochemical machinery to drive protein synthesis and metabolize sugars. They are extremely diverse in terms of their structure and genetic complexities – some have RNA genomes encoding only a few genes, and others have DNA genomes encoding up to 200 genes. Structurally, a virus is little more than a bag of protein and nucleic acid. However, life-forms even simpler than this have been identified:

- **Viroids** are infectious agents of plants which consist of nucleic acid alone, encoding no protein.

- **Prions** are essentially 'infectious proteins' associated with degenerative neurological diseases of animals and man, including scrapie, bovine spongiform encephalopathies (BSE) and Creutzfeld–Jakob disease (CJD).

A typical virus infection of a cell is shown in *Figure 16.1*. Viruses bind to host cells via specific receptors. This specificity identifies the tropism of a virus for a particular host or cell. Examples of cellular receptors used by viruses are shown in *Figure 16.2*. Following entry the virus uncoats, nucleic acid is released, and transcription occurs followed by the production of viral proteins. The viral genome is replicated and new 'progeny' virus particles (virions) are assembled and

Infection and replication of viruses

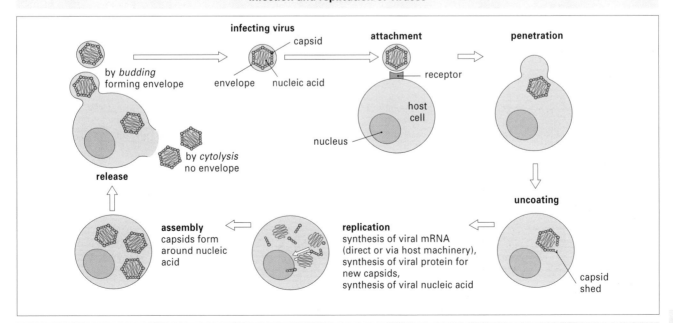

Fig. 16.1 Viruses must infect a host cell before they can replicate.

released to infect neighbouring cells and tissues. The details of this process depend on the particular virus and on the metabolic state of the host cell. For example, picornaviruses (small RNA viruses) take around eight hours to produce new virions, whereas human cytomegalovirus (a DNA virus) may take up to 48 hours.

Viruses are extremely diverse in their ability to infect, persist and initiate disease in a host. Entry is commonly at mucosal surfaces; puncturing skin (e.g. by insect bites or needles) is another, very efficient means of introducing virus directly into the blood stream. Replication usually occurs at epithelial surfaces, followed in some cases by viraemia (bloodborne spread) to infect other tissues. Recovery from the infection can involve the elimination of the virus from the host. Some viruses however (e.g. herpes virus) persist in a latent (non-infectious) form after the acute infection is resolved, and can reactivate to produce new infectious virions. Other viruses can persist in an infectious form despite the presence of the immune response (e.g. hepatitis B virus and lymphocytic choriomeningitis virus). In scrapie and CJD there is no acute stage; these agents persist as a slow infection, producing disease after many years. Unlike viruses, prions do not provoke an immune response nor is interferon produced following infection. A summary of the different forms of infection is shown in *Figure 16.3*.

■ INNATE IMMUNE RESPONSE TO VIRUSES

The early stage of an infection is often a race between the virus and the host's defence system. The initial defence against virus invasion is the integrity of the body surfaces. Once breached, early 'non-specific' or innate immune defences such as interferon, natural killer (NK) cells and macrophages become active.

Interferon (IFN) stimulates inhibition of viral replication

There are three types of interferon:
- IFNα (leucocyte interferon) is encoded by a family of some 20 genes on chromosome 9
- IFNβ (fibroblast interferon) is encoded by a single gene on chromosome 9
- IFNγ (immune interferon) is encoded by a single gene on chromosome 12.

Virus infection of a cell leads to the production of IFNα/β, which activates antiviral mechanisms in neighbouring cells enabling them to resist virus infection (*Fig. 16.4*). Interferons activate a number of genes, including two with direct anti-viral activity: a 67 kD protein kinase which inhibits the phosphorylation of e1F-2 and blocks translation of proteins; and a 2'5'-oligoadenylate synthetase which activates a latent endonuclease involved in degrading viral RNA.

Other anti-viral mechanisms exist which have a more specific action. The Mx gene, for example, inhibits the primary transcription of influenza virus genes, but has no effect against other viruses. In addition to the direct inhibition of virus replication, interferon-γ enhances the efficiency of the adaptive immune response by stimulating increased expression of MHC class I and II, and is also a potent activator of macrophages and NK cells (see below).

The importance of interferons *in vivo* is underlined by the increased susceptibility of mice to virus infection following the depletion of interferons by specific antibody treatment.

Natural Killer (NK) cells are cytotoxic for virally infected cells

Active NK cells are detected within two days of a virus infection. They have been identified as major effector cells against herpes viruses, and, in particular, cytomegalovirus (CMV). An

Virus receptors on host cells

virus	receptor	cell type infected
human immunodeficiency virus (HIV)	CD4	TH cells
Epstein–Barr virus	CR2 (complement receptor type 2)	B cells
influenza A virus	glycophorin A	many cell types
transmissible gastroenteritis virus	aminopeptidase N CD13	enterocytes
rhinovirus	ICAM-1	many cell types
polio virus	polio virus receptor (immunoglobulin superfamily)	neurons

Fig. 16.2 Viruses attach to cells via specific receptors and this partly determines which cell types become infected.

Different types of virus infection

initial infection	consequences	example
acute	recovery and elimination of virus	influenza virus, rotavirus
acute	latency (noninfectious virus); on reactivation, new viruses are shed	varicella zoster virus, herpes simplex virus
acute	persistence with continuance or intermittent shedding	hepatitis B virus, Epstein–Barr virus
not acute	persistent slow infection	Creutzfeld–Jakob disease, scrapie

Fig. 16.3 Virus infections can be acute or non-acute, and produce a variety of consequences.

absence or reduction of NK cell activity, as seen in Chediak–Higashi syndrome and beige mutant mice, correlates with an increased susceptibility to CMV infection. It is still unclear which molecules the NK cells recognize on the surface of virus infected cells. However, there is an inverse correlation between MHC class I expression and NK cell killing. This is an interesting feature since a number of viruses are now known to downregulate MHC class I expression; this is presumably a strategy to evade T cell recognition. Interferon-γ activates NK cell function and provides an important mechanism for focusing and activating cells at sites of infection. NK cells are also one of the main mediators of antibody-dependent cell-mediated cytotoxicity (ADCC).

◼ HOST DEFENCE INVOLVING B AND T CELLS

An absence of T cells renders the host highly susceptible to virus attack. For example, cutaneous infection of congenital athymic 'nude' mice (which lack mature T cells) with herpes simplex virus (HSV) results in a spreading lesion; the virus eventual-ly travels to the central nervous system, resulting in the death of the animal. The transfer of HSV-specific T cells shortly after infection is sufficient to protect the mice. The significance of T and B cells countering viral infections will now be discussed.

Antibodies and complement can limit viral spread or reinfection

Antibodies can neutralize the infectivity of viruses

As the infection proceeds the adaptive (specific) immune response unfolds, with the appearance of cytotoxic T cells, helper T cells and antiviral antibodies. Antibodies provide a major barrier to virus spread between cells and tissues and are particularly important in restricting virus spread in the blood stream. IgA production becomes focused at mucosal surfaces where it serves to prevent reinfection.

Antibodies may be generated against any viral protein in the infected cell, although only those against glycoproteins that are expressed on the virion envelope or on the infected cell membrane are of importance in controlling infection. Antibody-mediated immunity can be achieved in a number of ways, involving quite diverse mechanisms.

Defence against free virus particles involves neutralization of infectivity, which can occur in various ways (see *Fig. 16.5*). Such mechanisms are likely to operate *in vivo*, since injection of neutralizing monoclonal antibodies is highly effective at inhibiting virus replication. Clearly the presence of circulating virus-neutralizing antibodies is an important factor in the prevention of reinfection.

Complement is involved in the neutralization of some free viruses

Complement can also damage the virion envelope, a process known as virolysis. Some viruses can directly activate the classical and alternative complement pathways. However, complement is not considered to be a major factor in the defence against viruses since individuals with complement deficiencies are not predisposed to severe viral infection.

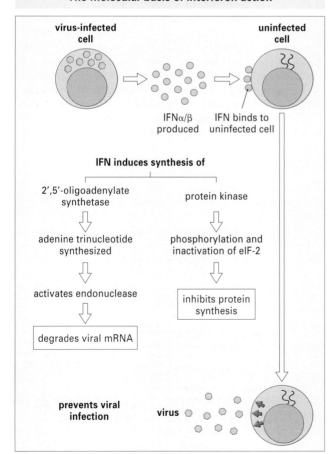

The molecular basis of interferon action

Fig. 16.4 The antiviral state develops within a few hours of interferon stimulation and lasts for 1-2 days.

Antiviral effects of antibody

target	agent	mechanism
free virus	antibody alone	blocks binding to cell blocks entry into cell blocks uncoating of virus
	antibody + complement	damage to virus envelope blockade of virus receptor
virus-infected cells	antibody + complement	lysis of infected cell opsonization of coated virus or infected cells for phagocytosis
	antibody bound to infected cells	antibody-dependent cell-mediated cytotoxicity by NK cells, macrophages and neutrophils

Fig. 16.5 Antibody acts to neutralize virus or kill virally-infected cells.

Antibodies mobilize complement and/or effector cells to destroy virus-infected cells

Antibodies are also effective in mediating the destruction of virus-infected cells. This can occur by antibody mediated activation of the complement system, leading to the assembly of the membrane attack complex and lysis of the infected cell (see Chapter 13). This process requires a high density of viral antigens on the membrane (about 5×10^6/cell) to be effective. In contrast, ADCC mediated by NK cells can recognize as few as 10^3 IgG molecules in order to bind and kill the infected cell. The IgG coated cells are bound using the FcγRIII (CD16), and are rapidly destroyed by a perforin-dependent killing mechanism (see Chapter 9). Just how important these mechanisms are *in vivo* is difficult to resolve. The best evidence in favour of ADCC comes from studying the protective effect of non-neutralizing monoclonal antibodies in mice. Although these antibodies fail to neutralize virus *in vitro*, they can protect C5-deficient mice from a high-dose virus challenge. (C5-deficient mice are used in this study to eliminate the role of the late complement components.)

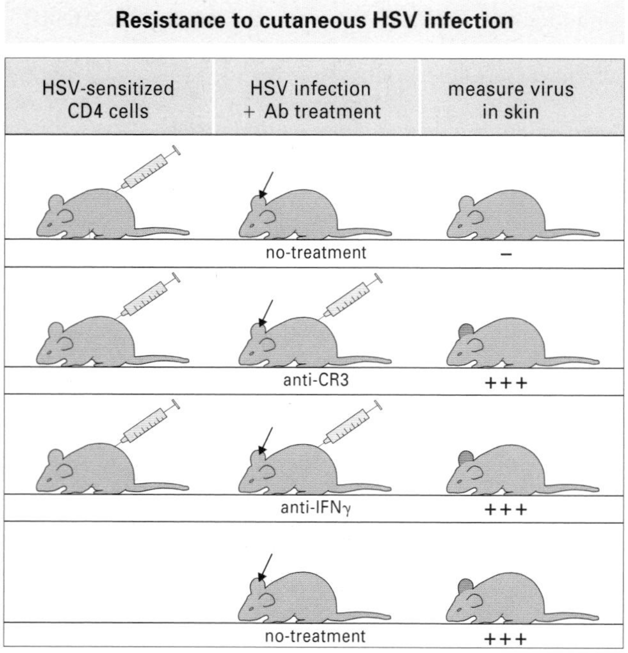

Resistance to cutaneous HSV infection

Fig. 16.6 CD4⁺ T cells, macrophages and IFNγ all have a protective role in cutaneous infections with HSV. CD4⁺ T cells were obtained from mice infected with HSV eight days previously. The cells were transferred to syngeneic mice infected with HSV in the skin. These mice were treated with anti-CR3 (to block macrophage migration to the site of infection), or anti-IFNγ (to block the activation of macrophages), or were untreated. An additional control group were infected but did not receive CD4⁺ T cells. The amount of infectious virus remaining after five days was then determined. The results demonstrate that the protective effects of CD4⁺ T cells are meditade by macrophages, and IFNγ.

T cells mediate viral immunity in several ways

T cells exhibit a variety of functions in antiviral immunity. Most of the antibody response is thymus-dependent, requiring the presence of CD4⁺ T cells for class switching and affinity maturation. CD4⁺ T cells also help in the induction of CD8⁺ cytotoxic T cells and in the recruitment and activation of macrophages at sites of virus infection.

CD8⁺ cytotoxic T cells

The principal T-cell surveillance system operating against viruses is highly efficient and selective. MHC class I restricted, cytotoxic CD8⁺ T cells focus at the site of virus replication and destroy virus-infected cells. Virtually all cells in the body express MHC class I molecules, making this an important mechanism for identifying and eliminating virus-infected cells.

Processing and presentation of virus proteins

Virtually any viral protein can be processed in the cytoplasm to generate peptides, which are then transported to the endoplasmic reticulum and are associated with MHC class I molecules. This has particular advantages for the host, since viral proteins expressed early in the replication cycle can be targeted, enabling T cell recognition to occur long before new viral progeny are produced. For example, T-cell mediated immunity against murine CMV is mediated by immediate early protein pp89. The epitope has been identified as a nonamer peptide presented by the MHC class I molecule L^d. Immunization of mice with a recombinant vaccinia containing pp89 is sufficient to confer complete protection from murine CMV induced disease; deletion of the DNA sequence encoding the nonapeptide abolishes the protective effect of the protein.

The importance of T cell mechanisms *in vivo* has been identified using various techniques:

- The adoptive transfer of specific T cell subpopulations or T cell clones to infected animals and monitoring of viral clearance.
- Depletion of T cell populations *in vivo* using monoclonal antibodies to CD4 or CD8.
- Creation of 'gene knockout' mice, in which genes such as CD4, CD8, and β₂ microglobulin are removed from the germline.

The continued ability of knockout mice that lack particular lymphocyte populations to mount a response against virus infections is a good illustration of the redundancy that can occur in the immune system. For example, in the absence of CD8⁺ T cells, CD4⁺ T cells or other mechanisms are able to compensate and bring the infection under control.

CD4⁺ T cells can have important effector functions against virus infections

CD4⁺ T cells are a major effector cell population in the immune response to HSV-1 infection of epithelial surfaces. In this instance recruitment of macrophages occurs as in delayed-type hypersensitivity (see Chapter 25) and an accelerated clearance of virus results. Macrophages are an important component in this process (*Fig. 16.6*). Key cytokines in this response include IFNγ, important in the activation of monocytes, and tumour necrosis factor (TNF). TNF has several antiviral activities; they are similar to those of IFNγ, but operate through a separate pathway.

CD4⁺ cytotoxic T cells

In measles virus infection, cytotoxic CD4⁺ T cells are generated which recognize and kill MHC class II positive cells infected with the virus. This suggests that measles virus peptides are generated by normal pathways of antigen presentation (i.e. following phagocytosis and degradation – see Chapter 7). However, other pathways have been implicated in which some measles proteins/peptides enter class II vesicles from the cytosol by an unknown mechanism.

A summary of antiviral defence mechanisms is illustrated in *Figure 16.7*, and the kinetics of their induction is shown in *Figure 16.8*.

■ STRATEGIES FOR EVADING IMMUNE DEFENCES

Viruses have evolved various strategies to evade recognition by antibody. Antigenic variation is the most effective ploy. It involves mutating regions on proteins that are normally targeted by antibody. Antigenic variation is seen in HIV and in foot and mouth disease virus, and is responsible for the antigenic shift and drift seen with influenza virus (*Fig. 16.9*). Humoral immunity to such diseases lasts only until the new virus strain emerges, making effective, long-lasting vaccinations difficult to produce.

Antibody can remove viral antigens from the plasma membrane by capping. This may possibly be a mechanism for forcing some viruses into a persistent intracellular infection. The

Response to a typical acute virus infection

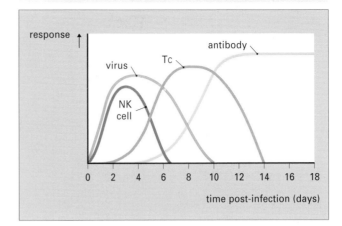

Fig. 16.8 Kinetics of host defences in response to a typical acute virus infection. Following an acute virus infection, for example by influenza or herpes virus, NK cells and interferon are detected in the blood stream, and locally in infected tissues. Cytotoxic T cells (Tc) then become activated in local lymph nodes or spleen, followed by the appearance of serum neutralizing antibodies. Although activated T cells are absent by the second to third week, T cell memory is established and lasts for many years.

Host defences against virus infection

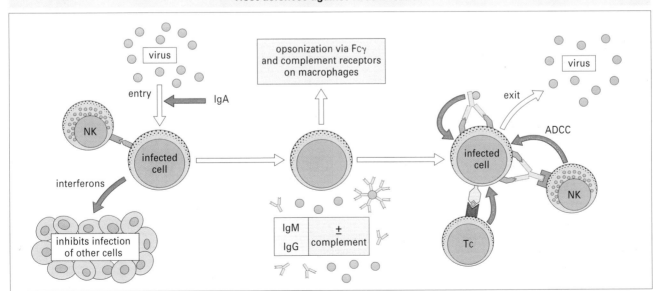

Fig. 16.7 Entry of virus at mucosal surfaces inhibited by IgA. Following the initial infection, the virus may spread to other tissues via the blood stream. Interferons produced by the innate (IFNα and IFNβ) and adaptive (IFNγ) immune responses make neighbouring cells resistant to infection by spreading virus. Antibodies are important in controlling free virus, whereas T cells and NK cells are effective at killing infected cells. (ADCC = antibody dependent cell-mediated cytotoxicity).

Antigenic shift and drift in influenza virus

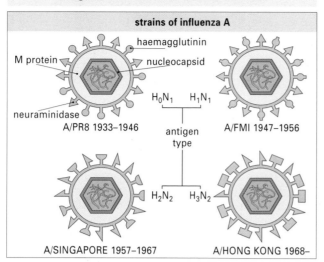

Fig. 16.9 The major surface antigens of influenza virus are haemagglutinin and neuraminidase. Haemagglutinin is involved in attachment to cells, and antibodies to haemagglutinin are protective. Antibodies to neuraminidase are much less effective. The influenza virus can change its surface slightly (antigenic drift) or radically (antigenic shift). Alterations in the structure of the haemagglutinin antigen render earlier antibodies ineffective and thus new virus epidemics break out. The diagram shows strains that have emerged by antigenic shift since 1933. The official influenza antigen nomenclature is based on the type of haemagglutinin (H_0, H_1 etc.) and neuraminidase (N_1, N_2 etc.) expressed on the surface of the virion. Note that although new strains replace old strains, the internal antigens remain unchanged.

herpesviruses (HSV and human CMV) encode glycoproteins with IgG-Fc receptor binding activity. This viral strategy could interfere with complement activation and block the action of antiviral antibodies.

Some viruses (e.g. Epstein–Barr virus and adenovirus) produce their own defences against the actions of interferon, producing short stretches of RNA that compete for the protein kinase and somehow inhibit the activation of the enzyme. Other viruses (e.g. adenovirus and CMV) encode proteins that are able to inhibit the transport of MHC class I molecules to the cell membrane. This strategy can give the virus a distinct advantage, helping it to avoid cytotoxic T cell recognition.

Some virus genes encode homologues of cytokine receptors or even cytokines. Soluble forms of the IL-1β, TNF and IFNγ receptors are secreted from infected cells and may subvert local cytokine activity. Epstein–Barr virus encodes an IL-10 homologue which mimics mammalian IL-10 activity *in vitro*. The full significance of these virus gene products *in vivo* has still to be elucidated.

A summary of virus encoded homologues of the host defence system is shown in *Figure 16.10*.

■ IMMUNOPATHOLOGY

Responses to viral antigens can cause tissue damage
Damage due to the formation of immune complexes
Immune complexes may arise in body fluids or on cell surfaces and are most common during persistent or chronic infections, for example with LCMV or hepatitis B virus. Antibody is ineffective (non-neutralizing) in the presence of large

---

Viral products that interfere with host defences

host defence effected	virus	virus product	mechanism
interferon	EBV	EBERS (small RNAs)	blocks protein kinase activation
	vaccinia	e1F-2α homologue	prevents phosphorylation of e1F-2α by protein kinase
complement	vaccinia	homologues of complement control proteins	blocks complement activation
	HSV-1	gC	binds Fcγ and blocks function
cytokines	myxoma	IFNγ receptor homologue	competes for IFNγ, blocks function
	shope fibroma virus	TNF receptor homologue	competes for TNF, blocks function
	EBV	IL-10 homologue	reduces IFNγ function
MHC class I	murine cytomegalovirus	early protein	prevents transport of peptide-loaded MHC
	adenovirus	E3	blocks transport of MHC to surface

Fig. 16.10 Viruses use a great variety of ingenious strategies to outwit the host defences.

amounts of the viral antigen; instead, immune complexes form and are deposited in the kidney or in blood vessels, where they evoke inflammatory responses leading to tissue damage, for example as glomerulonephritis (see Chapter 24).

An unusual pathological consequence of some virus–non-neutralizing antibody interactions is the Fc receptor-mediated uptake of the complex by macrophages and subsequent enhancement of virus infectivity. This is seen in Dengue virus infection and is implicated as the underlying mechanism of Dengue haemorrhagic fever and Dengue shock syndrome, which involves hyperactivation of the complement system.

T cell-mediated tissue damage

In any virus infection some tissue damage is likely to arise from the activity of T cells. However, in some situations this damage may be considerable, resulting in the death of the animal. The best example of this is the cytotoxic T cell response to LCMV in the central nervous system (see *Fig. 16.11*). Removal of T cells protects the animal from death, indicating that they, rather than the virus, are damaging the brain. A similar mechanism has been postulated for chronic active hepatitis in man.

Viruses can infect cells of the immune system

Some viruses (e.g. HIV) directly infect lymphocytes or macrophages, resulting in pathogenic effects. Immuno-competent cells are also favoured sites of virus persistence. In the resting state, leucocytes harbour the virus in a non-infectious form; on activation of the infected cells the virus may also be reactivated, to produce infectious virus particles. Examples of viruses infecting B cells, T cells and macrophages are shown in *Figure 16.12*.

Human immunodeficiency virus (HIV) infects CD4⁺ cells

Many of the points raised in previous sections are illustrated by HIV, the retrovirus that causes AIDS. Infection with HIV is characterized by prolonged clinical latency, ineffective immunity, continuous virus mutation, neuropathology, and a tendency to infect bone marrow-derived cells and lymphocytes (see Chapter 21).

HIV is taken up by T cells following binding of a viral glycoprotein (gp120) to CD4. It also enters macrophages and other APCs by this route. However, entry into cells bearing Fc receptors can be enhanced by antibody, suggesting that this provides an alternative route into phagocytic cells, or enhances entry when CD4 is scarce.

There is a long but variable period of clinical latency; in about 50% of patients, progression to AIDS does not occur for 10 years. During this latent period, HIV can exist as a provirus, integrated within the host's genomic DNA, without any transcription occurring. Numerous factors can lead to the activation of transcription. *In vitro* both TNF and IL-6 cause increased production of infectious virus from latently infected T cell lines. This may be important *in vivo*, because monocytes from individuals carrying HIV tend to release abnormally large quantities of these cytokines; it is possible that there is a cycle of TNF and IL-6 release, leading to enhanced virus transcription (*Fig. 16.13*). This could lead to infection of further cells, and release of more cytokine. Production is increased *in vitro* by other cytokines and lymphokines, and by mitogens and phorbol esters. Elimination of the virus does not occur for a variety of reasons, including latency, viral mutation (giving rapid antigenic drift), and progressive immunodeficiency.

Lymphocytic choriomeningitis virus (LCM) in mice

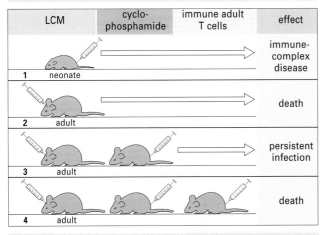

Fig. 16.11 The different effects of LCMV are related to differences in immune status. Infection of neonatal mice (1) produces chronic virus shedding and immune-complex disease, manifesting itself as glomerulonephritis and vasculitis. Intracerebral infection of adult mice (2) results in death. This is due to a T-cell reaction, since suppression of immunity with cyclophosphamide (3) leads to persistent infection, but prevents death. This 'protective' effect produced by cyclophosphamide can be reversed by T cells from an immune animal (4).

Virus infection of immunocompetent cells

B lymphocytes	Epstein–Barr virus murine gamma herpes virus infectious bursal disease virus
T lymphocytes	human T-lymphotrophic virus types 1 and 2 HIV measles virus herpes virus Saimiri human herpes virus 6
macrophages	Visna virus HIV lactate dehydrogenase virus cytomegalovirus

Fig. 16.12 Some viruses persist indefinitely in immunocompetent cells. Periodically, this infection may lead to pathological consequences, involving the death of the cell (HIV) or transformation leading to neoplasia (Epstein–Barr virus, HTLV–1).

Viral infection may provoke autoimmunity

Viruses may trigger autoimmune disease in a number of ways.

Virus induced damage – During the course of some virus infections tissues become damaged, provoking an inflammatory response during which 'hidden' antigens become exposed and can be processed and presented to the immune system. Examples of this include Theiler's virus (a murine picornavirus) and murine hepatitis virus infection of the nervous system, in which the constituents of myelin (the insulating material of axons) become targets for antibody and T cells.

In molecular mimicry – A sequence in a viral protein that is homologous to a 'self' protein becomes recognized, leading to a breakdown in immunological tolerance to cryptic self antigens in the consequent attack on host tissues by the immune system (see Chapter 27). Although experimental systems can be contrived to illustrate this mechanism, there is currently little evidence to suggest that it operates in natural virus infection.

Critical Thinking

■ What are the features of a virus that enable it to avoid host defence mechanisms?

■ A young boy was admitted to hospital suffering from a disseminated herpes virus infection. What immunotherapy would you prescribe and why?

Infection of lymphocytes and macrophages by HIV

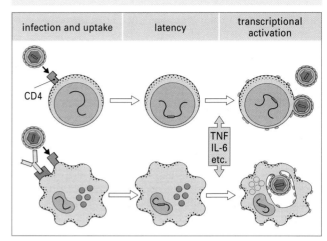

Fig. 16.13 The gp120 on the surface of HIV virions binds to CD4 on the lymphocyte membrane, and this triggers uptake. The virus can enter macrophages which express relatively low levels of CD4, but this may be assisted by binding through antibody to Fc receptors. The virus remains latent, integrated in the host cell's genomic DNA, until some stimulus (e.g. cytokines) causes transcriptional activation. Assembled viruses bud from the outer membrane of T cells, or into intracytoplasmic vacuoles of macrophages, where a large reservoir of potentially infectious particles can accumulate.

FURTHER READING

Borden EG, Rosenzweig IB, Byrne GI. Interferons: from virus inhibitor to modulator of amino acid and lipid metabolism. *Interferon Res* 1987;**7**:591.

Clements JE, Gdovin SL, Montelaro RC, Narayan O. Antigenic variation in lentiviral disease. *Annu Rev Immunol* 1988;**6**:139–59.

Doherty PC, Allan W, Eichelberger M, Carding SR. Roles of α/β and γ/δ T cell subsets in viral immunity. *Annu Rev Immunol* 1992;**10**:123–51.

Doherty PC. Cell-mediated cytotoxicity. *Cell* 1993;**75**:607.

Gooding LR. Virus proteins that counteract host immune defences. *Cell* 1992;**71**:5–7.

Levy JA. Pathogenesis of human immunodeficiency virus infection. *Microbio Rev* 1993;**57**:183–289.

Mims CA. Interactions of viruses with the immune system. *Clin Exp Immunol* 1986;**66**:1–16.

Nash AA, Cambouropoulos P. The immune response to herpes simplex virus. *Virology*, 1993;**4**:181–86

Oldstone MBA. Molecular mimicry and autoimmune disease. *Cell* 1987;**50**:819–20.

Ramsay AJ *et al.* A case for cytokines as effector molecules in the resolution of virus infection. *Immunol Today* 1993;**14**:155.

Sissons JG, Oldstone MBA. Antibody-mediated destruction of virus-infected cells. *Adv Immunol* 1980;**31**:1.

Smith GA. Virus strategies for evasion of the host response to infection. *Trends Microbiol* 1994;**2**:81–88.

Mechanisms of protection from a bacterial species can be deduced from the structure of the organism, particularly its cell wall, and its mode of pathogenicity.

Neutralizing antibody may be all that is needed for protection if the organism is pathogenic only because of a single toxin or adhesion molecule.

Non-specific, phylogenetically ancient recognition pathways for conserved bacterial structures can effect the rapid clearance of the vast majority of bacteria. These include phagocytosis, the alternative complement pathway and release of cytokines.

Complement can kill a few bacteria, particularly those with an exposed outer lipid bilayer, i.e. Gram-negative bacteria.

Phagocytes kill the majority of bacteria following a multistage process of chemotaxis, attachment, uptake and killing.

Successful pathogens have evolved a huge range of ways of avoiding the effects of complement, avoiding phagocyte function, or misdirecting the T-cell-dependent activation of phagocyte killing mechanisms.

Excessive release of cytokines caused by microorganisms can result in immunopathological syndromes, such as endotoxin shock and the Shwartzman reaction.

Chronic tissue-damaging immunopathology (as in tuberculosis) probably results from an imbalance of cytokine release patterns, leading to inappropriate effector functions.

Immunity to fungi is poorly understood but is apparently cell-mediated and similar to immunity to bacteria.

■ IMMUNITY TO BACTERIA

The defence mechanisms appropriate for a particular bacterial infection are related to the structure of the invading bacteria, and hence the immunological mechanisms to which they are susceptible, and to the mechanism of their pathogenicity.

Mechanisms of immunity are related to bacterial surface structure

There are four main types of bacterial cell wall (*Fig. 17.1*), belonging to the following groups:
- Gram-positive bacteria.
- Gram-negative bacteria.
- Mycobacteria.
- Spirochaetes.

The outer lipid bilayer of Gram-negative organisms is of particular importance because it is often susceptible to mechanisms that can lyse membranes, such as complement and certain cytotoxic cells. In contrast, killing of the other types of bacteria usually requires uptake by phagocytes.

The outer surface of the bacterium may also contain fimbriae or flagellae, or it may be covered by a protective capsule. These can impede the functions of phagocytes or complement, but they also act as targets for the antibody response, the role of which is discussed later (see p. 17.4)

Mechanisms of immunity are related to bacterial mechanisms of pathogenicity

The two extreme patterns of pathogenicity are:
- Toxicity without invasiveness.
- Invasiveness without toxicity (*Fig. 17.2*).

However, most bacteria are intermediate between these extremes, having some invasiveness assisted by some locally acting toxins and spreading factors (tissue-degrading enzymes).

Corynebacterium diphtheriae and *Vibrio cholerae* are examples of organisms that are toxic but not invasive. Since their pathogenicity depends almost entirely on toxin production, neutralizing antibody to the toxin is probably sufficient for immunity, although antibody, binding to the bacteria and so blocking their adhesion to the epithelium, could also be important.

In contrast, however, the pathogenicity of most invasive organisms does not rely so heavily on a single toxin, so immunity requires killing of the organisms themselves.

The first lines of defence are antibacterial mechanisms that do not depend on antigen recognition

The body's first line of defence against pathogenic bacteria consists of simple barriers to the entry or establishment of the infection. Thus, the skin and exposed epithelial surfaces have non-specific or innate protective systems which limit the entry of potentially invasive organisms (see *Fig. 1.1*). Intact skin is impenetrable to most bacteria. Additionally, fatty acids produced by the skin are toxic to many organisms. Indeed, the pathogenicity of some strains correlates with their ability to survive on the skin. Epithelial surfaces are cleansed, for example, by ciliary action in the trachea or by flushing of the urinary tract. Many bacteria are destroyed by pH changes in the stomach and vagina, both of which provide an acidic environment. In the vagina, the epithelium secretes glycogen, which is metabolized by particular species of commensal bacteria, producing lactic acid. More generally, commensals can limit pathogen invasion through production of antibacterial proteins termed colicins.

Bacterial cell walls

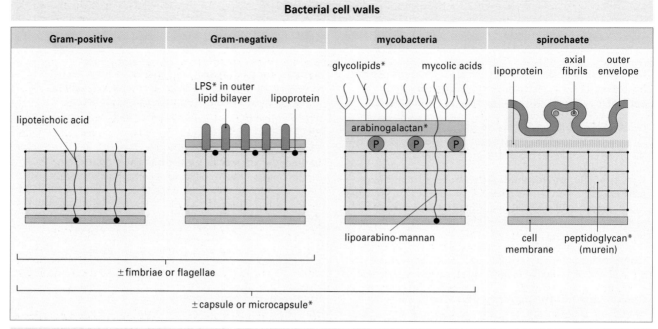

Fig. 17.1 Different immunological mechanisms have evolved to destroy the cell-wall structure of the different groups of bacteria. All types have an inner cell membrane and a peptidoglycan wall. Gram-negative bacteria also have an outer lipid bilayer in which lipopolysaccharide (LPS) is embedded. Lysosomal enzymes and lysozyme are active against the peptidoglycan layer, while cationic proteins and complement are effective against the outer lipid bilayer of the Gram-negative bacteria. The compound cell wall of the mycobacteria is extremely resistant to breakdown, and it is likely that this can only be achieved with the assistance of the bacterial enzymes working from within. Some bacteria also have fimbriae or flagellae, which can provide targets for the antibody response. Others have an outer capsule which renders the organisms more resistant to phagocytosis, or to complement. The components indicated with an asterisk (*) all have adjuvant properties; that is, they are recognized by the immune system as a non-specific signal that boosts immune activity.

Mechanisms of immunopathogenicity

Fig. 17.2 1. Some bacteria cause disease only because of a single toxin (e.g. *Corynebacterium diphtheriae, Clostridium tetani*) or because of an ability to attach to epithelial surfaces, without invading the host's tissues (e.g. in group A streptococcal sore throat). Immunity to such organisms may require only antibody to neutralize this critical function. 2. At the other extreme there are organisms which are not toxic, and cause disease by invasion of tissues and sometimes cells, where damage results mostly from the bulk of organisms, or from immunopathology (e.g. lepromatous leprosy). Where organisms invade cells, they must be destroyed and degraded by the cell-mediated immune response. 3. Most organisms fall between the two extremes, with some local

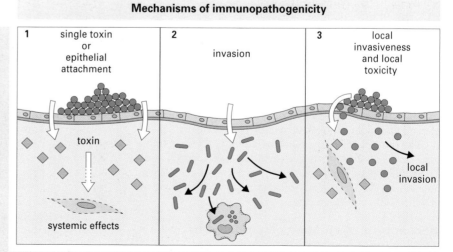

invasiveness assisted by local toxicity and enzymes which degrade extracellular matrix (e.g. *Staphylococcus aureus,* *Clostridium perfringens*). Antibody and cell-mediated responses are both involved in resistance.

Thus, when the normal flora are disturbed by antibiotics, infections by *Candida* or *Clostridium difficile* can occur.

In practice, only a minute proportion of the potentially pathogenic organisms around us ever succeed in gaining access to the tissues.

The second line of defence is mediated via recognition of common bacterial components

If the organisms do enter the tissues, they can be combated initially by further elements of the innate immune system. Numerous bacterial components are recognized in ways which do not rely on the antigen-specific receptors of either B cells or T cells. These types of recognition are phylogenetically ancient 'broad-spectrum' mechanisms that evolved before antigen-specific T cells and immunoglobulins, allowing protective responses to be triggered by common microbial components. Many organisms, such as non-pathogenic cocci, are probably removed from the tissues as a consequence of these pathways, without the need for a specific adaptive immune reaction. *Figure 17.3* shows some of the microbial components involved, and the host responses which are triggered. It is interesting to note that the 'Limulus assay', which is used to detect contaminating lipopolysaccharide (LPS) in preparations for use in man is based on one such recognition pathway found in an invertebrate species. In *Limulus polyphemus* (the horseshoe crab) tiny quantities of LPS trigger formation of fibrin which walls off the LPS-bearing infectious agent.

Lymphocyte-independent bacterial recognition pathways have several consequences

Activation of complement via the alternative pathway (see Chapter 13) – This may result in the killing of some bacteria, particularly those with an outer lipid bilayer susceptible to the lytic complex (C5b–9), i.e. Gram-negative bacteria. It also releases the chemotactic products, C3a and C5a. These cause smooth-muscle contraction and mast-cell degranulation, as well as attracting and activating neutrophils. The consequent release of histamine and leukotriene (LTB$_4$) contributes to further increases in vascular permeability (*Fig. 17.3*). Opsonization of the bacteria, by attachment of cleaved derivatives of C3, is important in subsequent interactions with phagocytes.

Chemotaxis – This attracts more phagocytes to the site of infection. It may be due both to complement activation and to direct chemotactic effects of bacterial products.

Release of cytokines from macrophages – The rapid release from macrophages of cytokines such as tumour necrosis factor

---

Protective mechanisms not involving antigen-specific B or T cells

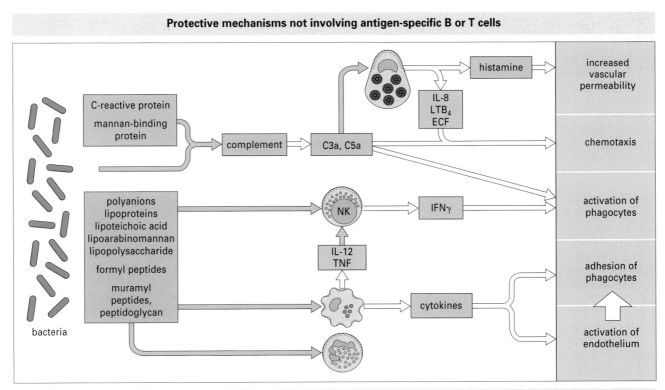

Fig. 17.3 Several common bacterial components are recognized by molecules present in serum, and by receptors on cells. These recognition pathways result in activation of the alternative complement pathway (Factors C3, B, D, P), with consequent release of C3a and C5a; activation of neutrophils, macrophages and NK cells; triggering of cytokine release; mast-cell degranulation, leading to increased blood flow in the local capillary network; increased adhesion of cells and fibrin to endothelial cells. These mechanisms, plus tissue injury caused by the bacteria, may activate the clotting system and fibrin formation, which limit bacterial spread.

(TNF) and interleukin-1 (IL-1) leads to systemic activation of phagocytic cells, and their increased adhesion to endothelium, facilitating their passage into inflamed tissue. There is also release of a family of small chemotactic peptides known as 'chemokines', which enhance the overall motility of cells (see Chapter 14).

Release of cytokines from natural killer (NK) cells – When murine NK cells are stimulated by IL-12 or TNF, they can release interferon-γ (IFNγ). This in turn can activate macrophages. This T-cell-independent pathway helps to explain the unexpected resistance of mice with SCID (severe combined immunodeficiency, a defect in lymphocyte maturation) to infections such as *Listeria monocytogenes.*

Adjuvant effects – 'Adjuvant' is derived from the Latin (*adiuvare,* to help). When given experimentally, soluble antigens evoke stronger T- and B-cell-mediated responses if they are mixed with bacterial components that act as adjuvants. Components with this property are indicated in *Figure 17.1.* The best known adjuvant in laboratory use, known as complete Freund's adjuvant, consists of killed *Mycobacterium tuberculosis* suspended in oil, which is then emulsified with the aqueous antigen solution. This effect probably reflects the fact that, when the antigen-specific immune response evolved, it did so in a tissue environment that already contained these pharmacologically active bacterial components. The response to a pure bacterial antigen, injected without adjuvant-active bacterial components, can be regarded as an artificial situation that does not occur in nature.

Selection of the appropriate lymphocyte-mediated response – 'Adjuvant' components of bacteria, and the early release of cytokines, play an important role in this. Different bacteria exert optimal adjuvant effects on different parameters of the immune system. This may reflect the need for the immune response to 'perform' some elementary 'taxonomy' on the infecting organism, so that it can activate the appropriate effector functions. Cytokine release by bacteria may also assist in this decision-making step, which is described in greater detail in Chapter 9.

Selection of inappropriate responses – Some microorganisms may exploit adjuvanticity to direct the immune response towards inappropriate mechanisms. Adjuvanticity is clearly an adaptation of the host. However, some microorganisms may exploit it to disturb immunoregulation, and so activate an inappropriate subset of helper T (TH) cells. This has been most clearly demonstrated in a model of infection of mice with the protozoan parasite *Leishmania major.* In this model, activation of TH2 cells leads to fatal disease, whereas activation of TH1 cells is fully protective (see Chapter 18).

Shock syndromes – If cytokine release is sudden and massive, several acute tissue-damaging syndromes can result and these are potentially fatal (see p. 17.14).

Antibody provides a further antigen-specific protective mechanism

The relevance to protection of interactions of bacteria with antibody depends on the mechanism of pathogenicity.

Antibody clearly plays a crucial role in dealing with bacterial toxins. It neutralizes diphtheria toxin by blocking the attachment of the binding portion of the molecule to its target cells. Similarly it may block locally acting toxins or extracellular matrix-degrading enzymes which act as spreading factors, and it can interfere with motility by binding to flagellae.

An important function on external and mucosal surfaces, often performed by secretory IgA (sIgA – see Chapter 3), is to stop bacteria binding to epithelial cells. For instance, antibody to the M proteins of group A streptococci gives type-specific immunity to streptococcal sore throats. It is also likely that some antibodies to the bacterial surface can block functional requirements of the organism such as binding of iron-chelating compounds or intake of nutrients (*Fig. 17.4*).

However, the most important role of antibody in immunity to non-toxigenic bacteria is the more efficient targeting of complement. With the aid of antibodies, even organisms that

The antibacterial roles of antibody

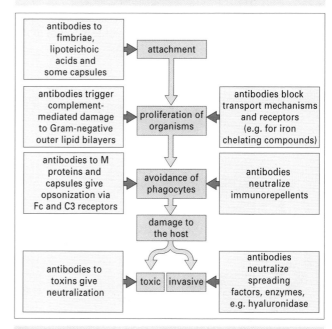

Fig. 17.4 This diagram lists the stages of bacterial invasion (blue) and indicates the antibacterial effects of antibody (yellow) that operate at the different stages. Antibodies to fimbriae, lipoteichoic acid and some capsules block attachment of the bacterium to the host-cell membrane. Antibody triggers complement-mediated damage to Gram-negative outer lipid bilayers. Antibody directly blocks bacterial surface proteins that pick up useful molecules from the environment and transport them across the membrane. Antibody to M proteins and capsules opsonizes the bacteria via Fc and C3 receptors for phagocytosis. Bacterial factors that interfere with normal chemotaxis or phagocytosis, are neutralized. Bacterial toxins may be neutralized by antibody, as may bacterial spreading factors that facilitate invasion (for example by the destruction of connective tissue or fibrin).

resist the alternative (i.e. innate) pathway (see below) are damaged by complement, or become coated with C3 products, which then enhance the binding and uptake by phagocytes (*Figs 17.5* and *17.6*). The most efficient complement-fixing antibodies in man are IgG1, IgG3 and IgM. IgG1 and IgG3 are also the subclasses with the highest affinity for Fc receptors.

Pathogenic bacteria can avoid the detrimental effects of complement

Some bacterial capsules are very poor activators of the alternative pathway (*Fig. 17.7*). Alternatively, long side-chains (O antigens) on bacterial LPS may fix C3b at a distance from the otherwise vulnerable lipid bilayer. Similarly, smooth-surfaced Gram-negative organisms (*Escherichia coli*, *Salmonella* spp., *Pseudomonas* spp.) may fix but then rapidly shed the C5b–C9 membrane lytic complex.

Other organisms exploit the physiological mechanisms that block destruction of host cells by complement. When C3b has attached to a surface it can either interact with factor B leading to further C3b amplification, or it can become inactivated by factors H and I. Capsules rich in sialic acid (as host-cell membranes are) seem to promote this interaction

Effect of antibody and complement on rate of clearance of virulent bacteria from the blood

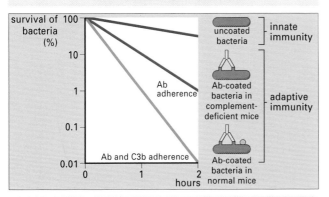

Fig. 17.5 Uncoated bacteria are phagocytosed rather slowly (unless the alternative pathway is activated by the strain of bacterium); on coating with antibody, adherence to phagocytes is increased many-fold. The adherence is somewhat less effective in animals temporarily depleted of complement.

The interaction between bacteria and phagocytic cells

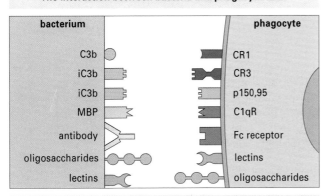

Fig. 17.6 A variety of molecules facilitate the binding of the organisms to the phagocyte membrane. The precise nature of the interaction may determine whether uptake occurs, and whether appropriate killing mechanisms are triggered. Note that apart from complement, antibody and mannan-binding protein (MBP) which bind to the bacterial surface, the other components are constitutive bacterial molecules.

Avoidance of complement-mediated damage

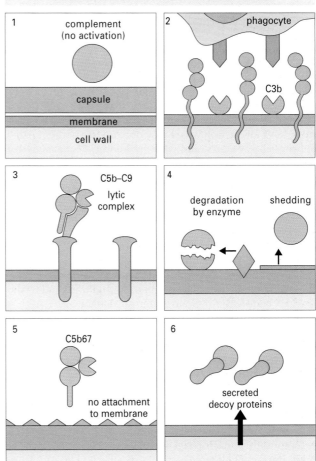

Fig. 17.7 Bacteria avoid complement-mediated damage by a variety of strategies. 1. An outer capsule or coat prevents complement activation. 2. An outer surface can be configured so that complement receptors on phagocytes cannot obtain access to fixed C3b. 3. Surface structures can be expressed which divert attachment of the lytic complex (MAC) from the cell membrane. 4. Membrane-bound enzyme can degrade fixed complement or cause it to be shed. 5. The outer membrane can resist the insertion of the lytic complex. 6. Secreted decoy proteins can cause complement to be deposited on them and not on the bacterium itself.

with H and I. *Neisseria meningitidis*, *E. coli* K1, and group B streptococci all resist complement attachment in this way. The M protein of group A streptococci acts as an acceptor for factor H, thus potentiating C3bB dissociation. These bacteria also have a gene for a C5a protease.

Ultimately most bacteria are killed by phagocytes

A few, mostly Gram-negative, bacteria are directly killed by complement, as stated earlier. There are also reports that some organisms, particularly Gram-negative bacteria, can be killed by mere contact with NK cells, or even cytotoxic T (Tc) cells. This probably involves the membrane-lysing mechanism of these cells (see Chapter 9), acting on the outer lipid bilayer that is characteristic of Gram-negative organisms.

However, most bacteria are killed by phagocytes. This process involves several steps (see *Fig. 1.15*).

Chemotaxis – Bacterial components such as f-Met-Leu-Phe (which is chemotactic for leucocytes), complement products such as C5a, and locally released chemokines and cytokines attract the phagocytes (see Chapter 14).

Attachment of the phagocyte to the organism – This is an important interaction which may determine whether uptake subsequently occurs, and whether killing mechanisms are triggered during uptake. The binding can be mediated by the following entities.

- **Lectins on the organism**, for example the mannose-binding lectin on the fimbriae of *E. coli*.
- **Lectins on the phagocyte.** Of particular interest in this respect are the complement receptors CR3 and p150,95 and the related molecule LFA-1 (leucocyte functional antigen-1 – a mediator of intercellular adhesion), which have multiple binding sites specific for different carbohydrate moieties. They can bind to β-glucans and to the LPS endotoxin of Gram-negative bacteria.
- **Complement deposited on the organism** via the alternative or classical pathways. It has recently been discovered that complement can also be fixed by mannan-binding protein present in serum, which can itself bind to C1q receptors.
- **Fc receptors on the phagocyte**, which link to antibody bound to the bacteria (see *Fig. 17.6*).

Triggering of uptake – The binding of an organism to a receptor on the macrophage membrane does not always lead to its uptake. For example, zymosan particles (derived from yeast) bind via the glucan-recognizing lectin-like site on the CR3 of the macrophage and are taken up, whereas erythrocytes coated with iC3b are not, even though the iC3b also binds to CR3.

Triggering of microbicidal activity – Just as the binding of an organism to membrane receptors does not guarantee uptake, so uptake does not guarantee the triggering of killing mechanisms. For example, *Yersinia pseudotuberculosis* induces its own uptake, but it also releases a gene product that modulates the uptake signal so that killing is not also triggered.

Phagocytic cells have many microbicidal mechanisms

Once the organism has been internalized by the phagocyte, it is exposed to an array of killing mechanisms.

One subset of killing mechanisms is dependent on oxygen

Reactive oxygen intermediates (ROIs) – This pathway involves an enzyme in the phagocyte membrane which reduces oxygen (O_2) to superoxide anion ($\cdot O_2^-$), a ROI which is toxic. This in turn generates other ROIs (*Fig. 17.8*). Cells from patients with chronic granulomatous disease lack this pathway, and so are unable to kill some microorganisms (see Fig. 21.16). The disease is characterized by chronic inflammatory lesions involving pyogenic organisms, for example staphylococci. If peroxidase is present, toxic bleach-like compounds are generated (*Fig. 17.8*); thus the monocytes of individuals with congenital myeloperoxidase deficiency may show defective microbicidal activity. Tissue macrophages do not contain peroxidase and thus do not carry out the peroxidase-dependent reactions.

Reactive nitrogen intermediates (RNIs) – This pathway (*Fig. 17.9*) results in the formation of nitric oxide (NO), which is toxic for bacteria and tumour cells. For optimal expression of this mechanism, macrophages need both activation by IFNγ, and triggering by TNF. This may be the mechanism which enables murine macrophages to kill mycobacteria, but human macrophages seem unable to generate significant quantities of NO. However, other human cell types can do so, and this may be one way in which they protect themselves from microbial invasion.

Oxygen-independent killing mechanisms may be important

These mechanisms may be more important than was previously thought. Many organisms can be killed by cells from patients with chronic granulomatous disease, which cannot produce reactive oxygen intermediates, or from patients with myeloperoxidase deficiency, which cannot produce hypohalous acids. Some of this killing may be due to NO, but many organisms can be killed anaerobically, so other mechanisms must exist. Some have been identified.

Cationic proteins with antibiotic-like properties – The defensins are cysteine- and arginine-rich cationic peptides of 30–33 amino acids, found in rabbit macrophages and human neutrophil polymorphs, where they comprise 30–50% of the granule proteins. They form ion-permeable channels in lipid bilayers. They are most effective at pH 7.0 so they probably act early after phagolysosome formation, before acidification takes place (*Fig. 17.10*). Defensins can kill organisms as diverse as *Staphylococcus aureus*, *Pseudomonas aeruginosa*, *E. coli*, *Cryptococcus neoformans* and the enveloped virus Herpes simplex. There are also cationic proteins with different pH optima, including cathepsin G and azurocidin, both of which are related to elastase but which have activity against Gram-negative bacteria; this is unrelated to their enzyme activity.

Other antimicrobial mechanisms – Following lysosome fusion there is a transient rise in pH before acidification (a fall in pH) of the phagolysosome takes place. This occurs

Oxygen-dependent microbicidal activity

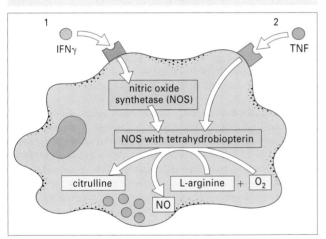

Fig. 17.8 1. An enzyme in the phagosome membrane reduces oxygen to superoxide anion ($\cdot O_2^-$). This can give rise to hydroxyl radicals ($\cdot OH$), singlet oxygen ($\Delta g^1 O_2$) and hydrogen peroxide (H_2O_2), all of which are potentially toxic. Lysosome fusion is not required for these parts of the pathway, and the reaction takes place spontaneously following formation of the phagosome. 2. If lysosome fusion occurs, myeloperoxidase may enter the phagosome. Myeloperoxidase (or under some circumstances, catalase from peroxisomes) acts on peroxides in the presence of halides (preferably iodide). Then additional toxic oxidants, such as hypohalite (HIO, HClO), are generated.

The nitric oxide pathway

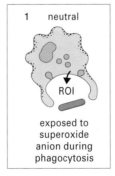

Fig. 17.9 Nitric oxide synthetase combines oxygen with the guanidino nitrogen of L-arginine to give nitric oxide, which is toxic for bacteria and tumour cells. Tetrahydrobiopterin is needed as a co-factor. IFNγ activates the pathway (1), which is then optimally triggered by TNF (2). Paradoxically, it is doubtful whether human macrophages can make tetrahydrobiopterin, but neutrophils and other human cell types can do so. This pathway may therefore be important for the self-defence of non-immunological tissue cells.

Mechanism involved in bacterial killing

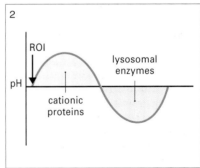

Fig. 17.10 During phagocytosis there is immediate exposure to reactive oxygen intermediates (ROIs) (1). This leads to a transient increase in pH, when cationic proteins may be effective (2). Subsequently the pH falls, as H^+ ions are pumped into the phagolysosome and lysosomal enzymes with low pH optima become effective. Lactoferrin acts by chelating free iron, and can do so at alkaline or acidic pH.

within 10–15 minutes. Killing of some organisms may be due to the acidification itself, though it is more likely to be related to the low pH optima of lysosomal enzymes. Certain Gram-positive organisms may be killed by lysozyme, which is active against their readily exposed peptidoglycan layer. A variety of other substances, such as lactoferrin (produced by

neutrophil polymorphs), have also been implicated in killing. Lactoferrin can bind iron and render it unavailable to bacteria even at an acid pH (thus, the ability of polymorphs to kill some bacteria is lost if they are loaded with iron). These mechanisms may all require phagolysosome fusion (*Figs 17.10* and *17.11*).

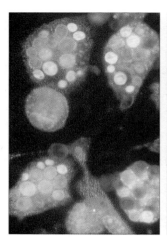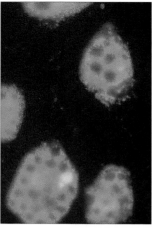

Fig. 17.11 Inhibition of fusion of secondary lysosomes with yeast-containing phagosomes by the addition of ammonium chloride. Mouse peritoneal macrophages were incubated in acridine orange, which concentrates in secondary lysosomes. Live baker's yeast was then added – these assume the appearance of 'holes' in the cell. Normally, the secondary lysosomes fuse with the phagosomes, and the acridine orange enters them, fluorescing green, yellow or orange depending on the concentration (left). However, in the presence of ammonium chloride, fusion does not occur and the 'holes' remain dark (right). Such blocking of lysosomal fusion may be employed by *M. tuberculosis* and some leishmania, which secrete ammonia. Some polyanions, such as polyglutamic acid or suramin, may also do this. (Courtesy of Mr R. Young and Dr P. D. Hart.)

Resting macrophages can kill, but killing can be enhanced, and new mechanisms can be expressed on activation

Activation occurs through exposure to microbial products, and to lymphokines derived from T cells. Similarly, the decline that usually occurs if the cells are kept in culture for a week can be reversed by treatment with suitable activating stimuli (*Fig. 17.12*).

Some microbial products can activate macrophages in the absence of lymphocyte recognition

A number of microbial products cause direct activation of monocytes and macrophages, or indirect activation by triggering cytokine release from them or from NK cells. The cytokines then activate the phagocytes. This was discussed earlier (p. 17.3) in relation to the non-lymphocyte-dependent recognition of bacteria.

Further activation of macrophages is mediated by lymphokines

In vivo, lymphokines released during T-cell-mediated responses are often required for phagocytes to become fully activated. The lymphokine most often implicated is IFNγ, which enhances both oxygen-dependent and oxygen-independent killing mechanisms. There are also reports implicating IL-2, granulocyte–macrophage colony stimulating factor (GM–CSF), TNF, and other cytokines. As discussed in greater detail in Chapter 9, activation of some functions requires combinations of cytokines.

Lymphokines *in vivo* have two effects on phagocytes – attracting them and activating them – and the relative importance of these two components differs for different organisms. Thus for immunity to *L. monocytogenes*, which can be killed by the baseline levels of oxygen-dependent mechanisms in both monocytes and neutrophils, it is the

Antibacterial function of human monocytes and macrophages

bacteria	cells at day 0 untreated	cultured for 7 days	
		untreated	treated with IFNγ
Escherichia coli	killed	killed	not affected
Salmonella typhimurium *Listeria monocytogenes*	killed	not killed	killed (this effect not blocked by glucocorticoids)
Legionella pneumophila	not killed	not killed	
Nocardia asteroides	killed	?	killed (this effect blocked by glucocorticoids)
Mycobacterium tuberculosis	not killed	not killed	variable (some stasis, but no killing by cells from some donors; 1,25-dihydroxycholecalciferol is more active than IFNγ in this system)
Chlamydia psittaci	killed	not killed	killed
Chlamydia trachomatis	killed	killed	not affected
C. trachomatis biovar *lymphogranuloma venereum*	killed	not killed	killed

Fig. 17.12 The table shows the ability of monocyte or macrophage preparations (from various donors) to kill the indicated organisms. These cells have an intrinsic ability to kill many bacteria. This may be partly lost after 7 days in culture, but it can often be restored by treatment with IFNγ. This lymphokine clearly activates several different killing pathways, some of which are inhibited by glucocorticoids, while others are not. Other organisms are killed only after lymphokine-mediated activation, while a few may not be killed at all. This emphasizes the complexity of the killing pathways.

attraction of the cells to the lesion which is most important. In contrast, for *M. tuberculosis*, which thrives inside neutrophils and monocytes, it is the activation of the cells which is critical.

Human and murine macrophages are different

This is important because much experimental work is based on murine macrophages. Mycobacteria illustrate the complexity of this topic. IFNγ can activate murine macrophages to destroy mycobacteria completely. This appears to be due to the nitric oxide pathway. However, IFNγ acting on human macrophages causes, at best, feeble inhibition of *M. tuberculosis* or, at worst, significantly increased growth. This may be because human macrophages, unlike murine ones, seem unable to make tetrahydrobiopterin, an essential co-factor for NO production (see *Fig. 17.9*).

On the other hand, human cells do something which has not been reported in murine cells. IFNγ causes human macrophages to express a 1-hydroxylase enzyme that converts the circulating inactive form of 25-hydroxycholecalciferol (vitamin D_3) into an active metabolite, 1,25-dihydroxycholecalciferol. This metabolite activates antimycobacterial mechanisms in the macrophages rather more efficiently than IFNγ itself (see *Fig. 17.12*).

Successful pathogens have evolved mechanisms for the avoidance of phagocyte-mediated killing

Since most organisms are ultimately killed by phagocytes, it is not surprising that successful pathogens have evolved an array of mechanisms to counteract this risk (see *Fig. 17.13*).

Intracellular pathogens may 'hide' in cells that have antimicrobial potential

Infected cells can be killed by Tc cells

Some organisms may thrive inside damaged or metabolically deranged host phagocytes, or escape killing by moving out of phagosomes into the cytoplasm. Other organisms, such as *Mycobacterium leprae*, can cause themselves to be taken up by cells that are not normally considered phagocytic, and have little antibacterial potential. Before they can be taken up by fresh activated phagocytes, or exposed to other killing mechanisms, the organisms may need to be released from such cells. Tc cells may perform this function by killing the infected cell. For instance mice become strikingly susceptible to *M. tuberculosis* if the β_2-microglobulin gene is knocked out so that Class I MHC cannot be recognized by the Tc cells. This is consistent with an essential role for cytotoxic CD8[+] T cells.

γδ T cells are usually cytotoxic, and may kill infected cells

A large proportion of T cells bearing γδ receptors seem to proliferate in response to bacterial antigens. Some subsets of these cells home to epithelial surfaces (see Chapter 2). Thus it seems likely that they have a role in infection, but this is not yet understood. In general they are cytotoxic, so they may destroy parasitized cells.

Some tissue cells can express antimicrobial mechanisms

Tissue cells which are not components of the immune system can also harbour bacteria such as *M. leprae*, invasive

Shigella and *Salmonella* species, or *Rickettsia* and *Chlamydia*. As mentioned earlier, these infected cells may be sacrificed by Tc. On the other hand, activation of fibroblasts by IFNγ can inhibit growth of intracellular organisms, probably via the NO pathway, which is not confined to phagocytic cells.

The response to bacteria can result in immunological tissue damage

Excessive cytokine release can lead to endotoxin shock

Endotoxin (septicaemic) shock occurs when there is massive production of cytokines, usually caused by bacterial products released during septicaemic episodes. Endotoxin (LPS) from Gram-negative bacteria is usually responsible, though Gram-positive septicaemia can cause a similar syndrome. There can

Evasion mechanisms of bacteria

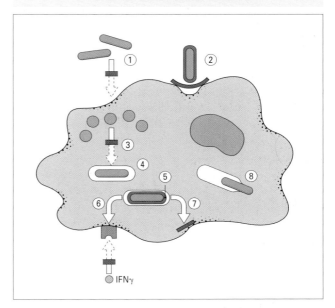

Fig. 17.13 Bacteria, particularly those which are successful intracellular parasites, have evolved the ability to evade different aspects of phagocyte-mediated killing. 1. Some can secrete repellents or toxins that inhibit chemotaxis. 2. Others have capsules or outer coats which inhibit attachment by the phagocyte. 3. Others permit uptake but release factors that block subsequent triggering of killing mechanisms. Once ingested some, such as *M. tuberculosis*, secrete molecules which inhibit lysosome fusion with the phagosome. 4. They may also secrete catalase which breaks down hydrogen peroxide. 5. Organisms such as *M. leprae* have highly resistant outer coats. *M. leprae* surrounds itself with a phenolic glycolipid which scavenges free radicals. 6. Mycobacteria also release a lipoarabinomannan, which blocks the ability of macrophages to respond to the activating effects of IFNγ. 7. Infected cells may also lose their efficacy as antigen-presenting cells. 8. Several organisms (e.g. *M. leprae*), can escape from the phagosome to multiply in the cytoplasm. Finally, the organism (e.g. *M. tuberculosis*) may kill the phagocyte.

be life-threatening fever, circulatory collapse, diffuse intra-vascular coagulation, and haemorrhagic necrosis, leading eventually to multiple organ failure (*Fig. 17.14*).

The Shwartzman reaction is a form of cytokine-dependent tissue damage occurring in inflammatory sites without a significant T-cell component

Shwartzman observed that if Gram-negative organisms were injected into the skin of rabbits, followed by a second dose given intravenously 24 hours later, haemorrhagic necrosis occurred at the prepared skin site. This is known as the Shwartzman reaction. He also noted that two intravenous injections 24 hours apart caused a systemic reaction, commonly involving circulatory collapse and bilateral necrosis of the renal cortex. Sanarelli had made similar observations and this is now known as the systemic Shwartzman or Sanarelli–Shwartzman reaction. These reactions can also be accompanied by necrosis in the pancreas, pituitary, adrenals and gut. There is marked diffuse intravascular coagulation and thrombosis.

Many other organisms are now known to 'prepare' the skin in the same way, including streptococci, mycobacteria, *Haemophilus* spp., corynebacteria and vaccinia virus. Endotoxin (LPS) is the active component of the intravenous 'triggering' injection. Early work implicated endothelial changes, fibrin deposition, neutrophil accumulation and degranulation, and platelets as mediating the damage. This is correct, but it is now clear that TNFα, IFNγ, IL-12 and IL-1 are the critical mediators (see Chapter 9). Direct injection of TNFα into sites of inflammation (evoked by a previous injection of bacteria) causes a similar type of necrosis; the injected TNFα may be doing the same work as the TNFα that arrives via the circulation after an intravenous dose of LPS.

This phenomenon explains the characteristic haemorrhagic rash seen in children with meningococcal meningitis. A first episode of septicaemia results in widespread inflammatory sites which are small and subclinical at the time, but which remain exquisitely cytokine-sensitive. A second, larger septicaemic episode triggers enough cytokine release to cause necrosis in those sites.

The Koch phenomenon is necrosis occurring in T-cell-mediated mycobacterial lesions and skin-test sites

This is a necrotic response to antigens of *M. tuberculosis*, originally demonstrated by Robert Koch in tuberculous guinea pigs (*Fig. 17.15*). It may be related to the necrosis, which also occurs in the lesions in this disease. It is at least partly due to the release of cytokines into a T-cell-mediated inflammatory site (delayed hypersensitivity site – see Chapter 25). Such sites can be extremely sensitive to the tissue-damaging effects of cytokines, as seen in the Shwartzman reaction, particularly when there is mixed TH1 and TH2 activity.

Figure 17.16 uses examples to illustrate the relationship between the nature of the organism, the disease and immunopathology caused, and the mechanism of immune response which leads to protection.

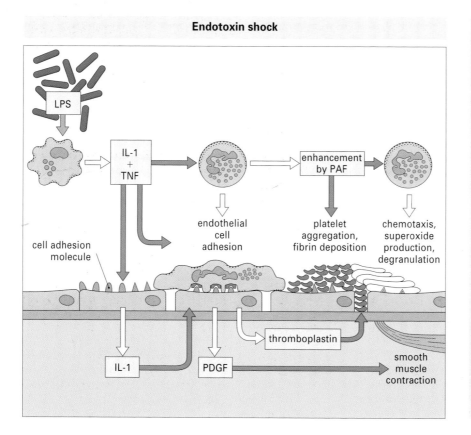

Endotoxin shock

Fig. 17.14 Excessive release of cytokines, often triggered by the endotoxin (LPS) of Gram-negative bacteria, can lead to diffuse intravascular coagulation with consequent defective clotting, changes in vascular permeability, loss of fluid into the tissues, a fall in blood pressure, circulatory collapse, and haemorrhagic necrosis, particularly in the gut. This figure illustrates some important parts of this pathway at the cellular level. The cytokines TNF and IL-1 cause endothelial cells to express cell adhesion molecules and tissue thromboplastin. These promote adhesion of circulating cells and deposition of fibrin, respectively. Platelet activating factor (PAF) enhances these effects. In experimental models, shock can be blocked by neutralizing antibodies to TNF, and greatly diminished by antibodies to tissue thromboplastin, or by inhibitors of PAF. Gram-positive bacteria can induce shock, for example by massive release of cytokines mediated by superantigens (see opposite). (PDGF = platelet-derived growth factor, produced by both platelets and endothelium.)

The Koch phenomenon

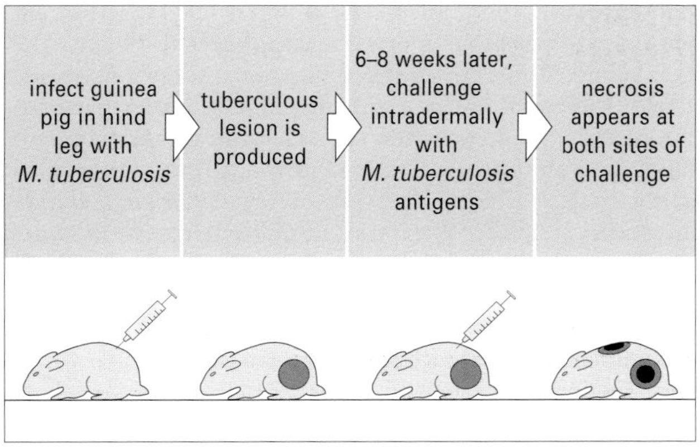

| infect guinea pig in hind leg with *M. tuberculosis* | tuberculous lesion is produced | 6–8 weeks later, challenge intradermally with *M. tuberculosis* antigens | necrosis appears at both sites of challenge |

Fig. 17.15 Robert Koch observed that injection of *Mycobacterium tuberculosis*, or soluble antigens from *M. tuberculosis*, into the skin of tuberculous guinea-pigs resulted in a necrotizing reaction both at the challenge site, and in the original tuberculous lesion. This is at least partly due to the fact that the delayed hypersensitivity reaction to mycobacterial antigens can, like the LPS-injected site in the Shwartzman reaction, be very sensitive to the toxicity of cytokines. These may be released locally in the skin-test site. A similar reaction is seen in humans who have, or have had, tuberculosis. Responses to the same antigen, in individuals who are skin-test positive as a result of BCG vaccination, do not usually show necrosis.

Immunity in some important bacterial infections

infection	pathogenesis	major defence mechanisms
Corynebacterium diphtheriae	non-invasive pharyngitis – toxin	neutralizing antibody
Vibrio cholerae	non-invasive enteritis – toxin	neutralizing and adhesion-blocking antibodies
Neisseria meningitidis (Gram-negative)	nasopharynx →bacteraemia →meningitis →endotoxaemia	killed by antibody and lytic complement; opsonized and phagocytosed
Staphylococcus aureus (Gram-positive)	locally invasive and toxic in skin etc.	osponized by antibody and complement; killed by phagocytes
Mycobacterium tuberculosis	invasive, evokes immunopathology, ? toxic	? macrophage activation by cytokines from T cells
Mycobacterium leprae	invasive, space-occupying and/or immunopathology	? macrophage activation by cytokines from T cells

Fig. 17.16 This table provides examples of how a knowledge of the organism, and the mechanism of disease, can lead to a prediction of the relevant protective mechanism.

New topics in bacterial immunology

Superantigens bypass antigen processing and presentation

These recently recognized bacterial components are so named because they bind directly (i.e. unprocessed) to the variable regions of β chains (Vβ) of antigen receptors on certain subsets of T cells, and cross-link them to the MHC of antigen-presenting cells (APCs) (see Fig. 2.30). As a result, all T cells bearing the relevant Vβ gene product are activated, without the processing and presentation of the antigen as peptides in the cleft of the MHC that is normally required for T-cell activation. Such superantigens have been found in staphylococci, streptococci, mycoplasmas and other species. The full biological significance of this bacterial adaptation is not yet clear, but one obvious effect can be the toxicity of the massive cytokine/lymphokine release that results from the simultaneous stimulation of a large subset of T cells. The staphylococcal toxins responsible for the toxic shock syndrome (TSST-1, etc.) appear to operate in this way.

Heat shock proteins (stress proteins) are highly conserved and prominent targets of immune responses

These proteins are found in all eukaryotic and prokaryotic cells, where they have essential roles in the assembly, folding and transport of other molecules. Cells exposed to abnormally elevated temperatures (or to other stresses) express higher levels of these proteins, which reflects their role in the stabilization of protein structure. Their amino acid sequences are very highly conserved and there is currently much speculation that, because bacterial heat shock proteins are so similar to human ones, they may be involved in the initiation of autoimmunity. Paradoxically, in spite of their similarity to host proteins, they seem to be target antigens in the protective response against many infectious organisms. This makes sense from an evolutionary point of view, because if the host possesses T cells that recognize a range of conserved heat shock protein epitopes, these T cells are likely to recognize any pathogen encountered.

▪ IMMUNITY TO FUNGI

There are four categories of fungal infection

Little is known of the precise mechanisms involved in immunity to fungal infections, but it is thought they are essentially similar to those involved in resistance to bacterial infections. The fungal infections of man fall into four major categories.

- **Superficial mycoses:** these are caused by fungi known as dermatophytes, and are usually restricted to the non-living keratinized components of skin, hair and nails.
- **Subcutaneous mycoses:** saprophytic fungi can cause chronic nodules or ulcers in subcutaneous tissues following trauma, for example chromomycosis, sporotrichosis and mycetoma.
- **Respiratory mycoses:** soil saprophytes produce subclinical or acute lung infections (rarely disseminated), or granulomatous lesions, e.g. histoplasmosis and coccidioidomycosis.
- **Candidiasis:** *Candida albicans* (a ubiquitous commensal) causes superficial (rarely systemic) infections of skin and mucous membranes.

Cell–mediated immunity is apparently the basis of resistance

Cutaneous fungal infections are usually self-limiting and recovery is associated with a certain limited resistance to re-infection. Resistance is apparently based on cell-mediated immunity, since patients develop delayed-type (Type IV) hypersensitivity reactions to fungal antigens, and the occurrence of chronic infections is associated with a lack of these

reactions. T-cell immunity is also implicated in resistance to other fungal infections, since resistance can sometimes be transferred with immune T cells. It is presumed that TH cells release cytokines that activate macrophages to destroy the fungi (*Fig. 17.17*). In respiratory mycoses, spectra of disease activity somewhat similar to the spectrum of activity in leprosy can be seen (see Chapter 25). Disturbance of normal physiology by immunosuppressive drugs, or of normal flora by antibiotics, can predispose to invasion by *Candida*. *Candida* infections are also common in immunodeficiency diseases (severe combined immunodeficiency, thymic aplasia, AIDS, etc.), implying that the immune system is involved in confining the fungus to its normal commensal sites.

There is also evidence for neutrophil polymorph involvement in immunity to some respiratory mycoses such as mucormycosis (*Fig. 17.18*). It is possible that the cationic proteins (defensins – see p. 17.7) are important for protection from fungi, since phagocytes from patients with defective oxygen reduction pathways nevertheless kill yeast and hyphae with near normal efficiency (*Fig. 17.19*). However, the nitric oxide pathway is effective against *Cryptococcus*, and this mechanism may turn out to be important for many fungi.

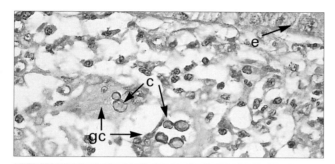

Fig. 17.17 Evidence for T-cell immunity in chromomycosis. The pigmented fungal cells of chromomycosis (a subcutaneous mycosis) (c) are visible inside giant cells (gc) in the dermis of a patient. The area is surrounded by a predominantly mononuclear cell infiltrate. The basal layer of epidermis (e) is visible at the top of the frame. H&E stain, × 400. (Courtesy of Prof R.J. Hay)

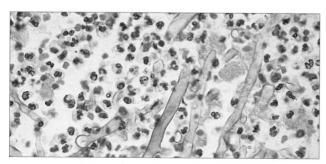

Fig. 17.18 Evidence for neutrophil-mediated immunity to mucormycosis. This is a section through a lung of a patient suffering from mucormycosis – an opportunistic infection in an immunosuppressed subject. The inflammatory reaction consists almost entirely of neutrophil polymorphs around the fungal hyphae. The disease is particularly associated with neutropenia (lack of neutrophils). Silver stain, × 400. (Courtesy of Prof R.J. Hay)

Monocyte/macrophage killing of fungi

organism	source of monocytes/macrophages		
	normal	chronic granulomatous disease	myeloperoxidase deficiency
Candida albicans	killed	sometimes killed	sometimes killed
Candida parapsilosis	killed	not killed	unknown
Cryptococcus neoformans	killed	unknown	killed
Aspergillus fumigatus conidia	killed	killed	unknown
Aspergillus fumigatus hyphae	killed	killed	unknown

Fig. 17.19 Many fungi are killed by monocytes or macrophages. Cells from patients with chronic granulomatous disease and individuals with myeloperoxidase deficiency can also effect killing, showing that non-oxygen-dependent mechanisms are important.

Critical Thinking

■ How many different microbicidal mechanisms do we know of, which are available to phagocytes?

■ What is the role of the massive load of bowel flora in autoimmune disease?

■ In what ways can bacteria distort the machinery of a phagocyte to evade destruction once they have been endocytosed? What examples are there of such evasion techniques?

■ How can we determine the roles of complement and phagocytes in the killing of different micro-organisms? What genetic or molecular biological techniques could be used to disect the mechanisms which allow organisms to evade these effector mechanisms?

■ What is the role of cytokines in activating macrophages to destroy phagocytosed bacteria? Is such activation always beneficial to the host?

FURTHER READING

General

Roitt IM, Delves PJ, eds. *Encyclopedia of Immunology*. London: Academic Press, 1992. (See numerous entries under names of individual fungi and bacteria.)

Bacteria

Catterall JR, Black CM, Leventhal JP, Rizk NW, Wachtel JS, Remington JS. Nonoxidative microbicidal activity in normal human alveolar and peritoneal macrophages. *Infect Immun* 1987;**55**:635.

Chan J, Xing Y, Magliozzo RS, Bloom BR. Killing of virulent *Mycobacterium tuberculosis* by reactive nitrogen intermediates produced by activated murine macrophages. *J Exp Med* 1992;**175**:1111.

Cohen IR, Young DB. Autoimmunity, microbial immunity and the immunological homunculus. *Immunol. Today* 1991;**12**:105.

De Libero G, Kaufmann SHE. Antigen-specific Lyt2 cytolytic T lymphocytes from mice infected with the intracellular bacterium *Listeria monocytogenes*. *J Immunol* 1986;**137**:2688.

Falkow S, Isberg RR, Portnoy DA. The interaction of bacteria with mammalian cells. *Annu.Rev.Cell.Biol* 1992;**8**:333.

Fleischer B. Superantigens. APMIS (1994) **102**:3–12

Kagan BL, Ganz T, Lehrer RI. Defensins: a family of antimicrobial and cytotoxic peptides. *Toxicology* 1994;**87**:131.

Kaufmann SH. Immunity to intracellular bacteria. *Annu Rev Immunol* 1993;**11**:129.

Lynn WA, Golenbock DT. Lipopolysaccharide antagonists. *Immunol Today* 1992;**13**(7):271.

Mims CA, Playfair JHL, Roitt IM, Wakelin D, Williams R, eds. *Medical Microbiology*. London: Mosby, 1993.

Moffitt MC, Frank MM. Complement resistance in microbes. *Springer Semin Immunopathology* 1994;**15**:327.

Ofek I, Sharon N. Lectinophagocytosis: a molecular mechanism of recognition between cell surface's sugars and lectins in the phagocytosis of bacteria. *Infect Immun 1988*;**56**:539.

Orme I, Flynn JL, Bloom BR. The role of CD8+ T cells in immunity to tuberculosis. *Trends Microbiol* 1993;**1**(3):77.

Pierson DE, Falkow S. The *ail* gene of *Yersinia enterocolitica* has a role in the ability of the organism to survive serum killing. *Infect Immun* 1993;**61**:1846.

Rook GAW, Bloom BR. Mechanisms of pathogenesis in tuberculosis. In: Bloom BR, ed. *Tuberculosis; Pathogenesis, Protection and Control*. Washington DC: ASM Press, 1994: 485.

Rothstein JL, Schreiber H. Synergy between tumour necrosis factor and bacterial products causes haemorrhagic necrosis and lethal shock in normal mice. *Proc Natl Acad Sci USA* 1988;**85**:607.

Thiel S. Mannan-binding protein, a complement activating animal lectin. *Immunopharmacology* 1992;**24**:91. *Toxicology* 1994;**87**:131.

Yamamura M, Uyemura K, Deans RJ, *et al.* Defining protective responses to pathogens: cytokine profiles in leprosy lesions. *Science* 1991;**254**:277–9.

Fungi

Jones HE. Immune response and host resistance of humans to dermatophyte infection. *J Am Acad Dermatol* 1993;**28**:S12.

Levitz SM. Overview of host defenses in fungal infections. *Clin Infect Dis* 1992;**14**:S37.

Murphy JW. Mechanisms of natural resistance to human pathogenic fungi. *Annu Rev Microbiol* 1991;**45**:509.

Parasites infect many millions of people. They are generally host-specific and most cause chronic infections. Many are spread by invertebrate vectors and have complicated life cycles. Their antigens are stage-specific.

Host resistance depends upon a number of mechanisms. Effector cells such as macrophages, neutrophils, eosinophils and platelets can kill both protozoa and worms. They secrete cytotoxic molecules such as reactive oxygen radicals and nitric oxide. All are more effective when activated by cytokines.

T cells are fundamental to the development of immunity. Antibody, alone or with complement, is effective against extracellular parasites. It enhances the phagocytic and cytotoxic potential of effector cells, and can prevent the invasion of new host cells.

Evasion of the host's immune response by parasites occurs in various ways. Some exploit the host response for their own development. Most interfere with it.

Worm infections are characteristically associated with an increase in eosinophil number and circulating IgE. TH1 and TH2 responses both play a role in immunity. TH2 cells are necessary for the elimination of intestinal worms. Mast cell products interact with eosinophils.

Both CD4$^+$ and CD8$^+$ T cells can be necessary for protection. TH1 cells provide protection against intracellular protozoa by secreting IFNγ, which activates macrophages.

Parasitic infections are associated with large amounts of non-specific antibody, splenomegaly and hepatomegaly. Much immunopathology may be T-cell mediated.

Parasitic infections typically stimulate a number of immunological defence mechanisms, both antibody- and cell-mediated, and the responses that are most effective depend upon the particular parasite and the stage of infection. The general principles of immunity to parasitic diseases are considered in this chapter, with special reference to some of the more important infections of man, which affect the host in diverse ways (*Fig. 18.1*).

Parasitic protozoa may live in the gut (e.g. amoebae), in the blood (e.g. African trypanosomes), within erythrocytes (e.g. *Plasmodium* spp.), in macrophages (e.g. *Leishmania* spp., *Toxoplasma gondii*), including those of the liver and spleen (e.g. *Leishmania* spp.), or in muscle (e.g. *Trypanosoma cruzi*). Parasitic worms that infect man include trematodes or flukes (e.g. schistosomes), cestodes (e.g. tapeworms) and nematodes or roundworms (e.g. *Trichinella spiralis*, hookworms, pinworms, *Ascaris* spp. and the filarial worms). Tapeworms and adult hookworms inhabit the gut, adult schistosomes live in blood vessels, and some filarial worms, for example, live in the lymphatics (*Fig. 18.2*). It is cleaar that there is widespread potential for damaging pathological reactions

Many parasitic worms pass through complicated life cycles, including migration through various parts of the host's body and the development of different stages in different tissues, before they reach the site where they finally mature and spend the rest of their lives (*Fig. 18.3*). Hookworms and schistosome larvae invade their hosts directly by penetrating the skin; tapeworms, pinworms and roundworms are ingested; and filarial worms depend upon an intermediate insect host or vector to transmit them from person to person. Most protozoa rely upon an insect vector apart from *Toxoplasma*, *Giardia* and amoebae, which are transmitted by ingestion. Thus, malarial parasites are spread by mosquitoes, trypanosomes by tsetse flies, *T. cruzi* by Triatomid bugs, and *Leishmania* by sandflies. The variety of methods of infection add to the problems of immunization.

▪ FEATURES OF PARASITIC INFECTIONS

Parasites infect very large numbers of people

Parasitic infections present a major medical problem, especially in tropical countries (*Fig. 18.1*). Malaria, for example, kills 1–2 million people every year. Intestinal worms infect a third of the world's population; the severity of disease depends upon the worm burden, but in children even moderate intensities of infection may be associated with stunted growth and slow mental development. Anaemia and malnutrition are also associated with parasitic disease.

Parasitic infections have some common features

Protozoan parasites and worms are considerably larger than bacteria and viruses (*Fig. 18.4*), and consequently contain a greater variety and a greater quantity of antigens. Some species can also change their surface antigens, a process known as antigenic variation. Parasites that have complicated life histories may express certain antigens only at a particular stage of development, giving rise to a stage-specific response. Thus, the protein coat of the sporozoite (the infective stage of the malarial parasite transmitted by the mosquito) induces the production of antibodies that do not react with the erythrocytic stage; the different stages of the worm *T. spiralis* also display different surface antigens.

Protozoa that are small enough to live inside human cells have evolved a special mode of entry. The merozoite, the invasive form of the blood stage of the malarial parasite, binds to certain receptors on the surface of the erythrocyte and uses a specialized organelle, the rhoptry, to enter the cell. *Leishmania* spp. parasites, which inhabit macrophages, use complement receptors to encourage the cells to engulf them. These parasites can also gain entry to the cell by using the mannose–fucose receptor on the macrophage surface.

Important parasitic infections of man

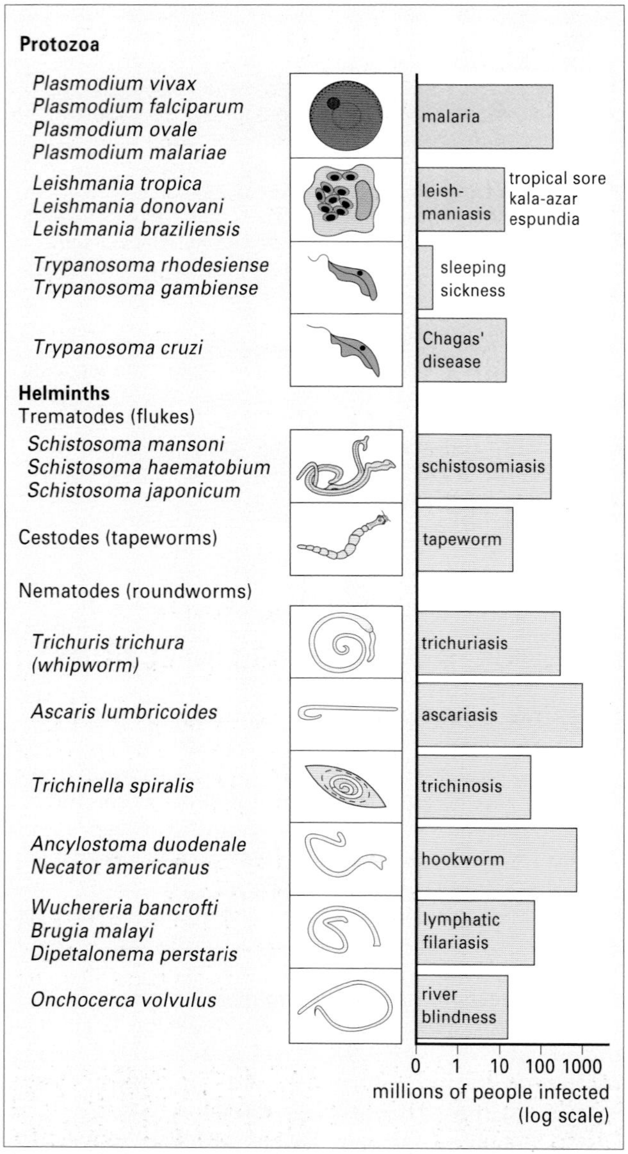

Protozoa

Plasmodium vivax
Plasmodium falciparum
Plasmodium ovale
Plasmodium malariae — malaria

Leishmania tropica
Leishmania donovani
Leishmania braziliensis — leishmaniasis — tropical sore / kala-azar / espundia

Trypanosoma rhodesiense
Trypanosoma gambiense — sleeping sickness

Trypanosoma cruzi — Chagas' disease

Helminths
Trematodes (flukes)
Schistosoma mansoni
Schistosoma haematobium
Schistosoma japonicum — schistosomiasis

Cestodes (tapeworms) — tapeworm

Nematodes (roundworms)

Trichuris trichura (whipworm) — trichuriasis

Ascaris lumbricoides — ascariasis

Trichinella spiralis — trichinosis

Ancylostoma duodenale
Necator americanus — hookworm

Wuchereria bancrofti
Brugia malayi
Dipetalonema perstaris — lymphatic filariasis

Onchocerca volvulus — river blindness

0   1   10 100 1000
millions of people infected
(log scale)

Fig. 18.1 Including data from the World Health Organization (1993).

Most parasites are host-specific

Over millions of years of evolution, parasites have become well adapted to their hosts and show marked host specificity. For example, the malarial parasites of birds, rodents or man can each multiply only in their own particular kind of host. There are some exceptions to this general rule: for example, the protozoan parasite *T. gondii* is not only able to invade and multiply in all nucleated mammalian cells, but can also infect immature mammalian erythrocytes, insect cell cultures, and the nucleated erythrocytes of birds and fish. Similarly, the tapeworm of the pig can also infect humans.

Sites of infection of medically important parasites

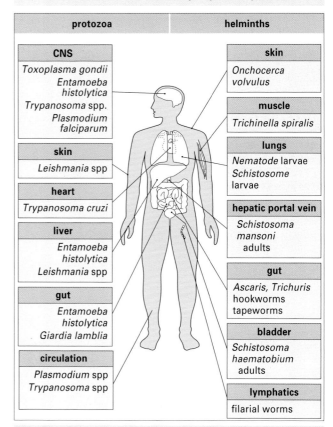

protozoa	helminths
CNS *Toxoplasma gondii* *Entamoeba histolytica* *Trypanosoma* spp. *Plasmodium falciparum*	**skin** *Onchocerca volvulus*
skin *Leishmania* spp	**muscle** *Trichinella spiralis*
heart *Trypanosoma cruzi*	**lungs** *Nematode* larvae *Schistosome* larvae
liver *Entamoeba histolytica* *Leishmania* spp	**hepatic portal vein** *Schistosoma mansoni* adults
gut *Entamoeba histolytica* *Giardia lamblia*	**gut** *Ascaris, Trichuris* hookworms tapeworms
circulation *Plasmodium* spp *Trypanosoma* spp	**bladder** *Schistosoma haematobium* adults
	lymphatics filarial worms

Fig. 18.2 Sites of infection of medically important parasites.

Host resistance to parasite infection may be genetic

The resistance of individual hosts to infection varies, and may be controlled by a number of immune response genes. Strains of mice – and some people – carrying certain MHC genes are less able to make antibody to one of the peptides of the malarial sporozoite coat because their T cells do not become sensitized. Similarly, the possession of certain HLA antigens, widespread in native West Africans but rare in Caucasians, appears to correlate with protection against severe malaria.

Non-MHC genes can also be important:
- The susceptibility of mice to infection by *Leishmania donovani*, and to several other parasites, is determined by a single dominant gene controlling macrophage activation (see Chapter 11).
- Merozoites of the malarial parasite *Plasmodium vivax* use a particular blood group substance on the erythrocyte surface, the Duffy antigen, as a receptor to effect their entry into the cell. Certain African populations lack this antigen – presumably from the pressures of natural selection – and are totally resistant to infection by the parasite.

In most helminth infections a heavy worm burden occurs in comparatively few individuals, but it should not be assumed

Parasite helminths in the human host

parasite and disease	lifespan (years)	eggs or larvae produced per adult per day	mode of entry	migratory pathway of larvae	final site of adult
Ascaris lumbricoides roundworm	1–2	>200 000	ingestion of eggs	gut→blood→lung→ trachea→pharynx →	small intestine
Trichuris trichura whipworm	1–2		ingestion of eggs	gut →	caecum
Ancylostoma duodenale hookworm	2–3	10 000–20 000	skin penetration by larvae in soil	blood→lung→ trachea→pharynx →	gut
Schistosoma mansoni bilharzia	2–3	100–300	skin penetration by larvae from water snail	blood→lung→blood →	hepatic portal vein
Schistosoma haematobium bladder fluke	3–5	500–3000	skin penetration by larvae from water snail	blood→lung→blood →	veins of bladder
Wuchereria bancrofti filariasis	3–5		mosquito bite	blood →	lymphatics

Fig. 18.3 Longevity, fertility and migratory pathways of parasitic helminths in the human host.

that this is necessarily due to genetic differences in resistance. Studies of human behaviour suggest that even in a small community people may vary greatly in their risk of infection through differences in their exposure to the invasive parasite.

Comparative size of various parasites

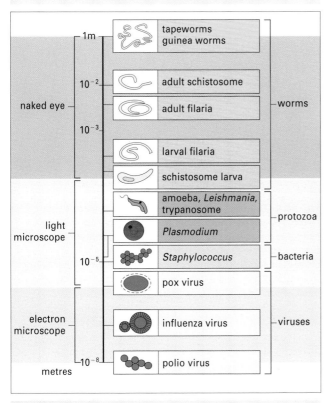

Fig. 18.4 Comparative size of various parasites.

Many parasitic infections are chronic

It is not in the interest of a parasite to kill its host, at least not until transmission to another host has been ensured. During the course of a chronic infection the type of immune response changes and is influenced by the presence of circulating antigens, persistent antigenic stimulation and the formation of immune complexes (*Fig. 18.5*). Immunosuppression and immunopathological effects are common.

Host defence depends upon a number of immunological effector mechanisms

The development of immunity is a complex process arising from the interactions of many different kinds of cells over a period of time. Effects are often local and many cell types secreting

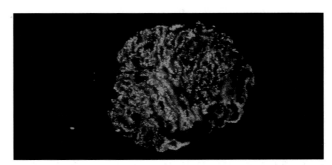

Fig. 18.5 Immune-complex deposition in quartan malaria nephrotic syndrome. Low power fluorescence micrograph of a renal glomerulus in a biopsy specimen from a Nigerian child with the syndrome. People infected with *Plasmodium malariae* may develop glomerulonephritis as a result of the deposition of immune complexes. The section was stained with FITC conjugated anti-human IgG and shows granular deposition of immunoglobulin throughout the capillary loops of the glomerulus. (Courtesy of Dr V. Houba.)

several different mediators may be present at sites of immune rejection. Moreover, the processes involved in controlling the multiplication of a parasite within an infected individual may differ from those responsible for the ultimate development of resistance to further infection. In some helminth infections a process of 'concomitant immunity' occurs, whereby an initial infection is not eliminated but becomes established, and the host then acquires resistance to invasion by new worms.

In general, antibody is most effective against extracellular parasites in blood and tissue fluids; cell-mediated responses are required to eliminate intracellular parasites. However, the type of response conferring most protection varies with the parasite. For example, antibody, alone or with complement, can damage some extracellular parasites, but is better when acting with an effector cell. As emphasized above, within a single infection different effector mechanisms act against different developmental stages of parasites. Thus in malaria, antibody against extracellular forms blocks their capacity to invade new cells and cell-mediated responses prevent the development of the liver stage within hepatocytes. Protective immunity to malaria does not correlate simply with antibody levels and can even be induced in the absence of antibody. This was shown in mice immunized with genetically engineered *Salmonella typhimurium* carrying a gene coding for a malaria sporozoite surface antigen and then challenged with sporozoites. Although the mice did not make specific antibody, they developed immunity to the parasite.

■ EFFECTOR MECHANISMS

Before a parasite succeeds in establishing itself within a new host and before specific immunity has been initiated or achieved, the parasite must overcome the host's pre-existing defence mechanisms. Complement plays a role here, as several types of parasite, including the adult worms and infective larvae of *T. spiralis* and the schistosomules of *Schistosoma mansoni*, carry molecules in their surface coats that activate the alternative pathway.

Macrophages, neutrophils, eosinophils and platelets form the first line of defence

Antibody and cytokines produced specifically in response to parasite antigens enhance the anti-parasitic activities of all these effector cells. However, tissue macrophages, monocytes and granulocytes all have some intrinsic activity, even before enhancement. The point of entry of the parasite is obviously important, for example:

- The cercariae of *S. mansoni* enter through the skin – experimental depletion of macrophages, neutrophils and eosinophils from the skin of mice increases their susceptibility to infection.
- Trypanosomes and malarial parasites entering the blood are removed from the circulation by phagocytic cells in the spleen and liver.
- Comparison of strains of mice with various immunological defects for their resistance to infection by Trypanosoma rhodesiense shows that the African trypanosomes are destroyed by macrophages. Later in infection, when opsonized with antibodies and complement C3b, they are taken up by macrophages in the liver more quickly still.

Before acting as antigen-presenting cells initiating an immune response, macrophages act as effector cells to inhibit the multiplication of parasites or even to destroy them. They also secrete molecules which regulate the inflammatory response. Some – IL-1, IL-12, TNFα and the colony-stimulating factors (CSFs) – enhance immunity by activating other cells or stimulating their proliferation. Others, like IL-10, IL-12, prostaglandins and TGFβ, may be anti-inflammatory and immunosuppressive.

Macrophages can kill extracellular parasites

Phagocytosis by macrophages provides an important defence against the smaller parasites; however, these cells also secrete many cytotoxic factors, enabling them to kill parasites without ingesting them. When activated by cytokines, macrophages can kill both relatively small extracellular parasites, such as the erythrocytic stages of malaria, and also larger ones, such as the larval stages of the schistosome.

Macrophages also act as killer cells through antibody-dependent cell-mediated cytotoxicity (ADCC); specific IgG and IgE, for instance, enhance their ability to kill schistosomules. They also secrete cytokines, such as TNFα and IL-1, that interact with other types of cell, for example, rendering hepatocytes resistant to malarial parasites.

Reactive oxygen intermediates (ROIs) are generated by macrophages and granulocytes following phagocytosis of *T. cruzi*, *T. gondii*, *Leishmania* spp. and malarial parasites, for instance; filarial worms and schistosomes also stimulate the respiratory burst (*Fig. 18.6*). When activated by cytokines, macrophages release more superoxide and hydrogen perox-

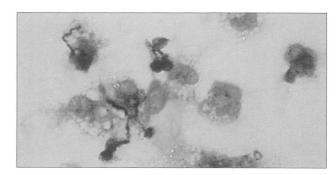

Fig. 18.6 The triggering of the respiratory burst of macrophages by *Leishmania donovani*. This picture shows a culture of resident peritoneal macrophages that have ingested promastigotes of *L. donovani* in the presence of nitroblue tetrazolium (NBT). The development of a black precipitate shows that the NBT has been reduced by products of the respiratory burst, which was triggered by contact with the parasites. More than 80% of promastigotes (the stages injected by the insect vector) are destroyed by normal macrophages but some escape from the phagolysosomes to become amastigotes. Amastigotes do not trigger the respiratory burst as effectively as promastigotes and survive well in normal macrophages. They can, however, be eradicated in vitro by incubation of the cells with cytokines. Both stages are killed by H_2O_2 but not by the other oxygen metabolites. (Courtesy of Dr J. Blackwell.)

ide than normal resident macrophages, and their O_2–independent killing mechanisms are similarly enhanced.

Nitric oxide (NO), a product of L-arginine metabolism, is one of the potent O_2–independent toxins. Its synthesis by macrophages is induced by the cytokines IFNγ and TNFα and is greatly increased when they act together. Nitric oxide can also be produced by endothelial cells. It contributes to host resistance in leishmaniasis, schistosomiasis and malaria, and is probably important in the control of most parasitic infections (*Fig. 18.7*). For instance, the innate resistance to infection by *T. gondii* that is lost in immunocompromised individuals, appears to be due to the inhibition of parasite multiplication by such an O_2–independent mechanism.

Activation of macrophages is a general feature of the early stages of infection

All macrophage effector functions are enhanced soon after infection. Although their specific activation is by cytokines secreted by T cells (e.g. IFNγ, GM-CSF, IL-3 and IL-4), they can also be activated by T cell-independent mechanisms, for example:

- NK cells secrete IFNγ when stimulated by IL-12 produced by macrophages.
- Macrophages secrete TNFα in response to some parasite products (e.g. phospholipid-containing antigens of malarial parasites and some *T. brucei* antigens); this TNFα then activates other macrophages.

Although TNFα may be secreted by several other cell types, activated macrophages are the most important source of this molecule, which is necessary for protective responses to several species of protozoa (e.g. *Leishmania* spp.) and helminths. Thus TNFα activates macrophages, eosinophils and platelets to kill the larval form of *S. mansoni,* its effects being enhanced by IFNγ.

Note that TNFα may have harmful as well as beneficial effects on the infected host, depending upon the amount produced and whether it is free in the circulation or locally confined. Administration of TNFα cures a susceptible strain of mice infected with the rodent malarial parasite *P. chabaudi,* but kills a genetically resistant strain. Presumably the latter can already make enough TNFα to control parasite replication, and any more has toxic effects.

Neutrophils can kill large and small parasites

The effector properties displayed by macrophages are also seen in neutrophils. Neutrophils are phagocytic and can kill by both O_2–dependent and O_2–independent mechanisms, including nitric oxide. They produce a more intense respiratory burst than macrophages and their secretory granules contain highly cytotoxic proteins (see Chapter 2). They can be activated by cytokines, such as IFNγ, TNFα, and GM-CSF. Extracellular destruction by neutrophils is mediated by H_2O_2, whereas granular components are involved in intracellular destruction of ingested organisms. Neutrophils are present in parasite-infected inflammatory lesions and probably act to clear parasites from bursting cells. Like macrophages, neutrophils bear Fc receptors and complement receptors and can participate in antibody-dependent cytotoxic reactions, to kill the larvae of *S. mansoni* for example. In this mode, they can be more destructive than eosinophils against several species

of nematode, including *T. spiralis,* although the relative effectiveness of the two types of cell may depend upon the isotype and specificity of antibody.

Eosinophils are characteristically associated with worm infections

It has been suggested that the eosinophil evolved specifically as a defence against the tissue stages of parasites that are too large to be phagocytosed, and that the IgE-dependent mast-cell reaction has evolved primarily to localize eosinophils near the parasite and enhance their anti-parasitic functions.

The importance of these effector cells *in vivo* has been shown by experiments using antiserum against eosinophils. Mice infected with *T. spiralis* and treated with the antiserum develop more cysts in their muscles than the controls: without the protection offered by eosinophils, the mice cannot eliminate the worms and so encyst the parasites to minimize damage.

However, recent work has shown that although eosinophils can help the host to control a worm infection, particularly by limiting migration through the tissues, they do not always do so. For instance, their removal does not abolish the immunity of mice infected with *S. mansoni,* nor does it diminish the parasite load in a tapeworm infection.

Eosinophils can kill helminths by both O_2-dependent and O_2-independent mechanisms

Eosinophils are less phagocytic than neutrophils. They degranulate in response to perturbation of their surface membrane and their activities are enhanced by cytokines such as TNFα and GM-CSF. Most of their activities, however, are controlled

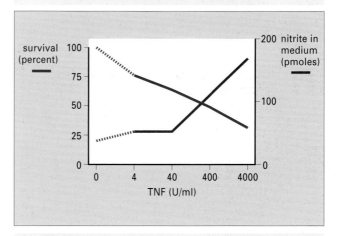

Toxic effect of NO on *Leishmania* in vitro

Fig. 18.7 Evidence that the killing of *Leishmania major* by activated macrophages is correlated with the release of nitric oxide. Macrophages in culture are activated by recombinant TNFα in a dose-related fashion, the highest doses decreasing parasite survival to about a third of that in control cultures. At the same time, the amount of NO released, measured as nitrite present in the culture medium, increases. Interference with NO production allows parasites to survive. (Based on data from Liew, Li, Millott. *Immunol* 1990;**71**:556.)

by antigen-specific mechanisms. Thus their binding *in vitro* to the larvae of worms coated with IgE or IgG (e.g. *S. mansoni* and *T. spiralis*) increases the release of their granular contents onto the surface of the worms. Damage to schistosomules can be caused by the major basic protein (MBP) of the eosinophil crystalloid core (*Figs 18.8 and 18.9*). MBP is not specific for any particular target, but since it is confined to a small space between the eosinophil and the schistosome, there is little damage to nearby host cells.

Eosinophils and mast cells act together

The killing of *S. mansoni* larvae by eosinophils is enhanced by mast cell products, and when studied *in vitro*, eosinophils from patients with schistosomiasis are more effective than those from normal subjects. The antigens released cause local IgE-dependent degranulation of mast cells and the release of mediators. These selectively attract eosinophils to the site and

further enhance their activity. Other products of eosinophils later block the mast cell reactions. That these effector mechanisms may function *in vivo* has been shown in monkeys, where schistosome killing is associated with eosinophil accumulation (*Fig. 18.10*).

Platelets can kill many types of parasite

Potential targets for platelets include the larval stage of flukes, *T. gondii* and *T. cruzi*. Like other effector cells, their cytotoxic activity is enhanced by treatment with cytokines (e.g. IFNγ and TNFα). In rats infected with *S. mansoni*, platelets become larvicidal when acute-phase reactants appear in the serum but before antibody can be detected. Incubation of normal platelets in such serum can cause their activation. Platelets, like macrophages and the other effector cells, also bear Fcε receptors on their surface membrane, by which they mediate antibody-dependent cytotoxicity associated with IgE.

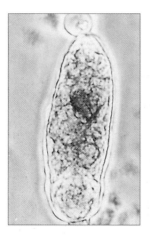
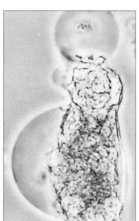
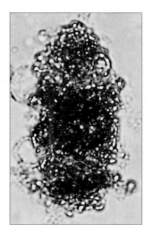

Fig. 18.8 Effect of major basic protein of eosinophils on schistosome larvae. The killing of schistosomules by eosinophils can be effected by the major basic protein of the eosinophil granule. These pictures show the progressive surface damage and disruption of a larva caused by incubation within this cell product: intact worm (left); initial stage of damage to the tegument and worm surface (middle); total destruction of the worm (right). (Courtesy of Dr D. McLaren.)

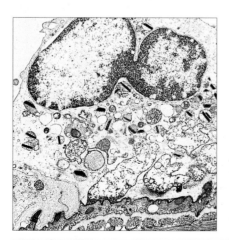
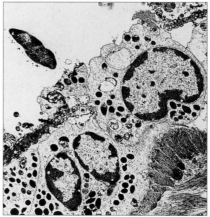
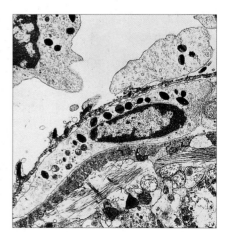

Fig. 18.9 Killing of schistosome larvae by eosinophils. Eosinophils can adhere to schistosomules and kill them. The damage is associated with degranulation of the eosinophils and the release of the contents of the granules onto the surface of the worm. This series of electron micrographs shows adherence of the eosinophils and degranulation onto the surface of the worm larva (left), and stages in the breakup of the worm tegument and migration of eosinophils through the lesions (middle and right). (Courtesy of Dr D. McLaren.)

T CELLS ARE FUNDAMENTAL TO THE DEVELOPMENT OF IMMUNITY

In most parasitic infections, protection can be conferred experimentally on normal animals by the transfer of spleen cells, especially T cells, from immune animals. The T cell requirement is also demonstrable by the way in which nude (athymic) or T-deprived mice fail to clear otherwise non-lethal infections of protozoa such as *T. cruzi* or *P. yoelii*, and by the way T-deprived rats fail to expel the intestinal worm *Nippostrongylus brasiliensis* (*Fig. 18.11*). However, it should be noted that in some cases transfer of T cells from acutely infected animals can suppress the protective response and cause the death of the recipients. This is because these T cells secrete IL-4 and IL-10, which inhibit the production and activity of the IFNγ required to activate macrophages and eliminate the parasite.

The role of cytokines in parasitic infections has been elucidated by administering the cytokine to infected animals, or eliminating it with monoclonal antibodies. More information is now emerging from the analysis of various infections in mice made transgenic for a particular cytokine, and from mice in which the cytokine gene has been inactivated ('knock-out' mice). We now know that many cytokines not only act on effector cells to enhance their cytotoxic or cytostatic capabilities but also act as growth factors to increase cell numbers. Thus in malaria, the monocytosis and the characteristic enlargement of the spleen, caused by an enormous increase in cell numbers, are T-cell dependent. Other examples include the accumulation of macrophages in the granulomas that develop in the liver in schistosomiasis, the eosinophilia characteristic of helminth infections, and the recruitment of eosinophils and mast cells into the gut mucosa that occurs in worm infections of the gastrointestinal tract. Mucosal mast cells and eosinophils, both important in determining the outcome of some helminth infections, proliferate in response to the products of T cells: IL-3 and GM-CSF, and IL-5, respectively.

However, an increase in cell number can itself harm the host. Thus administration of IL-3 to mice infected with *Leishmania major* can exacerbate the local infection and increase the dissemination of the parasites, probably through the proliferation of bone marrow precursors of the cells the parasites inhabit.

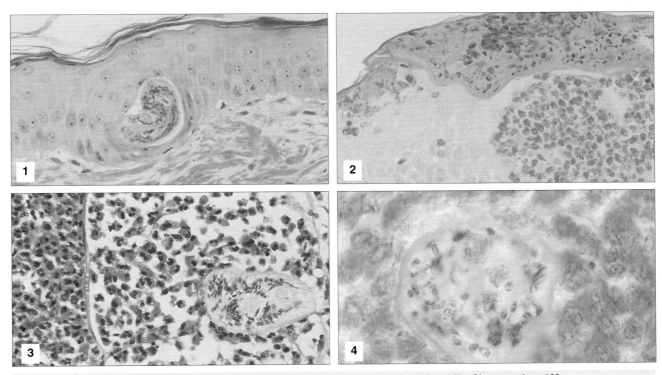

Fig. 18.10 Immunity to *Schistosoma mansoni* in vivo.
Normal or previously infected baboons were infected percutaneously with 1000 cercariae of *S. mansoni*.
1. In control animals at 72 hours after challenge, there is no inflammatory or immune reaction and the schistosomes lie just above the basement membrane. H&E stain, × 160.
2. In animals infected 2 years previously, an inflammatory infiltrate surrounds the schistosome by 24 hours after the challenge, and is predominantly eosinophilic. Giemsa stain, × 160.
3. In the immune animal 24 hours after challenge, the schistosomule is trapped in an abscess of adherent eosinophils. Giemsa stain, × 250.
4. A further biopsy from the same animal as (3) which shows a killed parasite, in which the interior of the schistosome has been invaded by eosinophils. × 640. (Courtesy of Dr B. J. Cottrell and Dr H. M. Seitz.)

Fig. 18.11 The first two graphs plot the increase in number of blood-borne protozoa (parasitaemia) following infection. **A** *Trypanosoma cruzi* multiplies faster (and gives fatal parasitaemia) in mice that have been thymectomized and irradiated to destroy T cells (Thym x). In normal mice, parasites are cleared from the blood by day 16. Reconstitution of T-deprived mice with T cells from immune mice (immune-T) restores their ability to control the parasitaemia. In these experiments both thymectomized groups were given fetal liver cells to restore vital haematopoietic function. **B** *Plasmodium yoelii* causes a self-limiting infection in normal mice and the parasites are cleared from the blood by day 20. In nude mice the parasites continue to multiply, killing the mice after about 30 days. **C** This graph illustrates the time course of the elimination of the intestinal nematode

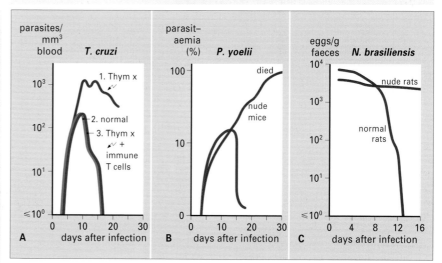

Parasitic infections in T-deprived mice

Nippostrongylus brasiliensis from the gut of rats. In normal rats the worms are all expelled by day 13, as determined by the number of worm eggs present in the rats'

faeces. T cells are necessary for this expulsion to occur, as shown by the establishment of a chronic infection in the gut of nude rats.

Both CD4+ and CD8+ T cells are needed for protection against some parasites

The type of T cell responsible for controlling an infection varies with the parasite and the stage of infection, and depends upon the kinds of cytokine they produce. For example, CD4+ and CD8+ T cells protect against different phases of *Plasmodium* infection: CD4+ T cells mediate immunity against blood stage *P. yoelii* while CD8+ cells protect against the liver stage of *P. berghei*. The action of CD8+ cells is twofold: they secrete IFNγ, which inhibits the multiplication of the parasites within hepatocytes, and they destroy infected hepatocytes. The hepatocytes express MHC class I but not MHC class II, so CD4+ T cells do not recognize them and are not stimulated to secrete IFNγ. Similarly, CD8+ cells do not affect the blood stage parasites because erythrocytes do not express MHC class I.

The immune response against *T. cruzi* depends not only upon CD4+ and CD8+ T cells, but also on NK cells and antibody production; the same is true for the immune response against *T. gondii*. In experiments, CD8+ cells confer protection in mice depleted of CD4+ T cells, both through their production of IFNγ and because they are cytotoxic for infected macrophages. NK cells, stimulated by IL-12 secreted by the macrophages, are another source of IFNγ. Chronic infections are associated with reduced production of IFNγ. These observations probably underlie the high incidence of toxoplasmosis in AIDS patients, who are short of CD4+ T cells.

CD4+ T cells act in different ways in different infections

T-helper cells can be divided into TH1 and TH2 subsets (see Chapter 9). In the early stages of an infection there may be a mixture of the two subsets; the balance may change with time or with age, polarizing after prolonged infection. As TH1 and TH2 cytokines are mutually antagonistic, the T cell subset that finally predominates will decide the outcome of the infection – this depends very much on the particular parasite species and may be unpredictable. Because the relative importance of TH1 and TH2 cells is generally different in infections caused by protozoa and even varies in different worm infections, these are best considered separately. (For a discussion of the cytokines produced by these subsets and their role in immunity see Chapter 9.)

TH1 and TH2 cells control malarial infection

TH1 cells act against the liver stage of malaria: administration of IFNγ (a TH1 cytokine) directly to chimpanzees infected with sporozoites of *P. vivax* diminishes parasitaemia. Furthermore, the ability of immune mice to withstand challenge by sporozoites of *P. berghei* can be overcome by treatment with an antibody against IFNγ. TH2 cells generally help to produce antibodies to add specificity to the immune reaction. For example, elimination of the blood stage of malaria occurs in the spleen via activated effector cells and antibody-dependent cytotoxicity. An intact but modified spleen is necessary for maintenance of immunity.

The TH1 subset enhances protective responses against intracellular protozoa

IFNγ activates macrophages to kill the protozoa that live within them, such as *L. major, T. cruzi* and *T. gondii* (*Figs 18.12 and 18.13*). It also enhances effector responses against other parasites. IFNγ effects are nicely illustrated by studies on *Leishmania*, in which resistant strains of mice are shown to control the development of cutaneous lesions caused by *L. major* through their production of IFNγ (a TH1 cytokine). In susceptible mice, which develop progressive disease, TH2 cells predominate; their secretion of IL-4 inhibits the production of IFNγ. Administration of antibody against IL-4 cured the infection by diminishing TH2 cell activity and allowing expansion of the TH1 cell population. Administration of recombinant IFNγ to susceptible mice was not itself enough to effect a cure, indicating that their susceptibility was due to excessive TH2 cell activity rather than deficient TH1 cell activity. However, IL-12 (produced by macrophages and B cells), which promotes the growth of activated TH1 cells and NK cells and the synthesis of a range of anti-Leishmanial cytokines, as well as IFNγ, suppressed the development of TH2 cells and cured the disease when given to the susceptible mice early in infection.

In people, diffuse cutaneous leishmaniasis and progressive visceral leishmaniasis are characterized by deficient IFNγ synthesis and increased expression of IL-10, the TH2-associated cytokine that suppresses the proliferation and function of TH1 cells. *In vitro*, IL-4 inhibits the IFNγ-induced activity of human monocytes against *L. donovani* (*Fig. 18.14*). These findings suggest that it might be possible to use IL-12 therapeutically in established leishmaniasis, provided that the antagonistic cytokines IL-4, IL-10 and TGFβ are neutralized at the same time.

Action of TH1 and TH2 cells in *Leishmania* infection

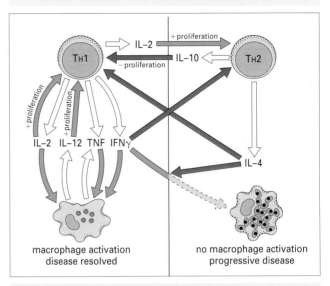

Fig. 18.14 Development of the immune response to *Leishmania* infection illustrating the cytokines secreted by the different subsets of T cells and their effect on the resolution of the disease. Note that IL-12, which is also produced by B cells, promotes the growth of NK cells as well as TH1 cells, and these cells are also a source of IFNγ, the cytokine which is essential for elimination of the parasite.

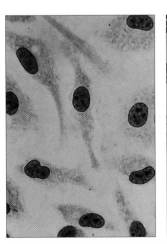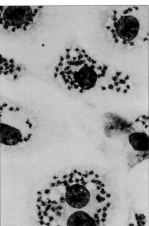

Fig. 18.12 Inhibition of parasite multiplication in macrophages treated with cytokines. Peritoneal macrophages from BALB/c mice, infected 72 hours previously with 10⁷ amastigotes of *Leishmania donovani*, were treated with either a supernatant from activated T cells (containing cytokines) or a control supernatant. Cells treated with cytokines do not contain any parasites following culture (left) whereas untreated macrophages contain many parasites (right). Subsequent studies using recombinant IFNγ and monoclonal antibody against IFNγ showed that the inhibition was mediated by this cytokine. (Courtesy of Dr H. Murray, with permission from *J Immunol* 1982;**129**:344–357, © American Association of Immunologists.)

Protective effect of IFNγ

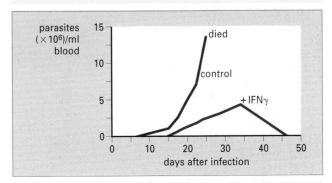

Fig. 18.13 The effect of administration of the T cell cytokine IFNγ on acute infection caused by *Trypanosoma cruzi*. In this strain of mice, the parasites multiply to kill their host in about 3 weeks. Administration of recombinant mouse IFNγ controls their multiplication and is followed ultimately by their elimination.

Both TH1 and TH2 responses are important in helminth infections

IgE and eosinophilia are the hallmarks of the immune response to worm infections, and depend upon cytokines secreted by TH2 cells. However, the relative contribution of the TH1 and TH2 subsets in the development of immunity to these parasites is still uncertain. To complicate matters further, responses in mice and rats and people differ, in schistosomiasis at least: in man, TH2 effects appear to be important, as resistance to reinfection after drug treatment is correlated with the production of IgE. In the mouse, TH1 cells and IFNγ are needed for vaccine-induced protection and TH2 cells are associated with egg-related immunopathology. The switch to TH2 is triggered by egg antigens.

The pattern of cytokine production in infected hosts may be different from that in vaccinated hosts. For example, in mice infected with *S. mansoni*, IL-5 producing TH2 cells predominate. In mice that have been immunized, IgE levels and eosinophil numbers are low and TH1 cells predominate. Secretion of IFNγ by TH1 cells activates effector cells that destroy lung stage larvae, via the production of nitric oxide. However, when adult worms start to produce eggs, a soluble egg antigen is released that has an effect only in susceptible mice. The antigen reduces TH1 function and levels of IFNγ and increases TH2 production of IL-5.

In some parasitic infections, the immune system cannot completely eliminate the parasite, and the body reduces damage by walling off the parasite behind a capsule of inflammatory cells. This reaction, which is TH1-dependent, is a chronic cell-mediated response to locally released antigen, and is mediated by cytokines, especially TNFα and IFNγ. Macrophages accumulate and release fibrogenic factors that stimulate the formation of granulomatous tissue and ultimately lead to fibrosis. In schistosomiasis, granuloma formation occurs in response to a particular soluble antigen secreted by or around worm eggs that have become trapped in the liver. Although this reaction may benefit the host, in that it insulates the liver cells from toxins secreted by the worm eggs, it is also the major source of pathology, causing irreversible changes in the liver and the loss of liver function. In the absence of T cells, there is no granuloma formation and no subsequent fibrous encapsulation (*Fig. 18.15*).

Different mechanisms may affect the worms that inhabit different anatomical sites, such as the gut (e.g. *Trichuris*) or the tissues (e.g. *Onchocerca volvulus*), and at different stages of the life cycle (e.g. schistosome larvae in the lungs and adult worms in the veins).

TH2 cells are clearly necessary for elimination of intestinal worms

Experiments have shown that TH2 cells are important in intestinal worm infections. For example, mice normally resistant to infection by a murine whipworm develop persistent infection if the TH2 cytokine IL-4 is neutralized. Conversely, susceptible mice expel the worms if IL-4 activity is promoted by administration of neutralizing antibody against IFNγ. Similarly, administration of IL-12 to rats soon after infection with the intestinal worm *N. brasiliensis* stimulates IFNγ production, and delays expulsion of the worms. IL-12 acts by inhibiting the production of TH2 cytokines, in particu-

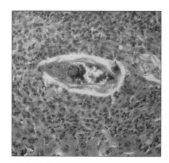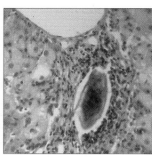

Fig. 18.15 T-cell-dependence of granuloma formation around schistosome eggs in the liver. Many of the eggs of schistosome worms are carried to the liver where they become insulated behind a capsule of inflammatory cells. In normal mice, the granulomas consist predominantly of eosinophils and are the result of a T cell-dependent reaction (left). In T cell-deficient mice, eggs of *Schistosoma mansoni* do not induce much granuloma formation and as a result toxic products of the eggs can diffuse out and cause damage to the surrounding liver tissue (right). (Courtesy of Dr M. Doenhoff.)

lar IL-4 and IL-5, and thus prevents the production of IgE and the hypertrophy of intestinal mast cells, mediated by IL-4, and the development of the eosinophilia, which is mediated by IL-5.

The mechanism of worm expulsion involves mucosal mast cells induced by antigen-activated T cells. Their products enhance the activity of other effector processes, interact with eosinophils and also accelerate expulsion (*Fig. 18.16*). The cytoplasmic granules of mast cells contain a number of preformed mediators (see Chapter 22). They are also a source of many different cytokines, including IL-3, IL-4, GM-CSF and TNFα, and a protease. They cause changes in the permeability of the gut and shedding of the epithelium which may also help eject some protozoan parasites. In intestinal nematode infections, the goblet cells coat the worms in mucus just before expulsion. We know this is a specific response because it occurs only in immune animals. By altering mucosal permeability, mast-cell mediators allow complement and serum antibodies to leak into the gut lumen. The mediators can also act on intestinal smooth muscle to facilitate expulsion by peristalsis.

Parasites induce non-specific and specific antibody production

Many parasitic infections provoke a non-specific hypergammaglobulinaemia, much of which is probably due to substances released from the parasites acting as B-cell mitogens. Levels of total immunoglobulins are raised: IgM in trypanosomiasis and malaria, IgG in malaria and visceral leishmaniasis. The relative importance of antibody-dependent and antibody-independent responses varies with the infection (*Fig. 18.17*). The mechanisms by which specific antibody can control parasitic infections and its effects are summarized in *Fig. 18.18* and are as follows:

Fig. 18.16 The expulsion of some intestinal nematodes occurs spontaneously a few weeks after primary infection. There seem to be 2 stages in the expulsion, which is achieved by a combination of T-dependent and T-independent mechanisms.
1. T cells (predominantly TH2 cells) respond to parasite antigens and induce (a) the production of antibody by B cells that have proliferated in response to IL-4 and IL-5, (b) the proliferation of mucosal mast cells, in response to IL-3, IL-4, IL-9 and IL-10, and (c) hyperplasia of mucus-secreting goblet cells in the intestinal epithelium. The worms are damaged by antibody together with products of IgE-senstized mast cells which degranulate following contact with antigen, and so release histamine which increases the permeability of the intestinal epithelium. These processes are not sufficient to eliminate the worms.
2. Non-specific inflammatory molecules secreted by macrophages, including TNF and IL-1, contribute to goblet cell proliferation and cause increased secretion of mucus. The mucus coats the worms and leads to their expulsion. The numbers of goblet cells in the jejunal epithelium and the secretion of mucus increase in proportion to the worm burden. The antigen-specific effector T cells are generated early in infection and the rate-limiting step is the onset of antibody damage. The relative importance of these various processes varies with the infecting nematode.

Processes involved in expulsion of nematodes from the gut

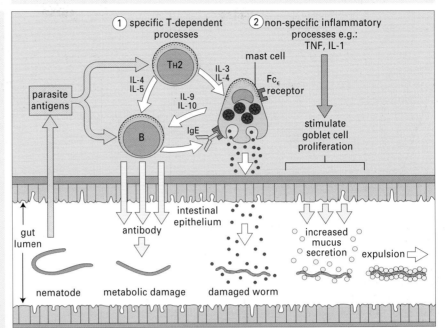

Relative importance of antibody-dependent and -independent responses in protozoal infections

parasite and habitat		antibody–dependent			antibody–independent	
		importance	mechanism	means of evasion	importance	mechanism
T. brucei free in blood	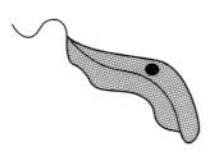	+ + + +	lysis with complement which also opsonizes for phagocytosis	antigenic variation	–	
Plasmodium inside red cell	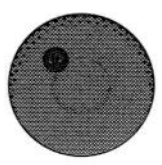	+ + +	blocks invasion, opsonizes for phagocytosis	intracellular; antigenic variation	liver stage + + + blood stage + + +	cytokines macrophage activation
T. cruzi inside macrophage	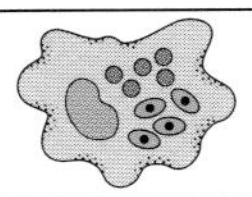	+ +	limits spread in acute infection, sensitizes for ADCC	intracellular	+ + + (chronic phase)	macrophage activation by IFNγ and TNFα, and killing by NO and metabolites of O_2
Leishmania inside macrophage	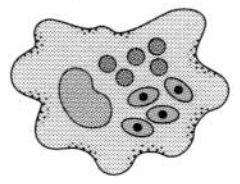	+	limits spread	intracellular	+ + + +	

Fig. 18.17 This table summarizes the relative importance of the two immune responses, the mechanisms involved and, for antibody, the means by which the protozoan can evade damage by antibody. Antibody is the most important part of the immune response against those parasites that live in the bloodstream, such as African trypanosomes and malarial parasites, whereas cell-mediated immunity is active against those like *Leishmania* that live in the tissues. Antibody can damage parasites directly, enhance their clearance by phagocytosis, activate complement or block their entry into their host cell and so limit the spread of infection. Once inside, the parasite is safe from its effects. *Trypanosoma cruzi* and *Leishmania* are both susceptible to the action of oxygen metabolites released by the respiratory burst of macrophages, and to nitric oxide. Treating macrophages with cytokines enhances release of these products and diminishes entry and survival of the parasites. Malarial parasites within the red cell may be destroyed by some secreted products of activated macrophages, including hydrogen peroxide and other cytotoxic factors.

Mechanisms by which specific antibody controls some parasitic infections

parasite	*Plasmodium* sporozoite, intestinal worms, trypanosome	*Plasmodium* sporozoite and merozoite, *Trypanosoma cruzi*, *Toxoplasma gondii*	*Plasmodium*, trypanosome	schistosomes, *Trichinella spiralis*, filarial worm larvae
mechanism	1 complement protein	2	3	4 larval worm
effect	direct damage or complement-mediated lysis	prevents spread by neutralizing attachment site, prevents escape from lysosomal vacuole, prevents inhibition of lysosomal fusion	enhancement of phagocytosis	antibody-dependent cell-mediated cytotoxicity (ADCC)

Fig. 18.18 1. Direct damage. Antibody activates the classical complement pathway, causing damage to the parasite membrane and increasing susceptibility to other mediators.
2. Neutralization. Parasites such as *Plasmodium* spp. spread to new cells by specific receptor attachment; blocking the merozoite binding site with antibody prevents attachment to the receptors on the erythrocyte surface and hence prevents further multiplication.

3. Enhancement of phagocytosis. Complement C3b deposited on parasite membrane opsonizes it for phagocytosis by cells with C3b receptors (for example macrophages). Macrophages also have Fc receptors.
4. Eosinophils, neutrophils, platelets and macrophages may be cytotoxic for some parasites when they recognize the parasite via specific antibody (ADCC). The reaction is enhanced by complement.

- Antibody can act directly on protozoa to damage them, either by itself or by activating the complement system (*Fig. 18.19*).
- Antibody can neutralize a parasite directly by blocking its attachment to a new host cell, as with *Plasmodium* spp., whose merozoites enter red blood cells through a special receptor: their entry is inhibited by specific antibody (*Fig. 18.20*). Antibody may also act to prevent spread, for example in the acute phase of infection by *T. cruzi*.
- Antibody can enhance phagocytosis by macrophages. Phagocytosis is increased even more by the addition of complement. These effects are mediated by Fc and C3 receptors on the macrophages, which may increase in number as a result of macrophage activation.
- Antibody is also involved in antibody-dependent cell-mediated cytotoxicity, for example, in infections caused by *T. cruzi*, *T. spiralis*, *S.mansoni* and filarial worms. Cytotoxic cells such as macrophages, neutrophils and eosinophils adhere to antibody-coated worms by means of their Fc and C3 receptors and exocytose in apposition to the parasite.

Different antibody isotypes may have different effects. As mentioned previously, in individuals infected with schistosomes parasite-specific IgE is associated with resistance to infection and there is an inverse relationship between the amount of IgE in their blood and reinfection. IgG4 appears to block the action of IgE; reinfection is more likely in children who have high levels of IgG4. The development of immunity seems to depend upon a switch from IgG4 to IgE that occurs with age; infection rates are highest in 10- to 14-year-olds, when IgG4 levels are also at their highest.

In many infections it is difficult to distinguish between cell-mediated and antibody-mediated responses, since both act in concert against the parasite. This is illustrated in *Figure 18.21* which summarizes the immune reactions that can be mounted against schistosome larvae.

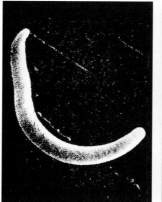 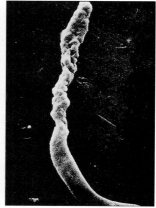

Fig. 18.19 Direct effect of specific antibody on sporozoites of malarial parasites. These scanning electron micrographs show a sporozoite of *Plasmodium berghei*, which causes malaria in rodents, before (left) and after (right) incubation in immune serum. The surface of the sporozoite is damaged by the antibody which perturbs the outer membrane, causing leakage of fluid. Specific antibody protects against infection with *Plasmodium* spp. at several of the extracellular stages of the life cycle. The antibody is stage-specific in each case. (Courtesy of Dr R. Nussenzweig.)

■ ESCAPE MECHANISMS

It is a necessary characteristic of all successful parasitic infections that they can evade the full effects of their host's immune responses; parasites have developed many different ways of doing this. Some even exploit cells and molecules of the immune system to their own advantage: *Leishmania* parasites, by using complement receptors to effect their entry into macrophages, avoid triggering the oxidative burst and thus destruction by its toxic products.

Despite their protective role in the immune response to many different parasites, host TNFα actually stimulates egg production by adult worms of *S. mansoni*, while IFNγ is used as a growth factor by *T. brucei*.

Parasites can resist destruction by complement

In the case of *Leishmania*, such resistance correlates with virulence. *L. tropica*, which is easily killed by complement, causes a localized self-healing infection in the skin, whereas *L. donovani*, which is ten times more resistant to complement, becomes disseminated throughout the viscera, causing a disease that is often fatal.

The mechanisms whereby parasites can resist the effect of complement differ. The lipophosphoglycan surface coat of *L. major* activates complement, but the complex is then shed so the parasite avoids lysis. The trypomastigotes of *T. cruzi* bear a surface glycoprotein which has activity resembling the decay accelerating factor (DAF) that limits the complement reaction (see Chapter 13). The resistance schistosomules acquire as they mature is also correlated with the appearance of a surface molecule similar to DAF.

Effect of antibody on malarial parasites

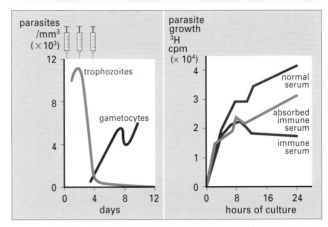

Fig. 18.20 Left: Transfer of γ-globulin from immune adults to a child infected with *Plasmodium falciparum* caused a sharp drop in parasitaemia. Specific antibody acts at the merozoite stage in the life of the parasite and prevents the initiation of further cycles of multiplication in the blood. The development of gametocytes from existing intracellular forms is unaffected.
Right: In culture, the presence of immune serum blocks the continued increase in number of *P. knowlesi* (a malarial parasite of monkeys), as measured by incorporation of ^{3}H-leucine. It stops multiplication at the stage after schizont rupture by preventing the released merozoites from invading fresh red blood cells. The inhibitory activity of the immune serum can be reduced by prior absorption of the specific antibody with free schizonts.

Possible effector responses to schistosomules

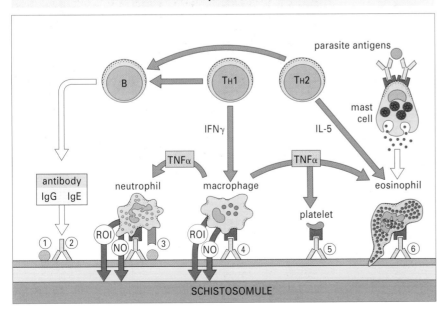

Fig. 18.21 This diagram illustrates the various effector mechanisms that have been shown to damage schistosomes *in vitro*. Complement alone damages worms (1) and also does so in combination with antibody (2). Antibody sensitizes neutrophils (3), macrophages (4), platelets (5) and eosinophils (6) for antibody-dependent cell-mediated cytotoxicity. Neutrophils and macrophages probably act by releasing toxic oxygen and nitrogen metabolites, whereas eosinophils damage the worm tegument by release of major basic protein. The response is potentiated by cytokines (e.g. TNFα). IgE antibody is important both in sensitizing eosinophils and local mast cells, which release a variety of mediators, including those that activate the eosinophils.

Intracellular parasites avoid destruction by various means

Those that live inside macrophages have evolved different ways of avoiding being killed by oxygen metabolites and lysosomal enzymes (*Figs 18.22 and 18.23*). *T. gondii* penetrates the macrophage by a non-phagocytic pathway and so avoids triggering the oxidative burst; *Leishmania* organisms can enter by binding to complement receptors, another way of avoiding stimulating the respiratory burst. In addition, *Leishmania* spp. possess enzymes that inhibit the progression of the burst, superoxide dismutase which protects them against the action of oxygen radicals, and a lipophosphoglycan surface coat (LPG) that acts as a scavenger of oxygen metabolites and affords protection against enzymatic attack. A glycoprotein, Gp63 (*Fig. 18.24*), inhibits the action of the macrophage's lysosomal enzymes. *Leishmania* spp. can also downregulate the expression of MHC Class II on the macrophages they inhabit, thus reducing their capacity to stimulate TH cells. These escape mechanisms, however, are less efficient in the immune host.

Extracellular parasites can disguise themselves

Parasites that are vulnerable to specific antibody have evolved different methods of evading its effects. The African trypanosome undergoes antigenic variation: the molecule that forms its surface coat, the variable surface glycoprotein (VSG) changes to protect the underlying surface membrane from the host's defence mechanisms. New populations of parasites are antigenically distinct from previous ones (*Fig. 18.25*). Several antigens of malarial parasites also undergo antigenic variation.

Other parasites, such as schistosomes, acquire a surface layer of host antigens, so that the host does not distinguish them from 'self' (*Fig. 18.26*). Schistosomules cultured in

The different means by which protozoa that multiply within macrophages escape digestion by lysosomal enzymes

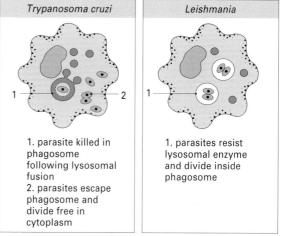

Fig. 18.22 *Toxoplasma gondii*. Live parasites coated with host laminin enter the cell actively into a membrane-bound vacuole, by binding to a member of the integrin family of receptors on the surface of the macrophage. They are not attacked by enzymes because lysosomes do not fuse with this vacuole. Dead parasites, however, are taken up by normal phagocytosis into a phagosome (by interaction with the Fc receptors on the macrophage if they are coated with antibody) and they are then destroyed by the enzymes of the lysosomes which fuse with it.
Trypanosoma cruzi. Survival of these parasites depends upon their stage of development; trypomastigotes escape from the phagosome and divide in the cytoplasm whereas epimastigotes do not escape and are killed. The proportion of parasites found in the cytoplasm is decreased if the macrophages are activated.
Leishmania spp. These parasites multiply within the phagosome and the presence of a surface protease helps them resist digestion. If the macrophages are first activated by cytokines the number of parasites entering the cell and the number that replicate diminish.

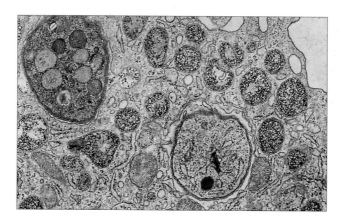

Fig. 18.23 Electron micrograph showing part of a macrophage infected with *Toxoplasma gondii*. Following infection, the macrophages were treated with thorotrast to make the contents of the secondary lysosomes electron dense. The live parasite has inhibited fusion of secondary lysosomes with its phagosome. Several dead parasites lie in a phagosome that contains thorotrast; it can be seen that a phagosome has just fused with the vacuole and emptied its contents into it. ×14000. (Courtesy of Prof. T. C. Jones.)

Two surface antigens of *Leishmania*

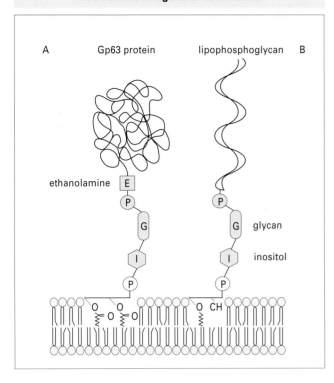

Fig. 18.24 Schematic representation of two surface antigens of *Leishmania* that are anchored to the membrane by phosphatidylinositol tails (GPI anchors).

A This protein antigen, Gp63, has protease activity. That of *L. mexicana*, together with a lipophosphoglycan (LPG), binds complement. This enables the promastigote to enter the macrophage through the C3 complement receptor.

B This glycolipid antigen, a lipophosphoglycan, imparts resistance to complement-mediated lysis. That of *L. major* binds C3b, the third component of complement, enabling the promastigote to enter through the CR1 complement receptor. Antibodies to both antigens confer protection against murine cutaneous leishmaniasis.

Note that many coat proteins of parasites, such as the variable surface glycoprotein (VSG) of *T. brucei*, are now known to be bound to the surface membrane by a GPI anchor.

Antigenic variation in African trypanosomes

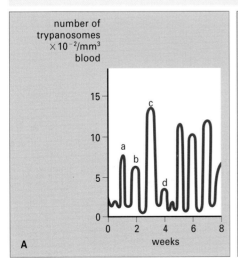

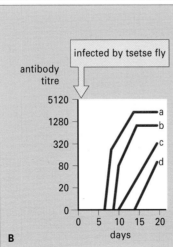

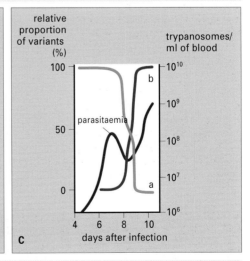

Fig. 18.25 Trypanosome infections may run for several months giving rise to successive waves of parasitaemia.

Graph A shows a chart of the fluctuation in parasitaemia in a patient with sleeping sickness. Although infection was initiated by a single parasite, each wave is caused by an immunologically distinct population of parasites (a,b,c,d); protection is not afforded by antibody against any of the preceding variants. There is a strong tendency for new variants to appear in the same order in different hosts. Variation does not occur in immunologically compromised animals (that is, animals treated to deprive them of some aspect of immune function).

Graph B shows the time-course of production of antibody against four variants in a rabbit bitten by a tsetse fly carrying *Trypanosoma brucei*. Antibody to successive variants appears shortly after the appearance of each variant and rises to a plateau. The appearance of antibody drives the parasite towards another variant type.

Graph C shows the kinetics of one cycle of antigenic variation. A rat was infected with a homogeneous population of one variant (a) of *T. brucei*. The second wave of parasitaemia develops as the new variant (b) emerges and predominates.

medium containing human serum and red blood cells can acquire surface molecules containing A, B and H blood-group determinants. They can also acquire MHC molecules. However, schistosomules maintained in medium devoid of host molecules also become resistant to attack by antibody and complement, as mentioned before.

Some extracellular parasites hide from immune attack

Some species of protozoa (e.g. *Entamoeba histolytica*) and of helminths (e.g. *T. spiralis*) form protective cysts, while adult worms of *O. volvulus* in the skin induce the host to surround them with collagenous nodules. Intestinal nematodes and tapeworms are preserved from many host responses simply because they are in the gut.

Some extracellular parasites can withstand immune attack

There are numerous examples of simple, physical protective strategies in parasites: nematodes have a thick extracellular cuticle which protects them from toxic onslaught; the tegument of schistosomes thickens during maturation to offer similar protection; the loose surface coat of many nematodes may slough off under immune attack; tapeworms actually prevent attack by secreting an elastase inhibitor, which stops them attracting neutrophils.

Many parasitic worms have evolved methods of resisting the oxidative burst. For instance, filarial worms in the lymphatics can secrete a surface-associated glutathione peroxidase, schistosomes have surface-associated glutathione S-transferases, and *Onchocerca* can secrete superoxide dismutase. Some nematodes and trematodes have evolved an elegant method of disabling antibodies by secreting proteases which cleave immunoglobulins, removing the Fc portion.

Most parasites interfere with the immune response

Immunosuppression is a universal feature of parasite infection (*Fig. 18.27*) and has been demonstrated for both antibody and cell-mediated responses. Whereas some parasites can cause disruption of lymphoid cells or tissue directly (e.g. newly hatched larvae of *T. spiralis*, which release a soluble lymphocytotoxic factor), much of the suppression may be due to interference with macrophage function. These cells may become overloaded with free antigen as many worms secrete quantities of polysaccharides and glycoconjugates which interfere with antigen processing. Certainly, macrophages from mice infected with schistosomes are defective at presenting antigen. Similarly, in mice infected with African trypanosomes, antigen presentation is diminished and IL-1 secretion reduced. In malaria, macrophages accumulate the pigment haemozoin, a breakdown product of haemoglobin, which interferes with many of their functions. Many parasite products stimulate macrophages to release prostaglandins and other suppressive molecules which subdue inflammatory reactions. Interestingly, filarial worms and tapeworms are themselves able to secrete prostaglandins, which also act to suppress inflammatory reactions.

Soluble parasite antigens released in huge quantities may impair the host's response by a process termed immune distraction. Thus the soluble antigens (S- or heat-stable antigens) of *P. falciparum* are thought to mop up circulating antibody, providing a 'smokescreen' and diverting the antibody from the body of the parasite. Many of the surface antigens that are shed are soluble forms of molecules inserted into the parasite membrane by a GPI anchor, including the VSG of *T. brucei*, the LPG or 'excreted factor' of *Leishmania* (*Fig. 18.24*) and several surface antigens of schistosomules. These are released by endogenous phosphatidylinositol-specific phospholipases.

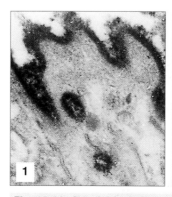
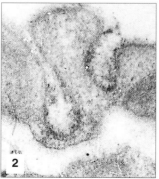
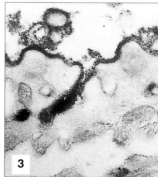
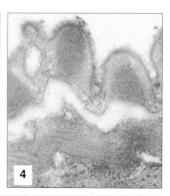

Fig. 18.26 Acquisition of host antigens by schistosomes. These electron micrographs show sections of the surface of schistosomes that have been incubated with labelled antibody against schistosome antigens or against mouse erythrocytes. Presence of each antigen is shown by the layer of electron-dense deposit of labelled antibody. Young 3-hour schistosomules bind parasite-specific antibody *in vitro* (1) but not after 4 days in a mouse host (2). Antibody against mouse antigens binds to the 4-day-old lung-stage parasite (3) but not to the newly transformed schistosomules (4). Thus, older worms express the species-specific antigens of their host but not their own antigens. Lung-stage worms are immune to attack by complement and antibody-mediated effectors *in vitro*. Worms transferred from one species to another die within 24 hours. They are only susceptible to attack by specific antibody in vitro if they are not coated with host protective antigens. (Courtesy of Dr D. McLaren.)

Interference with host's immune response by free antigens released by protozoa or worms

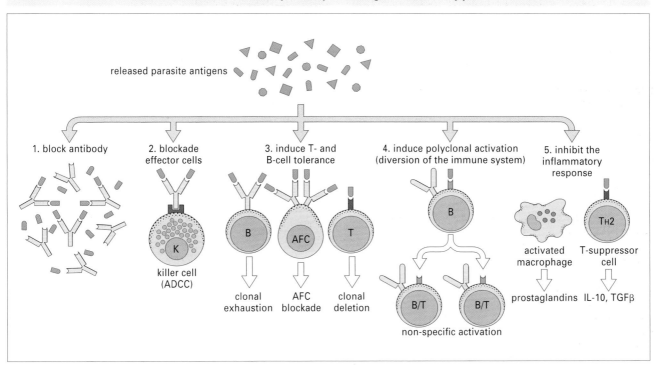

Fig. 18.27 Free antigens can:
1. Combine with antibody and divert it from the parasite. The variant surface glycoprotein of *Trypanosoma brucei* and the soluble antigens of *Plasmodium falciparum*, which are also polymorphic and contain repetitive sequences of amino acids, are thought to act in this way as a smokescreen or decoy.
2. Blockade effector cells, either directly or as immune complexes. Circulating complexes, for example, are able to inhibit the action of cytotoxic cells active against *Schistosoma mansoni*.
3. Induce T- or B-cell tolerance, presumably by blockage of antibody-forming cells (AFC) or by depletion of the mature antigen-specific lymphocytes through clonal exhaustion.
4. Cause polyclonal activation. Many parasite products are mitogenic to B or T cells, and the high serum concentrations of non-specific IgM (and IgG) commonly found in parasitic infections probably result from this polyclonal stimulation. Its continuation is believed to lead to impairment of B cell function, the progressive depletion of antigen-reactive B lymphocytes and thus immunosuppression.
5. Activate T cells, especially TH2 cells, or macrophages, or both, to release immunosuppressive molecules.

Antigen-specific suppression also occurs by suppression of delayed hypersensitivity. This may be selective, affecting only one of the CD4+ T cell subsets, but altering the balance between TH1 and TH2 lymphocytes to the parasite's advantage. Thus in leishmaniasis, T cells from patients infected with *L. donovani* when cultured with specific antigen do not secrete IL-2 or IFNγ. Their production of IL-1 and expression of MHC Class II is also decreased, and their secretion of prostaglandins is enhanced. Such patients benefit from treatment with IFNγ combined with pentavalent antimony. Similarly, in filariasis, TH1 cells do not proliferate in response to specific antigens though antibody responses remain intact. Indeed, patients heavily infected with filarial worms or schistosomes have large amounts of IgG4, which blocks protective IgE responses. In schistosomiasis, IgM and IgG2 antibodies against some schistosome carbohydrates inhibit the cytotoxic functions of granulocytes and are correlated with susceptibility to reinfection.

IL-2, another cytokine secreted by proliferating TH1 lymphocytes, is deficient in some protozoal infections, includ-ing malaria, African trypanosomiasis and Chagas' disease. In mice infected with *T. cruzi*, a parasite product appears to interfere with expression of the IL-2 receptor so that injection of IL-2 induces the receptor and restores T-helper cell activity, leading to more parasite-specific IgM and IgG, fewer parasites in the blood and longer survival time.

Some of the escape mechanisms discussed above are summarized in *Figure 18.28*.

■ IMMUNOPATHOLOGICAL CONSEQUENCES OF PARASITIC INFECTIONS

Apart from the directly destructive effects of some parasites and their products on host tissues, many immune responses themselves have pathological effects. In malaria, African trypanosomiasis and visceral leishmaniasis, the increased number and heightened activity of macrophages and lymphocytes in the liver and spleen lead to enlargement of those organs.

In schistosomiasis much of the pathology results from the T-cell dependent granulomas forming around eggs in the liver. The gross changes occurring in individuals with elephantiasis are probably caused by immunopathological responses to adult filariae in the lymphatics. The formation of immune complexes is common; they may be deposited in the kidney, as in the nephrotic syndrome of quartan malaria, and may give rise to many other pathological changes. For example, tissue-bound immunoglobulins have been found in the muscles of mice infected with African trypanosomes and in the choroid plexus of mice with malaria.

The IgE of worm infections can have severe effects on the host due to release of mast-cell mediators. Anaphylactic shock may occur when a hydatid cyst ruptures. Asthma-like reactions occur in *Toxocara canis* infections, and in tropical pulmonary eosinophilia when filarial worms migrate through the lungs.

Autoantibodies, which probably arise as a result of polyclonal activation, have been detected against red blood cells, lymphocytes and DNA (e.g. in trypanosomiasis and in malaria). Antibodies against the parasite may cross-react with host tissues. For example, the chronic cardiomyopathy, enlarged oesophagus and megacolon that occur in Chagas' disease are thought to result from the autoimmune effects on nerve ganglia of antibody and of cytotoxic T cells that cross-react with *T. cruzi*. Similarly *O. volvulus*, the cause of river blindness, possesses an antigen which cross-reacts with a protein in the retina.

Some mechanisms by which parasites avoid host defences

parasite	habitat	main host effector mechanism	method of avoidance
Trypanosoma brucei	bloodstream	antibody + complement	antigenic variation
Plasmodium spp.	hepatocyte, blood cell	antibody, cytokines	intracellular, antigenic variation
Toxoplasma gondii	macrophage	O$_2$ metabolites, NO, lysosomal enzymes	failure to trigger, inhibits fusion of lysosomes
Trypanosoma cruzi	many cells	O$_2$ metabolites, NO, lysosomal enzymes	escapes into cytoplasm, so avoiding digestion
Leishmania	macrophage	O$_2$ metabolites, NO, lysosomal enzymes	O$_2$ burst impaired and products scavenged, avoids digestion
Trichinella spiralis	gut, blood, muscle	myeloid cells, antibody + complement	encystment in muscle development of DAF
Schistosoma mansoni	skin, blood, lungs, portal vein	myeloid cells, antibody + complement	acquisition of host antigens, blockade by antibody, soluble antigens and immune complexes, antioxidants
Wuchereria bancrofti	lymphatics	myeloid cells, antibody + complement	thick extracellular cuticle, antitoxidants

Fig. 18.28 A summary of the various methods which parasites have evolved to avoid host defence mechanisms.

Possible causes of development of anaemia in malaria

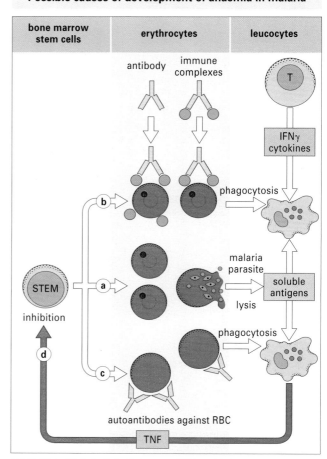

Fig. 18.29 There is more destruction of erythrocytes in malaria than can be accounted for by the number of infected by parasites. In addition to those lost by lysis when the schizont ruptures (a), immunopathological mechanisms probably contribute to the anaemia. Parasite antigens, or immune complexes containing parasite antigens, may bind to unparasitized erythrocytes and accelerate their clearance by cells of the macrophage/monocyte lineage in the spleen and liver (b). There is also some autoantibody produced against normal erythrocytes which again accelerates their removal (c). TNFα released in response to infection inhibits red blood cell development from bone marrow stem cells and alters the kinetics of red cell turnover (d).

Excessive production of some cytokines may contribute to some of the manifestations of disease. Thus the fever, anaemia, diarrhoea and pulmonary changes of acute malaria closely resemble the symptoms of endotoxaemia and are probably caused by TNFα. The severe wasting of cattle with trypanosomiasis may also be mediated by TNFα. Several immunological mechanisms may combine in producing pathological effects, as is likely in the anaemia of malaria (*Fig. 18.29*).

Lastly, the non-specific immunosuppression that is so widespread probably explains why people with parasitic infections are especially susceptible to bacterial and viral infections (e.g. measles). It may also account for the association of Burkitt's lymphoma with malaria.

■ VACCINES

Some vaccines that are composed of attenuated living parasites have proved successful in veterinary practice. However, so far there are none in use against human parasites, although much effort has been directed towards the development of subunit vaccines against malarial parasites and schistosomes in particular. Some clinical trials are in progress of vaccines against malaria, based on combinations of putatively protective peptides. For further details, see Chapter 19.

Critical Thinking

■ Parasites well adapted to existence within their host. What sort of evidence is there for effective immunity?

■ How would a naive host and an immune host differ in their defence mechanisms?

■ What is meant by 'stage-specific immunity' and why does it occur?

■ Why should T cells matter? How could they exacerbate an infection? How do they affect the expulsion of a parasitic worm from the gut?

■ How do TNFα and IFNγ affect parasite survival?

■ How do mechanisms involved in protection against intracellular and extracellular parasites differ?

■ How can protozoa living inside a macrophage escape destruction by enzymes or other cytotoxic molecules?

■ How do parasites living free in the blood or body fluids evade the immune response?

■ How do parasites induce immunopathology?

FURTHER READING

Brophy PM, Pritchard DI. Immunity to helminths: ready to tip the biochemical balance. *Parasitol Today* 1992;**8**:419.

Capron AR. Immunity to schistosomes. *Curr Opin Immunol* 1992;**4**:419.

Colley DG, Nix NA. Do schistosomes exploit the host pro-inflammatory cytokine TNF-α for their own survival? *Parasitol Today* 1992;**8**:355.

Cox FEG, Liew EY. T-cell subsets and cytokines in parasitic infections. *Parasitol Today* 1992;**8**:371.

Cox FEG. Vaccination against parasites. In: Behnke JM. *Parasites: Immunity and Pathology. The consequences of parasitic infection in mammals.* London: Taylor & Francis, 1990:396–416.

James SL. The effector functions of nitrogen oxides in host defense against parasites. *Exp Parasitol* 1991;**73**:223.

Kwiatkowski D. Malaria: becoming more specific about non-specific immunity. *Curr Opin Immunol* 1992;**4**:425.

Locksley RM, Louis JA. Immunology of leishmaniasis. *Curr Opin Immunol* 1992;**4**:413.

Non-specific immunization, for example by cytokines, may be of use in selected conditions when it is desirable to boost general immune activity.

Adjuvants, substances that enhance antibody production, are usually required with non-living vaccines.

Recombinant DNA technology will probably be the basis for the next generation of vaccines.

Adaptive immunity and the ability of lymphocytes to develop memory for a pathogen's antigens underlie vaccination.

A wide range of antigen preparations are in use as vaccines, from whole organisms to simple peptides and sugars.

Living and non-living vaccines have important differences, living vaccines being generally more effective.

Active immunization is known as vaccination.

Passive immunization, the direct administration of antibodies, still has a role to play in certain circumstances, for example when tetanus toxin is already in the circulation.

Vaccination is the best-known and the most successful application of immunological principles to human health. The first vaccine was named after vaccinia, the cowpox virus. Jenner pioneered its use 200 years ago. It was the first deliberate scientific attempt to prevent an infectious disease (smallpox), but it was done in complete ignorance of viruses (or indeed any kind of microbe) and immunology.

It was not until the work of Pasteur 100 years later that the general principle governing vaccination emerged: altered preparations of microbes could be used to generate enhanced immunity against the fully virulent organism. Thus Pasteur's dried rabies-infected rabbit spinal cords and heated anthrax bacilli were the true forerunners of today's vaccines, while Jenner's animal-derived (i.e. 'heterologous') vaccinia virus has had no real successors.

Even Pasteur did not have a proper understanding of immunological memory or the functions of the lymphocyte, which had to wait another half century. Finally, with Burnet's clonal selection theory (1957) and the discovery of T and B lymphocytes (1965), the key mechanism became clear. The antigen(s) of a vaccine must induce clonal expansion in specific T and/or B cells, leaving behind a population of memory cells. These enable the next encounter with the same antigen(s) to induce a secondary response which is more rapid and effective than the normal primary response. The primary response is so often too slow to prevent serious disease (see Fig. 1.20).

Vaccination, therefore, involves *adaptive* immunity, the art of vaccination being to produce antigenic preparations from the pathogen that:
- Are safe to administer.
- Induce the right sort of immunity.
- Are affordable by the population at which they are aimed.
For many diseases, this has been achieved with brilliant success, but for others there is no vaccine whatsoever. This chapter is mainly concerned with the reasons for this disparity.

■ ANTIGENS USED AS VACCINES

The type of antigen used in a vaccine depends on many factors. In general, the more antigens of the microbe retained in the vaccine, the better, and living organisms tend to be more effective than killed ones (see later). Exceptions to this rule are diseases where a toxin is responsible for the pathology. In this case the vaccine can be based on the toxin alone. Another example is a vaccine in which microbial antigens are expressed in another type of cell, which acts as a vector.

Figure 19.1 lists the main antigenic preparations currently available.

The main antigenic preparations

type of antigen		vaccine examples
living organisms	natural	vaccinia (for smallpox) vole bacillus (for TB; historical)
	attenuated	*polio (Sabin; oral polio vaccine) *measles.*mumps.*rubella yellow fever 17D varicella-zoster (human herpes virus 3) *BCG (for TB)
intact but non-living organisms	viruses	*polio (Salk), rabies, influenza, hepatitis A, typhus
	bacteria	*pertussis, typhoid, cholera, plague
subcellular fragments	capsular polysaccharides	pneumococcus meningococcus *Haemophilus influenzae*
	surface antigen	*hepatitis B
toxoids		*tetanus, *diphtheria
recombinant DNA-based	gene cloned and expressed	*hepatitis B (yeast-derived)
	genes expressed in vectors	experimental
	naked DNA	experimental
anti-idiotype		experimental
* Standard in most countries		

Fig. 19.1 A wide range of antigenic preparations are used as vaccines.

Live vaccines can be natural or attenuated organisms

Natural live vaccines have rarely been used

Apart from vaccinia, no other completely natural organism has ever come into standard use. However bovine and simian rotaviruses have been tried in children, the vole tubercle bacillus was once popular against tuberculosis (TB), and in the Middle East and Russia *Leishmania* infection from mild cases is reputed to induce immunity. It is possible that another good heterologous vaccine will be found, but the safety problems will be considerable.

Attenuated live vaccines have been highly successful

The preferred strategy has been to *attenuate* a human pathogen, with the aim of diminishing its virulence while retaining the desired antigens. This was first done successfully by Calmette and Guérin with a bovine strain (*M. bovis*) of *Mycobacterium tuberculosis*, which during 13 years (1908–

1921) of culture *in vitro* changed to the much less virulent form now known as BCG (bacille Calmette–Guérin), which has at least some protective effect against TB. The real successes have been with viruses, starting with the 17D strain of yellow fever virus obtained by passage in mice and chicken embryos (1937), and followed by a roughly similar approach with polio, measles, mumps and rubella (*Fig. 19.2*). Just how successful the latter vaccines are is shown by the decline in these four diseases in the last two to three decades (*Fig. 19.3*).

Attenuation can be achieved by mutation. – What is meant by 'changed'? With these pioneer attenuated organisms, it meant a purely random series of mutations, induced by the unfavourable conditions of growth, constantly monitored and selected for antigen retention and loss of virulence. This a tedious process which has been aptly termedn 'genetic roulette'. When the sequencing of viral genomes became possible, it emerged that the results were widely divergent. An example of this is the differences between the three types of live (Sabin) polio vaccine. The Type 1 polio vaccine contains 57 mutations, and has almost never reverted to wild type (i.e. virulence), while the Type 2 and 3 vaccines depend for their safety on only two key mutations. In these later types frequent reversions to the wild type have occurred, some of which have led to outbreaks of paralytic poliomyelitis. One outbreak, in Sweden, was sufficient to persuade the health authorities there to discontinue the live vaccine in favour of the killed (Salk) one (see below). In favour of the live vaccine is the fact that in many parts of the USA it has now replaced the wild-type virus in the water supplies, no doubt protecting some individuals who were never vaccinated – a perfect example of 'herd immunity'. With the sophisticated recombinant DNA technology now available, it seems likely that future attenuated vaccines, both viral and bacterial, will have 'site-directed' rather than random mutations.

Killed vaccines are intact but non-living organisms

These are the successors of Pasteur's killed vaccines mentioned earlier. Some are very effective (rabies and the Salk polio vaccine), some moderately so (typhoid, cholera and influenza), some are of debatable value (plague and typhus) and some

Live attenuated vaccines

	disease	remarks
viruses	polio	Types 2, 3 may revert; also killed vaccine
	measles	80% effective
	mumps	
	rubella	now given to both sexes
	yellow fever	stable since 1937
	varicella-zoster	mainly in leukaemia
	hepatitis A	also killed vaccine
bacteria	tuberculosis	stable since 1921; also some protection against leprosy

Fig. 19.2 Attenuated vaccines are available for many, but not all, infections. In general it has proved easier to attenuate viruses than bacteria.

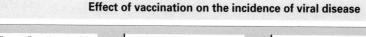

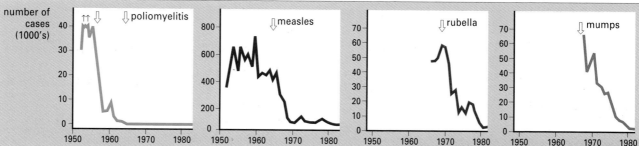

Fig. 19.3 The effect of vaccination on the incidence of various viral diseases in the USA has been that most infections have shown a dramatic downward trend after the introduction of a vaccine (arrows).

are controversial on the grounds of toxicity (pertussis). *Figure 19.4* lists the main killed vaccines in use today. It is hoped that some of these may eventually be replaced by attenuated versions, because these would be more effective, and there is some prospect of this for rabies and (genetically engineered) typhoid and cholera.

Inactivated toxins and toxoids are the most successful bacterial vaccines

The most successful of all bacterial vaccines – tetanus and diphtheria (*Fig. 19.5*) – are based on inactivated exotoxins (*Fig. 19.6*), and in principle the same approach can be used for several other infections.

Tetanus toxoid can be used as a 'carrier' for other vaccines

Tetanus toxoid has another useful role, as a 'carrier' for small peptide vaccines that would otherwise be non-immunogenic.

This works because most people have been vaccinated against tetanus and therefore have memory T cells that recognize the toxin. It is better to use as a carrier a protein from the organism against which vaccination is being directed (pneumococcus, malaria, etc.).

Subcellular fragments and surface antigens are safe and effective vaccines

It is the surface antigens of most organisms that the immune system sees first and responds to, particularly in the case of B cells and antibody. With organisms that can be controlled by a brisk antibody response, the surface antigens constitute a

Killed (whole-organism) vaccines

disease		remarks
viruses	polio	preferred in Scandinavia; safe in immunocompromised
	rabies	can be given post-exposure, with passive antiserum
	influenza	strain-specific
	hepatitis A	also attenuated vaccine
bacteria	pertussis	potential to cause brain damage (controversial)
	typhoid	about 70% protection
	cholera	protection dubious; may be combined with toxin subunit
	plague	short-term protection only
	Q fever	good protection

Fig. 19.4 The principal whole-organism, killed vaccines.

Toxin-based vaccines

organism	vaccine	remarks
Clostridium tetani	inactivated toxin (formalin)	3 doses, alum-precipitated; boost every 10 years
Corynebacterium diphtheriae		usually given with tetanus
Vibrio cholerae	toxin, B subunit	sometimes combined with whole killed organisms
Clostridium perfringens	inactivated toxin (formalin)	newborn lambs

Fig. 19.6 The principal toxin-based vaccines. Note that there are no vaccines against the numerous staphylococcal and streptococcal exotoxins, or against bacterial endotoxins such as lipopolysaccharides.

Success of immunization against diphtheria

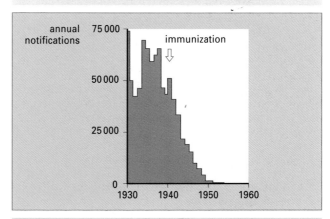

Fig. 19.5 Annual notifications of diphtheria demonstrate the great success of vaccines based on inactivated toxin: the number of cases dropped dramatically after vaccination was introduced in 1940. (Courtesy of Professor J. R. Pattison, Ch. 26 in Brostoff J. *et al.*, eds, *Clinical Immunology*, London: Mosby, 1991.)

Vaccines based on subcellular microbial fragments

	organism	remarks
bacteria	Neisseria meningitidis	groups A and C; effective group B: non-immunogenic
	Streptococcus pneumoniae	84 serotypes; vaccines contain at least 23
	Haemophilus influenzae B	all polysaccharide vaccines require conjugation to a protein carrier
	Neisseria gonorrhoeae	not very effective
	Escherichia coli	veterinary
virus	hepatitis B virus	>95% protective

Fig. 19.7 The principal vaccines based on subcellular microbial fragments.

safe and effective vaccine (*Fig. 19.7*). The major successes have been with capsulated bacteria, whose capsular polysaccharides can be obtained in commercial quantities, and the hepatitis B virus, which has the unusual feature of massively over-producing its surface coat (HBs).

Small antigens can be made synthetically or by gene cloning

Where it can be shown that a small peptide is protective, which is by no means always the case, it may be more convenient to make it synthetically or by cloning its gene into a suitable expression vector. This approach has been highly successful with the HBs antigen, cloned into yeast and now replacing the first-generation HBs vaccine which was laboriously purified from the blood of HB carriers; it has also brought down the cost of the vaccine.

An attractive feature of this approach is that further sequences can be added – for example selected B- and T-cell epitopes can be combined in various ways to optimize the resulting immune response. It is important to remember that, whereas B cells respond to the 3-dimensional *shape* of antigens, T cells recognize *linear sequences* of amino acids (see Chapter 7). Thus peptides can function well as T-cell epitopes but cannot readily mimic the discontinuous B-cell epitope. Even where a B-cell determinant is linear, antibodies raised against the free flexible peptide do not bind optimally to the sequence in the way that they do when it is present as a more rigid structure with the native protein molecule.

Future vaccines will use genes and vectors to deliver antigen *in situ*

A further development of the use of gene-cloning is to put the desired gene into some vector which can then be injected into the patient and allowed to replicate, express the gene and deliver large amounts of the antigen *in situ* (*Fig. 19.8*). It was originally proposed that vaccinia, although occasionally toxic, would be a suitable vector. Against this is the fact that many people are already immune to it and would eliminate it too rapidly. Almost all the available attenuated viral vaccines have been suggested as alternatives.

Another approach is to use attenuated bacteria as vectors. BCG seems a natural candidate, as it has been calculated that its genome is large enough to accommodate genes from all the other vaccine candidate organisms. There is also a range of mutant salmonellae that can be given by mouth and immunize the gut lymphoid tissues before being eliminated; these would be ideal for inducing local gut immunity – a very desirable aim in view of the fact that infantile diarrhoeal disease is the world's number one killer. A further advantage is that the attenuated organism may be taken up by macrophages, thereby inducing a systemic immune response through dissemination to other parts of the body.

An even more recent development is to inject the DNA itself, coupled to a suitable promoter, into the muscles of the individual to be vaccinated. Surprisingly, this gives rise to excellent immunity, both antibody- and cell-mediated, and no evidence for the tolerance that might have been expected to result from the potentially unlimited source of foreign antigen. There is tremendous interest and activity in this new field.

Anti-idiotype vaccines could be used when the original antigen is unsuitable

This is the only type of vaccine for which immunological thinking has been entirely responsible. The idea is to use

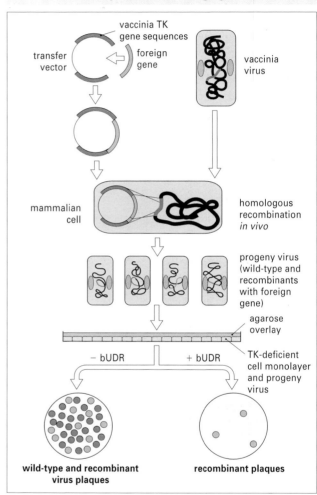

Generation of recombinant vaccinia virus for expression of a foreign gene

Fig. 19.8 Recombinant vaccinia virus can be generated to express a foreign gene. The foreign gene is inserted into vaccinia's thymidine kinase (TK) gene so that recombinant virus plaques can be distinguished from wild-type. TK is used by virus to take up thymidine from the culture medium or intracellular pool for DNA synthesis: the recombinant virus cannot produce TK, because the gene has been interrupted and so must use the separate pathway for *de novo* synthesis of thymidine. In the presence of bromodeoxyuridine (bUDR), a thymidine analogue that blocks DNA synthesis when it is incorporated into DNA, wild-type virus replication is blocked by bUDR but recombinant virus replication continues, using *de novo* synthesis of thymidine. The cell monolayer must be TK deficient so that recombinant virus cannot use the cells' TK to take up bUDR. (Courtesy of Dr D. J. Rowlands, Ch. 26 in Brostoff J. *et al.*, eds, *Clinical Immunology*, London: Mosby, 1991.)

monoclonal antibody (mAb) technology to make large amounts of anti-idiotype (anti-Id) against the V region (idiotype) of an antibody of proven protective value. The anti-Id, if properly selected, would then have a 3-dimensional shape similar to the original immunizing antigen and could be used in place of it (*Fig. 19.9*). Though often dismissed as 'armchair immunology', this strategy could have real value where the original antigen is not itself suitable, i.e. is not immunogenic. Polysaccharides are one example, and the lipid A region of bacterial endotoxin (LPS) is another. The advantage of the mAb would be that since it is a protein it should induce memory, which polysaccharides and lipids normally do not.

■ EFFECTIVENESS OF VACCINES

To be introduced and approved, a vaccine must obviously be effective, and the efficacy of all vaccines is reviewed from time to time. Many factors affect it. An effective vaccine must:

- **Induce the right sort of immunity:** antibody for toxins and extracellular organisms such as *Streptococcus pneumoniae*; cell-mediated immunity for intracellular organisms such as the tubercle bacillus. Where the ideal type of response is not clear (as in malaria, for instance), designing an effective vaccine becomes correspondingly more difficult.
- **Be stable on storage:** this is particularly important for living vaccines, which normally require to be kept cold, i.e. a complete 'cold chain' from manufacturer to clinic, by no means always easy to maintain.
- **Have sufficient immunogenicity:** with non-living vaccines it is often necessary to boost their immunogenicity with an *adjuvant* (see later).

Live vaccines are generally more effective than killed ones

Induction of appropriate immunity depends on the properties of the antigen. Living vaccines have the great advantage of providing an increasing antigenic challenge that lasts days or weeks, and inducing it in the right site – which in practice is most important where mucosal immunity is concerned (*Fig. 19.10*). Live vaccines are likely to contain the greatest number of microbial antigens. Killed vaccines may suffer from two other inconveniences: T-cell independence and major histocompatibility complex (MHC) restriction (see Chapter 9).

Anti-idiotype antibodies as vaccines

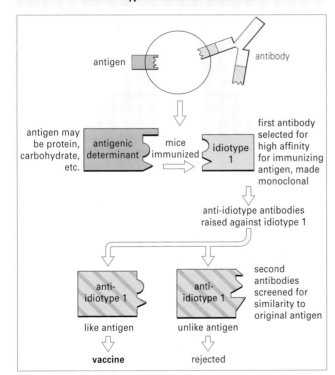

Fig. 19.9 Monoclonal antibody technology and the discovery of the 'idiotype network' (see Chapter 11) has meant that immunoglobulins can now be used as 'surrogate' antigens. In the case of a carbohydrate or lipid antigen, this allows a protein 'copy' to be made, which may have some advantages as a vaccine.

Antibody responses to live and killed polio vaccine

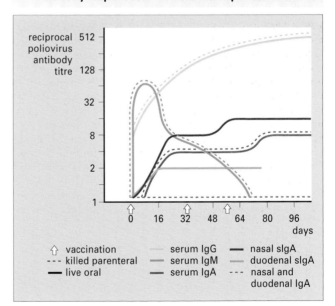

Fig. 19.10 The antibody response to orally administered live-attenuated polio vaccine (solid lines) and intramuscularly administered killed polio vaccine (broken lines). The live vaccine induces production of secretory IgA (sIgA) in addition to serum antibodies. As sIgA is the immunoglobulin of the mucosa-associated lymphoid tissue (MALT) system (see Chapter 3), the live vaccine confers protection at the portal of entry of the virus, the gastrointestinal mucosa. (Courtesy of Professor J. R. Pattison, Ch. 26 in Brostoff J. *et al.*, eds, *Clinical Immunology*, London: Mosby, 1991.)

Polysaccharides are typically thymus independent, since they do not bind to MHC and so do not immunize T cell. The present strategy for inducing memory is to couple them either to a standard protein carrier such as tetanus toxoid (see p. 19.2) or to a protein from the immunizing organism such as the outer membrane protein of pneumococci, *Haemophilus*, etc. MHC restriction affects small peptides in the 10–20 amino acid range, and shows up as 'genetic unresponsiveness' because the peptides bind only to certain MHC molecules. This is probably more hypothetical than real, since most candidate vaccines are considerably larger than this. Nevertheless, even the most effective vaccines often fail to immunize every individual; for example, about 5% fail to seroconvert after the full course of hepatitis B vaccine.

■ VACCINE SAFETY

Having been somewhat ignored in the early days, safety has now become an overriding consideration. It is of course a relative term, minor local pain or swelling at the injection site, and even mild fever, being generally acceptable, although the public (led by the legal profession) is becoming increasingly aware of the possibilities of profitable litigation. This is not surprising when one remembers that, unlike antibiotics, etc., most vaccinations are given to people who have previously been perfectly well.

Some more of the serious complications may stem from the vaccine or from the patient (*Fig. 19.11*). Vaccines may be contaminated with unwanted proteins or toxins, or even live viruses. Supposedly killed vaccines may not have been properly killed; attenuated vaccines may revert to the wild type. The patient may be hypersensitive to minute amounts of contaminating protein, or immunocompromised, in which case any living vaccine is usually contraindicated.

Safety problems with vaccines

type of vaccine	potential safety problems	examples
attenuated vaccines	reversion to wild type	especially polio Types 2 and 3
	severe disease in immunodeficient patients	vaccinia, BCG, measles
	persistent infection	varicella-zoster
	hypersensitivity to viral antigens	measles
	hypersensitivity to egg antigens	measles, mumps
killed vaccines	vaccine not killed	polio, BCG accidents in the past
	yeast contaminant	hepatitis B
	contamination with animal viruses	polio
	contamination with endotoxin	pertussis

Fig. 19.11 The potential safety problems encountered with vaccines emphasize the need for continuous monitoring of both production and administration.

■ COST OF VACCINATION

Although vaccination can safely be considered the most cost-effective treatment for infectious disease, individual vaccines may still be too expensive for the people they are designed for. A good example is hepatitis B; even the gene-cloned vaccine, at $80 per person, is out of reach of 90% of the world's population. At the other end of the scale, BCG can be delivered at a few cents per dose. Given the low profitability of vaccines compared to antibiotics, one should perhaps be grateful that there are any vaccine manufacturers are left!

■ CURRENT VACCINES

Vaccines in general use have variable success rates

Figure 19.12 lists the vaccines in standard use worldwide. Four of them – polio, measles, mumps and rubella – are so successful that these diseases are earmarked for eradication early in the 21st century. If this happens, it will be an extraordinary achievement, because mathematical modelling suggests that they are all more 'difficult' targets for eradication than smallpox was. However, for a number of reasons, other vaccines are less likely to lead to eradication of disease:

- **The carrier state:** eradication of hepatitis B would be a major triumph, but it will require the breaking of the carrier state, especially in the Far East, where mother to child is the normal route of infection.
- **Suboptimal effectiveness:** effectiveness of BCG varies markedly from country to country (tuberculosis is on the increase, especially in patients with immune deficiency syndrome, or AIDS), and the pertussis vaccine is only about 70% effective.
- **Side-effects:** the pertussis vaccine is suspected of having side-effects, reducing the public's willingness to be vaccinated.
- **Free-living forms and animal hosts:** the free-living form of tetanus will presumably survive indefinitely, and it will not be possible to eradicate diseases that also have an animal host, such as yellow fever.

One of the future problems is going to be maintaining

Vaccines in general use

disease	vaccine	remarks
tetanus	toxoid	given together in 3 doses between 2 and 6 months; tetanus and diphtheria boosted every 10 years
diphtheria	toxoid	
pertussis	killed whole	
polio	killed (Salk) or attenuated (Sabin)	
measles	attenuated	given together ('MMR') at 12–18 months
mumps		
rubella		
Haemophilus	polysaccharide	new; may be added to above

Fig. 19.12 Vaccines that are currently given, as far as is possible, to all individuals.

awareness of the need for vaccination against diseases that seem to be disappearing. Another problem is that as the reservoir of infection diminishes, cases tend to occur at a later age, which with measles and rubella could actually lead to worse clinical consequences.

Some vaccines are reserved for special groups only

In the developed world BCG and hepatitis B fall into this category, but some vaccines will probably always be confined to selected populations – travellers, nurses, the elderly, etc. (*Fig. 19.13*). In some cases this is because of geographical restrictions (e.g. yellow fever) or the rarity of exposure (e.g. rabies), while in others it is due to problems in producing sufficient vaccine in time to meet the demand. For example, each influenza epidemic is caused by a different strain, requiring a new vaccine. A vaccine effective against all strains of influenza would be of tremendous value; unfortunately, however, both the haemagglutinin and neuraminidase antigens, which together make up the outer layer of the virus and are the antigens of importance in the vaccine, are subject to variation.

For parasitic and some other infections, there are only experimental vaccines

Some of the most intensely researched vaccines are those for the major tropical protozoal and worm infections. However, none has come into standard use, and some have argued that none will, since none of these diseases induces effective immunity and 'you cannot improve on nature'. Nevertheless, extensive work in laboratory animals has shown that vaccines against malaria, leishmaniasis and schistosomiasis are perfectly feasible, and there is a moderately effective vaccine against babesia in dogs. In cattle an irradiated vaccine against the lungworm has been in veterinary use for decades.

It remains possible, however, that the parasitic diseases of humans are uniquely difficult to treat, partly because of the polymorphic and rapidly changing nature of many parasitic antigens. For example, none of the small animal models of malaria shows such extensive antigenic variation as does *Plasmodium falciparum*, the protozoan causing malignant tertian malaria in humans. Similarly, rats appear to be much easier to immunize against schistosomiasis than other animals, including possibly humans. Part of the problem is that these parasites are usually not in their natural host in the laboratory.

Three trials of clinical malaria vaccine have been published, and the results of a fourth are awaited at the time of writing. Malaria is unusual in that its life cycle offers a variety of possible targets for vaccination (*Fig 19.14*). The trials show that at least some protection is possible against both the liver and the blood stages. A trial of killed leishmania parasites combined with BCG gave no less than 90% protection in Venezuela.

A problem with these chronic parasitic diseases is that of immunopathology. For example, the symptoms of *Trypanosoma cruzi* infection (Chagas' disease) are largely due to the immune system, i.e. autoimmunity. A bacterial parallel is

Vaccines restricted to certain groups

disease	vaccine	eligible groups
tuberculosis	BCG	tropics: at birth UK: 10–14 years USA: at-risk only
hepatitis B	surface antigen	at-risk (medical, nursing staff, etc.) drug addicts; male homosexuals known contacts of carriers
rabies	killed	at-risk (animal workers) post-exposure
meningitis yellow fever typhoid, cholera hepatitis A	polysaccharide attenuated killed; mutant killed/attenuated	travellers
influenza	killed	at-risk; elderly
pneumococcal pneumonia	polysaccharide	elderly
varicella-zoster	attenuated	leukaemic children

Fig. 19.13 Vaccines that are currently restricted to certain groups.

Malaria vaccine strategies

stage	vaccine strategy
sporozoites	sporozoite vaccine to induce blocking antibody, already field-tested in humans
liver stage	sporozoite vaccine to induce cell-mediated immunity to liver stage
merozoites	merozoite (-antigen) vaccine to induce blocking antibody
asexual erythrocyte stage	asexual stage (-antigen) vaccine to induce other responses to red-cell stage, and against toxic products ('anti-disease' vaccine)
gametocytes gametes	vaccines to interrupt sexual stages – 'transmission-blocking' vaccine

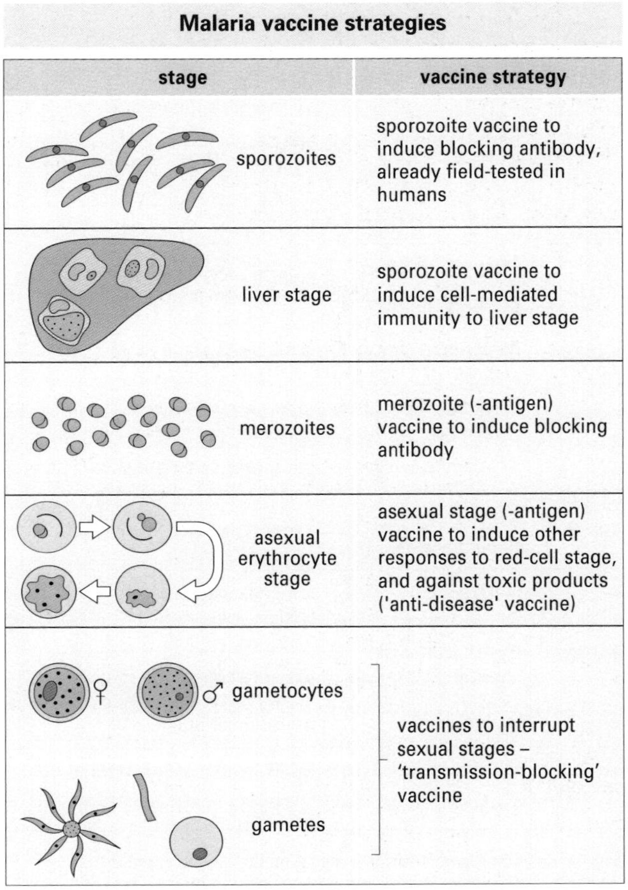

Fig. 19.14 A number of different approaches to malaria vaccines are being investigated, reflecting the complexity of both the life cycle of malaria and immunity to it.

leprosy, where the symptoms are due to the (apparent) over-reactivity of TH1 or TH2 cells. A vaccine that boosted immunity without clearing the pathogen could make these conditions worse. Another example of this unpleasant possibility is with dengue, where certain antibodies enhance the infection by allowing the virus to enter cells via Fc receptors. Enhancing antibodies have also been reported in an experimental model of a transmission-blocking anti-malarial vaccine.

Other experimental vaccines
Some other viral and bacterial vaccines are also in the experimental category (cholera toxin, attenuated *Shigella*, 'nursery' strains of rotavirus, Epstein–Barr virus surface glycoprotein).

For many diseases there is no vaccine available
There remains a long list of serious infectious diseases where no vaccine is currently available (*Fig. 19.15*). Headed by human immunodeficiency virus (HIV), these represent the major challenge for research and development in the coming decade.

Major diseases for which no vaccines are available

	disease	problems
viruses	HIV	antigenic variation; immunosuppression?
	herpes viruses	risk of reactivation? (but varicella-zoster appears safe)
	adenoviruses, rhinoviruses	multiple serotypes
bacteria	staphylococci	early vaccines ineffective (antibiotics originally better)
	group A streptococci	
	Mycobacterium leprae	(BCG gives some protection)
	Treponema pallidum (syphilis)	ignorance of effective immunity
	Chlamydia	early vaccines ineffective
fungi	*Candida*	ignorance of effective immunity
	Pneumocystis	
protozoa	malaria	antigenic variation (trials encouraging)
	trypanosomiasis: sleeping sickness Chagas' disease leishmaniasis	extreme antigenic variation immunopathology; autoimmunity trials encouraging
worms	schistosomiasis	(trials in animals encouraging)
	onchocerciasis	ignorance of effective immunity

Fig. 19.15 For some serious diseases there is currently no effective vaccine. The predominant problem is the lack of understanding of how to induce effective immunity.

■ ADJUVANTS

During work in the 1920s on the production of animal sera for human therapy, it was discovered that certain substances, notably aluminium salts, added to or emulsified with an antigen, greatly enhance antibody production; that is, they act as *adjuvants*. Aluminium hydroxide is still widely used with, for example, diphtheria and tetanus toxoids. With modern understanding of the processes leading to lymphocyte triggering and the development of memory, considerable efforts have been made to produce better adjuvants, particularly for T-cell-mediated responses. *Figure 19.16* gives a list of these, but it should be stressed that none of the new adjuvants is yet accepted for routine human use.

Adjuvants either concentrate antigen at appropriate sites or induce cytokines
It appears that the effect of adjuvants is due mainly to two activities: the concentration of antigen in a site where lymphocytes are exposed to it (the 'depot' effect) and the induction of cytokines which regulate lymphocyte function. Aluminium salts probably have a predominantly depot function, inducing small granulomas in which antigen is retained. Newer devices such as liposomes and immune-stimulating complexes (ISCOMs) achieve the same purpose by ensuring that antigens trapped in them are delivered to antigen-presenting cells. Bacterial products such as mycobacterial cell walls, endotoxin,

Adjuvants

adjuvant type	routinely used in man	experimental* or too toxic for human use†
inorganic salts	aluminium hydroxide (alhydrogel) aluminium phosphate calcium phosphate beryllium hydroxide	beryllium hydroxide
delivery systems		liposomes* ISCOMS* block polymers slow release formulations* BCG
bacterial products	*Bordetella pertussis* (with diphtheria, tetanus toxoids)	*Mycobacterium bovis* and oil† (complete Freund's adjuvant) muramyl dipeptide (MDP†)
natural mediators (cytokines)		IL-1 IL-2 IFNγ

Fig. 19.16 A variety of foreign and endogenous substances can act as adjuvants, but only aluminium and calcium salts and pertussis are routinely used in clinical practice.

etc., probably act mainly by stimulating the formation of the appropriate cytokines. This theory is supported by the fact that cytokines themselves have been shown to be effective adjuvants, particularly when coupled directly to the antigen. Cytokines may be particularly useful in immunocompromised patients (*see Fig. 19.18*), who often fail to respond to normal vaccines. It is hoped that they might also be useful in directing the immune response in the desired direction – for example in diseases where only TH1 (or TH2) cell memory is wanted.

PASSIVE IMMUNIZATION

Driven from use by the advent of antibiotics, the idea of injecting preformed antibody to treat infection is still valid for certain situations (*Fig. 19.17*). It can be life-saving where toxins are already circulating (e.g. in tetanus, diphtheria and snake-bite), and where high-titre specific antibody is required, generally made in horses but occasionally obtained from recovered patients. At the opposite end of the scale, normal pooled human immunoglobulin contains enough antibody against common infections for a dose of 100–400 mg of IgG to protect hypogammaglobulinaemic patients for a month. Over 1000 donors are used for each pool, and the sera must be screened for HIV and hepatitis B and C.

The use of specific monoclonal antibodies, though theoretically attractive, has not yet proved to be an improvement on traditional methods, and their chief application to infectious disease at present remains in diagnosis. This may change as human monoclonal antibodies become more readily available (and less expensive) either through cell culture or protein engineering (see Chapter 28).

NON-SPECIFIC IMMUNOTHERAPY

Many of the same compounds that act as adjuvants for vaccines have also been used on their own in an attempt to boost the general level of immune activity (*Fig. 19.18*). The best results have been obtained with cytokines, and among these interferon-α (IFNα) is the most widely used, mainly for its anti-viral properties (but also for certain tumours – see below and Chapter 20). Perhaps the most striking clinical effect of a cytokine has been that of granulocyte–colony-stimulating factor (G–CSF) in restoring bone-marrow function after anti-cancer therapy, with benefit to both bleeding and infection.

Finally cytokine inhibitors can be used for severe or chronic inflammatory conditions. Various ways of inhibiting tumour necrosis factor (TNF) and interleukin-1 (IL-1) have proved valuable in rheumatoid arthritis and, more controversially, in septic (Gram-negative) shock and severe malaria. In a few years, one would expect the clinical pharmacology of cytokines and cytokine inhibitors to be clarified so that these communication molecules of the immune system can be fully exploited, in the same way as vaccination has exploited the properties of the lymphocyte.

VACCINATING AGAINST CANCER

The idea of non-specifically stimulating the immune system to reject tumours goes back almost a century to the work of Coley, who used bacterial filtrates with considerable success, possibly through the induction of cytokines such as TNF and

Passive immunization

disease	source of antibody	indication
diphtheria tetanus	human, horse	prophylaxis, treatment
varicella-zoster	human	treatment in immunodeficiencies
gas gangrene botulism snake bite scorpion sting	horse	post-exposure
rabies	human	post-exposure (plus vaccine)
hepatitis B	human	post-exposure
hepatitis A measles	pooled human immunoglobulin	prophylaxis (travel) post-exposure

Fig. 19.17 Although not so commonly used as 50 years ago, injections of specific antibody can still be a life-saving treatment in specific clinical conditions.

Non-specific immunotherapy

	source	remarks
microbial	filtered bacterial cultures	used by Coley (1909) against tumours
	BCG	some activity against tumours
cytokines	IFNα	effective in chronic: hepatitis B, hepatitis C, herpes zoster, wart virus, prophylactic against common cold (also some tumours)
	IFNγ	effective in some cases of: chronic granulomatous disease, lepromatous leprosy, leishmaniasis (cutaneous)
	IL-2	leishmaniasis (cutaneous)
	GCSF	bone marrow restoration after cytotoxic drugs
cytokine inhibitors	TNF antagonists	septic shock
	IL-1 antagonists	severe (cerebral) malaria?
	IL-10	

Fig. 19.18 Non-specific stimulation or inhibition of particular components of the immune system may sometimes be of benefit.

IFN. However, attempts to equal his results with purified cytokines or immunostimulants (e.g. BCG) have been successful only in a restricted range of tumours, and current efforts are mainly directed at the induction of *specific* immunity – just as for infectious microbes – encouraged by the evidence that tumours may sometimes be spontaneously rejected as if they were foreign grafts. This subject is dealt with more fully in Chapter 20.

■ ANTI-FERTILITY VACCINES

In principle, conception and implantation can be interrupted by inducing immunity against a wide range of pregnancy hormones. The target of the most successful experimental trials has been human chorionic gonadotropin (hCG), the embryo-specific hormone responsible for maintaining the corpus luteum. Vaccines based on the β chain of hCG, coupled to tetanus or diphtheria toxoid, have been extremely successful in preventing conception in baboons and, more recently, humans. In the human trial, infertility was only temporary, and no serious side-effects were observed. Clearly this represents a powerful new means of safely limiting family size, though there are of course cultural and ethical aspects to consider too.

Critical Thinking

■ Why have attenuated vaccines not been developed for all viruses and bacteria?

■ 'A vaccine cannot improve on nature.' Is this unduly pessimistic?

■ 'The smallpox success story is unlikely to be repeated.' Is this true?

■ Will vaccines eventually replace antibiotics?

■ BCG: vaccine, adjuvant, or non-specific stimulant?

■ Why could an anti-worm vaccine do more harm than good?

■ By what means, other than their reaction with antibodies, might you identify antigens that could be used as vaccines?

FURTHER READING

Immunisation against Infectious Disease. London: HMSO, 1988.
Modern Vaccines. London: Edward Arnold, 1990.
Vaccination in: *Medical Microbiology*, Mims CA, Playfair JHL, Roitt IM, Wakelin D, Williams R. London: Mosby, 1993.

Vaccine Design. Brown F, Dougan G, Hoey EM, Martin SJ, Rima BK, Trudgett A. Chichester: John Wiley & Sons, 1993.

Immune surveillance is a concept that envisages prevention of the development of most tumours, through early destruction of abnormal cells by the host's immune system.

Surveillance probably acts against viruses not tumours. The evidence for this is provided by the fact that, although there is an increased incidence of tumours in immunosuppressed individuals, the most dramatic increase is in tumours associated with oncogenic viruses.

Cellular responses to tumour-associated antigens occur; the antigens may be virus coded, or they may be altered or over-expressed host gene products.

Differentiation antigens expressed on tumours can be detected by monoclonal antibodies. Although these are not restricted to tumour cells alone, they are useful in diagnosis and may be targets for antibody-mediated therapy.

Passive immunotherapy with monoclonal antibodies is promising when single cells are targeted or the problem of poor penetration into tumour masses can be circumvented.

Immunotherapy by active immunization or by passive transfer of cells is still largely experimental. Cytokines are active against a few tumour types.

■ THE TUMOUR AS A TISSUE GRAFT

The idea that there might be immune responses to tumours is an old one. At the turn of the century, Paul Ehrlich suggested that in humans there was a high frequency of 'aberrant germs' (tumours), which would overwhelm us if they were not kept in check by the immune system. Thus tumours came to be regarded as being similar to grafted tissue and recognizable by the immune system. This led to attempts to stimulate the immune system to reject them. Occasional regressions of tumours after treatment with bacterial vaccines (Coley's toxin), or occurring spontaneously, were taken as evidence of an effective immune response.

Early in the century, experimentalists began to investigate tumour immunity and noted that transplanted tumours usually regressed, proposing that this revealed immune responses to tumours. However, much of this early work fell into disrepute when it was realized that the regression was simply a consequence of the genetic disparity of host and tumour. So it was only in the post-war years, when genetically homogeneous inbred rodents became available, that it became possible to investigate the immune responses of tumour-bearing animals. An added impetus to these studies was provided by Burnett and Thomas, who developed Ehrlich's idea of immune responses to 'aberrant germs', elaborating it into the theory of Immune Surveillance.

■ IMMUNE SURVEILLANCE

Surveillance is most effective against viruses not tumour cells

Burnett and Thomas proposed that the immune system continually surveyed the body for the presence of abnormal cells, which were destroyed when recognized. The immune response to a tumour was therefore thought to be an early event, leading to the destruction of the majority of tumours before they became clinically apparent. It was also proposed that the immune system played an important role in delaying the growth, or causing regression of established tumours. A variety of evidence was cited to support these ideas:

- Postmortem data suggest that there may be more tumours than become clinically apparent.
- Many tumours contain lymphoid infiltrates and in some tumours this may be a favourable sign.
- Spontaneous regression of tumours occurs.
- Tumours occur more frequently in the neonatal period and in old age, when the immune system functions less effectively.
- Tumours arise frequently in immunosuppressed individuals.

Although at first sight this appears impressive evidence in favour of the theory, on closer examination the strongest point – the association between immunosuppression and increased tumour incidence – is less conclusive. The largest body of data comes from the study of kidney transplant recipients, many of whom have been followed for over 20 years. The frequency of many tumour types is increased in this immunosuppressed population, and for several types there is strong evidence that a virus may be involved (*Fig. 20.1*). However, there is also a slight but definite increased risk for many other cancers in which viruses are not known to play a role. This suggests that the immune response is probably most important in preventing the spread of potentially oncogenic viruses and that surveillance against other tumours is relatively ineffective. Certainly, normal humans who become infected with Epstein–Barr virus (EBV) carry the virus for life and show a strong cytotoxic T (Tc) cell response to the virus. Furthermore, increased virus replication and shedding of viral particles in secretions has been demonstrated in immunodeficient individuals. So it is clear that the immune response limits virus replication under normal circumstances (*Fig. 20.2*).

Data from animal experiments support the view that immune surveillance is largely directed towards viruses rather than tumours. Studies of athymic nude mice or mice immunosuppressed with anti-lymphocyte serum, showed no general increase in tumour frequency. However, a high proportion of the mice developed tumours caused by the small DNA

Tumour viruses and immunodeficiency

cause of immunodeficiency	common tumour types	viruses involved
inherited immunodeficiency	lymphoma	EBV
immunosuppression for organ transplants or due to AIDS	lymphoma	EBV
	cervical cancer	papilloma viruses
	skin cancer	probably papilloma viruses
	liver cancer	hepatitis B virus
	Kaposi's sarcoma	not known
malaria	Burkitt's lymphoma	EBV

Fig. 20.1 In all forms of immunodeficiency, the greatest increase is in tumours of the lymphoid system. Epstein–Barr virus (EBV) is involved in many of these. Most normal adults carry EBV throughout life with no ill effects. Most epithelial cancers, which show no viral association, are not increased in patients who are immunosuppressed or immunodeficient.

polyoma virus, which seldom causes tumours in normal animals. This does not imply that there is no immune response whatsoever to the majority of tumours but it does suggest that, for the majority of tumours, the immune response may be relatively late and ineffective.

Tumour antigens may be detected by immune cells or antibodies

In man few tumour types are known to be caused by viruses (*Fig. 20.3*) but, among those that are, liver and cervical cancer do cause many deaths worldwide. Viral antigens may be targets for immune responses but there is also abundant evidence of genetic alterations (mutation, gene amplification, chromosomal deletion or translocation) in most, if not all, tumours. Some of these lead to the expression of altered molecules in tumour cells and others to over-expression of normal molecules. These changes may be demonstrated either by detecting the host immune response or experimentally by deliberately immunizing other species with tumour.

■ TUMOUR-ASSOCIATED ANTIGENS DETECTED BY IMMUNE CELLS

Tumour antigens were first demonstrated by transplantation tests. When a tumour was grafted onto an animal previously immunized with inactivated cells of the same tumour, resistance to the graft was seen. Tumour resistance, subsequently shown to be mediated by immune cells, was directed at tumour-associated transplantation antigens (TATAs) of two types. The first are antigens which are shared by many tumours (T antigens), even though these may not be even of the same tissue of origin. The second are antigens which are specific to an individual tumour (tumour-specific transplantation antigens – TSTAs). Tumours may express both specific and shared antigens.

Role of EBV in tumorigenesis

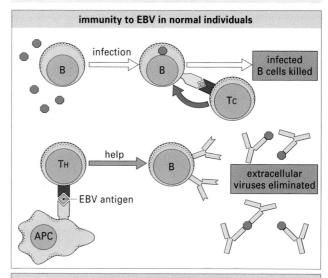

immunity to EBV in normal individuals

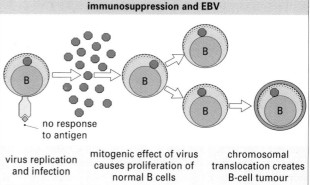

immunosuppression and EBV

Fig. 20.2 In normal individuals EBV infects B lymphocytes but spread of infection is prevented by Tc cells and antibody, which eliminate infected cells and virus. In immunosuppressed individuals, and in some patients receiving the immuno-suppressant cyclosporin, the virus replicates and infects more B cells. The virus is also mitogenic for B cells, so in an immunosuppressed individual infected B cells tend to proliferate more rapidly. A chromosomal translocation in an infected B cell can then lead to malignant transformation.

Shared tumour antigens are of viral origin

These antigens are found on tumours induced by viruses such as the small DNA polyoma and SV40 viruses, which can cause tumours in experimental animals, and the papillomaviruses, which are implicated in human cervical cancer. These viruses code for T (tumour) antigens which are shared by other viruses of the same group. T antigens are nuclear proteins, which play a role in the maintenance of the transformed (cancerous) state.

In animals infectious RNA tumour viruses cause leukaemias and sarcomas, and at least one human leukaemia virus (HTLV-1) has been discovered (*Fig. 20.3*). These viruses bud from the cell membrane of infected cells, and the viral envelope's glycoprotein can be detected at the host cell membrane. There are strong humoral and cell-mediated responses to the shared antigens of DNA- and to those of RNA-tumour viruses, which can protect against tumour challenge. Since tumours produced by a given oncogenic virus all share the same antigen, inbred mice immunized, say, by repeated injection of irradiated SV40 virus-induced tumour cells reject a different SV40 tumour, whereas they are susceptible to a tumour induced by polyomavirus.

In some strains of mice, activation of endogenous RNA-tumour viruses occurs regularly, leading to leukaemia. In others, when carcinogenic chemicals are given, the resulting tumours may express viral antigens and produce infectious mouse leukaemia virus (MuLV). Such tumours express common tumour-associated antigens as well as the tumour-specific antigens discussed below. However, host immune responses to endogenous RNA viruses are weak, perhaps because of immunological tolerance (see Chapter 12).

Specific tumour antigens are due to alterations in tumour genes or gene expression

Specific tumour antigens are those which can provoke an immune response to injected tumour cells, but only if the animal has been previously immunized with the same tumour (*Fig. 20.4*). These antigens were first detected using tumours that had been induced in inbred mice by chemical carcinogens, and their nature has now been elucidated, as will be described here.

A transplantable (therefore poorly immunogenic) tumour of inbred mice was exposed *in vitro* to a powerful mutagen. This produced mutant tumour subclones, some of which would no longer grow *in vivo* unless very large numbers of tumour cells were implanted. The mutants had clearly become more immunogenic than the parent tumour. One of these so-called tumour-negative (tum–) variant clones was used to immunize genetically identical mice. This generated Tc cells that would kill only the immunizing tumour and not the parental tumour line or other tum– variants (*Fig. 20.5*). The Tc cells were then used as probes to identify the presence of the mutated tumour antigen during molecular cloning of the

tumour antigen gene. Ultimately, the mutant gene coding for the tumour antigen (the tum– gene) was identified and sequenced. Comparison of this gene with the homologous gene from the parental tumour showed a single amino acid difference. Formal proof that this mutation could generate the immunogenic antigen recognized by the Tc cells was then obtained: parental tumour cells incubated with a 10 amino acid peptide having the tum– sequence could be killed by the Tc cells, but if they were incubated with the homologous peptide from parental cells they could not (*Fig. 20.6*). Remembering that Tc cells are MHC class I restricted, it seems likely that the tumour-specific protein is processed within the cell to generate a peptide which then becomes associated with MHC class I and is transported to the cell surface.

Tumour antigen genes cloned from other tum– variants were sometimes identical to the parental gene. In these tum– variants, the difference from the parent tumour was that the antigen was over-expressed in the tum– variant cells. There is

Viruses and human tumours

tumour	virus
liver cancer	hepatitis B
cervical cancer	human papillomaviruses (HPV 16, 18 and others)
Burkitt's lymphoma and other lymphomas in immunosuppression	EBV
nasopharyngeal cancer	EBV
adult T-cell leukaemia	human T leukaemia virus I (HTLV-I)

Fig. 20.3 EBV is associated with Burkitt's lymphoma in Africa and nasopharyngeal cancer in China, suggesting that co-factors, either genetic or environmental, are required to cause the tumours. Adult T-cell leukaemia is found mainly in Japan and the Caribbean.

Demonstration of tumour-specific antigens of chemically induced tumours

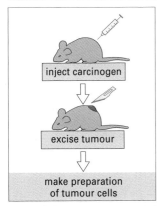
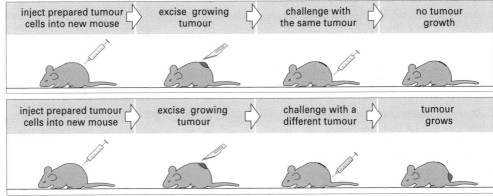

Fig. 20.4 Mice were induced to produce tumours by the injection of a chemical carcinogen (methyl cholanthrene). Tumour cells from these mice were then injected subcutaneously into genetically identical mice. Later, the growing tumours were removed surgically. Mice challenged with the same tumour were able to reject it, but those challenged with a different tumour (induced with the same carcinogen) were not. The ability to reject the tumour could be transferred with lymphoid cells.

Specificity of tumour immunity

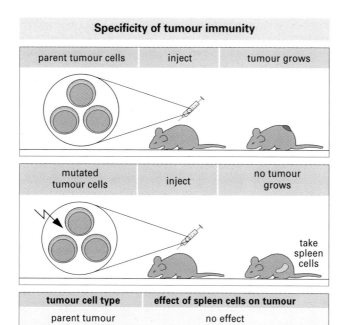

tumour cell type	effect of spleen cells on tumour
parent tumour	no effect
tum− variant	cytotoxic

Fig. 20.5 The production of a highly immunogenic (tum−) variant tumour in DBA2 mice and Tc cells specific for it are shown. After inducing mutations in the parent tumour cells, subclones were obtained, some of which would no longer grow in DBA2 mice. Spleen Tc cells from mice injected with these tum− cells could kill tum−, but not the parent tumour, *in vitro*.

Specificity of Tc cells for a tumour antigen peptide

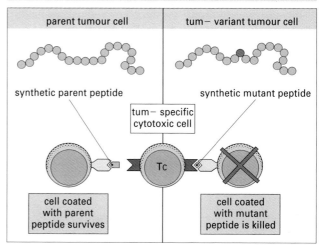

Fig. 20.6 Tc cells were taken from a mouse immunized with a tum− variant tumour. *In vitro*, they killed tumour cells coated with a peptide from the tum− gene sequence, but not cells coated with the homologous peptide from the parental tumour. The two peptides differ by a single amino acid.

good evidence that there are class II restricted responses at least to human tumours, but much less is known about tumour antigens recognized in association with MHC class II.

■ TUMOUR-ASSOCIATED ANTIGENS DETECTED BY ANTIBODIES

Few antigens are unique to tumours

There have been many attempts to detect antigens unique to tumours, using either serum from the tumour-bearing host (autologous typing) or sera derived from animals deliberately immunized with tumour material (heterologous typing). Recent work has relied on monoclonal antibodies, derived from either autologous or heterologous B cells. Although there is very little evidence for molecules uniquely expressed in tumours, several types of antigen associated with tumours in some way have been identified.

Sera from patients with tumours detect widely distributed antigens

Sera from tumour-bearing patients, or monoclonal antibodies derived from them, usually detect antigens that are widely distributed on, or more often in, both tumour and normal cells. The antibodies are often IgM and therefore of low affinity. Similar monoclonal antibodies can be derived by immortal-izing B cells from normal individuals. These antibodies detect autoantigens, and their importance in the host response to tumours (if any) is unclear.

Tumours may express normal differentiation antigens that have a restricted distribution in normal cells

Most tumour cells represent the clonal progeny of a single cell, and cells of that type may be relatively rare. Tumour cells may therefore express antigens that are present on only a few normal cells. The common acute lymphoblastic leukaemia antigen (CALLA or CD10) is an example (*Fig. 20.7*). Other examples are the oncofetal antigens, which are differentiation antigens expressed during fetal development but normally not expressed (or expressed at very low levels) in adult life. Examples of this are α-fetoprotein (AFP), which is produced by liver cancer cells, and carcinoembryonic antigen (CEA), produced by colon cancer cells and other epithelial tumours.

Normal antigens expressed in tumours may be altered by glycosylation

Glycosylation is altered in many tumours. This may give rise to the expression of new carbohydrate epitopes, such as the Thomsen–Friedenreich antigen, a disaccharide which is usually hidden on normal cells. Aberrant blood groups can also be created in this way. Alterations in glycosylation may also reveal epitopes on the protein backbone which are rarely detected in normal cells. For example, polymorphic epithelial mucins are produced by many normal epithelial cells. They are high molecular weight glycoproteins with a repeating core peptide carrying the carbohydrate side chains. In epithelial tumours, a new protein epitope can be detected in the repeating core structure.

HUMAN TUMOUR IMMUNE RESPONSES AND ESCAPE MECHANISMS

Most tumours have lymphoid infiltrates

Histological studies of human tumours have shown that the majority contain a marked infiltrate of inflammatory cells (*Fig. 20.8*). Lymphocytes and macrophages usually predominate but other cells can be detected including dendritic cells, granulocytes and mast cells. The use of monoclonal antibodies (mAbs) to detect lymphoid cell subtypes has allowed a more refined analysis of cell types within tumours (*Fig. 20.9*), and has shown that most major lymphocyte subtypes can be found in tumours.

The state of activation of the cells can also be analysed using mAbs specific for the interleukin-2 (IL-2) receptor, MHC class II molecules and other activation markers. However, no very clear associations have yet emerged between the presence of particular subtypes of lymphoid cells and the cancer patient's prognosis. This may be because only a small fraction of the infiltrating cells observed are actually recruited specifically to the the tumour site. This difficulty in interpretation has led to attempts to analyse the function of tumour-infiltrating lymphocytes *in vitro*. These studies are discussed in the next section.

Mixed lymphocyte–tumour cultures reveal anti-tumour responses *in vitro*

The realization that responses of antigen-primed helper T (TH) and Tc cells can be revealed by re-stimulating them with specific antigen *in vitro* led to experiments in which lymphocytes from patients were stimulated by inactivated tumour cells in mixed lymphocyte–tumour culture (MLTC) (*Fig. 20.10*), to see whether the patient's immune system could react to the tumour. The lymphocytes might be taken from peripheral blood, from tumour-draining lymph nodes or from the tumour itself (the latter are known as tumour-infiltrating lymphocytes).

MLTC can stimulate TH (CD4+) cells, which proliferate and secrete effector cytokines, but in these cultures Tc (CD8+) cells are also generated, and it is possible to measure their cytotoxic activity by the ^{51}Cr-release assay (see Fig. 28.26).

Expression of CALLA in normal cells and lymphomas

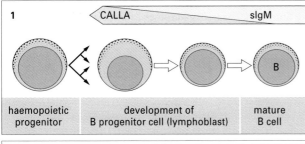

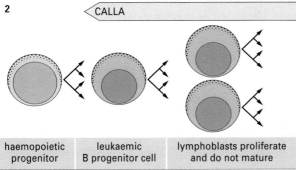

Fig. 20.7 1. CALLA is normally expressed only on B-cell progenitors or lymphoblasts, which make up < 1% of normal bone marrow cells. 2. CALLA becomes much more abundant in the commonest form of childhood leukaemia.

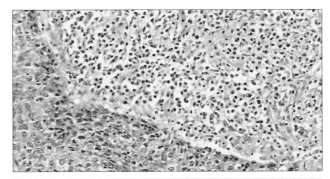

Fig. 20.8 Immunological reaction to a breast carcinoma. The section shows a tumour surrounded by a heavy infiltrate of mononuclear cells. Such inflammation suggests that tumours may be recognized by cells of the immune system which are potentially active in slowing tumour growth or eliminating tumour cells. Haematoxylin and eosin stain.

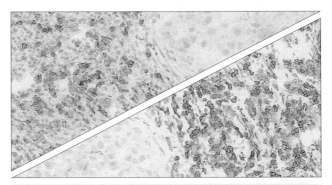

Fig. 20.9 CD4+ and CD8+ T cells in carcinoma of the breast. CD4+ and CD8+ cells were detected by the immunoalkaline phosphatase technique (pink stain) using monoclonal antibodies. The sections are counterstained with haematoxylin. CD4 (upper), and fewer CD8 cells (lower), were seen surrounding the tumour but few lymphocytes were within the tumour itself.

Mixed lymphocyte–tumour culture (MLTC)

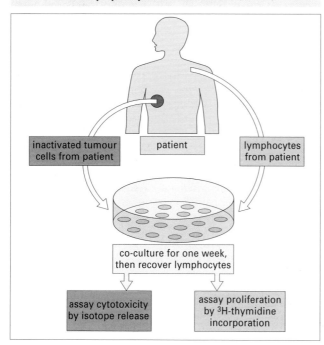

Fig. 20.10 Lymphocytes taken from blood, from draining lymph nodes or directly from tumour tissue, are co-cultured with autologous tumour cells, which have been inactivated by X-irradiation or treatment with mitomycin-C. After a suitable period of culture, the lymphocytes can be assayed for proliferation by incorporation of ^{3}H–thymidine (from the culture medium). They can be assayed for their ability to lyse target cells in isotope release assays.

Patterns of response generated in MLTC

target cell	responder lymphocytes			
	tumour-specific Tc	autoreactive Tc	tumour-specific MHC-unrestricted cytotoxic cells	NK cells ± T cells
NK target	–	–	–	+
allogeneic tumour	–	–	+	+
autologous normal cell	–	+	–	+
autologous tumour	+	+	+	+

Fig 20.11 Lymphocytes harvested from MLTC have been assayed in a ^{51}Cr-release assay on several different tumour or normal cells. Killing is detected by release of isotope into the supernatant of the cultures. Several patterns of specificity can be detected in the lymphocytes from different patients, varying from lysis of the autologous tumour only, to non-specific lysis of all target cells. The latter may be due to either activated NK cells or T cells. Among the T cells, CD4$^+$ and CD8$^+$ cells behave in a similar way, both showing the same variety of responses.

Tc cells can also be obtained by culturing them in IL-2 to expand any effector cells generated *in vivo*. The activity of Tc cells must be distinguished from that of natural killer (NK) cells, which can be done by assaying the expanded lymphocyte population on appropriate reference target cells.

Many different T-cell specificities are generated in MLTC

The specificities of both TH and Tc cells are similar and show a variety of patterns of reactivity against different targets in different patients (*Fig. 20.11*).

- In both cases, a minority of cloned T cells are specific for autologous tumour.
- Some clones react to autologous tumour and all, or a proportion, of autologous tissues tested.
- Some clones show reactivity to autologous and some allogeneic tumours.
- The remaining cells show broad reactivity to many tumour targets.

Tumour-specific T cells have been detected in patients with several different types of human tumour. Melanoma appears to be particularly immunogenic and several different target molecules have been defined using the strategy outlined for mouse TSTA. The Tc-cell target molecules include melanoma antigens (MAGEs), which are expressed in few normal cells, and tyrosinase, an enzyme associated with pigment cells. Neither the MAGE nor tyrosinase gene shows any mutations in the tumour cells. Responses to mutated *ras* oncogene protein and p53, the tumour suppressor gene product, have also been detected in human tumour patients.

The third type of clone has been isolated from breast and ovarian cancer patients. Recent data suggest that this type of clone may respond in a specific but unrestricted fashion to the repeating core peptide of mucin. It is not yet clear whether the peptide is presented by MHC molecules or in some other fashion (for example acting as a superantigen). Mucin-responsive cells may be of TH or Tc (CD4$^+$ or CD8$^+$) type.

The significance *in vivo* of the cytotoxic responses which have been detected *in vitro* remains uncertain. In animal model experiments, however, cloned anti-tumour cytolytic cells can cause tumour regression.

Tumours have multiple mechanisms for evading immune responses

Since spontaneous tumours grow and kill the host, many tumours must escape the host immune response. Many mechanisms have been proposed. The most obvious is that the tumour is non-immunogenic. This may be not because potential tumour antigens are lacking but because the tumour cells are poor antigen-presenting cells (APCs). Induction of immune responses requires co-stimuli, which may be cell-surface molecules or cytokines secreted by APCs. The B7 molecule, present on specialized APCs, is now known to be a key co-stimulus acting via its counter-receptor CD28 on the T-cell surface (see Chapter 8). Experimentally, presentation of MHC–peptide antigen complexes to the T-cell receptor in the absence of B7 co-stimulation may lead to anergy and there is evidence that tumour-infiltrating lymphocytes may sometimes be anergic. Additionally, if the tumour lacks MHC class II, initiation of TH responses will depend on processing of tumour antigens by specialized APC (*Fig. 20.12*).

Tumour cells may also lack other molecules required for adhesion of lymphocytes such as LFA-1 and -3 or ICAM-1 (see Chapter 14), or they may express molecules such as mucins, which can be anti-adhesive. They may also secrete immunosuppressive cytokines such as TGFβ. A particularly important escape mechanism is loss of MHC antigens, leading to inability to present tumour antigen peptides. More than 50% of tumours may lose one or more MHC class I alleles, and sometimes all class I is lost (*Fig. 20.13*).

■ IMMUNODIAGNOSIS

Although few molecules are exclusive to tumour cells, antibodies to tumour-associated molecules can be very useful in tumour diagnosis, by detecting either increased amounts of an antigen or the presence of an antigen in an abnormal site. For this reason the antigens need not be tumour specific to be used for diagnosis.

In vivo – Radiolabelled antibodies against tumour-associated molecules have been used for detection of tumours (*Fig. 20.14*) but the method is seldom more sensitive than modern methods of computerized tomography (CT) or nuclear magnetic resonance imaging (MRI). In addition, immunoscintigraphy has the dis-advantage that antibodies need to be freshly labelled for each patient, and different antibodies are optimal for different tumour types. The development of recombinant fragments of high-affinity antibodies may improve the sensitivity of immunoscintigraphy in the future.

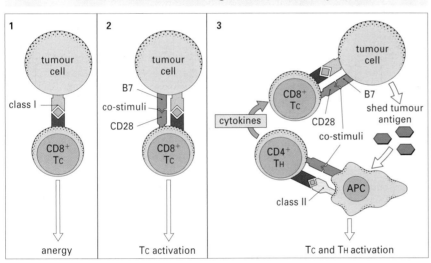

Presentation of tumour antigen to the immune system

Fig. 20.12 Tumour antigen may be presented to T cells in a number of ways. 1. Directly in the absence of necessary co-stimuli, resulting in anergy. 2. Directly by a tumour which expresses co-stimulatory molecules, resulting in Tc cell activation. 3. Directly by tumour cells and indirectly via specialized APCs, resulting in activation of both Tc and TH cells.

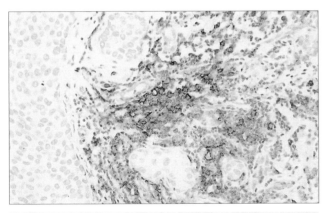

Fig. 20.13 Breast cancer tissue reactive with a monoclonal antibody to a monomorphic determinant of HLA class I antigens. Only stromal cells are stained (brown colour), as malignant epithelial cells fail to express normal MHC class I antigens. Some 50% of primary human cancers fall into this category. Aberrant class II expression may also occur on some tumours. (Indirect immunoperoxidase technique, counterstained with haematoxylin.)

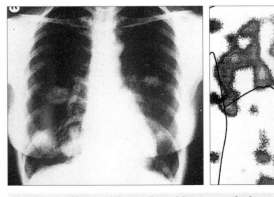

Fig. 20.14 Chest radiograph and immunoscintigraphy scan of a patient with carcinoma of the colon who has lung and liver metastases. The monoclonal antibody YPC2/12.1, raised against human colorectal cancer, binds to CEA. (It reacts with a glycoprotein of 180 kDa.) The antibody was radiolabelled with ^{131}I and administered intravenously. Scintigrams were obtained after 48 hours. The image is that obtained after a subtraction procedure to eliminate background blood-borne antibody. (Courtesy of Professor K. Sikora.)

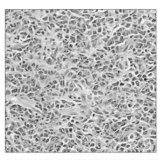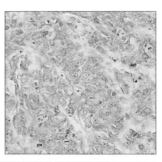

Fig. 20.15 Identification of the cell of origin of an undifferentiated tumour. Conventional histology of a biopsy of this tumour (left) showed a sheet of undifferentiated tumour cells which could not be identified. When the tumour was stained by the indirect immunoperoxidase method (right) with an antibody against CD45 (the leucocyte common antigen), it was found to be strongly positive, identifying it as a lymphoma.

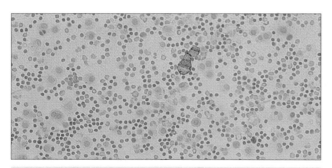

Fig 20.16 Detection of micrometastases using a monoclonal antibody. The figure shows an aspirate of bone marrow taken from a patient with small cell cancer of the lung. The section is stained by the immunoalkaline phosphatase method with an antibody against a cytokeratin. Carcinoma cells express cytokeratins and are clearly stained pink. Scattered tumour cells, such as are present in this bone marrow sample, are easily missed by conventional cytological examination.

In vitro – Antibodies are useful for identifying the cell of origin of undifferentiated tumours (*Fig. 20.15*) and for the detection of micrometastases in bone marrow, cerebrospinal fluid, lymphoid organs or elsewhere (*Fig. 20.16*). There are also immunoassays available for several tumour-associated molecules that can be detected in the serum. These include CEA and AFP. Raised levels of either of these molecules may be useful in diagnosis, but neither is associated with only one tumour type, so they are generally more useful in following the course of treatment (*Fig. 20.17*).

■ IMMUNOTHERAPY

Immunotherapy has a limited role at present

Immunotherapy has a long history but it is rarely the treatment of first choice. Intervention may be active or passive, specific or non-specific, or even combined. *Figure 20.18* summarizes several possibilities.

Active immunotherapy is still largely experimental

Specific active immunization – Using inactivated tumour cells, this approach has shown some success in animal models where immunization is performed before tumour challenge. Attempts to induce regression of established tumours have been much less successful. While much effort has been expended in designing means of making tumour cells more immunogenic (*Fig. 20.19*), most of these have been empirical. More recently, the knowledge that T-cell epitopes are presented by MHC molecules, and that induction of immune responses is dependent on co-stimuli, has led to development of more rational strategies.

Transfection of the genes for the co-stimulator B7 or cytokines such as IL-2, IL-4, interferon-γ (IFN-γ) or granulocyte–macrophage colony stimulating factor (GM–CSF) into tumour cells has been shown to increase greatly their

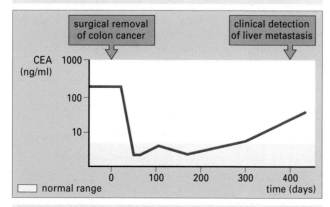

Monitoring serum CEA level in colon carcinoma

surgical removal of colon cancer — clinical detection of liver metastasis

CEA (ng/ml)

□ normal range

time (days)

Fig. 20.17 The relationship of serum CEA level to clinical course in a patient with carcinoma of the colon is shown. At presentation there is a high CEA level, which falls following surgery. A rise is found well before the clinical detection of metastatic tumour.

Immunotherapy of tumours

active	non-specific	BCG, *Corynebacterium parvum*, levamisole
	specific	preventive vaccines of tumour cells, cell extracts, purified or recombinant antigens, or idiotypes
passive	non-specific	LAK cells, cytokines
	specific	antibodies alone or coupled to drugs, pro-drugs, toxins or radioisotopes bi-specific antibodies T cells
	combined	LAK cells and bi-specific antibody

Fig. 20.18 Non-specific agents boost specific and non-specific immune mechanisms probably via release of cytokines. Alternatively cytokines or cells (such as lymphokine-activated killer cells, LAK) may be given alone or together with bi-specific antibody, to target the cells to the tumour (see p. 20.11).

Specific active immunotherapy augmenting the host response

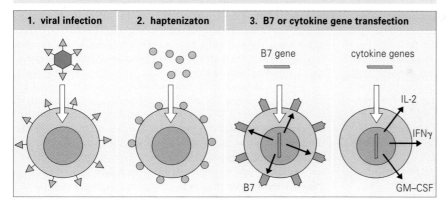

Fig. 20.19 1. and 2. Vaccination against tumours has been investigated for many years, using empirical methods to boost the immunogenicity of tumour cells. 3. More recently, molecules such as B7 or cytokines, known to be important co-stimuli for induction of immune responses, have been introduced into tumour cells by transfection of DNA. Once activated, the primed T cells can now attack the parent tumour cells since they no longer need the co-stimulating molecules for triggering.

immunogenicity in animal tumour protection experiments. Similarly, immunization with defined peptide epitopes in novel adjuvants can induce Tc cells able to cause rejection of experimental tumours. DNA constructs coding for tumour antigens and co-stimuli can also be used directly to immunize animals, avoiding problems of genetic restriction inherent in using tumour cells themselves. While all these methods can protect animals against subsequent tumour challenge they are much less successful in treating established tumours and there is little evidence that specific active immunization has been effective so far in man.

Non-specific stimulation of immune responses – A variety of agents have been used (*Fig. 20.20*). Most attempts at systemic

therapy in man have not been conspicuously successful, but intralesional BCG can cause regression of melanoma and non-specific local immunization with BCG is effective against bladder tumours.

Immunization against oncogenic viruses – As there is increasing evidence for a role of viruses in some human cancers, the most promising avenue for active immunization may be in preventing infection with potentially oncogenic agents. Successful mass immunization against hepatitis B virus will certainly decrease the incidence of primary hepatoma. It may be possible eventually to vaccinate at-risk populations against papillomaviruses, HTLV-1 or EBV.

Passive immunotherapy with mAbs shows some promise but has limitations

Early attempts at passive immunotherapy with polyclonal antisera were limited because of the difficulty of achieving high titre and specificity. The advent of mAbs promises to overcome these difficulties. Although no antigens unique to tumours have yet been discovered (with the exception of B- and T-cell idiotypes on lymphomas), some antigens do show increased expression on certain tumour cells and damage to normal body cells carrying the same antigen may be unimportant or tolerable, opening the way for mAb treatment. Monoclonal antibodies may be used either alone, or coupled to drugs, pro-drugs, toxins, cytokines or isotopes (*Fig. 20.21*). There are, however, a number of limitations to antibody therapy, as follows.

- **Antibody penetration into large tumour masses is often poor:** in principle this might be overcome by smaller molecules that retain specific antigen binding, such as Fab fragments, or by engineered single-domain antibodies. Alternatively, it may be possible to target therapy to the endothelium of tumour blood vessels.
- **Antibodies are bound by other cells:** any normal cells expressing the target antigen, and non-specifically by cells bearing Fc receptors or receptors for immunoglobulin carbohydrates. Chemical modification or genetic engineering of the antibody molecules may partially overcome these difficulties. Better discrimination between tumour and normal cells might be obtained with a bi-specific antibody against two different antigens that are both present on the tumour cells but are only found separately on normal cells.

Non-specific active immunotherapy: biological response modifiers (BRMs)

type of BRM	examples	major effect
bacterial products	BCG, *C. parvum*, muramyl dipeptide, trehalose dimycolate	activate macrophages and NK cells
synthetic molecules	pyran copolymer, MVE, poly I:C, pyrimidines	induce IFN production
cytokines	IFNα, IFNβ, IFNγ, IL-2, TNF	activate macrophages and NK cells
hormones	thymosin, thymulin, thymopoietin	modulate T-cell function

Fig. 20.20 Biological response modifiers (BRMs) are used to enhance immune responses to tumours and fall into four major groups. Broadly speaking, bacterial products have adjuvant effects on macrophages (see Chapters 17 and 19); a variety of synthetic polymers, nucleotides and polynucleotides induce IFN production and release; the cytokines administered directly act on macrophages and NK cells, and a variety of hormones including the thymic hormones can be used to enhance T-cell function. (MVE = maleic anhydride divinyl ether; TNF = tumour necrosis factor; poly I: C = polyinosinic–polycytidylic acid.)

- **Antibodies are immunogenic:** they may therefore be attacked by the immune system. Even chimeric or humanized antibodies may induce an immune response to their idiotype. The use of different mAbs for successive courses of therapy might solve this problem.

In spite of these difficulties there have been some encouraging results. In a randomized study, mAb has been used to treat colon cancer following surgery to remove the primary tumour. Here the aim was to target micrometastases, avoiding the problem of poor penetration into large tumour masses. The treated group showed significantly improved survival. Similarly, radiolabelled anti-B cell antibodies show promise against lymphomas resistant to conventional therapy.

Antibodies may also be used *in vitro* either to purge tumour cells from bone marrow for autografting (*Fig. 20.22*) or to remove T cells for prevention of graft-versus-host disease in allotransplants.

The effectiveness of passive immunotherapy with lymphocytes is uncertain

When human peripheral blood mononuclear cells are cultured *in vitro* with IL-2, they become highly cytotoxic to a wide variety of tumour targets, many of which are resistant to freshly isolated NK cells. Initial animal and human experiments, in which these lymphokine-activated killer (LAK) cells were re-infused, gave some good results, especially when IL-2 was given at the same time. However, controlled trials have given less encouraging results and the therapy, involving high-dose IL-2, has significant toxicity. It seems likely that few LAK cells localize in tumours, and this may contribute to the poor results. To overcome this, bi-specific mAbs have been used. In these, one antibody is directed against a tumour molecule and the other against surface markers on effector cells, such as CD3 on Tc cells and CD16 on NK cells. In theory, these antibodies should help to localize the LAK cells on the tumour. While such strategies certainly work *in vitro*, their effectiveness *in vivo* is less clear.

T cells extracted from tumour sites can also be grown *in vitro* using IL-2 and eventually re-infused. In a proportion of cases the cultured T cells show relative specificity for the tumour from which they were derived. In animal model systems there is no doubt that tumour-specific cytotoxic T cells can cause dramatic regression of tumour. The tumour toxicity of such tumour-infiltrating lymphocytes may be increased by transfecting into them genes coding for cytokine production. However, the real efficacy of such strategies in humans remains to be tested. In humans large numbers of EBV-specific Tc cells have been grown *in vitro* using IL-2 and infused into patients who have developed lymphoma following bone marrow transplantation. Remission of tumour occurred. In this case the strong viral antigens of EBV are the target but although these results are encouraging, the efficacy of this strategy against common epithelial malignancies remains to be tested.

Passive immunotherapy with cytokine can cause tumour regression

Many cytokines have been cloned, expressed and used for tumour therapy. *Figure 20.23* gives information on those which have been most thoroughly investigated to date.

Therapeutic modification of monoclonal antibodies

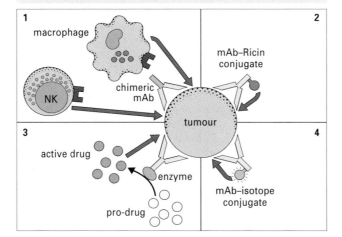

Fig. 20.21 1. Genetically engineered chimeric antibodies with a human Fc portion attached to a mouse Fab′2 reduce the risk of an immune response to the mAb. Human Fc will also recruit human effector mechanisms. Alternatively, various molecules can be coupled to mAbs for targeting to tumour cells. These include toxins (2), cytotoxic drugs or enzymes capable of activating pro-drugs (3) or radioactive isotopes (4).

In vitro purging of tumour-infiltrated bone marrow

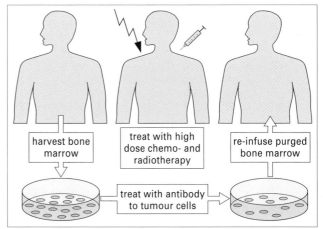

Fig. 20.22 Bone marrow containing tumour cells can be purged using mAbs and complement, antibody–toxin conjugates or antibodies coupled to magnetic beads. The purged marrow is stored while the patient is given high-dose chemo- and radiotherapy. The purged marrow is then returned to the patient. This therapy has given encouraging results in some leukaemia and lymphoma patients who were not helped by their conventional therapy.

Successes have so far been few and far between, though IFNα can induce prolonged remission of the rare hairy-cell leukaemia and IL-2 is effective in a proportion of melanomas and renal carcinomas. There are also encouraging results in treatment of intraperitoneal ovarian tumours with IFNγ and

TNFα. However, it is possible that cytokines have so far been used in an inappropriate way. Generally they have been used in a similar fashion to cytotoxic drugs – i.e. in the highest tolerable dose. Recent data on head and neck cancer suggest that lower doses may be equally, if not more, effective. Used in this way, cytokines also have far fewer adverse effects.

Some cytokines are finding a useful role in supportive therapy. For example, colony stimulating factors can shorten the period of aplasia after bone marrow transplantation or cytotoxic therapy, and erythropoietin can relieve the anaemia.

Cytokine therapy for tumours

cytokine	tumour type and results	cytokine effects and possible anti-tumour mechanisms
IFNα	prolonged remissions of hairy-cell leukaemia	possible cytostatic effect on tumour
	weak effects on some carcinomas	increased expression of MHC class I, cytostasis
IFNγ	ineffective systemically, remissions of peritoneal carcinoma of the ovary	increased MHC class I and II macrophage activation, Tc activation, cytostasis
IL-2	remissions in renal cancer and melanoma	T-cell activation and proliferation, NK-cell activation
TNFα	can reduce malignant ascites	?increased tumour cell adhesion, macrophage and lymphocyte activation

Fig 20.23 Most cytokines have been given systemically in high doses. The mechanism of the anti-tumour effect is uncertain in most cases. *In vitro*, IFNs and TNFα are cytostatic for some tumour cells, but *in vivo* any effects seen may be indirect because many cytokines induce production of other cytokines (the cytokine cascade). The fact that some patients treated with IL-2 suffer transient autoimmune thyroiditis provides some evidence that cytokine administration does potentiate immune responses.

Critical Thinking

■ There is evidence that there is a host immune response to tumour-associated antigens in many patients. Nevertheless, if they are not treated, most cancers grow and eventually kill their host. How can this paradox be accounted for?

■ Tumour immunology is often discussed as almost a separate subject. Are there special features of immune responses to tumours which set them apart?

■ Immunotherapy for cancer has been attempted over the last 100 years. Why has success been very limited so far and what is the likelihood of greater success in the future?

■ Prophylactic immunization against infectious diseases has been highly effective. Will this be the greatest contribution of immunology to oncology?

FURTHER READING

Boon T, Cerottini J-C, Van den Eynde B, van der Bruggen P, Van Pel A. Tumour antigens recognised by T lymphocytes. *Annu Rev Immunol* 1994;**12**: 337–66.

Franks LM, Teich N. *Introduction to the Cellular and Molecular Biology of Cancer.* Oxford: Oxford University Press, 1991.

Finke JH, Zea AH, Stanley J, *et al.* Loss of T-cell receptor ζ chain and p56[lck] in T-cells infiltrating human renal cell carcinoma. *Cancer Res* 1993;**53**:5613–16.

Kedar E, Klein E. Cancer immunotherapy: are the results discouraging? Can they be improved? *Adv Cancer Res* 1992;**59**:245–94.

Pardoll DM. New strategies for enhancing the immunogenicity of tumours. *Curr Opinion Immunol* 1993;**5**:719–25.

Riethmuller G, Schneider-Gädicke E, Schlimok G, *et al.* German Cancer Aid 17-1A Study Group. Randomised trial of monoclonal antibody for adjuvant therapy of resected Dukes' C colorectal carcinoma. *Lancet* 1994;**343**:1177–83.

Sheil AGR. Development of malignancy following renal transplantation in Australia and New Zealand. *Transplant Proc* 1992;**24**:275–79.

Sulitzeanu D. Immunosuppressive factors in human cancer. *Adv Cancer Res* 1993;**60**:247–62.

Vlasveld LT, Rankin EM. Recombinant interleukin-2: basic and clinical aspects. *Cancer Treat Rev* 1994;**20**:275-311.

Defective antibody responses result in increased susceptibility to pyogenic infections and are due to failure of B-cell function, such as occurs in X-linked agammaglobulinaemia, or from failure of proper T-cell signals to B cells such as occurs in hyper-IgM syndrome, common variable immunodeficiency (CVID) and transient hypogammaglobulinaemia of infancy.

Defective cell-mediated immunity results in increased susceptibility to opportunistic infections and is due to failure of T-cell function such as occurs in severe combined immunodeficiency (SCID), MHC class II deficiency, ataxia–telangiectasia, the Wiskott–Aldrich syndrome and the DiGeorge anomaly.

Secondary immunodeficiency may result from extrinsic causes such as irradiation, malnutrition, drugs or infections, and may involve B cells, T cells or both. The most prominent cause of acquired immunodeficiency at present is infection with human immunodeficiency virus (HIV), which causes Acquired Immunodeficiency Syndrome (AIDS).

HIV infects CD4$^+$ T cells and leads to their destruction with concomitant loss of cell-mediated immunity, overwhelming opportunistic infections and death (AIDS).

Hereditary complement component defects are found in a number of clinical syndromes, the most common of which is that of the C1 inhibitor, which results in hereditary angioedema.

Hereditary complement deficiencies of the terminal complement components (C5, C6, C7 and C8) and the alternative pathway proteins (Factor H, Factor I and properdin) lead to extraordinary susceptibility to infections with the two *Neisseria* species, *N. gonorrhoeae* and *N. meningitidis*.

Defects in the oxygen reduction pathway of phagocytes, so that the phagocytes cannot assemble NADPH oxidase and produce the hydrogen peroxide and oxygen radicals that kill bacteria, are the basis of chronic granulomatous disease. The resulting persistence of bacterial products in phagocytes leads to abscesses or granulomas depending on the pathogen.

Leucocyte adhesion deficiency is associated with a persistent leucocytosis because phagocytic cells with defective integrin molecules cannot migrate through the vascular endothelium from the blood stream into the tissues.

Immunodeficiency disease results from the absence, or failure of normal function, of one or more elements of the immune system. Specific immunodeficiency diseases involve abnormalities of T or B cells, the cells of the adaptive immune system. Non-specific immunodeficiency diseases involve abnormalities of elements such as complement or phagocytes, which act non-specifically in immunity. Primary immunodeficiency diseases are due to intrinsic defects in cells of the immune system and are for the most part genetically determined. Secondary immunodeficiency diseases result from extrinsic factors such as drugs, irradiation, malnutrition or infection. Thus, AIDS is a secondary immunodeficiency resulting from a virus infection.

Immunodeficiency diseases cause increased susceptibility to infection in patients. The infections encountered in immunodeficient patients fall, broadly speaking, into two categories. Patients with defects in immunoglobulins, complement proteins or phagocytes are very susceptible to recurrent infections with encapsulated bacteria such as *Haemophilus influenzae*, *Streptococcus pneumoniae* and *Staphylococcus aureus*. These are called pyogenic infections, because the bacteria give rise to pus formation. On the other hand, patients with defects in cell-mediated immunity, i.e. in T cells, are susceptible to overwhelming, even lethal, infections with microorganisms that are ubiquitous in the environment and to which normal people rapidly develop resistance. For this reason, these are called opportunistic infections; opportunistic microorganisms include yeast and common viruses such as chickenpox.

■ B-CELL DEFICIENCIES

Patients with common defects in B-cell function (*Fig. 21.1*) have recurrent pyogenic infection such as pneumonia, otitis media and sinusitis. If untreated, they develop severe obstructive lung disease (bronchiectasis) from recurrent pneumonia, which destroys the elasticity of the airways.

In X-linked agammaglobulinaemia (X-LA) early B-cell maturation fails

The model B-cell deficiency is X-linked agammaglobulinaemia. It was the first immunodeficiency disease to be understood in detail, the underlying deficiency being discovered in 1952. Affected males have few or no B cells in their blood or lymphoid tissue; consequently their lymph nodes are very small and their tonsils are absent. Their serum usually contains no IgA, IgM, IgD or IgE, and only small amounts of IgG (less than 100 mg/dl). For the first 6–12 months of life, they are protected from infection by the maternal IgG that crossed the placenta into the fetus. As this supply of IgG is exhausted, affected males develop recurrent pyogenic infections. If they are infused intravenously with large doses of gammaglobulin they remain healthy.

The X-LA gene is on the long arm of the X-chromosome (*Fig. 21.2*). This is the site of many other hereditary immunodeficiency diseases, and the localization of these genes facilitates prenatal diagnosis. The gene that is defective in X-LA has recently been identified as a B-cell cytoplasmic

Primary B-cell deficiencies

X-linked agammaglobulinaemia
IgA deficiency
IgG subclass deficiency
immunodeficiency with increased IgM
common variable immunodeficiency
transient hypogammaglobulinaemia of infancy

Fig. 21.1 The range of B-cell deficiencies varies from a delayed maturation of normal immunoglobulin production, through single isotype deficiencies to X-linked agammaglobulinaemia, where affected male children have no B cells and no serum immunoglobulins.

The X-linked immunodeficiencies

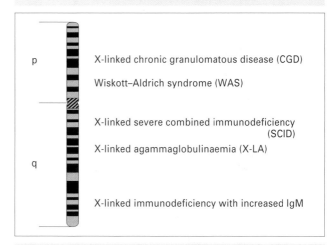

Fig. 21.2 The genes for many immunodeficiency diseases are located on the X-chromosome. The genetic defects have been identified for all these diseases (Adapted from Schwaber J, Rosen FS. *Immunodeficiency Rev* 1990:**2**;235.)

tyrosine kinase (*btk*) belonging to the *src* oncogene family. Its role in B-cell maturation is not yet understood, but it is obviously vital for the process of B-cell maturation. Bone marrow of males with X-LA contains normal numbers of pre-B cells but, as a result of mutations in the *btk* gene, they cannot mature into B cells (*Fig. 21.3*).

In IgA and IgG subclass deficiency terminal differentiation of B cells fails

IgA deficiency is the most common immunodeficiency. One in 700 Caucasians have the defect, but it is not found, or is found only rarely, in other ethnic groups. People with IgA deficiency tend to develop immune-complex disease (Type III hypersensitivity). About 20% of IgA-deficient individuals also lack IgG2 and IgG4, and so are very susceptible to pyogenic infections. In humans, most antibodies to the capsular polysaccharides of pyogenic bacteria are in the IgG2 subclass; a deficiency in IgG2 alone therefore also results in recurrent pyogenic infections. For reasons that are unclear, individuals with deficiency of only IgG3 are also susceptible to recurrent infections. These class and subclass deficiencies result from failures in terminal differentiation of B cells (*see Fig. 21.3*).

In immunodeficiency with increased IgM (HIGM) isotype switching does not occur

A peculiar immunodeficiency results in patients who are IgG- and IgA-deficient but synthesize large amounts (more than 200 mg/dl) of polyclonal IgM. They are susceptible to pyogenic infections and should be treated with intravenous gammaglobulin. They tend to form IgM autoantibodies to neutrophils, platelets and other elements of the blood, as well as to tissue antigens, thereby adding the complexities of autoimmune disease to the immunodeficiency. The tissues, particularly of the gastrointestinal tract, become infiltrated with IgM-producing cells (*Fig. 21.4*). In HIGM the B cells cannot make the switch from IgM to IgG, IgA and IgE synthesis that normally occurs in B-cell maturation. In normal B cells, this switch is induced by two factors: IL-4 must bind to the B-cell receptor for IL-4, and the CD40 molecule on the B-cell surface must bind to the CD40 ligand on activated T cells. In 70% of cases HIGM is inherited as an X-linked recessive that

results from mutations in the CD40 ligand, whose gene maps to precisely the same location on the long arm of the X–chromosome as HIGM.

In common variable immunodeficiency (CVID) there are defects in T-cell signalling to B cells

Individuals with CVID have acquired agammaglobulinaemia in the second or third decade of life, or later. Both males and females are equally affected and the cause is generally not known, but may follow infection with viruses such as Epstein–Barr virus (EBV). Patients with CVID, like males with X-LA, are very susceptible to pyogenic organisms and to the intestinal protozoan, *Giardia lamblia* (*Fig. 21.5*), which causes severe diarrhoea. Most patients (80%) with CVID have B cells that do not function properly and are immature. The B cells are not defective; instead, they fail to receive proper signals from the T cells. However, the T-cell defects have not been defined well in CVID. Patients with CVID should be treated with intravenous gammaglobulin as it provides protection against recurrent pyogenic infections. Many patients develop autoimmune diseases, most prominently pernicious anaemia, and the reason for this is not known. CVID is not hereditary, but is commonly associated with the MHC haplotypes HLA-B8 and HLA-DR3.

IgG production is delayed in transient hypogammaglobulinaemia of infancy

As mentioned in *Fig. 21.3*, infants are protected initially by their mother's IgG. The maternal IgG is catabolized, with a half-life of approximately 30 days. By 3 months of age, normal infants begin to synthesize their own IgG, although formation of antibody to bacterial capsular polysaccharides does not commence in earnest until the second year of life. In some infants, the onset of normal IgG synthesis can be delayed for as long as 36 months and,

B-cell maturation in X-linked immunodeficiencies

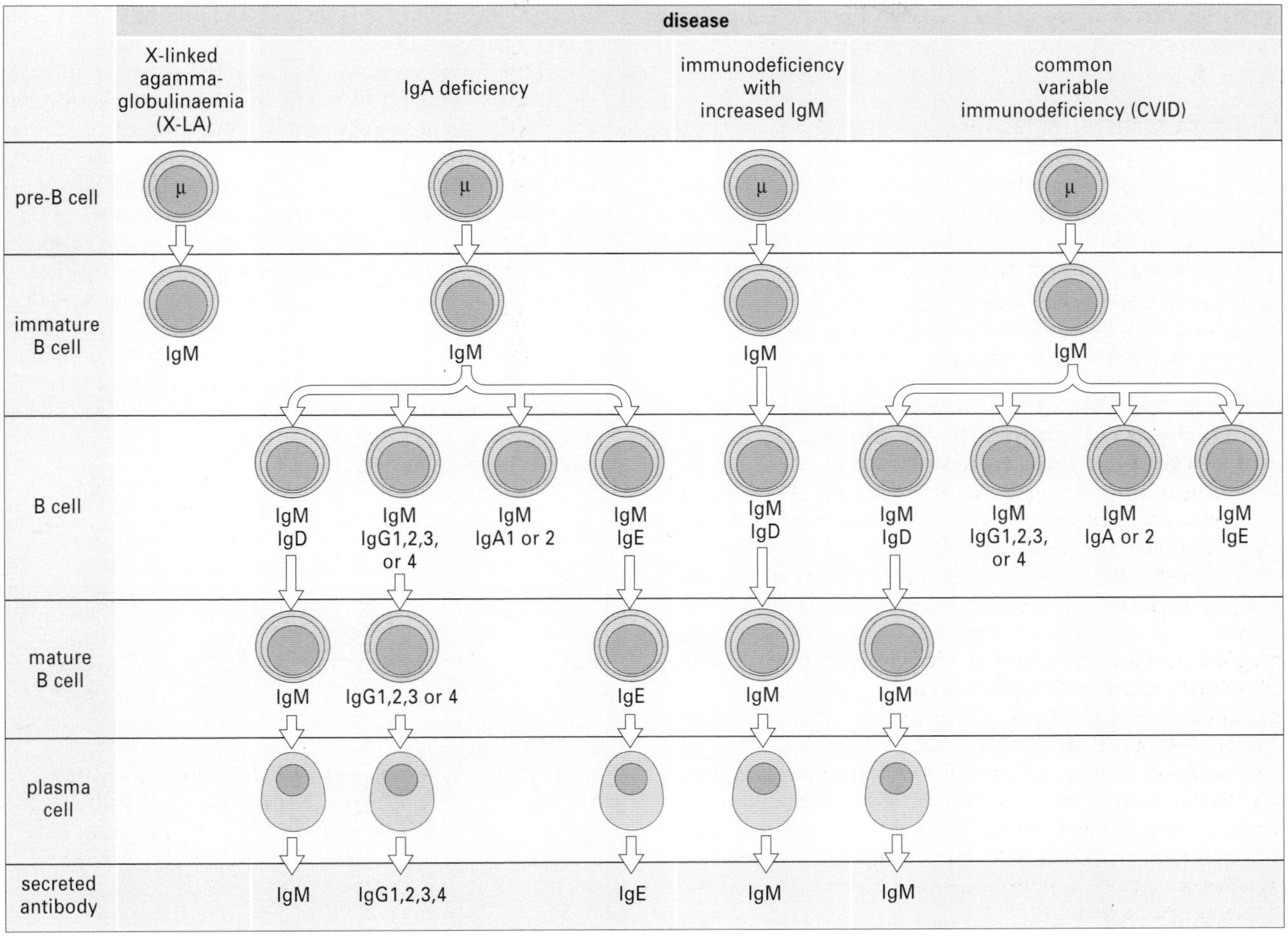

	disease			
	X-linked agamma-globulinaemia (X-LA)	IgA deficiency	immunodeficiency with increased IgM	common variable immunodeficiency (CVID)
pre-B cell	μ	μ	μ	μ
immature B cell	IgM	IgM	IgM	IgM
B cell	IgM IgD	IgM IgG1,2,3, or 4	IgM IgA1 or 2 · IgM IgE	IgM IgD	IgM IgD · IgM IgG1,2,3, or 4 · IgM IgA or 2 · IgM IgE
mature B cell	IgM · IgG1,2,3 or 4	IgE	IgM	IgM
plasma cell				
secreted antibody	IgM · IgG1,2,3,4	IgE	IgM	IgM

Fig. 21.3 In X-LA, affected male infants have no B cells and no serum immunoglobulins, except for small amounts of maternal IgG. In IgA deficiency, IgA-bearing B cells and in some cases IgG2- and IgG4-bearing B cells, are unable to differentiate into plasma cells. People with immunodeficiency with increased IgM lack IgG and IgA. In CVID, B cells of most isotypes are unable to differentiate into plasma cells.

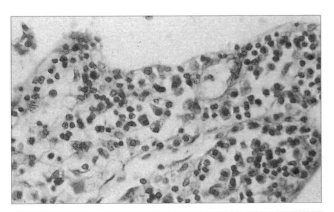

Fig. 21.4 Gall bladder from a patient with immunodeficiency with increased IgM. The submucosa is filled with cells with pink-staining cytoplasm and eccentric nuclei. The cells are synthesizing and secreting IgM.

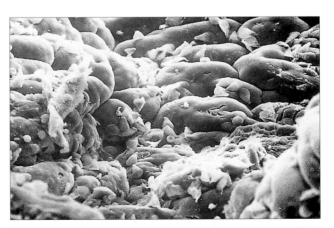

Fig. 21.5 *Giardia lamblia.* Innumerable *Giardia* parasites can be seen swarming over the mucosa of the jejunum of a patient with CVID.

until then, such infants are susceptible to pyogenic infections. The B cells of these infants are normal but they appear to lack help from CD4⁺ T cells in synthesizing antibodies.

■ T-CELL DEFICIENCIES

The major T-cell deficiencies are shown in *Fig. 21.6*. Patients with no T cells, or poor T-cell function, are susceptible to opportunistic infections. Since B-cell function in humans is largely T-cell dependent, T-cell deficiency also results in humoral immunodeficiency; in other words, T-cell deficiency leads to a combined deficiency of both humoral and cell-mediated immunity.

In severe combined immunodeficiency (SCID) there is lymphocyte deficiency and the thymus does not develop

The most profound hereditary deficiency of cell-mediated immunity occurs in infants with SCID who develop recurrent infections early in life (in contrast to X-LA). They have prolonged diarrhoea due to rotavirus or bacterial infection of the gastrointestinal tract and develop pneumonia, usually due to the protozoan, *Pneumocystis carinii*. The common yeast organism *Candida albicans* grows luxuriantly in their mouth or on their skin (*Fig. 21.7*). If they are vaccinated with live organisms, such as poliovirus or bacille Calmette–Guérin (BCG) (used for immunization against tuberculosis), they die of progressive infection from these ordinarily benign organisms. SCID is incompatible with life and affected infants usually die within the first 2 years unless they are rescued with transplants of bone marrow. In this case they become lymphocyte chimeras and can survive and live normally.

Infants with SCID have very few lymphocytes in their blood (fewer than 3 000/ml). Their lymphoid tissue also contains no or few lymphocytes. The thymus has a fetal appearance (*Fig. 21.8*), containing the endodermal stromal cells derived embryonically from the third and fourth

pharyngeal pouch. Lymphoid stem cells, which normally populate the thymus by 6 weeks of human gestation (see Chapter 10), fail to appear and the thymus does not become a lymphoid organ.

SCID is more common in male than female infants (3:1) because over 50% of SCID cases are caused by a gene defect on the X-chromosome. The defective gene encodes the γ chain of the IL-2 receptor. This γ chain also forms part of the receptors for IL-4, 7, 11 and 15. Thus, the lymphoid stem cells are incapable of receiving a number of signals for growth and maturation. The remaining cases of SCID are due to recessive genes on other chromosomes. Of these, half have a genetic deficiency of adenosine deaminase (ADA) or purine nucleoside phosphorylase (PNP). Deficiency of these purine degradation enzymes results in the accumulation of metabolites that are toxic to lymphoid stem cells, namely dATP and dGTP (*Fig. 21.9*). These metabolites inhibit the enzyme ribonucleotide reductase, which is required for DNA synthesis and,

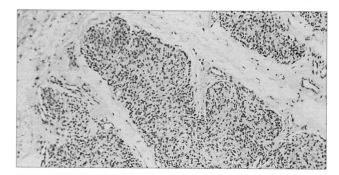

Fig. 21.7 *Candida albicans* in the mouth, in a patient with SCID. This organism grows luxuriantly in the mouth and on the skin of SCID patients.

Primary T-cell deficiencies
severe combined immunodeficiency
adenosine deaminase deficiency
purine nucleoside phosphorylase deficiency
MHC class II deficiency
DiGeorge anomaly
hereditary ataxia telangiectasia
Wiskott–Aldrich syndrome

Fig. 21.6 There is a wide range of causes for T-cell deficiencies, ranging from absence of lymphocytes, to enzyme deficiency, through to MHC deficiency. All affect the ability of T cells to function, which leads to combined T- and B-cell deficiency.

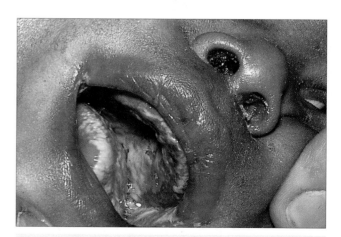

Fig. 21.8 Thymus of SCID. Note that the thymic stroma has not been invaded by lymphoid cells and no Hassall's corpuscles are seen. The gland has a fetal appearance.

Possible role of ADA and PNP deficiency in SCID

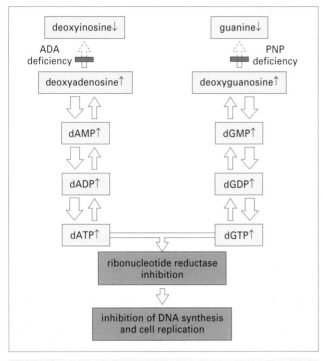

Fig. 21.9 It is thought that deficiencies of ADA and PNP lead to accumulations of dATP and dGTP respectively. Both of these metabolites are powerful inhibitors of ribonucleotide reductase, an essential enzyme for DNA synthesis.

therefore, for cell replication. Since ADA and PNP are found in all mammalian cells, why should these defects only affect lymphocytes? The explanation appears to lie in the relative deficiency of 5'-nucleotidase in lymphoid cells; in other cells, this enzyme compensates for defective ADA or PNP by preventing dAMP and dGMP accumulation.

The optimal treatment for SCID is a bone-marrow transplant from a completely histocompatible donor, usually a normal sibling. About 70% of patients do not have a histocompatible sibling, in which case parental marrow, which would have one haplotype identical, has sometimes been transplanted successfully. Recently a retroviral vector, into which the ADA gene had been inserted, has been used to transfect the lymphocytes of children who are ADA deficient. This was the first example of successful 'gene therapy'.

In MHC class II deficiency TH-cell deficiency results

The failure to express class II MHC molecules on antigen-presenting cells (macrophages and B cells) is inherited as an autosomal recessive characteristic, which is not linked to the MHC locus on the short arm of chromosome 6. Affected infants have recurrent infections, particularly of the gastrointestinal tract. Because the development of CD4$^+$ TH cells (T-helper cells) depends on positive selection by MHC class II molecules in the thymus (see

Chapter 12), MHC class II deficient infants have a deficiency of CD4$^+$ T cells. This lack of TH cells leads to a deficiency in antibodies as well. The MHC class II deficiency results from defects in promoter proteins that bind to the 5' untranslated region of the class II genes.

The DiGeorge anomaly arises from a defect in thymus embryogenesis

As previously mentioned, the thymic epithelium is derived from the third and fourth pharyngeal pouches by the sixth week of human gestation. Subsequently the endodermal anlage is invaded by lymphoid stem cells that undergo development into T cells. The parathyroid glands are also derived from the same embryonic origin. A congenital defect in the organs derived from the third and fourth pharyngeal pouches results in the DiGeorge anomaly. The T-cell deficiency is variable, depending on how badly the thymus is affected. Affected infants have distinctive facial features (*Fig. 21.10*) in that their eyes are widely separated (hypertelorism), the ears are low set, and the philtrum of the upper lip is shortened. They also have congenital malformations of the heart or aortic arch and neonatal tetany from the hypoplasia or aplasia of the parathyroid glands.

In hereditary ataxia–telangiectasia (AT) chromosomal breaks occur in TCR and immunoglobulin genes

AT is inherited as an autosomal recessive trait. Affected infants develop a wobbly gait (ataxia) at about 18 months. Dilated capillaries (telangiectasia) appear in the eyes and on the skin by 6 years of age. AT is accompanied by a variable T-cell deficiency. About 70% of AT patients are also IgA deficient and some also have IgG2 and IgG4 deficiency. They develop severe sinus and lung infections. Their cells exhibit chromosomal breaks, usually in chromosome 7 and chromosome 14, at the sites of the T-cell receptor (TCR) genes and the genes encoding the heavy chains of immunoglobulins. AT patients, as well as the cells from AT patients *in vitro*, are very susceptible to ionizing irradiation; they appear to have a defect in DNA repair, but the reason for this is not known.

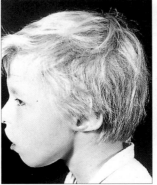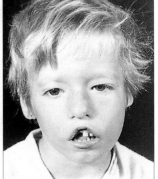

Fig. 21.10 DiGeorge anomaly. Note the wide-set eyes, low-set ears and shortened philtrum of upper lip. Congenital malformations of the cardiovascular may also occur.

In Wiskott–Aldrich syndrome (WAS) there are T-cell defects and abnormal Ig levels

WAS is an X-linked immunodeficiency disease. Affected males have small and profoundly abnormal platelets, which are also few in number (thrombocytopenia). Boys with WAS develop severe eczema as well as pyogenic and opportunistic infections. Their serum contains increased amounts of IgA and IgE, normal levels of IgG and decreased amounts of IgM. Their T cells are defective in function and this malfunction of cell-mediated immunity gets progressively worse. The T cells have a uniquely abnormal appearance, as shown by scanning electron microscopy, reflecting a cytoskeletal defect. They have fewer microvilli on the cell surface than do normal T cells. The sialoglycoproteins in the membranes of both platelets and T cells are abnormal, but the cause of this is at present not known.

■ SECONDARY IMMUNODEFICIENCIES

Secondary immunodeficiencies are those that result from extrinsic or environmental causes. For example, most drugs used in cancer chemotherapy are cytotoxic for T cells. Worldwide, protein malnutrition is probably the leading cause of immunodeficiency in children; it leads to a profound T-cell deficiency and susceptibility to opportunistic infections. Loss of immunoglobulin into the bowel, in inflammatory bowel disease, may lead to a humoral immunodeficiency. Burns can also lead to a severe loss of immunoglobulins through damaged skin. Infections may cause immunodeficiency by parasitizing cells of the immune system, as in AIDS.

Acquired Immunodeficiency Syndrome (AIDS)

AIDS is caused by infection with the human immuno-deficiency virus (HIV). HIV can be transmitted by sexual contact, or from mother to child through the placenta or milk, or by transfusion of whole blood or blood products. There are no other well-established modes of transmission of HIV. Exposure to HIV by one of these routes may or may not result in infection.

Clinical manifestations – When an individual is first infected with HIV he or she may develop a transient illness characterized by fever, swollen lymph nodes, a rash and inflammation of the meninges. This occurs in about 15% of infected individuals. The remainder are asymptomatic at the time of initial infection. As time passes, an individual with HIV infection may develop swollen lymph nodes; this is called progressive generalized lymphadenopathy (PGL). Patients with PGL, as well as asymptomatic individuals, may have progression of the infection to fever, night sweats, weight loss and perhaps minor infections such as yeast organisms in the mouth (thrush due to *Candida albicans*). After a varying length of time, the patient develops major opportunistic infections, such as *Pneumocystis carinii* pneumonia, *Mycobacterium avium-intracellulare*, *Toxoplasma gondii*, or cryptosporidial diarrhoea, or genital and anal herpes simplex. One of the bizarre malignancies associated with AIDS may develop.

The most prominent malignancies observed in patients with AIDS are Kaposi's sarcoma, a tumour of endothelial cells that gives rise to prominent purplish spots on the skin, and B-cell lymphomas. At any time in the course of HIV infection, patients may develop thrombocytopenia (low platelet count), or diseases of the nervous system leading to dementia and paralysis.

HIV life cycle and the immune system – The structure of HIV-1 is shown schematically in *Fig. 21.11*. Its membrane envelope contains two linked glycoproteins, gp120 and gp41, cleaved from a common precursor, gp160. The gp120 protein binds to CD4 and the virus enters cells carrying this marker. These include CD4$^+$ T cells (TH cells), and cells of the monocyte/macrophage lineage, such as the dendritic cells of lymphoid tissue and skin (Langerhans' cells), and the microglia of the central nervous system.

The nucleocapsid of HIV contains four proteins, p24, p17, p9 and p7, which are cleaved from the 53 kDa molecule (p53) encoded by the *gag* gene of the virus. Individuals infected with HIV make antibodies to gp120, gp41 and, most prominently of the *gag* proteins, to p24. Because of difficulties in detecting the virus itself, infection is defined by the appearance in the serum of antibodies to

Human immunodeficiency virus (HIV)-1

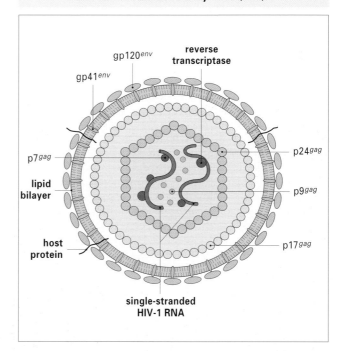

Fig. 21.11 There are two proteins contained in the membranous envelope (*env*), and four in the nuclear region (*gag*) with the single-stranded RNA genome. Also in the nuclear region is reverse transcriptase, a DNA polymerase that uses RNA as a template. (Adapted from Greene WC. *New Engl J Med* 1990:**324**;309.)

any or all of these proteins. The appearance of antibodies (called seroconversion) can take up to 3 months from the initial infection.

The life cycle of the virus is depicted in *Fig. 21.12.* Having entered a CD4$^+$ cell, HIV loses its coat, and a single-stranded DNA copy of the viral RNA is made. This is mediated by the viral enzyme HIV reverse transcriptase. Ultimately, a complementary strand of DNA is made, to give a double-stranded DNA replica of the viral genome. This is incorporated into the host genome. A DNA copy of the viral RNA may remain dormant within the cell for months or years. Infectious viral particles are subsequently made, particularly when an infected T cell is activated. Shortly after the primary infection, as many as 1 in 100 T cells may contain HIV. Host defence mechanisms decrease the viral burden at first, but ultimately the virus overcomes them and progressively infects more and more T cells.

HIV-2 is fundamentally similar in lifecycle and structure to HIV-1 although there is little if any serological cross-reaction between the envelope antigens. HIV-2 is less pathogenic in the sense that patients stay healthy and alive for longer than individuals infected with HIV-1. Enumeration of CD4$^+$ cells in the patient's blood is the best indicator of the progress of the infection. When the

absolute number of CD4$^+$ T cells falls below 600/ml, the patient begins to lose cell-mediated immunity and opportunistic infections ensue. Among the many organisms that can affect the immunocompromised host, especially patients with AIDS, are *Pneumocystis carinii, Candida albicans, Mycobacterium avium-intracellulare, Toxoplasma gondii, Cryptosporidium* spp. and genital and anal herpes simplex. During the early phases of the infection there is polyclonal expansion of B cells and the serum contains large amounts of IgG, IgM and IgA. In the late stages of AIDS, the amount of immunoglobulin in the serum falls dramatically and the antibody titres to gp120 and p24 decrease concomitantly.

Therapy – The only therapy for HIV infection thus far which has had some measure of success, has been the use of dideoxynucleosides, principally azidothymidine (AZT or zidovudine). These compounds inhibit the reverse transcriptase of HIV, so impairing the production of DNA replicas of the virus.

Resistance to AZT develops and renders AZT of limited usefulness. However AZT given to infected pregnant women effectively reduces transplacental virus transmission by 75%.

Life cycle of HIV-1

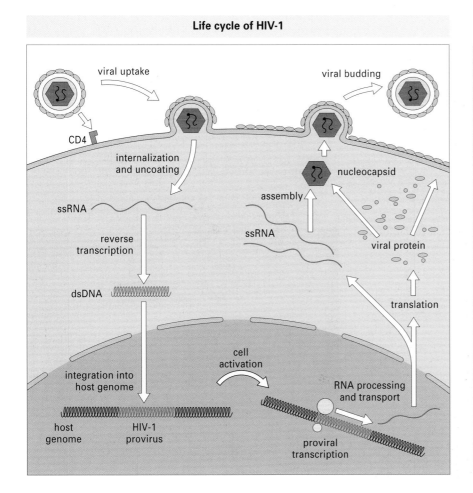

viral uptake

viral budding

CD4

internalization and uncoating

nucleocapsid

assembly

ssRNA

ssRNA

reverse transcription

viral protein

dsDNA

translation

cell activation

integration into host genome

RNA processing and transport

host genome

HIV-1 provirus

proviral transcription

Fig. 21.12 After the interaction of gp120^{env} with the CD4 membrane receptor, gp41-mediated membrane fusion occurs, leading to the entry of HIV-1 into the cell. After uncoating, reverse transcription of viral RNA begins, and this results in the production of the double-stranded DNA form of the viral genome. In turn, the HIV-1 integrase promotes the insertion of this viral DNA duplex into the host genome, giving rise to the HIV-1 provirus. The expression of the HIV-1 genome is stimulated initially by the action of particular inducible and constitutive host transcription factors with binding sites in the genome's long terminal repeat. Stimulation leads to the sequential production of various viral mRNAs. The first mRNAs produced are the multiply spliced species of approximately 2.0 kb encoding the Tat, Rev, and Nef regulatory proteins. The structural proteins of the virus are then produced, allowing the assembly of virions. The free HIV-1 virions produced by viral budding from the host cell can then reinitiate the retroviral life cycle by infecting other CD4$^+$ target cells. (Adapted from Greene WC. *New Engl J Med* 1990:**324**;309.)

DEFECTS IN COMPLEMENT PROTEINS

The proteins of the complement system and their interactions with the immune system are discussed in Chapter 13. Genetic deficiencies of almost all the complement proteins have been found in human beings (*Fig. 21.13*) and these deficiencies reveal much about the normal function of the complement system.

In clearance of immune complexes, inflammation, phagocytosis and bacteriolysis

Deficiencies of the classical pathway components, C1q, C1r and C1s, C4 or C2, result in a propensity to develop immune-complex diseases such as systemic lupus erythematosus. This correlates with the known function of the classical pathway in the dissolution of immune complexes. Deficiencies of C3, Factor H or Factor I result in increased susceptibility to pyogenic infections; this correlates with the important role of C3 in opsonization of pyogenic bacteria. Deficiencies of the terminal components, C5, C6, C7 and C8, and of the alternative pathway components, Factor D and properdin, result in remarkable susceptibility to infection with the two pathogenic species of the *Neisseria* genus: *N. gonorrhoeae* and *N. meningitidis*. This clearly demonstrates the importance of the alternative pathway and the macromolecular attack complex in the bacteriolysis of this genus of bacteria.

All these genetic complement component deficiencies are inherited as autosomal recessive traits, except for properdin deficiency, which is inherited as an X-linked recessive, and C1 inhibitor deficiency, which is inherited as an autosomal dominant.

Hereditary angioneurotic oedema (HAE) is due to C1 inhibitor deficiency

Clinically, the most important deficiency of the complement system is that of the C1 inhibitor. This molecule is responsible for dissociation of activated C1, by binding to $C1r_2C1s_2$. The deficiency results in the well-known disease, hereditary angioneurotic oedema (HAE) (*Fig. 21.14*). This disease is inherited as an autosomal dominant trait. Patients with HAE have recurrent episodes of circumscribed swelling of various parts of the body (angioedema). When the oedema involves the intestine, excruciating abdominal pains and cramps result, with severe vomiting. When the oedema involves the upper airway, the patients may choke to death from respiratory obstruction. Angioedema of the upper airway therefore presents a medical emergency, which requires rapid action to restore normal breathing.

C1 inhibitor not only inhibits the classical pathway of complement but also joint elements of the kinin, plasmin and clotting systems. The oedema is mediated by two peptides generated by uninhibited activation of the complement and contact systems: a peptide derived from the activation of C2, called C2 kinin, and bradykinin derived from the activation of the contact system (*Fig. 21.15*). The effect of these peptides is on the post-capillary venule, where they cause endothelial cells to contract, forming gaps that allow leakage of plasma (see Chapter 14).

There are two genetically determined forms of HAE. In type I, the C1 inhibitor gene is defective and no transcripts are formed. In type II, there are point mutations in the C1 inhibitor gene with the consequence that defective molecules are synthesized. This distinction is important because the diagnosis of type II disease cannot be made by quantitative measurement of serum C1 inhibitor alone.

Genetic deficiencies of human complement

group	type	deficiency	heredity AR	AD	XL
I	immune-complex deficiency	C1q	•		
		C1s, or C1r + C1s	•		
		C2	•		
		C4	•		
II	angioedema	C1 inhibitor		•	
III	recurrent pyogenic infections	C3	•		
		Factor H	•		
		Factor I	•		
IV	recurrent *Neisseria* infections	C5	•		
		C6	•		
		C7	•		
		C8	•		
		properdin			•
		Factor D	?	?	?
V	asymptomatic	C9	•		

Fig. 21.13 Genetic deficiencies of human complement. (AR = phenotypically autosomal recessive; AD = autosomal dominant; XL = X-linked recessive.)

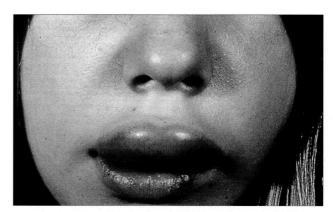

Fig. 21.14 Hereditary angioneurotic oedema. This clinical photograph shows the transient localized swelling which occurs in this condition.

Simultaneous measurements of C4 must also be done. C4 is always decreased in the serum of HAE patients, because of its destruction by uninhibited, activated C1.

C1 inhibitor deficiency may be acquired later in life. In some cases an autoantibody to C1 inhibitor is found. In others, there is a monoclonal B-cell proliferation such as occurs in chronic lymphocytic leukaemia, multiple myeloma or B cell lymphoma. Such patients make an anti-idiotype to their over-produced immunoglobulin; the idiotype –anti-idiotype interaction, for unknown reasons, causes consumption of C1, C4 and C2 and of C1 inhibitor without formation of an effective C3 convertase (which would cause C3 deposition and removal of the complement complex.

■ DEFECTS IN PHAGOCYTES

Phagocytic cells – polymorphonuclear leucocytes and cells of the monocyte/macrophage lineage – are important in host defence against pyogenic bacteria and other intracellular microorganisms. A severe deficiency of poly- morphonuclear leucocytes (neutropenia) can result in overwhelming bacterial infection. Two genetic defects of phagocytes are clinically important in that they result in susceptibility to severe infections and are often fatal: chronic granulomatous disease and the leucocyte adhesion deficiency.

Chronic granulomatous disease is due to a defect in the oxygen reduction pathway

Patients with CGD have defective NADPH oxidase which catalyses the reduction of O_2 to O_2^- by the reaction:

$$NADPH + 2O_2 \rightarrow NADP^+ + 2O_2^- + H^+$$

Thus, they are incapable of forming superoxide anions (O_2^-) and hydrogen peroxide in their phagocytes, following ingestion of microorganisms and so cannot readily kill ingested bacteria or fungi, particularly catalase-producing organisms (see Chapter 17). As a result, microorganisms remain alive in phagocytes of patients with CGD. This gives rise to a cell-mediated response to persistent intracellular microbial antigens, and granulomas form. Children with CGD develop pneumonia, infections in the lymph nodes (lymphadenitis), and abscesses in the skin, liver and other viscera.

The diagnosis of CGD is made by the inability of phagocytes to reduce nitroblue tetrazolium (NBT) dye after a phagocytic stimulus. NBT, a pale, clear, yellow dye, is taken up by phagocytes when they are ingesting a particle. When NBT accepts H and is reduced, as a result of NADPH oxidation, it forms a deep purple precipitate inside the phagocytes; precipitation does not occur in the phagocytes of CGD patients (*Fig. 21.16*).

The NADPH oxidase reaction is complicated and the enzyme complex has many subunits. In resting phagocytes the membrane contains a phagocyte-specific cytochrome, cytochrome b_{558}. This cytochrome is composed of two chains, one of 91 kDa, encoded by a gene on the short arm of the X-chromosome, and one of 22 kDa, encoded by a gene on chromosome 16. When phagocytosis occurs, several proteins from the cytosol become phosphorylated,

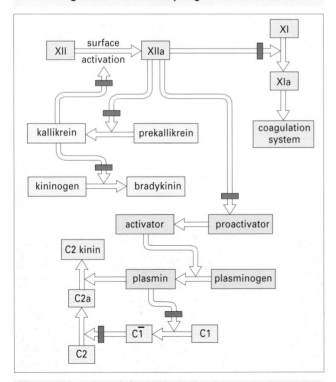

Fig. 21.15 C1 inhibitor is involved in inactivation of elements of the clotting, kinin, plasmin and complement systems, which may be activated following the surface dependent activation of Factor XII (Hageman factor). The points at which C1 inhibitor acts are shown in red. Uncontrolled activation of these pathways results in the formation of bradykinin and C2 kinin, which induce oedema formation.

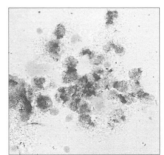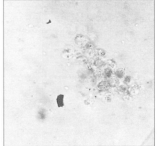

Fig. 21.16 Nitroblue tetrazolium (NBT) test. Left: In normal polymorphs and monocytes, reactive oxygen intermediates (ROIs) are activated by phagocytosis, and yellow NBT is converted to purple-blue formazan. Right: Patients with CGD cannot form ROIs and so the dye stays yellow. (Courtesy of Professor A. R. Hayward.)

move to the membrane and bind to cytochrome b_{558}. The complex that is formed acts as an enzyme, NADPH oxidase, catalysing the NADPH oxidation reaction and thereby activating oxygen radical production (*Fig. 21.17*). The most common form of CGD is X-linked and involves a defect in the 91 kDa chain of cytochrome b_{558}. Three types of CGD are autosomal recessive and result from defects in the 22 kDa chain of the cytochrome b_{558}, or from defects in one or other of two proteins, called p47*phox* or p67*phox* (*phox* is an abbreviation for phagocytic oxidase).

Leucocyte adhesion deficiency (LAD) is due to integrin gene defects

The receptor in the phagocyte membrane that binds to C3bi on opsonized microorganisms is critical for the ingestion of bacteria by phagocytes. This receptor, an integrin called complement receptor 3 (CR3), is deficient in patients with LAD and consequently they develop severe bacterial infections, particularly of the mouth and gastrointestinal tract.

CR3 is composed of two polypeptide chains: an α chain of 165 kDa (CD11b), and a β chain of 95 kDa (CD18). In LAD, there is a genetic defect of the β chain, encoded by a gene on chromosome 21. Two other integrin proteins share the same β chain, namely lymphocyte function associated antigen (LFA-1) and p150,95 (see Chapter 14). Although they have unique α chains (CD11a and CD11c, respectively), these proteins are also defective in LAD. LFA-1 is important in cell adhesion and interacts with intercellular adhesion molecule-1 (ICAM-1) on endothelial cell surfaces and other cell membranes. Because of the defect in LFA-1, phagocytes from patients with LAD cannot adhere to vascular endothelium and thus cannot migrate out of blood vessels into areas of infection. Thus patients with LAD cannot form pus efficiently; this allows the rapid spread of bacterial invaders.

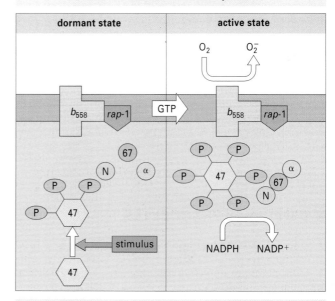

NADPH oxidase and its components

Fig. 21.17 Prevailing knowledge of the NADPH oxidase suggests that, in its dormant state, some of its component parts are in the membrane (cytochrome b_{558} and possibly *rap-1*) while others are in the cytosol (p47*phox*, p67*phox*, the NADPH-binding component, N, and a putative fourth component, α). After the stimulus provided phagocytosis, the cytosolic components associate and move to the membrane, an event possibly mediated by phosphorylation (P) of p47*phox*. Once the cytosol components are associated with the membrane components, the oxidase becomes catalytically active and p47*phox* is phosphorylated further. In the different forms of CGD, there are defects in the genes for different components of the oxidase. (Adapted from Curnutte JT. *Blood* 1991:**77**;673, with permission.)

Critical Thinking

■ Males with X-linked agammaglobulinaemia have a clinical course that is indistinguishable from hereditary deficiency of the third component of complement (C3), in that both groups of patients have increased susceptibility to pyogenic infections. How do you explain this?

■ Patients with MHC class II deficiency lack CD4+ T cells. There are rare patients with MHC class I deficiency. What T-cell subpopulation do you expect would be deficient in these patients?

■ Patients with early complement component deficiencies (C1, C2, C4 and C1 inhibitor) may not be particularly susceptible to pyogenic infections, in contrast to patients with C3 deficiency. How do you explain this?

■ Immunity to HIV is probably mediated by antibodies and cytotoxic CD8+ T cells. HIV infects CD4+ T cells and macrophages. How does the depletion of CD4+ cells by HIV affect antibody formation and cytotoxic CD8+ T cell function?

FURTHER READING

Conley ME. Molecular approaches to analysis of X-linked immunodeficiencies. *Ann Rev Immunol* **10**;215 1992.

Curnutte JT,. Orkin SH, Dinauer MC. Genetic disorders of phagocyte function. In: Stamatoyannopoulos G, Nienhuis AW, Majerus PW, Varmus H. *The Molecular Basis of Blood Diseases*. Philadelphia, PA, Saunders 1994, p. 443

Rosen FS, Seligman M. *Immunodeficiency Reviews*, Vols 1–3. London: Gordon Breech, 1988–1992.

Von Andrian UH, Berger EM, Chambers JD, Ramezani L, Ochs H, Harlan JM, Paulson JD, Etzioni A, Arfors K-E. *In vivo* behaviour of neutrophils from two patients with distinct inherited leukocyte adhesion deficiency syndromes. *J Clin Invest* **91**;2893, 1993.

In atopic/allergic individuals IgE is produced after contact with low levels of innocuous environmental allergens, e.g. pollen, animal dander and house-dust mite.

IgE binds to mast cells via specific receptors (FcεRI). Interaction of bound IgE with allergen leads to the release of mast cell mediators (autocoids, cytokines), that produce the clinical symptoms of allergy.

Typical examples of allergic reactions are hay fever, asthma, atopic eczema, drug allergy and anaphylaxis. Therapies include antihistamines, bronchodilators, adrenaline, corticosteroids and specific immunotherapy.

Epidemiological studies on families, and particularly on twins through concordance studies, show that IgE production is due to a genetic predisposition to make TH2/IL-4 type immune responses to allergen.

Environmental factors such as allergen load, viral infections and exposure to pollutants modify and enhance the IgE response and clinical symptoms.

IgE may have originally evolved as a defence against parasitic worm infections. Its production in response to allergens produces allergic reactions which can be considered an unfortunate side effect of its activity.

When an adaptive immune response occurs in an exaggerated or inappropriate form, the term hypersensitivity is applied. Hypersensitivity reactions are the result of normally beneficial immune responses acting inappropriately, and sometimes cause inflammatory reactions and tissue damage. They can be provoked by many antigens; the cause of a hypersensitivity reaction will vary from one individual to the next. Hypersensitivity is not manifested on first contact with the antigen, but usually appears on subsequent contact. Coombs and Gell described four types of hypersensitivity reaction (Types I, II, III and IV), but in practice these types do not necessarily occur in isolation from each other. The first three are antibody-mediated; the fourth is mediated mainly by T cells and macrophages.

Type I (immediate) hypersensitivity occurs when an immunoglobulin E (IgE) response is directed against innocuous environmental antigens, such as pollen, house-dust mites or animal dander. The resulting release of pharmacological mediators by IgE-sensitized mast cells produces an acute inflammatory reaction with symptoms such as asthma or rhinitis. Type II, or antibody-dependent cytotoxic hypersensitivity, occurs when antibody binds to either self antigen or foreign antigen on cells, and leads to phagocytosis, killer cell activity or complement-mediated lysis (see Chapter 23). Type III hypersensitivity develops when immune complexes are formed in large quantities, or cannot be cleared adequately by the reticuloendothelial system, leading to serum-sickness type reactions (see Chapter 24). Type IV or delayed type hypersensitivity (DTH), is most seriously manifested when antigens (for example those on tubercle bacilli) are trapped in a macrophage and cannot be cleared. T cells are then stimulated to elaborate cytokines which mediate a range of inflammatory responses. Other aspects of DTH reactions are seen in graft rejection and allergic contact dermatitis (see Chapter 25). These four types of hypersensitivity reaction are summarized in *Figure 22.1*.

The four types of hypersensitivity reaction

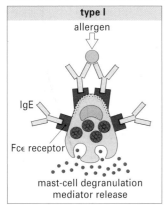

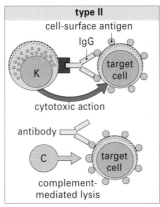

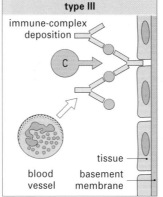

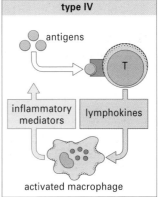

Fig. 22.1 There are four types of hypersensitivity reaction. **Type I** Mast cells bind IgE via their Fc receptors. On encountering allergen the IgE becomes cross-linked, inducing degranulation and release of mediators that produce allergic reactions. **Type II** Antibody is directed against antigen on an individual's own cells (target cell) or foreign antigen, such as transfused red blood cells. This may lead to cytotoxic action by K cells, or by complement-mediated lysis.

Type III Immune complexes are deposited in the tissue. Complement is activated and polymorphs are attracted to the site of deposition, causing local tissue damage and inflammation. **Type IV** Antigen-sensitized T cells release lymphokines following a secondary contact with the same antigen. Cytokines induce inflammatory reactions and activate and attract macrophages, which release inflammatory mediators.

■ TYPE I – IMMEDIATE HYPERSENSITIVITY

Type I hypersensitivity is characterized by an allergic reaction (*Fig. 22.2*) that occurs immediately following contact with the antigen, referred to as the allergen. The term 'allergy', meaning 'changed reactivity' of the host when meeting an 'agent' on a second or subsequent occasion, was originally coined in 1906 by von Pirquet. He made no strictures as to the type of immunological response made by the host. It is only in recent years that 'allergy' has become synonymous with Type I hypersensitivity.

Atopy – the umbrella term covering asthma, eczema, hay fever and food allergy

Originally described by Coca and Cooke in 1923, the term 'atopy' describes the clinical presentations of Type I hypersensitivity, which include asthma, eczema, hay fever, urticaria and food allergy. These usually occur in subjects with a family history of these or similar conditions, and who also show immediate wheal-and-flare skin reactions to common environmental allergens.

It had already been suggested that the anaphylaxis in animals, discovered by Portier and Richet in 1902, was related to hay fever and asthma in humans, but whereas 90% of animals develop precipitating antibodies to injected foreign proteins or toxins, only 10–20% of the human population become sensitized following exposure to an airborne allergen. Another important difference was the strong hereditary linkage seen in human allergy but not (at the time) in animal anaphylaxis. Thus, originally, allergic reactions in animals and atopy in man appeared distinct.

Allergy is mediated by immunoglobulin E

The first description of the mechanism of the allergic reaction was presented by Prausnitz and Küstner in 1921. They

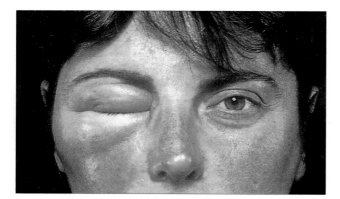

Fig. 22.2 The anaphylactic response to bee venom. The immediate reaction is a clear cut example of Type I hypersensitivity due to the release of pharmacological mediators, including histamine, from mast cells. This is a localized reaction to a facial sting. The reaction can also produce generalized anaphylaxis and even death, as the allergen is injected into the patient rather than being inhaled. The reaction can be aggravated by mellitin in the venom, which can trigger mast cells non-immunologically.

took serum from Küstner (who was allergic to fish) and injected it into the skin of Prausnitz. When fish antigen was subsequently injected into the sensitized site, there was an immediate wheal-and-flare reaction. (This is similar to the PCA test, used for the assay of IgE production in experimental animals.) Prausnitz and Küstner proposed the existence of an 'atopic reagin' in the serum of allergic subjects. Some 45 years later, Ishizaka and colleagues isolated this 'atopic reagin' and showed that it was a new class of immunoglobulin – IgE.

Type I hypersensitivity reactions follow the triggering of IgE-sensitized mast cells by allergen

The reactions characteristic of Type I hypersensitivity are dependent on the specific triggering of IgE-sensitized mast cells by allergen. The mast cells release pharmacological mediators that produce the inflammatory responses typical of Type I hypersensitivity reactions (*Fig. 22.3*).

Important new research has shown that several multifunctional cytokines are also released as a result of IgE-mediated mast cell activation. IL-3 and IL-4 may have significant autocrine effects on the mast cell itself, and with other cytokines may facilitate IgE production by B cells. In addition, several cytokines, including IL-5 and products of the IL-8 and IL-9 gene families, may be important in the chemotaxis and activation of inflammatory cells at sites of allergic reaction. However, it is important to note that the role of the mast cell-derived cytokines *in vivo* still remains to be elucidated.

■ IMMUNOGLOBULIN E

The initial contact of an allergen with the mucosa is followed by a complex series of events, leading to the production of IgE. The IgE response is a local event occurring at the site of the allergen's entry into the body, i.e. at mucosal surfaces and/or at local lymph nodes. IgE production by B cells depends on allergen presentation by antigen-presenting cells (APCs) and cooperation between the B cells and TH2 cells (see *Fig. 22.3*). Locally produced IgE first sensitizes local mast cells; 'spill-over' IgE then enters the circulation and binds to specific receptors on both circulating basophils and tissue-fixed mast cells throughout the body.

An important characteristic of IgE is its ability to bind to mast cells and basophils with high affinity through its Fc portion. Thus, although the serum half-life of free IgE is only a few days, mast cells may remain sensitized by IgE for many months due to the high affinity of binding to the IgE receptor FcεRI, which protects IgE from destruction by serum proteases (FcεRII has a much lower affinity for IgE). Early experiments by Stanworth demonstrated this elegantly. He sensitized twelve separate skin sites on his own arm with atopic serum. He then challenged a fresh set once a week, every week for three months with the specific antigen. When the last site was challenged, there was still an immediate wheal-and-flare reaction, showing that adequate amounts of IgE were still attached to local skin mast cells three months after sensitization.

Induction and effector mechanisms in Type I hypersensitivity

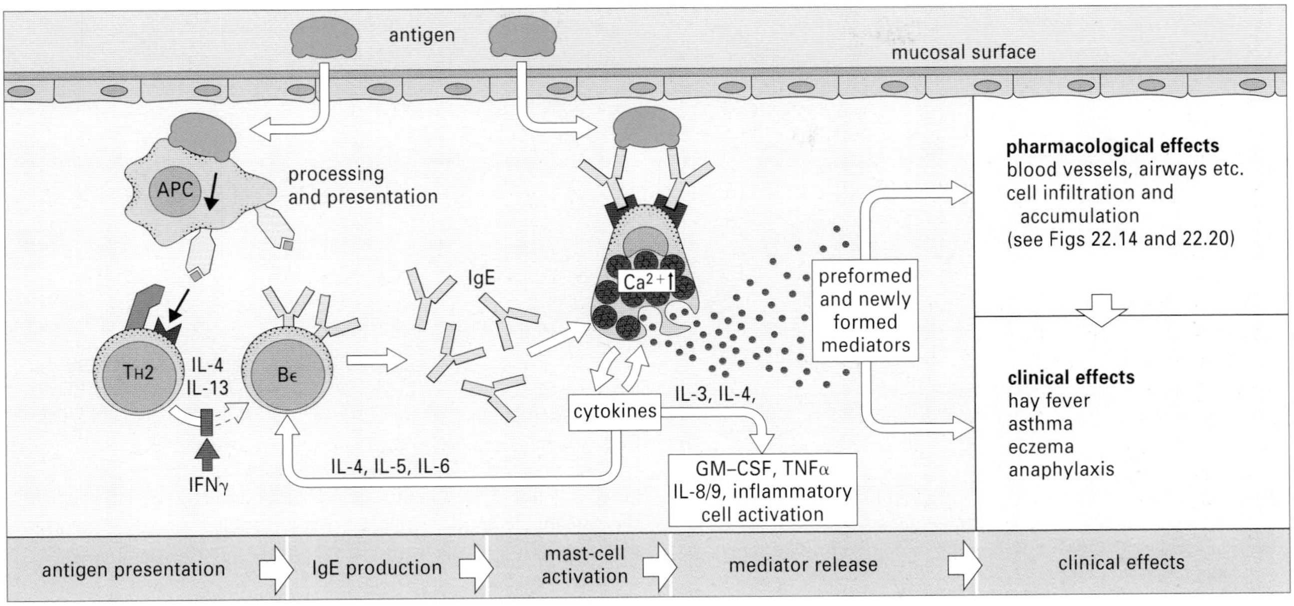

Fig. 22.3 Innocuous environmental antigens (allergens) enter via mucosal surfaces and are taken up by local antigen-presenting cells (APCs), which process and present them to TH cells. TH2 cells secrete cytokines that induce B cell proliferation and favour the production of an allergen specific IgE response. The IgE binds, via FCε receptors (FCεRI), to mast cells thus sensitizing them. When allergen subsequently reaches the sensitized mast cell it cross-links surface-bound IgE, causing an increase in intracellular calcium (Ca²⁺) that triggers the release of pre-formed mediators, such as histamine and proteases, and newly synthesized, lipid-derived mediators such as leukotrienes and prostaglandins. These autocoids produce the clinical symptoms of allergy.

Cytokines are also released from degranulating mast cells and may augment the inflammatory and IgE response.

IgE levels are elevated in allergic diseases

IgE levels are often raised in allergic disease and grossly elevated in parasitic infestations. When assessing children or adults for the presence of atopic disease a raised level of IgE aids the diagnosis, although a normal IgE level does not exclude atopy (*Fig. 22.4*). Note that the determination of IgE alone will not predict an allergic state, since genetic and environmental factors also play an important part in the expression of clinical symptoms. Nevertheless, if a patient does have a very high IgE and no evidence of a worm infection, allergy does become increasingly likely.

When skin tests are performed on large numbers of subjects, many more have positive skin test reactions than actually complain of symptoms. A recent survey has shown that up to 30% of a random group of 5000 subjects had a positive skin test reaction to one or more common allergens. Thus, these subjects can produce specific IgE but lack some factor (factor X, see *Fig. 22.27*), which precipitates the expression of the clinical symptoms of atopy.

IgE production is controlled by helper T cells
Early studies suggested a regulatory role for a 'suppressor' T cell

Studies by Tada and colleagues in the early 1970s using rats clearly demonstrated the importance of T cells in controlling IgE production. Animals immunized with the antigen DNP-*Ascaris* (with *Bordetella pertussis* as adjuvant) showed a rise in IgE titres which peaked after five to ten days and returned to normal over the next six weeks. If the animals were first thymectomized or irradiated, the IgE response was enhanced and prolonged. If, during this phase of enhanced IgE production, the thymectomized animal was passively given thymocytes or spleen cells from *Ascaris*-primed animals, IgE production was suppressed (*Fig. 22.5*). The suppression of the IgE response was considered to be due to the activity of suppressor T cells in the transferred cell population, an activity that was reduced by thymectomy or irradiation treatment. The IgG and IgM levels were unchanged by the cell transfer, showing that IgE responses were particularly sensitive to the effects of the proposed suppressor T cells.

Other experiments have shown that neonatal thymectomy completely abolishes the capacity of rats to produce IgE to DNP-*Ascaris*, showing the need for TH cells in the induction of an IgE response. In several clinical conditions an association has been suggested between low suppressor T-cell numbers and high levels of IgE, indicating that T-cell control of IgE production is also important in man.

The suppressor effect is provided by TH1 cells

It is now known that subsets of TH cells that produce particular profiles of cytokines are responsible for the regulation of

IgE levels and atopic disease

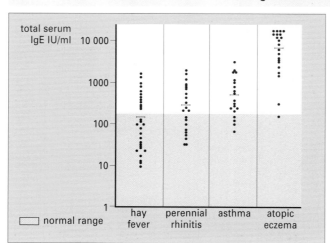

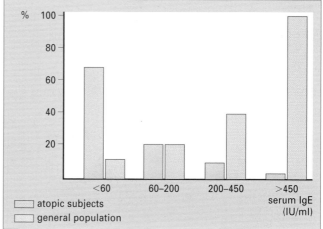

Fig. 22.4 Left: The serum concentration of IgE (which is around 100 IU/ml) is 10^5 times less than that of IgG (around 10 mg/ml) and comprises less than 0.001% of the total immunoglobulin. Levels of atopic patients tend to be raised, and this is especially so in atopic eczema (1 IU = 2 ng) **Right:** The higher the level of IgE the smaller the percentage of the population, but the greater the likelihood of atopy. Where the level is greater than 450 IU/ml the majority of subjects are atopic.

IgE production observed by Tada. The cellular and molecular mechanisms involved in this regulation are outlined in *Figure 22.6*. Note that the profile of cytokines produced by

T-cell control of the IgE response–early studies

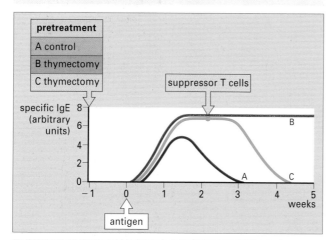

Fig. 22.5 The IgE response is under both T-helper (TH) and T-supressor (Ts) cell control. This experiment uses three groups of rats – a control group (A), receiving no pretreatment 1 week before antigen challenge, and two groups which are first thymectomized (B and C). Following antigen challenge the IgE response is measured regularly. On immunization with antigen there is a transient rise in antigen-specific IgE in the controls. Thymectomy (or irradiation) causes a prolonged response (B) which can be curtailed by the addition of antigen-stimulated spleen cells containing suppressor T cells (C). In neonatally thymectomized rats, no IgE response is seen, indicating the basic requirement for TH cells.

TH2 cells (IL-3, 4, 5, 9, 13) is encoded in a gene cluster on chromosome 5 in humans and chromosome 13 in mice. The crucial role of these cytokines *in vivo* has been shown in mice, where neutralizing antibodies to IL-4, or administration of IFNγ, both lead to an inhibition of IgE responses. Also, transgenic mice homozygous for a mutation that inactivates the IL-4 gene cannot produce IgE after a nematode infection. In patients with hyper-IgE syndrome, giving IFNα (in preference to IFNγ because it has fewer adverse effects) also leads to a reduction in serum IgE levels. The molecular mechanisms by which IL-4/IL-13 cause B-cell switching to IgE production remain to be elucidated.

It is noteworthy that TH2 cells also produce IL-5, which promotes the synthesis and secretion of IgA from B cells and is also crucial in eosinophil development and survival at inflammatory sites. This may explain the eosinophilia that is so frequently associated with IgE-mediated allergic reactions (see also *Figs 22.20–22.22*). Clearly, influencing the profile of cytokine production, or the effect of cytokines, could be a useful strategy for the future treatment of IgE-mediated disorders.

■ GENETICS OF THE ALLERGIC RESPONSE IN MAN

Studies in the 1920s showed that allergic parents tended to have a higher proportion of allergic children than parents who were not allergic. In fact, with two allergic parents there is a greater than 50% chance of the children having allergy; even with one allergic parent the chances are almost 30%. Thus, a parental history of allergy is a risk factor for atopy (*Fig. 22.7*).

Note that a variety of non-genetic factors may also play an important role, such as the level of allergen exposure, the nutritional status of the individual and the presence of chronic underlying infections or acute viral illnesses. As regards the quantity of exposure, the annual challenge of individuals by airborne pollens is in the order of 1 µg. It is perhaps surprising that some 20% of the population respond to this exceptionally low-dose challenge.

Genetic mechanisms regulate three aspects of the allergic response:

- Total IgE levels
- The allergen-specific response
- General hyperresponsiveness.

Total IgE levels are determined by genetic factors

It is clear from the study of families and twins that total IgE levels are determined by genetic factors. Since TH2 cells and the cytokines they produce provide an environment that favours IgE responses, it was perhaps logical to search for a linkage between genetic markers in the 'IL-4 cytokine gene cluster' region, and total and specific IgE levels. The group

Cytokine control of the IgE response

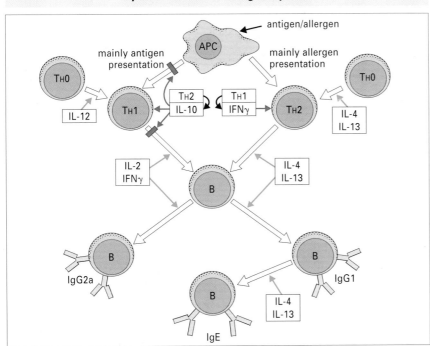

Fig. 22.6 The cytokine environment determines which T-cell subset is produced from TH0 cells, and therefore which pathway B cells will take.

Thus a cytokine environment dominated by IL-4 and IL-13 favours TH2 development and B cell switching to IgE. TH2 production of IL-10 inhibits TH1 cell responses via an effect on APCs and maintains and augments the 'TH2-ness' of the response. Thus, TH2 responses promote the production of IgE to allergens. Conversely, TH1 responses to typical antigens such as tetanus toxoid are favoured by the production of IFNγ and IL-2, which also suppress TH2 cell development. TH1 responses promote the production of IgG2a and T-cell immunity.

Heredity and environment in atopy

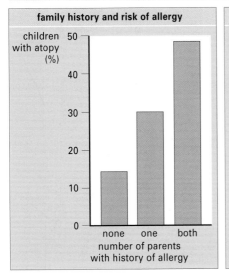

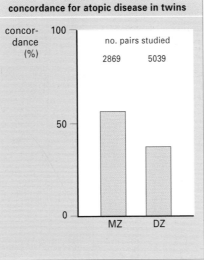

Fig. 22.7 Left: There is often a strong family history of atopy in allergic subjects. Large studies confirm that the greater the parental history of allergy, the greater the likelihood of the children being atopic. **Right**: The concordance of atopic disease in dizygotic (DZ; non-identical) twins is slightly greater than that found in the general population (approximately 20%). However, the concordance in monozygotic (MZ; identical) twins is well below the 100% that might be expected if the genotype was the sole factor in determining the development of atopy. These two findings suggest that both genetic and environmental factors are important in the expression of atopic disease.

of David Marsh performed such a study and confirmed that a linkage does indeed exist. They showed that IL-4 and/or another gene in this region regulates total (but not specific) IgE levels.

Genes controlling the allergen-specific response are linked to HLA

The major control of allergen-specific IgE responses appears to reside in the HLA-linked immune response (IR) genes. This is most striking for very low-dose allergen exposure and especially for low molecular weight minor determinants. For example, more than 90% of IgE responders to the ragweed allergen *Amb a* V (5 kDa) are HLA-Dw2 (*Fig. 22.8*). IgE responders to the larger, more abundant, allergen *Amb a* I (38 kDa) have no known HLA association.

The association is greater with IgE antibody and immediate hypersensitivity skin tests than with IgG antibody. However, following hyposensitization to ragweed it is only the HLA-Dw2, *Amb a* V+ subjects who make a good IgG response, showing that immune response to *Amb a* V is not restricted to IgE, but includes other immunoglobulin classes as well.

Lastly, there is a higher degree of HLA linkage when the subject has a low total IgE. For example, of patients who are allergic to ragweed, only 1 in 6 respond to the minor determinant *Amb a* III. Of the *Amb a* III+ patients with low levels of total IgE, 90% of subjects carry HLA-A2 (*Fig. 22.9*). With increasing total IgE levels, that HLA association disappears.

General and specific hyperresponsiveness is HLA-linked

A patient who gives positive skin tests to a broad range of antigens is said to demonstrate general hyperresponsiveness. Experiments have shown that such patients carry HLA-B8 and HLA-Dw3, but not HLA-A1, at significantly higher frequencies than normal subjects.

A more specific hyperresponsiveness can also be seen in those already making anti-ragweed IgE antibodies, where patients with HLA-B8 have higher titres of antibody and also higher levels of total IgE.

HLA-B8 is also strongly associated with other forms of immune 'hyperactivity', for example autoimmune diseases. This raises the possibility that HLA-B8 is linked to suppressor T-cell control of immune responses, since depressed suppressor cell activity is thought to be involved in the development of both autoimmune and IgE responses.

■ MAST CELLS

It has long been recognized that there are species differences in mast-cell morphology. These morphological differences may be seen not only in the staining properties of the cells

Atopy: IgE levels and HLA type

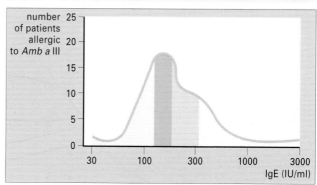

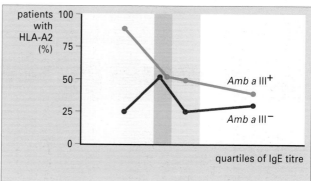

Fig. 22.9 Upper: Graph showing the number of ragweed-allergic patients (*Amb a* III+) with given levels of total IgE; quartiles of the range are indicated in different shades. **Lower:** Graph showing the percentage of patients in the four quartiles possessing HLA-A2. This is shown for both *Amb a* III+ and *Amb a* III− individuals. It appears that a person is more likely to be sensitive to *Amb a* III if she or he possesses HLA-A2. This association is most marked (i.e. the linkage is tightest) where the IgE level is low. HLA-A2 is present in 47% of the general population.

Allergens and HLA associations

systematic name	old name	mol.wt (daltons)	primary association	p value
Ambrosia (Ragweed) spp.				
Amb a I	AgE	37 800	none	–
Amb a III	Ra3	12 300	A2	0.01
Amb a VI	Ra6	11 500	DR5	<10⁻⁷
Amb a V	Ra5	5000	DR2/Dw2	<10⁻⁹
Amb t V	Ra5G	4400	DR2/Dw2	<10⁻³
Lolium (ryegrass) spp.				
Lol p I	Rye I	27 000	DR3/Dw3	<10⁻³
Lol p II	Rye II	11 000	DR3/Dw3	<10⁻³
Lol p III	Rye III	11 000	DR3/Dw3	<10⁻⁴

Fig. 22.8 HLA association of IgE responses to allergens from ragweed and ryegrass. (Courtesy of Dr D. Marsh.)

and the outer structure of their granules, but also in the detailed mechanism of the degranulation process. This last point can be clearly demonstrated; in man, the membranes surrounding the mast-cell granules fuse before exocytosis (compound exocytosis), whereas in rats the granules are expelled singly (*Fig. 22.10*).

Two types of mast cells – connective tissue mast cells (CTMC) and mucosal mast cells (MMC) – have been defined based on their tissue distribution, staining characteristics and the proteases they contain (*Fig. 22.11* and *22.12*).

There are also functional differences in the way that particular mast-cell populations respond to drugs that stimulate mast-cell degranulation (Ca^{2+} ionophores, compound 48/80 etc.) or that inhibit histamine release (sodium cromoglycate).

Classification of mast cells is based on their location and morphology

CTMCs are found around blood vessels in most tissues. Although CTMCs from different sites have similar properties, the gross morphology of CTMCs from the peritoneum and the skin for example, may be quite different in terms of the number and size of the granules, the density of staining and their pharmacological properties (see *Figs. 22.11* and *22.12*). MMCs have a different distribution; in man the highest concentrations are found in the mucosa of the midgut and in the lung.

During parasitic infections, for example in rats infected with *Nippostrongylus brasiliensis*, there is a marked increase in MMCs in the gut mucosa. This increase is also seen in Crohn's disease and in ulcerative colitis. There is a similar increase of CTMCs in the synovium of patients with rheumatoid arthritis. However, the role that mast cells play in these diseases is not clear.

It has been suggested that the precursors of gut MMCs arise in the mesenteric lymph nodes that drain the gut, and then migrate via the thoracic duct into the intestine. It is clear that MMC proliferation after a parasitic infection is dependent on T-cell derived cytokines including IL-3 and IL-4. CTMC clones arise in culture from fibroblast layers, independent of T cells or T-cell factors.

Recent evidence suggests that MMCs and CTMCs are derived from the same precursor cell, with the end-cell phenotype depending on factors found in the local microenvironment.

CTMCs and MMCs have characteristic granule proteases

A number of mast-cell granule proteases have recently been cloned and sequenced. Two of these, tryptase and chymase, have been used to further define the CTMC and MMC mast-cell subpopulations (see *Fig. 22.12*).

These proteases are of clinical interest in that tryptase can cause bronchial hyperresponsiveness and chymase stimulates

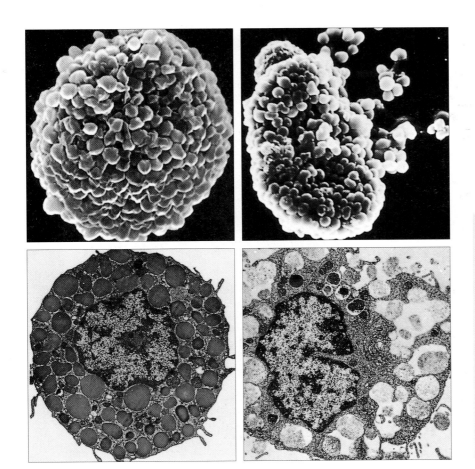

Fig. 22.10 Electron micrograph study of rat mast cells. Upper left: An intact rat peritoneal mast cell with the cell membrane shrunk onto the granules. Scanning electron micrograph, ×1500. **Upper right:** A rat peritoneal mast cell degranulating following incubation with anti-IgE for 30 seconds. Scanning electron micrograph, ×1500. (Courtesy of Dr T. S. C. Orr.) **Lower left:** Rat peritoneal mast cells showing electron-dense granules. **Lower right:** Following incubation with anti-IgE, vacuolation with exocytosis of the granule contents has occurred. Transmission electron micrographs, ×2700. (Courtesy of Dr D. Lawson.)

Differences between mast-cell populations – I

	mucosal mast cell	connective tissue mast cell
location *in vivo*	gut and lung	ubiquitous
life span	<40 days (?)	>40 days (?)
T-cell-dependent	+	–
number of Fcε receptors	25×10^5	3×10^4
histamine content	+	+ +
cytoplasmic IgE	+	–
major AA metabolite $LTC_4:PGD_2$ ratio	25:1	1:40
DSCG/theophylline inhibits histamine release	–	+
major proteoglycan	chondroitin sulphate	heparin

Fig. 22.11 There are at least two subpopulations of mast cells, the mucosal mast cells (MMCs) and the connective tissue mast cells (CTMCs). The differences in their morphology and pharmacology suggest different functional roles *in vivo*. MMCs are associated with parasitic worm infections and, possibly, allergic reactions. In contrast to the CTMC, the MMC is smaller, shorter lived, T-cell dependent, has more Fcε receptors and contains intracytoplasmic IgE. Both cells contain histamine and serotonin in their granules; the higher histamine content of the CTMC may be accounted for by the greater number of granules. Major arachidonic acid (AA) metabolites (prostaglandins and leukotrienes) are produced by both mast-cell types, but in different amounts. For example, the ratios of production of the leukotriene LTC_4 to the prostaglandin PGD_2 are 25:1 in the MMC and 1:40 in the CTMC. The effect of drugs on degranulation is different between the two cell types. Sodium cromoglycate (DSCG) and theophylline both inhibit histamine release from the CTMC but not from the MMC. (This may have important implications in the treatment of asthma.) Note that many of these data come from rodent studies and may not apply to man.

Differences between mast-cell populations – II

cell type	location	amount per cell (pg)	
		tryptase	chymase
MC_T (MMC)	lung and nasal cavity, intestinal mucosa	10	<0.04
MC_TC (CTMC)	skin, blood vessels, intestinal submucosa	35	4.5
Basophil	circulation	0.04	<0.04

Fig. 22.12 Tryptase is a tetramer of 134 kDa which may comprise as much as 25% of the mast-cell protein. Chymase is a monomer of 30 kDa. The relative proportions of these proteases in mast cells define MC_T and MC_{TC} populations, which have different distributions in human tissues. Basophils have very low amounts of both proteases. (The suffixes T and TC represent the content of tryptase and chymase in the respective cells.)

bronchial mucus secretion – both of which are hallmarks of asthma (see *Fig. 22.2*). Both proteases can also degrade vasoactive intestinal peptide (VIP), a mediator of bronchial relaxation. Furthermore, tryptase is a potent fibroblast growth factor and may provide a molecular link between mast-cell activation and fibrosis.

Clinical studies of mast cells in asthma and hay fever

A number of recent clinical studies have demonstrated that MMCs infiltrate the nasal epithelium in patients with hay fever during, but not before, the pollen season. Similarly, increased numbers of mast cells (which have not been characterized) are found in the bronchoalveolar lavage fluid of asthmatics.

Since the bronchial mucosal surface is the first site of contact for inhaled allergen, the interaction of the superficial mast cells with allergen will lead to the release of mediators and result in increased permeability of the mucosa to allergen. This leads to further mediator release by submucosal mast cells, thereby amplifying the clinical symptoms. (Degranulation may

be assessed by measuring the serum level of tryptase. Due to its stability, tryptase is a more reliable marker of mast-cell degranulation than histamine.

Drugs targeting mast cells can have important clinical effects

A better understanding of the nature of these superficial, bronchoalveolar mast cells and their responsiveness to anti-allergic drugs could have important therapeutic implications. For instance, in rats infested with the nematode parasite *Nippostrongylus brasiliensis*, the accumulation of MMCs in the gut is rapidly and dramatically suppressed by treatment with corticosteroids.

Interestingly, locally applied corticosteroids also suppress the increase in nasal mast-cell numbers seen in hay fever patients during the pollen season. The mechanism of this suppression is not clear, but it is known that corticosteroids inhibit cytokine production by TH cells, including the cytokines IL-3 and IL-4, both of which have mast-cell growth factor activity.

The effect of drugs on mast-cell degranulation is crucial, both functionally and clinically. In the rat, sodium cromoglycate and theophylline both inhibit histamine release from CTMCs but not from MMCs. Because of mast-cell heterogeneity and species differences, it is unsafe to extrapolate these results to man. The development of 'pure' human mast cell lines could be of great use in developing drugs for the management of allergic diseases in man.

Other immune cells can also bind IgE

Normal eosinophils and platelets, when sensitized with IgE, have enhanced cytotoxicity against some parasites, including schistosomes. In addition, these cells may become sensitized by circulating immune complexes containing IgE in allergic patients. These cell types could contribute to the allergic response, since they both contain a variety of mediators and inflammatory proteins capable of exacerbating allergic reactions. Recent evidence shows that eosinophils, macrophages, platelets and Langerhans' cells express both the high and low affinity receptors for IgE (*Fig. 22.13*).

Interestingly, Langerhans' cells in the skin of patients with atopic eczema have surface-bound IgE which may be important in antigen/allergen presentation to skin infiltrating T cells, thereby inducing inflammatory reactions in the skin. Such IgE-binding Langerhans' cells are not seen in normal skin or in atopic subjects without eczema.

Mast-cell degranulation can be triggered in several ways

Once IgE has bound to FcεRI on mast cells and basophils, degranulation can be triggered by IgE cross-linking. This is achieved by allergen or other molecules, and leads to aggregation of the Fcε receptors. This causes an influx of calcium ions into the cell, followed by degranulation.

Degranulation is also effected by manoeuvres that directly cross-link the receptors (*Fig. 22.14*). For example, lectins such as PHA and ConA can cross-link IgE by binding to carbohydrate residues on the Fc region. This might be an explanation for the urticaria induced in some individuals by strawberries, which contain large amounts of lectin.

Other compounds are extremely active in degranulating mast cells. Probably the most important of these *in vivo* are the breakdown products of complement activation, C3a and C5a. These anaphylatoxins also affect many other cells, including neutrophils, platelets and macrophages. Other compounds that can directly activate mast cells include calcium ionophores, mellitin and compound 48/80, and drugs such as synthetic ACTH, codeine and morphine. All of these compounds lead to the activation of mast cells by causing an influx of calcium ions. The anaphylactic response induced by these agents is identical to that seen in IgE-mediated reactions although, of course, they act by IgE-independent mechanisms.

Degranulation releases preformed mediators and induces the synthesis of others from arachidonic acid

The antigen-induced calcium ion influx into mast cells has two main results. Firstly, there is an exocytosis of granule contents with the release of preformed mediators, the major one in man being histamine. Secondly, there is the induction of synthesis of newly formed mediators from arachidonic acid, leading to the production of prostaglandins and leukotrienes, which have a direct effect on the local tissues. In the lung they cause immediate bronchoconstriction, mucosal oedema and hypersecretion, leading to asthma (see *Figs. 22.14* and *22.20*).

It is becoming clear that different profiles of newly formed mediators are produced by distinct populations of mast cells. For example, antihistamines are effective clinically in rhinitis and urticaria but not in asthma, where leukotrienes play a more important role.

Drugs may block the release of mediators either by increasing the intracellular levels of cAMP (e.g. isoprenaline, which stimulates β-adrenergic receptors) or by preventing the breakdown of cAMP by phosphodiesterase (e.g. theophylline). The mode of action of sodium cromoglycate in preventing histamine release from mast cells is not clear, but may involve inhibition of the initial allergen-induced calcium influx, and may also affect mediator release from other cells.

IgE binding on cells other than mast cells

receptors	cells		comment
FcεRIIa	B cells		expressed in normal B cells functions as cell growth and adhesion molecule
FcεRIIb	T cells	B cells	macrophages	induced by IL-4 on normal cells expressed routinely by some T and B cells, monocytes and eosinophils, Langerhans' cells and follicular dendritic cells, and may also express FcεRI
	Langerhans' cells	follicular dendritic cells	

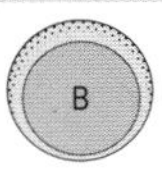

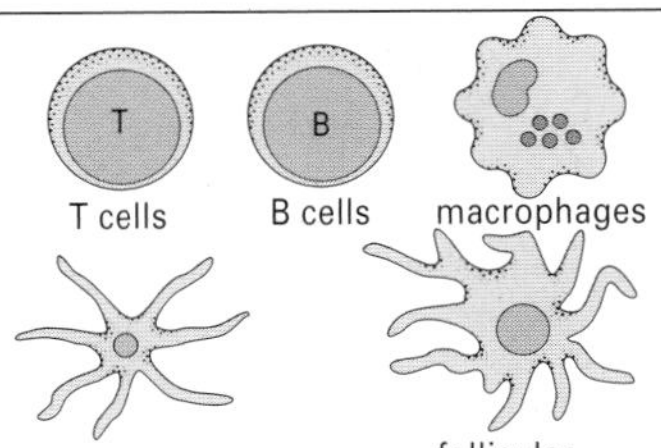

Fig. 22.13 Compared to the FcεRI on mast cells and basophils, receptors on other cells (FcεRII) have a much lower affinity for IgE. FcεRIIa is constitutively expressed on normal B cells whereas FcεRIIb expression is induced on various cell types by IL-4. T cells, B cells, monocytes and macrophages express FcεRIIb, as do Langerhans' cells in skin. Langerhans' cells, macrophages, platelets and eosinophils may also express the high affinity FcεRI.

Mast-cell activation and physiological effects of mast-cell derived mediators

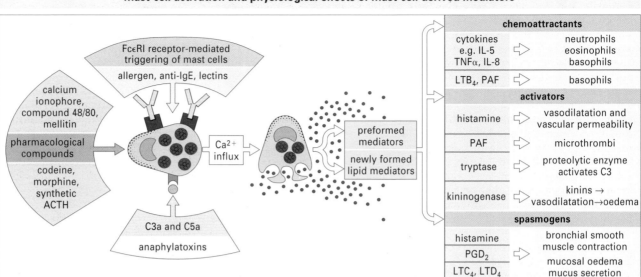

Fig. 22.14 Mast-cell activation can be produced by immunological stimuli which cross-link Fcε receptors, and by other agents such as anaphylatoxins and secretagogues (e.g. compound 48/80, mellitin, calcium ionophore, A23187). Some other drugs such as codeine, morphine and synthetic ACTH have also been found to act on mast cells directly. The common feature in each case is the influx of Ca^{2+} ions into the mast cell, which is crucial for degranulation. Microtubule formation and movement of the granules to the cell membrane lead to fusion of the granule with the plasma membrane, and the release of preformed granule-associated mediators. Changes in the plasma membrane, associated with activation of phospholipase A_2, release arachidonic acid; this can then be metabolized by lipoxygenase or cyclooxygenase enzymes, depending on the mast-cell type. These newly formed lipid metabolites include prostaglandins (PGD_2) and thromboxanes, produced by the cyclooxygenase pathway, and leukotrienes (LTC_4, LTD_4 and chemotactic LTB_4), produced by the lipoxygenase pathway. Both the preformed, granule-associated lipid mediators and the newly formed lipid mediators have three main areas of action.

Chemotactic agents A variety of cells are attracted to the site of mast-cell activation, in particular eosinophils, neutrophils and mononuclear cells including lymphocytes. In addition, recent evidence suggests that certain of the preformed cytokines released from degranulating mast cells are also chemotactic for inflammatory cells.

Inflammatory activators can cause vasodilatation, oedema and, via platelet activating factor (PAF), microthrombi, leading to local tissue damage. Tryptase, the major neutral protease of human lung mast cells, can activate C3 directly; this function is inhibited by heparin. Kininogenases are also released and these affect small blood vessels by generating kinins from kininogens, again leading to inflammation.

Spasmogens have a direct effect on bronchial smooth muscle, but could also increase mucus secretion leading to bronchial plugging.

■ CUTANEOUS REACTIONS

The skin prick test – It is remarkable that the skin prick test, the most simple diagnostic test for allergy, tells us so much about the immunopathology of allergic reactions. The classical skin test in atopy is the immediate wheal-and-flare reaction, in which allergen introduced into the skin leads to the release of preformed mediators; these cause increased vascular permeability, local oedema and itching (*Fig. 22.15*). A positive skin test usually correlates with a positive radioallergosorbent test (RAST) for allergen-specific IgE in serum, and a positive provocation test of the relevant area (challenge of the nasal or bronchial mucosa, for example, with the allergen). The late response following skin testing is not often seen because it is rarely looked for. When it does occur it has the appearance of a lump in the skin which is painful rather than itchy.

The fact that patients with a variety of atopic disorders show the classical immediate wheal-and-flare response following skin prick tests demonstrates that IgE is bound to skin mast cells, even though their allergic symptoms may be in the nose or bronchi. However, there is a small group of patients

Immediate and late skin reactions

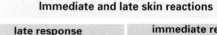
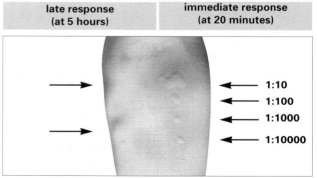

late response (at 5 hours)	immediate response (at 20 minutes)

1:10
1:100
1:1000
1:10000

Fig. 22.15 Skin tests were performed 5 hours (**left**) and 20 minutes (**right**) before the photograph was taken. The tests on the right show the typical endpoint result of an immediate (Type 1) wheal-and-flare reaction. The late phase skin reaction (**left**) can be clearly seen at 5 hours, especially where a large immediate response has preceded it. Figures for dilution of the allergen extract are given.

who give a clear-cut history of, for example, allergic rhinitis, but in whom skin tests and RAST are negative. Despite the absence of IgE in both skin and serum, these patients do make a local mucosal IgE response. This can be shown by a positive nasal provocation test, and by the detection of the relevant specific IgE in the nasal secretion using RAST. If the lymphocytes of these patients are stimulated with allergen *in vitro*, lymphocyte transformation and cytokine production result, indicating that their T cells respond to the allergen. This does not necessarily imply that delayed hypersensitivity is contributing directly to the disease process. However, it does indicate that allergen-specific TH2 cells are present in these patients and may be providing 'help' in the IgE response.

The skin patch test – The skin patch test involves the application of allergen to lightly abraded, 'normal' skin. For example, patients with atopic eczema (*Fig. 22.16*) who have IgE antibodies to the house dust mite give positive patch test results for mite allergen (*Fig. 22.17*). It is interesting that a proportion of patients with allergic rhinitis due to house dust mite (*Fig. 22.18*), also show house dust mite-positive patch tests with basophil infiltration, suggesting that the infiltration is not specific to atopic eczema.

When the late-phase skin reaction was originally described, it was thought that the mechanism might have been a Type III hypersensitivity reaction (immune-complex mediated) due to a precipitating IgG antibody, as occurs in bronchopulmonary aspergillosis. However, precipitating antibodies have not generally been found with this late reaction and further research has confirmed that the late-phase response is IgE-dependent.

■ BRONCHIAL REACTIONS

Bronchial reactions to allergens also show both an immediate and late-phase response (*Fig. 22.19*). Sodium cromoglycate is a very effective treatment in allergic asthma and prevents both the immediate and late phase responses that follow bronchial provocation with allergen. This implies that the development of a late reaction in the lung depends upon an initial allergen–IgE–mast cell interaction; preventing degranulation with sodium cromoglycate prevents all subsequent events. If the patients are pretreated with corticosteroids or prostaglandin synthetase inhibitors, late reactions alone are abolished, leaving the immediate response quite unchanged. This indicates a role for mast-cell-derived arachidonic acid metabolites, for example prostaglandins and leukotrienes, in the late response (see *Fig. 22.14*).

Most asthmatics with reversible airway obstruction benefit from treatment with inhaled corticosteroids, which reduces the inflammatory cell infiltration seen in the bronchi, especially associated with the late phase reaction (*Fig. 22.20*).

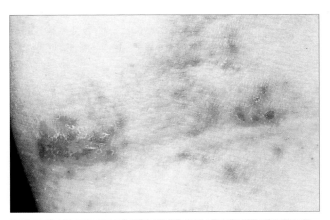

Fig. 22.16 The appearance of atopic aczema on the hand of a child allergic to rice and eggs.

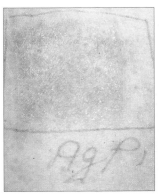
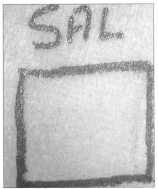

Fig. 22.17 Skin patch tests in a patient with atopic eczema using purified house dust mite (Dermatophagoides pteronyssinus) antigen. Left: The surface keratin of an unaffected area is removed by gentle abrasion and the extract is placed on the skin and occluded for 48 hours, at which time the site is examined. The lesions are macroscopically eczematous and microscopically contain infiltrates of eosinophils and basophils. **Right**: A saline control. (Courtesy of Dr E. B. Mitchell.)

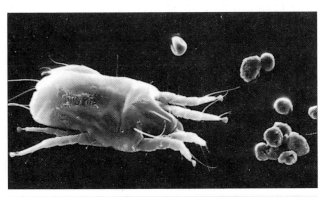

Fig. 22.18 House dust mite – a major allergen. Electronmicrograph showing a house dust mite, Dermatophagoides pteronyssinus, and faecal pellets (bottom right) which represent the major source of allergen. Biconcave pollen grains (top right) are shown for size comparison. It is the faecal pellets rather than the mite itself becomes airborne and reaches the lungs. (Courtesy of Dr R. Tovey.)

Immediate and late-phase bronchial reactions

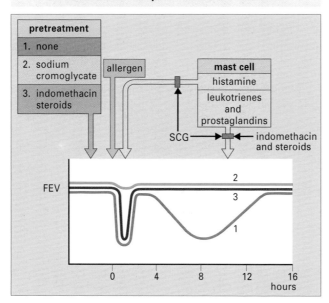

Fig. 22.19 This graph plots the forced expiratory volume (FEV), a measure of lung function, in three groups of individuals prior to and several hours after bronchial provocation with allergen. In the control (group 1) there is a biphasic (initial and late) bronchial constriction. The initial reaction lasts for 1 hour and is followed by a late-phase reaction (LPR) lasting several hours. Histamine released from degranulating mast cells is thought to be the major mediator of the immediate reaction in man. The other two groups are pretreated differently. Pretreatment with sodium cromoglycate, SCG (group 2) inhibits mast-cell degranulation and is seen to prevent both early and late-phase reactions. Pretreatment with indomethacin or corticosteroids, which block arachidonic acid metabolic pathways, inhibits the late-phase reaction but not the immediate reaction (group 3). This implicates leukotrienes and prostaglandins in the development of the late-phase reaction. Although prolonged steroid treatment can blunt the immediate reaction, it abolishes the LPR. The first line of treatment for asthmatics is often inhaled corticosteroids, reducing the inflammatory cell infiltration. This suggests that the LPR, and its sequelae, are of major clinical importance in chronic asthma.

The inflammatory response in asthmatic bronchi

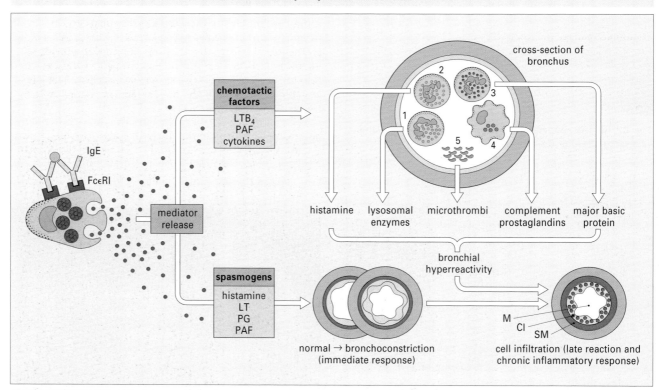

Fig. 22.20 Mast cell mediators include chemotactic and spasmogenic factors. Spasmogens produce the immediate response of bronchoconstriction and lead to increased small-vessel permeability, oedema and cell emigration. Chemotactic factors, and cytokines such as GM–CSF, IL-5 and TNFα, lead to active accumulation of neutrophils (1), basophils (2), eosinophils (3), macrophages (4) and platelets (5). Production of a further set of inflammatory molecules by these infiltrating cells leads to the late-phase response and a chronic inflammatory response typical of asthma. Many different factors, including hypersecretion of mucus (M), smooth muscle (SM) hypertrophy and cellular infiltration (CI), with associated bronchial hyperreactivity, combine to produce subacute or chronic asthma. Also, treatment with corticosteroids reduces cell infiltration and the production of nitric oxide (NO).

Bronchoalveolar mast cells are important in the asthma response

Asthmatics have increased numbers of mast cells in the lumen of the bronchi. These cells are uniquely situated to react with inhaled allergen and initiate IgE-mediated reactions in the lung. Studies on these cells, isolated by bronchoalveolar lavage (BAL), show that they have a low degranulation threshold (indicated by high levels of mediators in the BAL fluid). These cells are likely to be the major therapeutic target for the anti-asthmatic drug sodium cromoglycate, and perhaps other drugs such as cyclosporine. They are easily inhibited compared with those obtained from the lung parenchyma (*Fig. 22.19*). In addition, recent evidence shows that the predominant T-cell subtype in asthmatic BAL is TH2, reflecting the allergic IgE-linked nature of the immune response in the asthmatic lung. There is also a significant cellular infiltration of the bronchial mucosa, which must contribute to the chronicity of asthma.

Other factors are involved in chronic asthma

Eosinophils – Much evidence suggests a central role for inflammatory cell infiltration during the late-phase reaction. In particular, eosinophils are found in increased numbers in BAL and in the bronchial mucosa during the late (but not the early) phase of asthmatic reactions. The IL-5 released by TH2 cells and mast cells is chemotactic for eosinophils and enhances their release of mediators and cytokines (*Fig. 22.21*). Eosinophils damage the respiratory epithelium by the release of granule-derived basic proteins (*Fig. 22.22*). This may facilitate allergen entry and the access of inflammatory mediators to afferent nerve endings, causing bronchoconstriction through axon reflex pathways. The release of neurogenic peptides such as VIP, Substance P and calcitonin gene related peptide (CGRP) increase and extend the ongoing inflammatory response, so increasing the bronchial hyperreactivity.

Bronchial hyperreactivity – Asthma is associated with hyperreactivity of the bronchi to histamine and to non-specific stimuli such as cold air and water vapour. Thus, normal subjects

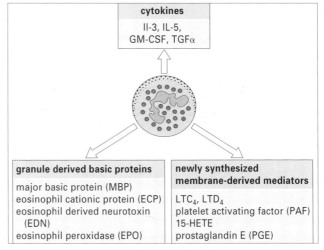

Eosinophil mediators

cytokines
Il-3, IL-5, GM-CSF, TGFα

granule derived basic proteins	newly synthesized membrane-derived mediators
major basic protein (MBP) eosinophil cationic protein (ECP) eosinophil derived neurotoxin (EDN) eosinophil peroxidase (EPO)	LTC$_4$, LTD$_4$ platelet activating factor (PAF) 15-HETE prostaglandin E (PGE)

Fig. 22.21 Eosinophil degranulation may be stimulated by allergen via IgE bound to the FcεRI and FcεRII or by soluble mediators such as PAF and LTB$_4$. Eosinophils release a variety of pro-inflammatory cytokines and newly synthesized membrane-derived mediators. In addition, they also release highly cytotoxic granule-derived basic proteins that are responsible for epithelial cell damage in chronic asthma.

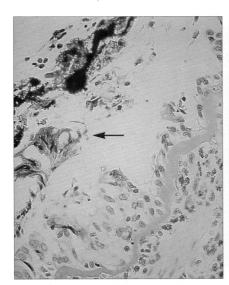
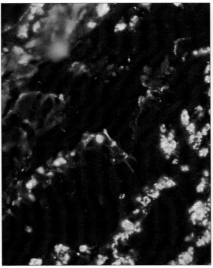
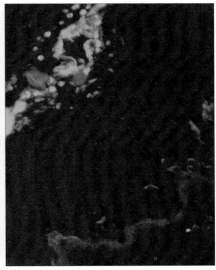

Fig. 22.22 Localization of MBP in the lung of a severe asthmatic. Left: Respiratory epithelium showing striking submucosal eosinophil infiltration and a cluster of desquamated epithelial cells in the bronchial lumen (arrowed) next to a 'stringy' deposit of soot. H&E stain. **Centre:** The same section stained for major basic protein (MBP) showing immunofluorescent localization in infiltrating eosinophils. MBP deposits are also seen on desquamated epithelial cells on the luminal surface. **Right:** A control section stained with normal rabbit serum does not stain eosinophils or bronchial tissue but does show some non-specific staining of the sooty deposit. (Courtesy of Dr G. Gleich, from *J Allergy Clin Immunol* 1982;**70**:160–69, with permission.)

become asthmatic following inhalation of 10 ng of histamine, whereas asthmatics respond to 0.5 ng or less. The idea that this hyperreactivity is a response to chronic allergen challenge is strongly supported by the data of Platts-Mills, who removed asthmatics from their home environment (house dust mite) to a clean hospital environment for up to three months. At the end of that time their sensitivity to histamine was either greatly reduced, or normal; their asthma was similarly improved.

Nitric oxide – The inducible form of nitric oxide synthase (iNOS) produces nitric oxide (NO) in many cell types in response to stimulation by cytokines. This enzyme has recently been found in high levels in the bronchial epithelium of asthmatics, but not in non-asthmatic subjects (*Fig. 22.23*).The NO produced by iNOS can be measured in the exhaled air of untreated asthmatics; it is reduced by treatment with inhaled corticosteroids (*Fig. 22.23*), which are known to downregulate the expression both of cytokines and iNOS. These results suggest that NO may play a role in the pathogenesis of asthma, and that measurement of exhaled NO may be useful clinically in the diagnosis, monitoring and management of the disease.

Nitric oxide in asthma

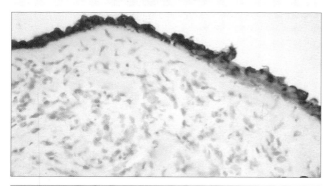

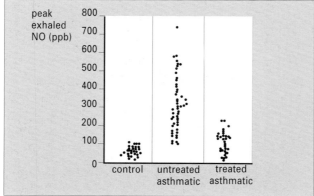

Fig. 22.23 Above: shows a biopsy from an asthmatic subject. Strong staining for iNOS is seen in the bronchial epithelium which shows signs of damage in some areas. **Below:** in untreated mild asthmatics NO is frequently elevated in exhaled air compared to controls. In corticosteroid treated asthmatics, exhaled NO levels are similar to controls.

FACTORS INVOLVED IN THE DEVELOPMENT OF ALLERGY

As well as the known genetic predisposition for developing allergy, it is now appreciated that other factors may also be important, and these are discussed below.

T-cell deficiency is associated with atopy

There is substantial evidence for a role for T cells in both the development and suppression of IgE responses (see *Figs. 22.5* and *22.6*). This led to the earlier suggestion that a defect in T cells, and in particular 'suppressor T cells', could be involved in the aetiology of atopy. Indeed it has been shown that there are reduced numbers of CD8+ suppressor T cells in patients with eczema (*Fig. 22.24*). In addition, T-cell mitogen responses are reduced in severe atopics (those with eczema). These reduced T-cell responses *in vitro* correlate with reduced cell-mediated immunity, which may be reflected *in vivo* as depressed delayed hypersensitivity skin responses.

Until recently it was not clear whether this T-cell deficiency was a cause or a consequence of atopic disease. However, there is now some evidence for a causal relationship between T-cell deficiency and atopy, but only in bottle-fed babies. Soothill and colleagues have shown that the incidence of eczema in children is reduced if they are breast fed, and work by other groups has shown a relationship between bottle feeding with cows' milk in infancy, reduced numbers of some subsets of regulatory T cells, and increased IgE levels (*Fig. 22.25*). However, it is not certain whether the bottle feeding itself affects T-cell numbers. Clearly, other environmental factors are also important in the expression of allergic disorders.

T cells in atopy

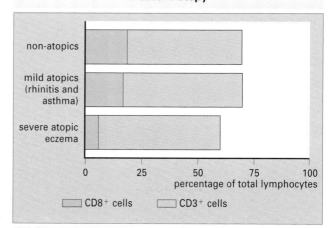

Fig. 22.24 Patients with severe atopic eczema, but not patients with rhinitis or asthma, have a reduced number of CD3+ T cells, which is almost wholly accounted for by fewer CD8+-staining T cells.These cells are thought to contain a 'suppressor' population and decreased numbers of these cells in the circulation are associated with the often grossly elevated serum IgE levels seen in patients with atopic eczema.

The exact relationship between differences in suppressor T-cell numbers observed in earlier studies, and the importance of TH1/TH2 balance in immune responses that are observed now, remains to be elucidated.

Environmental pollutants act to increase antigen-specific IgE

Environmental pollutants such as sulphur dioxide, nitrogen oxides, diesel exhaust particulates and fly ash may increase mucosal permeability and enhance allergen entry and IgE responsiveness. Diesel exhaust particulates (DEP) can act as a powerful adjuvant for IgE production (*Fig. 22.26*). They are less than 1 μm in diameter, are buoyant in the atmosphere of polluted districts and are inhaled. The concentration in urban air is approximately 2 μg/m^3, can reach 30 μg/m^3 on main roads , and during times of peak traffic can go as high as 500 μg/m^3. DEP given intranasally with antigen produces a marked increase in antigen-specific IgE. This adjuvant effect can be seen with low-dose antigen exposure, of the order that might be experienced in the environment.

The increased incidence of allergic rhinitis and asthma in the last three decades parallels an increase in air pollution and diesel exhaust. Thus, environmental pollutants may be facilitating IgE responses, thereby contributing to the increase in allergic disease. Note that family size also has some bearing in the incidence of atopy, as firstborn children are more likely to be affected.

The effect of smoking seems to be dose-dependent, giving an enhancement of IgE levels with low-level cigarette consumption, and suppression at high levels. Active smokers show a substantial reduction in the immune response to inhaled antigens; passive smoking may increase the risk of asthma in children.

■ THE CONCEPT OF ALLERGIC BREAKTHROUGH

It is evident that a number of factors must contribute to allergy. The hypothesis of allergic breakthrough suggests that the clinical symptoms of allergy are seen only when an arbitrary level of immunological activity is exceeded (*Fig. 22.27*). This will depend on a number of conditions, such as the level of exposure to allergen, genetic predisposition, the tendency to make IgE, and other factors such as the presence of upper respiratory tract viral infections, the relative contribution of TH1/TH2 cells to the immune response and transient IgA deficiency. The increasing prevalence of allergy is associated with environmental pollution, a further factor that must be taken into account in allergic breakthrough.

Effect of bottle feeding on T cells and IgE levels

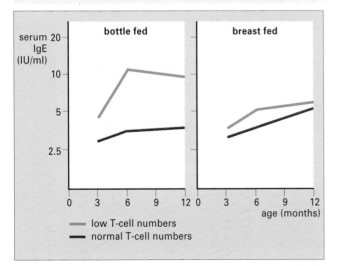

Effect of pollutants on IgE responses

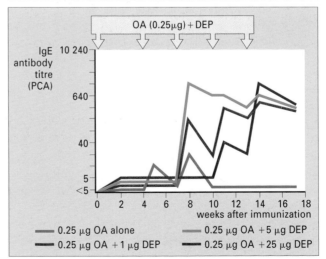

Fig. 22.25 Effect of bottle feeding on T cells and IgE. In a survey of infants with low numbers of circulating T cells, those who had been bottle fed with cows' milk showed higher serum IgE levels than those who had been breast fed. The latter children had similar IgE levels to those infants with normal levels of T cells who were breast or bottle fed. These data show that the type of feeding and T cell number affect IgE levels, and suggest that a T-cell defect in association with an environmental factor (feeding) may influence the development of the atopic state.

Fig. 22.26 The effects of pollutants, namely diesel exhaust particulates (DEP), on IgE anti-ovalbumin responses in mice. When mice are immunized intranasally with ovalbumin (OA), a small peak of IgE antibody is seen at weeks 5 and 8, and none thereafter. If DEPs are added to the OA, there is a dose-related increase in IgE persisting after immunization ceases. Thus, DEPs are good adjuvants for IgE production and may partially explain the increase in allergy in recent years. (Courtesy of Dr S. Takafuji, from *J Allergy Clin Immunol* 1987:**79**;639–45, with permission.)

HYPOSENSITIZATION

Hyposensitization therapy involves the injection of increasing doses of allergen. Although clinical benefit is often obtained, the exact mechanism(s) by which it occurs is unknown. Following treatment there is an increase in serum levels of allergen-specific IgG and suppressor T-cell activity, while specific IgE levels tend to fall (*Fig. 22.28*), although in most cases there is no clear-cut correlation between any of these findings and clinical improvement in the patient. However, it has been shown that allergen-specific suppressor T cells develop in successfully hyposensitized ragweed allergic patients; this may have a number of effects, such as suppression of the IgE response and of T-cell-dependent mast-cell recruitment. Again, this could also be explained as a shift from TH2 to TH1 dominance in the immune response to the allergen. In the case of people allergic to bee venom where IgG is produced by hyposensitization therapy, there is a good correlation between circulating levels of venom-specific IgG blocking antibodies and clinical protection from anaphylaxis.

Allergen structure can be modified to induce tolerance

Recent studies on the structure of allergens have shown that their T-cell epitopes can be defined by *in vitro* lymphocyte proliferation. Immunotherapy with these peptides has induced T cell tolerance and may be of use clinically. Another approach to controlling IgE responses in mice is to use glutaraldehyde-modified allergens, which shift the balance of T-cell responses from TH2 to TH1, and thereby change the antibody response from IgE to IgG2a (see *Fig. 22.6*). In both situations, IL-4 production decreases. The potential for these types of modified allergen specific immunotherapy remains to be evaluated in man. Similar modified allergens – so called allergoids – were used therapeutically in the 1950s and did show some clinical effect.

Tolerance induction suppresses IgE responses without deleting IgE B cells

There is now good evidence in experimental animals for the existence of very long-lived suppressor T cells and radiation-resistant (non-dividing) IgE memory B cells. For example, in normal rats and mice, repeated inhalation of antigen (ovalbumin) results in tolerance, with suppression of IgE responses.

Holt's group have shown that the IgE memory and IgE plasma cells of high-IgE-responder animals are very resistant to the effects of ovalbumin-specific suppressor T cells, and that their IgE responses to ovalbumin are unaffected. However, administration of such suppressor T cells to unimmunized high-responder animals prevents them mounting IgE responses to ovalbumin. These results are clearly relevant, since allergic humans are clinically diagnosed after sensitization; this may explain the relative lack of success of hyposensitization therapy in many subjects. A better understanding of the mechanism(s) by which these long-lived Bε cells are maintained, for example by continued presentation of allergen on dendritic cells or by the idiotypic network system, will undoubtedly be important in the future for therapy.

Interestingly, Holt's group has also shown that inhalation of noxious substances (nitrous oxide or histamine) before inhalation of antigen can induce significant IgE responses in low responder animals, supporting a role for environmental factors in promoting IgE responses, as discussed above.

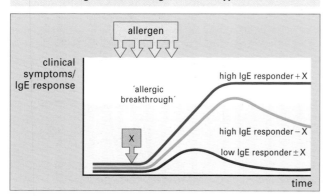

Allergic breakthrough in man: hypothesis

Fig. 22.27 On exposure to allergen an IgE response may develop transiently in low IgE responders before being controlled by suppressor T-cell activity and/or a change in the TH1/TH2 balance of the immune response. In high responders, the IgE response to allergen is much greater than in low responders, but the overt expression of clinical symptoms is only seen at the point of allergic breakthrough. This may depend on the presence of concomitant factors (X) such as viral infections of the upper respiratory tract, transient IgA deficiency or decreased suppressor T-cell activity, which augment IgE responses and the development of clinical symptoms. In the absence of factor X, the high responder subject may not show clinical symptoms after a short period of allergen exposure alone, but may be induced to express clinical symptoms of allergy by further exposure to allergen and factor X.

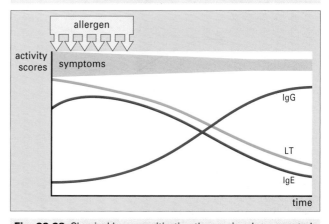

Effects of hyposensitization therapy

Fig. 22.28 Classical hyposensitization therapy involves repeated injection of increasing doses of allergen. There is an increase in antigen-specific IgG accompanied by a fall in antigen-specific IgE. This fall was thought to be due to an increase in activity of suppressor T cells, which is reflected in reduced antigen-induced lymphocyte transformation (LT) *in vitro*. It may also be due to a shift in the TH1/TH2 balance of the immune response to allergen.

THE BENEFICIAL ROLE OF IgE

With so many disadvantages inherent in the IgE response to innocuous environmental allergens, the question arises: why has IgE antibody evolved?

It has long been considered that IgE has evolved to play a major role in the defence against parasitic worms; the mechanisms involved are illustrated in Figure 18.9. Parasitic worms that reside in the gut release soluble allergens that stimulate phenomenal IgE (and IgG) responses in gut-associated lymphoid tissues (GALT). Mast cells maturing in the GALT are sensitized with IgE and migrate to the gut mucosa, where they are triggered to degranulate following contact with worm antigen, releasing mediators that increase vascular permeability and attract inflammatory cells, including eosinophils, to the area. IgE from the lymph node also sensitizes the worm to attack by eosinophils, which bear Fc receptors for IgE. Complement and worm-specific IgG also enter the site, due to increased vascular permeability caused by mediators such as histamine. There is also an associated increase in mucus production by goblet cells in the mucosa. All of these mechanisms lead to worm damage and expulsion.

Since approximately one-third of the world's population has parasitic worm infections, this may be the evolutionary pressure that initiated development of the IgE class, with allergies being an unfortunate by-product of this evolutionary step.

Critical Thinking

- TH2 cells (and the cytokines they produce) are the single most important factor in the development of allergies. Do you agree?

- If you could develop new strategies to treat allergies, what would they be?

- How would you intervene to specifically block late-phase reactions in the lung and would this have an effect on the asthmatic response?

- How would you test the relative importance of genetic compared with environmental influences on the development of allergy?

- Why has the prevalence of allergies in the population increased from 1–2% in the year 1900, to almost 30% today?

- Is allergic asthma really an example of delayed type hypersensitivity in the lung?

FURTHER READING

Beaven MA, Metzger H. Signal transduction by Fc receptors: the FcεRI case. *Immunol Today* 1993;**14**:222–26.

Bruynzeel-Koomen C, Wichen D, Toonstra J, Berren SL, Bruynzeel PLB. The presence of IgE molecules on epidermal Langerhans' cells in patients with atopic dermatitis. *Arch Dermatol Res* 1986;**278**:199–205.

Coca AF, Cooke RA. On the classification of the phenomenon of hypersensitiveness. *J Immunol* 1923;**8**:163.

Cooke RA, Vander-Veer A. Human sensitization. *J Immunol* 1916;**1**:201.

de Vries JE. Novel fundamental approaches to intervening in IgE-mediated allergic diseases. *J Invest Dermatol* 1994;**102**,141–44.

Galli SJ. New concepts about the mast cell. *N Engl J Med* 1993;**328**:257–65.

Geha RF. Regulation of IgE synthesis in humans. *J Allergy and Clin Immunol* 1992;**90**:143–50.

Gordon J. CD23: novel disease marker with a split personality. *Clin Exp Immunol* 1991;**86**:356–59.

Gordon JR, Burd PR, Galli SJ. Mast cells as a source of multifunctional cytokines. *Immunol Today* 1990;**11**:458–64.

Juto P. Elevated serum immunoglobulin E in T cell deficient infants fed cow's milk. *J Allergy Clin Immunol* 1980;**66**:402.

Kaliner MA. The late-phase reaction and its clinical implications. *Hosp Prac* 1987;**15(Oct)**:73–83.

Kharitonov SA, Yates D, Robbins RA, et al. Increased nitric oxide in exhaled air of asthmatic patients. *Lancet* 1994;**343**:133–35.

Marsh DG, Neely JD, Breazeale DR, *et al*. Linkage analysis of IL-4 and other chromosome 5q31.1 markers and total serum immunoglobulin E concentrations. *Science*, 1994;**264**:1152–56.

Miller JS, Schwartz LB. Human mast cell proteases and mast cell heterogeneity. *Curr Opin Immunol* 1989;**1**:637–42.

Montfort S, Robinson HC, Holgate ST. The bronchial epithelium as a target for inflammatory attack in asthma. *Clin Exp Immunol* 1992;**22**:511–20.

O'Hehir RE, Lamb JR. Strategies for modulating immunoglobulin E synthesis. *Clin Exp Allergy* 1992;**22**:7–10.

Prausnitz C, Küstner H. In: Gell PGH, Coombes RRA, eds. *Clinical Aspects of Immunology*. Oxford: Blackwell Scientific Publications, 1962:808–16 (Appendix).

Romagnani S. Human TH1 and TH2 subsets: Regulation of differentiation and role in protection and immunopathology. *Int Arch Allergy Immunol* 1992;**98**:279–85.

Sedgwick JD, Holt PG. Induction of IgE-secreting cells in the lymphatic drainage of the lungs of rats following passive antigen inhalation. *Int Arch Allergy Appl Immunol* 1986;**79**:329–31.

Shau-Ku H, Marsh DG. Genetics of allergy. *Annals of Allergy*, 1993;**70**:347–58.

Spry CJF, Kay AB, Gleich GJ. Eosinophils 1992. *Immunol Today* 1992;**13**:384–87.

Sutton BJ, Gould HJ. The human IgE network. *Nature* 1993;**366**:421–28.

Takafuji S, Suzukki S, Kolzumi K, *et al*. Diesel-exhaust particulates inoculated by the intranasal route have adjuvant activity for IgE production in mice. *J Allergy Clin Immunol* 1987;**79**:639–45.

Wide L, Bennich H, Johansson SGO. Diagnosis of allergy by an *in vitro* test for allergen antibodies. *Lancet* 1967;**ii**:1105.

Type II hypersensitivity reactions are caused by IgG or IgM antibodies against cell surface and extracellular matrix antigens. Antibodies to intracellular components also occur. These are not normally pathogenetic, although they may be diagnostically useful.

Transfusion reactions to erythrocytes are produced by antibodies to blood group antigens, which may occur naturally or may have been induced by previous contact with incompatible tissue or blood following transplantation, transfusion or during pregnancy.

The antibodies damage cells and tissues by activating complement, and by binding and activating effector cells carrying Fcγ receptors.

Haemolytic disease of the newborn occurs when maternal antibodies to fetal blood group antigens cross the placenta and destroy the fetal erythrocytes.

Damage to tissues may be produced by antibody to basement membranes, to intercellular adhesion molecules, or to receptors. The pathology depends on the molecules and tissues targeted by the antibodies.

Type II hypersensitivity reactions are mediated by IgG and IgM antibodies binding to specific cells or tissues. The damage caused is thus restricted to the specific cells or tissues bearing the antigens. In general, those antibodies which are directed against cell surface antigens are usually pathogenetic, while those against internal antigen usually are not so. The Type II reactions therefore differ from Type III reactions which involve antibodies directed against soluble antigens in the serum, leading to the formation of circulating antigen–antibody complexes. Damage occurs when the complexes are deposited non-specifically onto tissues and/or organs (see Chapter 24).

■ MECHANISMS OF DAMAGE

In Type II hypersensitivity, antibody directed against cell surface or tissue antigens interacts with complement and a variety of effector cells to bring about damage to the target cells (*Fig. 23.1*).

Once the antibody has attached itself to the surface of the cell or tissue, it can bind and activate complement component C1. The consequences of this activation are as follows (see Chapter 13):

- Complement fragments (C3a and C5a) generated by activation of complement attract macrophages and polymorphs to the site, and also stimulate mast cells and basophils to produce molecules that attract and activate other effector cells (see Chapter 8).
- The classical complement pathway and activation loop lead to the deposition of C3b, C3bi, and C3d on the target cell membrane.
- The classical complement pathway and lytic pathway result in the production of the C5b–9 membrane attack complex and insertion of the complex into the target cell membrane.

Effector cells – in this case macrophages, neutrophils, eosinophils, and K (killer) cells – bind either to the complexed antibody, via their Fc receptors, or to the membrane-bound C3b, C3bi and C3d, via their C3 receptors (see *Fig. 23.2* and Chapter 13). Antibody binding to Fc receptors stimulates phagocytes to produce more leukotrienes and prostaglandins; which are molecules involved in the inflammatory response

(see Chapter 14). Chemokines and chemotactic molecules, including C5a, leukotriene B₄ (LTB₄), and fibrin peptides may also activate incoming cells. The effector cells, firmly bound to the target cell and fully activated, can cause considerable damage (see Chapter 9).

The different antibody isotypes vary in their capacity to induce these reactions, depending on their ability to bind to C1q or to interact with Fc receptors on the effector cells. Complement fragments or IgG can act as opsonins bound to host tissues or to microorganisms, and phagocytes take up the opsonized particles. By enhancing the lysosomal activity of phagocytes, and potentiating their capacity to produce reactive oxygen intermediates, the opsonins not only increase the

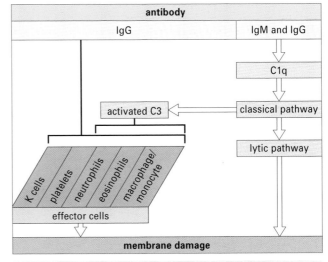

Antibody-dependent cytotoxicity

Fig. 23.1 Effector cells – K cells, platelets, neutrophils, eosinophils, and cells of the mononuclear phagocyte series – all have receptors for Fc, which they use to engage antibody bound to target tissues. Activation of complement C3 can generate complement-mediated lytic damage to target cells directly, and also allows phagocytic cells to bind to their targets via C3b, C3bi or C3d, which also activate the cells.

phagocytes' capacity to destroy pathogens but also increase their ability to produce immunopathological damage in Type II hypersensitivity reactions (*Fig. 23.3*). For example, neutrophils from the synovial fluid of a patient with rheumatoid arthritis produce more superoxide when stimulated than neutrophils from the patient's blood. This is thought to be due to neutrophil activation in the rheumatoid joint by mediators such as immune complexes and complement fragments.

The mechanisms by which the effector cells damage target cells in Type II hypersensitivity reactions reflect their normal methods of dealing with infectious pathogens (*Fig. 23.4*). Thus, unless they are resistant to phagocyte-mediated attack, most pathogens are killed inside the phagolysosome by a combination of oxygen metabolites, radicals, ions, enzymes, altered pH, and other factors that interfere with their metabolism. If the target is too large to be phagocytosed, the granule and lysosome contents are released in apposition to the sensitized target in a process referred to as exocytosis (*Fig. 23.4*). In some situations, such as the eosinophil reaction to schistosomes (see Chapter 18), exocytosis of granule contents is beneficial; but when the target is host tissue that has been sensitized by antibody, the result is damaging (*Fig. 23.5*).

Antibodies also mediate hypersensitivity by cross-linking K cells to target tissues. K cells are mainly found in the population of large granular lymphocytes, and bind antibody via their high-affinity Fc receptors. K-cell cytotoxicity has been demonstrated against a number of different cell types *in vitro*, and appears to follow the same mechanisms used by cytotoxic T cells. However, the impact of K-cell activity in Type II hypersensitivity reactions has proved difficult to assess. One reason for this is that no two target cells have the same range of susceptibilities to a given effector cell. This susceptibility depends on the amount of antigen expressed on the target cell's surface, and on the inherent ability of different target cells to sustain damage. For example, an erythrocyte may be lysed by a single active C5 convertase site, whereas it takes many such sites to destroy most nucleated cells.

The remainder of this chapter examines some of the instances where type II hypersensitivity reactions are thought to be of prime importance in causing target cell destruction or immunopathological damage.

■ REACTIONS AGAINST BLOOD CELLS AND PLATELETS

Some of the most clear-cut examples of Type II reactions are seen in the responses to erythrocytes. Important examples are:
- Incompatible blood transfusions, where the recipient becomes sensitized to antigens on the surface of the donor's erythrocytes.
- Haemolytic disease of the newborn, where a pregnant woman has become sensitized to the fetal erythrocytes.
- Autoimmune haemolytic anaemias, where the patient becomes sensitized to his own erythrocytes.

Reactions to platelets can cause thrombocytopenia and reactions to neutrophils and lymphocytes have been associated with systemic lupus erythematosus.

Neutrophil activation

neutrophil function	activator					
	IgG	C3	IgG + C3	C5a	C5b67	IgA
adherence	+	+	+ + +	+	−	+
oxygen metabolism	+	±	+ + + +	+ + +	+ +	+
lysosomal enzyme release	+	+	+ + + +	+ + +	+ +	+
chemotaxis	+	−	+	+ + +	+ +	?
phagocytosis	+	±	+ + + +	−	−	?

Fig. 23.3 Neutrophils are activated by complexed antibodies (IgG or IgA) and activated complement components. Each mediator has a particular spectrum of activity. Note how activated C3 (including C3b, C3bi and C3d, depending on the maturity of the cells involved) and activation via IgG potentiate each other. Together, they present a particularly powerful signal to the cells.

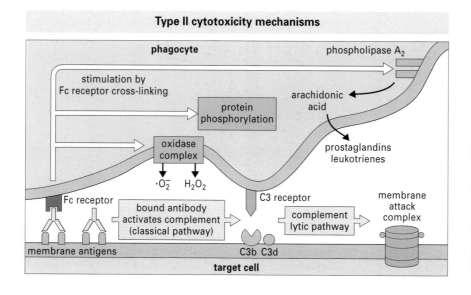

Type II cytotoxicity mechanisms

Fig. 23.2 Antibody bound to membrane antigens on target cells opsonizes them for phagocytes. Cross-linking of the Fc receptors in the phagocyte activates a membrane oxidase complex to secrete oxygen radicals; it causes increased protein phosphorylation and hence cellular activation; and also causes increased arachidonic acid release from membrane phospholipids (effected by phospholipase A_2). Immune complexes induce complement C3b deposition, which can also interact with receptors on phagocytes. Activation of the lytic pathway causes the assembly of the membrane attack complex (MAC) by components C5–C9.

Transfusion reactions occur when a recipient has antibodies that react against donor erythrocytes

More than 20 blood group systems, generating over 200 genetic variants of erythrocyte antigens, have been identified in man. A blood group system consists of a gene locus that specifies an antigen on the surface of blood cells (usually, but not always, erythrocytes). Within each system there may be two or more phenotypes. In the ABO system, for example, there are four phenotypes (A, B, AB and O), and thus four possible blood groups. An individual with a particular blood group can recognize erythrocytes carrying allogeneic (non-self) blood group antigens, and will produce antibodies against them. However, for some blood group antigens such antibodies can also be produced 'naturally', i.e. without prior sensitization by foreign erythrocytes (see below). Transfusion of allogeneic erythrocytes into an individual who already has antibodies against them may produce erythrocyte destruction and symptoms of a 'transfusion reaction'. Some blood group systems (e.g. ABO and Rhesus) are characterized by antigens that are relatively strong immunogens; such antigens are more likely to induce antibodies. When planning a blood transfusion, it is important to ensure that donor and recipient blood types are compatible with respect to these major blood groups, otherwise transfusion reactions will occur. Some major human blood groups are listed in *Figure 23.6*.

The ABO system – This blood group system is of primary importance. The epitopes concerned occur on many cell types in addition to erythrocytes and are located on the carbohydrate units of glycoproteins. The structure of these carbohydrates, and of those determining the related Lewis blood

Damage mechanisms

normal antimicrobial action

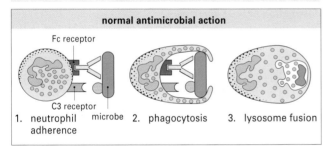

1. neutrophil adherence   2. phagocytosis   3. lysosome fusion

Type II hypersensitivity reaction

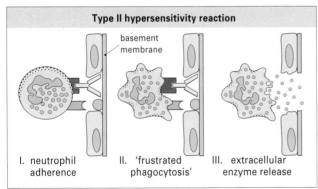

I. neutrophil adherence   II. 'frustrated phagocytosis'   III. extracellular enzyme release

Fig. 23.4 1. Neutrophil-mediated damage is a reflection of normal antibacterial action. Neutrophils engage microbes with their Fc and C3 receptors. 2. The microbe is then phagocytosed and destroyed as lysosomes fuse to form the phagolysosome (3). In Type II hypersensitivity reactions, individual host cells coated with antibody may be similarly phagocytosed, but where the target is large, for example a basement membrane (I), the neutrophils are frustrated in their attempt at phagocytosis (II). They exocytose their lysosomal contents, causing damage to cells in the vicinity (III).

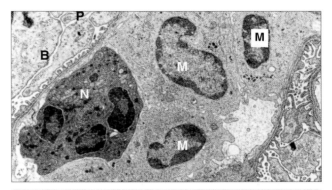

Fig. 23.5 Phagocytes attacking a basement membrane. This electronmicrograph shows a neutrophil (N) and three monocytes (M) binding to the capillary basement membrane (B) in the kidney of a rabbit containing anti-basement membrane antibody. P = podocyte. ×3500. (Courtesy of Professor G. A. Andres.)

Five major blood group systems involved in transfusion reactions

system	gene loci	antigens	phenotype frequencies	
ABO	1	A, B or O	A B AB O	42% 8% 3% 47%
Rhesus	3 closely linked loci: major antigen=RhD	C or c D or d E or e	RhD$^+$ RhD$^-$	85% 15%
Kell	1	K or k	K k	9% 91%
Duffy	1	Fy^a, Fy^b or Fy	Fy^{a}Fy^b Fy^a Fy^b Fy	46% 20% 34% 0.1%
MN	1	M or N	MM MN NN	28% 50% 22%

Fig. 23.6 Not all blood groups are equally antigenic in transfusion reactions: thus, RhD evokes a stronger reaction in an incompatible recipient than the other Rhesus antigens; and Fy^a is stronger than Fy^b. Frequencies stated are for Caucasian populations – other races have different gene frequencies.

group system, is determined by genes coding for enzymes that transfer terminal sugars to a carbohydrate backbone (*Fig. 23.7*). Most individuals develop antibodies to allogeneic specificities of the ABO system without prior sensitization by foreign erythrocytes; this sensitization occurs through contact with identical epitopes, coincidentally and routinely expressed on a wide variety of microorganisms. Antibodies to ABO antigens are therefore extremely common, making it particularly important to match donor blood to the recipient for this system.

The Rhesus system – This system is also of great importance, since it is a major cause of haemolytic disease of the newborn (HDNB). Rhesus antigens are lipid-dependent proteins and are sparsely distributed on the cell surface. They are generated by three closely linked genes, of which the Rhesus D locus is most important, due to its high immunogenicity. However, all people are tolerant to the O antigen, so that individuals are universal donors with respect to the ABO system

Minor blood group systems – MN system epitopes are expressed on the *N*-terminal glycosylated region of glycophorin A, a glycoprotein present on the erythrocyte surface. Antigenicity is determined by polymorphisms at amino acids 1 and 5. The related Ss system antigens are carried on glycophorin B. The relationship of the blood groups to erythrocyte surface proteins is listed in *Figure 23.8*. Transfusion reactions caused by the minor blood groups are relatively rare, unless repeated transfusions are given. Again, the risks are greatly reduced by accurately cross-matching the donor blood to that of the recipient.

Cross-matching – The aim of cross-matching is to ensure that the blood of a recipient does not contain antibodies that will be able to react with and destroy transfused (donor) erythrocytes. For example, antibodies to ABO system antigens cause incompatible cells to agglutinate in a clearly visible reaction. Minor blood group systems cause weaker reactions that may only be detectable by an indirect Coombs' test (see *Fig. 23.12*). If the individual is transfused with whole blood, it is also necessary to check that the donor's serum does not contain antibodies against the recipient's erythrocytes. However, transfusion of whole blood is unusual – most blood donations are separated into cellular and serum fractions, to be used individually.

Transfusion reactions involve extensive destruction of host blood cells

Transfusion of erythrocytes into a recipient who has antibodies to those cells produces an immediate reaction. The

---

ABO blood group reactives

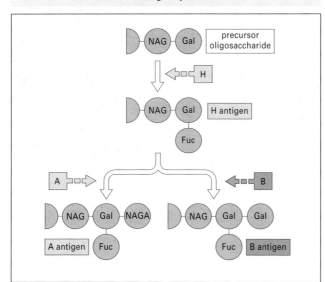

blood group (phenotype)	genotypes	antigens	antibodies to ABO in serum
A	AA, AO	A	anti-B
B	BB, BO	B	anti-A
AB	AB	A and B	none
O	OO	H	anti-A and anti-B

Fig. 23.7 The diagram shows how the ABO blood groups are constructed. The enzyme produced by the H gene attaches a fucose residue (Fuc) to the terminal galactose (Gal) of the precursor oligosaccharide. Individuals possessing the A gene now attach *N*-acetylgalactosamine (NAGA) to this galactose residue, while those with the B gene attach another galactose, producing A and B antigens, respectively. People with both genes make some of each. The table indicates the genotypes and antigens of the ABO system. Most people naturally make antibodies to the antigens they lack. (NAG = *N*-acetylglucosamine.)

Erythrocyte blood group antigens

erythrocyte surface glycoprotein	blood groups expressed	number of epitopes per cell
anion transport protein	ABO, Ii	10^6
glycophorin A	MN	10^6
glucose transporter	ABO, Ii	5×10^5
Mr 45 000–100 000	ABO } Rh	$1 \cdot 2 \times 10^5$
Mr 30 000	ABO }	
glycophorin B	N, Ss	$2 \cdot 5 \times 10^5$
glycophorins C & D	Gerbich (Ge)	10^5
DAF (delay accelerating factor)	Cromer	< 10 000
CD44 (80 kD)	Ina/Inh	3000–6000
Kell (93 kD)	Kell	3000–6000
Fg (40 kD)	Fg	12 000
lutheran (78 & 85 kD)	lutheran	1500–4000

Fig. 23.8 Note that blood group epitopes based on carbohydrate moieties, such as ABO and Ii (expressed on the precursor of the ABO polysaccharide), can appear on many different proteins, including Rh antigens. Antigens such as Rhesus and Cromer are proteins, so the epitope only appears on one type of molecule. In general, the most important blood group antigens are present at high levels on the erythrocytes, thus providing plenty of targets for complement-mediated lysis or Fc receptor-mediated clearance.

symptoms include fever, hypotension, nausea and vomiting, and pain in the back and chest. The severity of the reaction depends on the class and the amounts of antibodies involved.

Antibodies to ABO system antigens are usually IgM, and cause agglutination, complement activation and intravascular haemolysis.

Other blood groups induce IgG antibodies, which cause less agglutination than IgM. The IgG-sensitized cells are usually taken up by phagocytes in the liver and spleen, although severe reactions may cause erythrocyte destruction by complement activation. This can cause circulatory shock, and the released contents of the erythrocytes can produce acute tubular necrosis of the kidneys. These acute transfusion reactions are often seen in previously unsensitized individuals, and develop over days or weeks as antibodies to the foreign cells are produced. This can result in anaemia or jaundice.

Transfusion reactions to other components of blood may also occur, though their consequences are not usually as severe as reactions to erythrocytes.

Hyperacute graft rejection is related to the transfusion reaction

Hyperacute graft rejection occurs when a graft recipient has preformed antibodies against the graft tissue. It is only seen in tissue that is revascularized directly after transplantation, in kidney grafts for example. The most severe reactions in this type of rejection are due to the ABO group antigens that are expressed on kidney cells. The damage is produced by antibody and complement activation in the blood vessels, with consequent recruitment and activation of neutrophils and platelets. However, donors and recipients are now always cross-matched for ABO antigens, and this reaction has become extremely rare. Antibodies to other graft antigens (e.g. MHC molecules) induced by previous grafting can also produce this type of reaction.

Haemolytic disease of the newborn is due to maternal IgG antibodies which react against the child's erythrocytes *in utero*

Haemolytic disease of the newborn (HDNB) occurs when the mother has been sensitized to antigens on the infant's erythrocytes and makes IgG antibodies to these antigens.

These antibodies cross the placenta and react with the fetal erythrocytes, causing their destruction (*Figs 23.9* and *23.10*). Rhesus D (RhD) is the most commonly involved antigen.

A risk of HDNB arises when a Rh$^+$ sensitized Rh$^-$ mother carries a second Rh$^+$ infant. Sensitization of the Rh$^-$ mother to the Rh$^+$ erythrocytes usually occurs during birth of the first Rh$^+$ infant, when some fetal erythrocytes leak back across the placenta into the maternal circulation and are recognized by the maternal immune system. Thus the first incompatible child is usually unaffected, whereas subsequent children have an increasing risk of being affected, as the mother is re-sensitized with each successive pregnancy.

Reactions to other blood groups may also cause HDNB, the second most common being the Kell system K antigen. Reactions due to the latter are much less common than reactions due to RhD because of the relatively low frequency (9%) and weaker antigenicity of the K antigen.

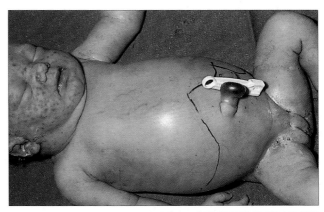

Fig. 23.10 The child is suffering from HDNB. There is considerable enlargement of the liver and spleen associated with erythrocyte destruction caused by maternal anti-erythrocyte antibody in the fetal circulation. The child had elevated bilirubin (breakdown product of haemoglobin). The facial petechial haemorrhaging was due to impaired platelet function. (Courtesy of Dr K. Sloper.) The most commonly involved antigen is RhD.

Haemolytic desease of the newborn – 1

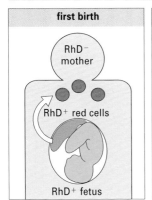
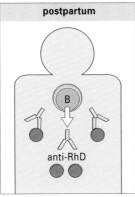
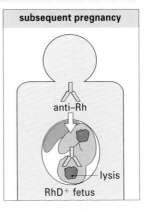

| first birth | postpartum | subsequent pregnancy |

Fig. 23.9 Erythrocytes from a Rhesus$^+$ (RhD$^+$) fetus leak into the maternal circulation usually during birth. This stimulates the production of anti-Rh antibody of the IgG class postpartum. During subsequent pregnancies, IgG antibodies are transferred across the placenta into the fetal circulation (IgM cannot cross the placenta). If the fetus is again incompatible the antibodies cause erythrocyte destruction.

The risk of HDNB due to Rhesus incompatibility is known to be reduced if the father is of a different ABO group to the mother. This observation led to the idea that these Rh⁻ mothers were destroying Rh⁺ cells more rapidly, because they were also ABO-incompatible. Consequently, fetal Rh⁺ erythrocytes would not be available to sensitize the maternal immune system to RhD antigen. This notion led to the development of Rhesus prophylaxis: pre-formed anti-RhD antibodies are given to Rh⁻ mothers immediately after delivery of Rh⁻ infants, with the aim of destroying fetal Rh⁺ erythrocytes before they can cause Rh⁻ sensitization. This practice has been successfully reduced the incidence of HDNB due to Rhesus incompatibility (*Fig. 23.11*).

Autoimmune haemolytic anaemias arise spontaneously as autoimmune diseases, or may be induced as reactions to drugs

Reactions to blood group antigens also occur spontaneously in the autoimmune haemolytic anaemias, in which patients produce antibodies to their own erythrocytes. Autoimmune haemolytic anaemia is suspected if a patient gives a positive result on an indirect antiglobulin test (*Fig. 23.12*), which identifies antibodies present on the patient's erythrocytes. These are usually antibodies directed towards erythrocyte antigens, or immune complexes adsorbed onto the erythrocytes' surface. The indirect antiglobulin test is also used to detect antibodies on red cells in mismatched transfusions, and in HDNB (see earlier). Autoimmune haemolytic anaemias can be divided into three types, depending upon whether they are due to:

- Warm-reactive autoantibodies, which react with the antigen at 37°C.
- Cold-reactive autoantibodies, which can only react with antigen at below 37°C.
- Antibodies provoked by allergic reactions to drugs.

Warm-reactive autoantibodies cause accelerated clearance of erythrocytes

Warm-reactive autoantibodies are frequently found against Rhesus system antigens, including determinants of the RhC and RhE loci as well as RhD. They differ from the antibodies responsible for transfusion reactions, in that they appear to react with different epitopes. Warm-reactive autoantibodies to other blood group antigens exist, but are relatively rare. Most of these haemolytic anaemias are of unknown cause, but

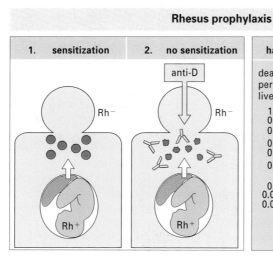
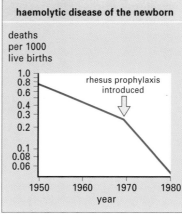

Rhesus prophylaxis

Fig. 23.11 1. Without prophylaxis, Rh⁺ erythrocytes leak into the circulation of a Rh⁻ mother and sensitize her to the Rh antigen(s) 2. If anti-Rh antibody (anti-D) is injected immediately postpartum it eliminates the Rh⁺ erythrocytes and prevents sensitization. The incidence of deaths due to HDNB fell during the period 1950–1966 with improved patient care. The decline in the disease was accelerated by the advent of Rhesus prophylaxis in 1969.

Indirect antiglobulin test

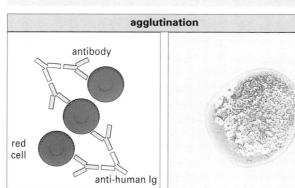
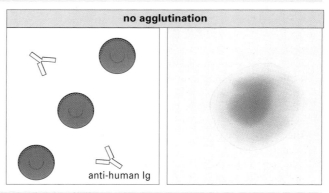

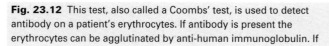

Fig. 23.12 This test, also called a Coombs' test, is used to detect antibody on a patient's erythrocytes. If antibody is present the erythrocytes can be agglutinated by anti-human immunoglobulin. If no antibody is present on the red cells, they are not agglutinated by anti-human immunoglobulin.

some are associated with other autoimmune diseases. The anaemia appears to be a result of accelerated clearance of the sensitized erythrocytes by spleen macrophages more often than being due to complement-mediated lysis.

Cold-reactive autoantibodies cause erythrocyte lysis by complement fixation

Cold-reactive autoantibodies are often present in higher titres than the warm-reactive autoantibodies. The antibodies are primarily IgM and fix complement strongly. In most cases they are specific for the Ii blood group system. The I and i epitopes are expressed on the precursor polysaccharides that produce the ABO system epitopes, and are the result of incomplete glycosylation of the core polysaccharide.

The reaction of the antibody with the erythrocytes takes place in the peripheral circulation (particularly in winter), where the temperature in the capillary loops of exposed skin may fall below 30°C. In severe cases, peripheral necrosis may occur due to aggregation and microthrombosis of small vessels of red cells caused by complement-mediated destruction in the periphery. The severity of the anaemia is therefore directly related to the complement-fixing ability of the patient's serum. (Fc-mediated removal of sensitized cells in the spleen and liver could not be involved, because these organs are too warm for the antibodies and erythrocytes to bind.)

Most cold-reactive autoimmune haemolytic anaemias occur in older people. Their cause is unknown, but it is notable that the autoantibodies produced are usually of very limited clonality, indicating that a limited number of auto-reactive clones are present. However, some cases may follow infection with *Mycoplasma pneumoniae*; and these are acute onset diseases of short duration with polyclonal autoanti-bodies. Such cases are thought to be due to cross-reacting antigens on the bacteria and the erythrocytes, producing a bypass of normal tolerance mechanisms (see Chapter 26).

Drug-induced reactions to blood components may be due either to antibodies binding to the drug adsorbed to cells, or to breakdown of self-tolerance

Drugs (or their metabolites) can provoke hypersensitivity reactions against blood cells, including erythrocytes and platelets. This can occur in three different ways (*Fig. 23.13*):
- The drug binds to the blood cells, and antibodies are produced against the drug. In this case it is necessary for both the drug and the antibody to be present to produce the reaction. This phenomenon was first recorded by Ackroyd, who noted thrombocytopenic purpura (destruction of platelets leading to purpuric rash) following administration of the drug Sedormid. Haemolytic anaemias have been reported following administration of a wide variety of drugs, including penicillin, quinine and sulphonamides. All these conditions are rare.
- Drug–antibody immune complexes are adsorbed on to the erythrocyte cell membrane. Damage occurs by complement-mediated lysis.
- The drug induces an allergic reaction, and autoantibodies are directed against the erythrocyte antigens themselves as is the case with 0.3% of patients given α-methyldopa. The antibodies produced are similar to those in patients with warm-reactive antibody. However, the condition remits shortly after the cessation of drug treatment.

Reactions against other blood cells have been associated with systemic lupus erythematosus and with thrombocytopenia

Antibodies to neutrophils and lymphocytes – Autoanti-bodies to neutrophils (*Fig. 23.14*) are truly tissue-specific; they bind neutrophils and nothing else. (Antibodies to ABO system antigens, by contrast, are highly non-tissue specific, because the same ABO antigens are found on erythrocytes, kidney, salivary gland; and many other tissues.) Antibodies to both neutrophils and lymphocytes are observed in systemic lupus erythematosus (SLE), but their contribution to the pathogenesis of the disease appears to be relatively small, possibly because these cells remove bound antibodies from their surface quite rapidly.

Drug-induced reactions to blood cells: ways in which drug treatment may induce damage

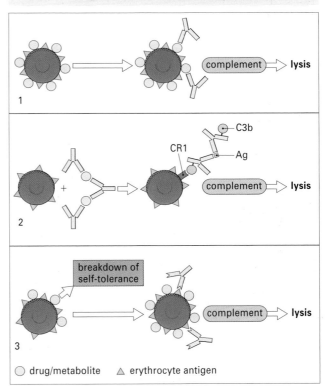

○ drug/metabolite   △ erythrocyte antigen

Fig. 23.13 Three ways that drug treatment can cause damage.
1. The drug adsorbs to cell membranes. Antibodies to the drug will bind to the cell and complement-mediated lysis will occur.
2. Immune complexes of drugs and antibody become adsorbed to the red cell. This could be mediated by an Fc receptor, but is more probably via the C3b receptor CR1. Damage occurs by complement-mediated lysis.
3. Drugs, presumably adsorbed onto cell membranes, induce a breakdown of self-tolerance, possibly by stimulating T-helper (TH) cells. This leads to formation of antibodies to other blood group antigens on the cell surface.
Note that in examples 1 and 2, the drug must be present for cell damage to occur, whereas in 3 the cells are destroyed whether they carry adsorbed drug or not.

Antibodies to platelets – Autoantibodies to platelets are seen in up to 70% of cases of idiopathic thrombocytopenic purpura, a disorder in which there is accelerated removal of platelets from the circulation, mediated primarily by splenic macrophages. The mechanism of removal is via the immune adherence receptors on these cells.

The condition most often develops after bacterial or viral infections, but may also be associated with autoimmune diseases including SLE. In SLE, antibodies to cardiolipin, which is present on platelets, can sometimes be detected. Autoantibodies to cardiolipin and other phospholipids can inhibit one aspect of blood clotting (lupus anticoagulant) and can be associated, in some cases, with venous thrombosis and recurrent abortions. Thrombocytopenia may also be induced by drugs, by similar mechanisms to those outlined in *Figure 23.13*.

■ REACTIONS AGAINST TISSUE ANTIGENS

A number of autoimmune conditions occur in which antibodies to tissue antigens cause immunopathological damage by activation of Type II hypersensitivity mechanisms. The antigens are extracellular, and may be expressed on structural proteins or on the surface of cells. Examples of such diseases – Goodpasture's syndrome, pemphigus and myasthenia gravis – are given below.

It is often possible to demonstrate autoantibodies to particular cell types, but in these cases the antigens are intracellular, and the importance of the Type II mechanisms is less well established. In these cases, recognition of autoantigen by T cells is probably more important pathologically, and the autoantibodies are of secondary importance.

Antibodies against basement membranes produce nephritis in Goodpasture's syndrome

A number of patients with nephritis are found to have antibodies to a glycoprotein of the glomerular basement membrane (see Fig. 24.3). The antibody is usually IgG and, in at least 50% of patients, it appears to fix complement. The condition usually results in severe necrosis of the glomerulus, with fibrin deposition.

The association of this type of nephritis with lung haemorrhage was originally noticed by Goodpasture (hence Goodpasture's syndrome). Although the lung symptoms do not occur in all patients, the association of lung and kidney damage is due to cross-reactive autoantigens in the two tissues.

A number of animal models for Goodpasture's syndrome have been developed. In nephrotoxic serum nephritis (Masugi glomerulonephritis) heterologous antibodies to glomerular basement membrane are injected into rats or rabbits. The injected antibody is deposited on to the basement membranes, and this is followed by further deposition of host antibodies to the injected antibody; this precipitates acute nephritis. Development of nephritis and proteinuria depends on the accumulation of neutrophils, which bind via complement-dependent and complement-independent mechanisms. Similar lesions can be induced by immunization with heterologous basement membrane (Stablay model).

Another animal model (Heymann nephritis), caused by raising autoantibodies to a protein present in the brush border of glomerular epithelial cells, resembles human membranous glomerulonephritis. In this model, the damage is mostly com-

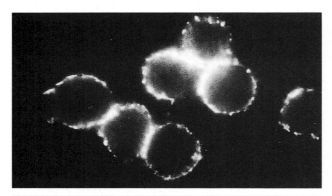

Fig. 23.14 Antibodies to neutrophils occur in SLE, as demonstrated by the immunofluorescence of these normal neutrophils. (Normal neutrophils have been exposed to serum from a patient with SLE, and then to anti-human-Fab' antibody labelled with a flourescent dye. This micrograph clearly shows the presence of anti-neutrophil antibodies). Acute transfusion reactions to neutrophils may cause pyrexia, presumably due to pyrogens released from the damaged neutrophils. This indicates that anti-neutrophil antibodies can damage neutrophils, although their role in the pathogenesis of SLE is uncertain. (Reproduced with permission from *J Clin Inv* 1979; **64**;902–12.)

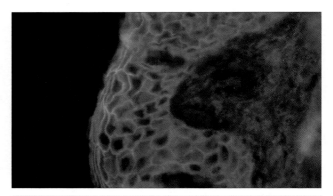

Fig 23.15 Autoantibodies in pemphigus are demonstrated on intercellular junctions between epidermal cells by immunofluorescence. The antigen forms part of the desmosome involved in cell adhesion. Immunofluorescence of human skin stained with anti-IgA. (Courtesy of Dr Mirakian and Mr P. Collins).

plement-mediated: complement depletion of the animals alleviates the condition.

Pemphigus is caused by autoantibodies to an intercellular adhesion molecule

Pemphigus is a serious blistering disease of the skin and mucous membranes. Patients have autoantibodies to one of the desmosome proteins, which form junctions between epidermal cells (*Fig 23.15*). The antibodies disrupt cellular adhesion leading to breakdown of the epidermis. The disease can be transferred to experimental animals with patients' serum, indicating that it is genuinely the antibodies which are pathogenic.

Myasthenia gravis and Lambert–Eaton syndrome are caused by antibodies that reduce the availability of acetylcholine at motor endplates

Myasthenia gravis, a condition in which there is extreme muscular weakness, is associated with antibodies to the acetylcholine receptors present on the surface of muscle membranes. The acetylcholine receptors are located at the motor endplate where the neuron contacts the muscle.

Transmission of impulses from the nerve to the muscle takes place by the release of acetylcholine from the nerve terminal and its diffusion across the gap to the muscle fibre.

It was noticed that immunization of experimental animals with purified acetylcholine receptors produced a condition of muscular weakness that closely resembled human myasthenia. This suggested a role for antibody to the acetylcholine receptor in the human disease. Analysis of the lesion in myasthenic muscles indicated that the disease was not due to an inability to synthesize acetylcholine, nor was there any problem in secreting it in response to a nerve impulse: it seemed that the released acetylcholine was less effective at triggering depolarization of the muscle (*Fig. 23.16*).

Examination of neuromuscular endplates by immunochemical techniques has demonstrated IgG and the complement proteins, C3 and C9, on the postsynaptic folds of the muscle (*Fig. 23.17*). (Further evidence for a pathogenetic role for IgG in this disease was furnished by the discovery of transient muscle weakness in babies born to myasthenic mothers. This is significant because it is known that IgG can and does

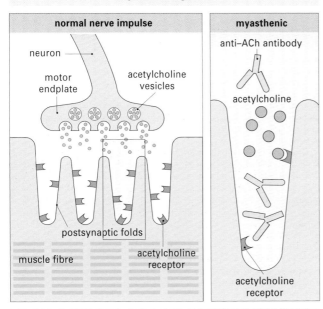

Fig. 23.16 Normally a nerve impulse passing down a neuron arrives at a motor endplate and causes the release of acetylcholine (ACh). This diffuses across the neuromuscular junction, binds ACh receptors on the muscle, and causes ion channels in the muscle membrane to open, which in turn triggers muscular contraction. In myasthenia gravis, antibodies to the receptor block binding of the ACh transmitter. The effect of the released vesicle is therefore reduced, and the muscle can become very weak. This is probably only one of the factors operating in the disease.

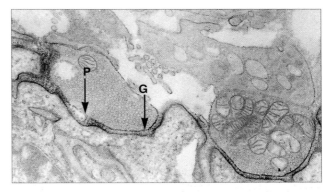
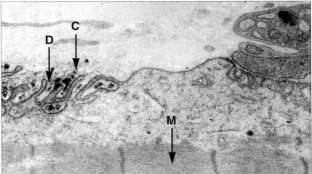

Fig. 23.17 Electronmicrographs showing IgG autoantibody (left) and complement C9 (right) localized at the motor endplate in myasthenia gravis. The upper micrograph shows IgG deposits (G) in discrete patches on the postsynaptic membrane (P). ×13 000. The lower micrograph illustrating C9 (C) shows the postsynaptic region denuded of its nerve terminal: it consists of debris and degenerating folds (D). There is a strong reaction for C9 on this debris. M = muscle fibre. ×9000. (Courtesy of Dr A. G.

cross the placenta, entering the bloodstream of the fetus.) IgG and complement are thought to act in two ways: by increasing the rate of turnover of the acetylcholine receptors, and by partial blocking of acetylcholine binding. Cellular infiltration of myasthenic endplates is rarely seen, so it is assumed that damage does not involve effector cells.

In a related condition, Lambert–Eaton syndrome, the muscular weakness is caused by defective release of acetylcholine from the neuron. If serum or IgG from patients with Lambert–Eaton syndrome is transfused into mice, the condition is also transferred, indicating the presence of autoantibody. The autoantigen is thought to be associated with an ion channel on the neuron itself, rather than the endplate. These two diseases exemplify conditions where autoantibodies to receptors block the normal function of the receptor. There are other diseases, however, where the autoantibody has an opposite effect; for example, in some forms of autoimmune thyroid disease antibodies to the TSH receptor mimic TSH (thyroid-stimulating hormone), thereby stimulating thyroid function (see Chapter 26).

Autoantibodies to tissue antigens do not necessarily produce a Type II hypersensitivity reaction

Although a great number of autoantibodies react with tissue antigens, their significance in causing tissue damage and pathology *in vivo* is not always clear. For example, although autoantibodies to pancreatic islet cells can be detected *in vitro* using sera from some diabetic patients (*Fig. 23.18*), most of the immunopathological damage in autoimmune diabetes is thought to be caused by autoreactive T cells.

The observation that many autoantibodies detected in autoimmune diseases are directed towards intracellular molecules, which are not normally accessible to antibodies, suggests that they may be formed only after tissue breakdown and release of autoantigens have occurred. Thus, although their pathogenetic significance is debatable, they often make excellent markers for particular autoimmune diseases.

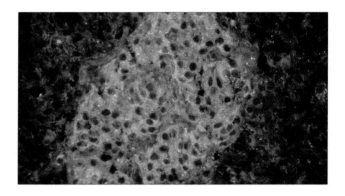

Fig. 23.18 Islet cell autoantibodies. Autoantibodies to the pancreas in diabetes mellitus may be demonstrated by immunofluorescence. The antibodies are diagnostically useful, and may contribute to the pathology. (Courtesy of Dr B. Dean.)

Critical Thinking

■ Which immune effector systems are activated during Type II hypersensitivity reactions?

■ What would happen to allogeneic erythrocytes, if they were transfused into an individual who was totally deficient in complement component C5 – on the first occasion or on a subsequent occasion?

■ Why do antibodies against cell surface antigens often produce pathological reactions, while antibodies against intracellular reactions do not?

■ Why does HDNB occur in only 1 in 20 maternal–fetal pairs that are Rhesus incompatible?

FURTHER READING

Anstee DJ. Blood group active substances of the human red blood cell. *Vox Sang* 1990;**58**:1.

Bloy C, Blanchard D, Lambin P, *et al*. Characterization of the D, C, E and G antigens of the Rh blood group system with human monoclonal antibodies. *Mol Immunol* 1988;**25**:926–30.

Burton DR. Immunoglobulin G: Functional sites. *Mol Immunol* 1985;**22**:161–206.

Druet P, Glotz D. Experimental autoimmune nephropathies: induction and regulation. *Adv Nephrol* 1984;**13**:115.

Hughes-Jones NC. Monoclonal antibodies as potential blood-typing reagents. *Immunol Today* 1987;**9**:68.

Lindstrom J. Immunobiology of myasthenia gravis, experimental autoimmune myasthenia gravis and Lambert–Eaton syndrome. *Annu Rev Immunol* 1985;**3**:109–31.

Naparstek Y, Plotz PH. The role of autoantibodies in autoimmune disease. *Annu Rev Immunol* 1993;**11**: 79–104.

Race R, Sanger R. *Blood Groups in Man*. 6th ed. Oxford: Blackwell Scientific Publications, 1975.

Watkin WM. Biochemical genetics of the blood group antigens: retrospect and prospect. *Biochem Soc Trans* 1987;**13**:614–24.

Yamamoto F–I, Clausen H, White T, Marhen J, Hakomori S-I. Molecular genetic basis of the histo-blood group ABO system. *Nature* 1990;**345**:229.

Immune complexes are formed every time antibody meets antigen and are removed by the mononuclear phagocyte system following complement activation.

Persistence of antigen from continued infection or in autoimmune disease can lead to immune-complex disease.

Immune complexes can form both in the circulation, leading to systemic disease, and at local sites such as the lung.

Complement helps to disrupt antigen–antibody bonds and keeps immune complexes soluble.

Primate erythrocytes bear a receptor for C3b and are important for transporting complement-containing immune complexes to the spleen for removal.

Complement deficiencies lead to formation of large, relatively insoluble complexes which deposit in tissues.

Charged cationic antigens have tissue-binding properties, particularly for the glomerulus, and help to localize complexes to the kidney.

Factors that tend to increase blood vessel permeability enhance the deposition of immune complexes in tissues.

Immune complexes are formed every time antibody meets antigen, and generally they are removed effectively by the mononuclear phagocyte system, but occasionally they persist and eventually deposit in a range of tissues and organs. The complement and effector-cell-mediated damage that follows is known as a Type III hypersensitivity reaction, or immune-complex disease. The sites of immune complex deposition are partly determined by the localization of the antigen in the tissues and partly by how circulating complexes become deposited.

■ TYPES OF IMMUNE-COMPLEX DISEASE

Diseases resulting from immune-complex formation can be divided broadly into three groups: those due to persistent infection, those due to autoimmune disease, and those caused by inhalation of antigenic material (*Fig. 24.1*).

Persistent infection – The combined effects of a low-grade persistent infection and a weak antibody response lead to chronic immune-complex formation, and eventual deposition of complexes in the tissues (*Fig. 24.2*). Diseases with this aetiology include leprosy, malaria, dengue haemorrhagic fever, viral hepatitis and staphylococcal infective endocarditis.

Autoimmune disease – immune-complex disease is a frequent complication of autoimmune disease, where the continued production of autoantibody to a self-antigen leads to prolonged immune complex formation. As the number of complexes in the blood increases, the systems that are responsible for the removal of complexes (mononuclear phagocyte, erythrocyte, and complement) become overloaded, and complexes are deposited in the tissues (*Fig. 24.3*). Diseases with this aetiology include rheumatoid arthritis, systemic lupus erythematosus (SLE) and polymyositis.

Inhalation of antigenic material – Immune complexes may be formed at body surfaces following exposure to extrinsic antigens. Such reactions are seen in the lungs following repeated

Three categories of immune-complex disease

cause	antigen	site of complex deposition
persistent infection	microbial antigen	infected organ(s), kidney
autoimmunity	self-antigen	kidney, joint, arteries, skin
inhaled antigen	mould, plant or animal antigen	lung

Fig. 24.1 This table indicates the source of the antigen and the organs most frequently affected.

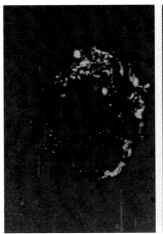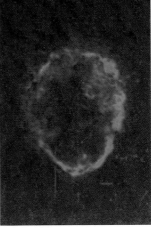

Fig. 24.2 Immunofluorescence study of immune complexes in infectious disease. These serial sections of the renal artery of a patient with chronic hepatitis B infection are stained with fluoresceinated anti-hepatitis B antigen (left) and rhodaminated anti-IgM (right). The presence of both antigen and antibody in the intima and media of the arterial wall indicates the deposition of complexes at this site. IgG and C3 deposits are also detectable with the same distribution. (Courtesy of Dr A. Nowoslawski.)

inhalation of antigenic materials from moulds, plants or animals. This is exemplified in Farmer's lung and pigeon fancier's lung, where there are circulating antibodies to actinomycete fungi (found in mouldy hay) or to pigeon antigens. Both diseases are forms of extrinsic allergic alveolitis, and only occur after repeated exposure to the antigen. (Note that the antibodies induced by these antigens are primarily IgG, rather than the IgE seen in Type I hypersensitivity reactions.) When

antigen again enters the body by inhalation, local immune complexes are formed in the alveoli leading to inflammation and fibrosis (*Fig. 24.4*). Precipitating antibodies to actinomycete antigens are found in the sera of 90% of patients with Farmer's lung. However, they are also found in some people with no disease, and are absent from some sufferers, so it seems that other factors are also involved in the disease process, including Type IV hypersensitivity reactions.

■ MECHANISMS IN TYPE III HYPERSENSITIVITY

Immune complexes are capable of triggering a wide variety of inflammatory processes:

- They interact with the complement system to generate C3a and C5a (anaphylatoxins). These complement fragments stimulate the release of vasoactive amines (including histamine and 5-hydroxytryptamine) and chemotactic factors from mast cells and basophils. C5a is also chemotactic for basophils, eosinophils and neutrophils.
- Macrophages are stimulated to release cytokines, particularly TNFα and IL-1, that are very important during inflammation.
- Complexes interact directly with basophils and platelets (via Fc receptors) to induce the release of vasoactive amines (*Fig. 24.5*).

The vasoactive amines released by platelets, basophils and mast cells cause endothelial cell retraction and thus increase vascular permeability, allowing the deposition of immune complexes on the blood vessel wall (*Fig. 24.6*). The deposited complexes continue to generate C3a and C5a.

Platelets also aggregate on the exposed collagen of the vessel basement membrane, assisted by interactions with the Fc regions of deposited immune complexes, to form microthrombi. The aggregated platelets continue to produce vasoactive amines and to stimulate the production of C3a and

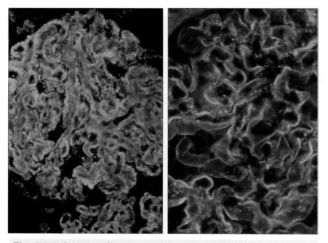

Fig. 24.3 Immunofluorescence study of immune complexes in autoimmune disease. These renal sections compare a patient with systemic lupus erythematosus (Type III hypersensitivity, left) and one with Goodpasture's syndrome (Type II hypersensitivity, right). In each case the antibody was detected with fluorescent anti-IgG. Complexes, formed in the blood and deposited in the kidney, form characteristic 'lumpy bumpy' deposits (**left**). The anti-basement membrane antibody in Goodpasture's syndrome forms an even layer on the glomerular basement membrane. (Courtesy Dr. S. Thiru.)

Extrinsic allergic alveolitis

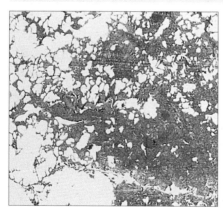

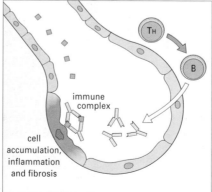

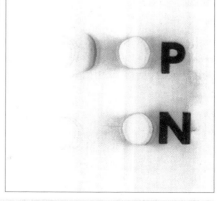

Fig. 24.4 When fungal antigen is inhaled into the lung of a sensitized individual, immune complexes are formed in the alveoli (**centre**). Complement fixation leads to cell accumulation, inflammation and fibrosis. The histological appearance of the lung

in extrinsic allergic alveolitis (**left**) shows consolidated areas due to cell accumulation. Precipitin antibody present in the serum of a patient with pigeon fancier's lung (**P; right**) are directed against the fungal antigen *Micropolyspora faeni*.

Deposition of immune complexes in blood vessel walls – I

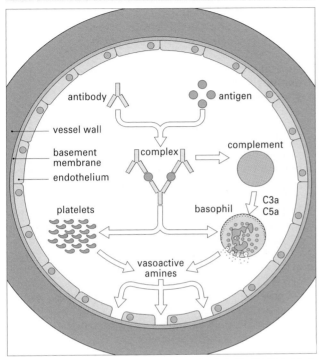

Fig. 24.5 Immune complexes act on complement to generate C3a and C5a, which in turn stimulate basophils to release vasoactive amines. The complexes also act directly on basophils and platelets (in humans) to produce vasoactive amine release. The amines released (e.g. histamine, 5-hydroxytryptamine) cause endothelial cell retraction and thus increase vascular permeability.

Deposition of immune complexes in blood vessel walls – II

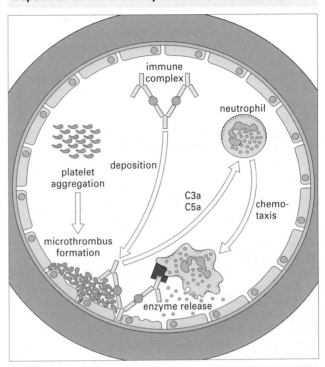

Fig. 24.6 Increased vascular permeability allows immune complexes to be deposited in the blood vessel wall. This induces platelet aggregation and complement activation. The aggregated platelets form microthrombi on the exposed collagen of the basement membrane of the endothelium. Neutrophils are attracted to the site by complement products, but cannot ingest the complexes. They therefore exocytose their lysosomal enzymes, causing further damage to the vessel wall.

C5a. (Platelets are also a rich source of growth factors – these may be involved in the cellular proliferation seen in immune-complex diseases such as glomerulonephritis and rheumatoid arthritis.)

Polymorphs are chemotactically attracted to the site by C5a. They attempt to engulf the deposited immune complexes, but are unable to do so because the complexes are bound to the vessel wall. They therefore exocytose their lysosomal enzymes onto the site of deposition (*Fig. 24.6*). If simply released into the blood or tissue fluids these lysosomal enzymes are unlikely to cause much inflammation, because they are rapidly neutralized by serum enzyme inhibitors. But if the phagocyte applies itself closely to the tissue-trapped complexes through Fc binding, then serum inhibitors are excluded and the enzymes may damage the underlying tissue.

■ EXPERIMENTAL MODELS OF IMMUNE-COMPLEX DISEASE

Experimental models are available for each of the three main types of immune-complex disease described above:

- Serum sickness, induced by injections of foreign antigen, mimics the effect of a persistent infection.
- The NZB/NZW mouse demonstrates autoimmunity.
- The Arthus reaction is an example of local damage by extrinsic antigen.

Care must be taken when interpreting animal experiments, as the erythrocytes of rodents and rabbits lack the receptor for C3b (known as CR1) which readily binds immune complexes that have fixed complement. This receptor is present on primate erythrocytes.

Serum sickness can be induced with large injections of foreign antigen

In serum sickness, circulating immune complexes deposit in the blood vessel walls and tissues, leading to increased vascular permeability and thus to inflammatory diseases such as glomerulonephritis and arthritis.

In the pre-antibiotic era, serum sickness was a complication of serum therapy, in which massive doses of antibody were given for diseases such as diphtheria. Horse anti-diphtheria serum was usually used, and some people made antibodies against the horse proteins.

Serum sickness is now commonly studied in rabbits by giving them an intravenous injection of a foreign soluble protein such as bovine serum albumin (BSA). After about one week antibodies are formed which enter the circulation and complex with antigen. Because the reaction occurs in antigen excess, the immune complexes are small (*Fig. 24.7*). These small complexes are only removed slowly by the mononuclear phagocyte system and therefore persist in the circulation. The formation of complexes is followed by an abrupt fall in total haemolytic complement; the clinical signs of serum sickness that develop are due to granular deposits of antigen–antibody and C3 forming along the glomerular basement membrane (GBM) and in small vessels elsewhere. As more antibody is formed and the reaction moves into antibody excess, the size of the complexes increases and they are cleared more efficiently, so the animals recover. Chronic disease is induced by daily administration of antigen.

Autoimmunity causes immune-complex disease in the NZB/NZW mouse

The F₁ hybrid NZB/NZW mouse produces a range of autoantibodies (including anti-erythrocyte, anti-nuclear, anti-DNA and anti-Sm) and suffers from an immune-complex disease similar in many ways to SLE in humans. An NZB/NZW mouse is born clinically normal, but within 2–3 months shows signs of haemolytic anaemia. Tests for anti-erythrocyte anti-body (the Coombs' test), anti-nuclear antibodies, lupus cells and circulating immune complexes are all positive, and there are deposits in the glomeruli and choroid plexus. The disease is much more marked in the females, who die within a few months of developing symptoms (*Fig. 24.8*).

Injection of antigen into the skin of presensitized animals produces the Arthus reaction

The Arthus reaction takes place at a local site in and around the walls of small blood vessels; it is most frequently demonstrated in the skin.

An animal is immunized repeatedly until it has appreciable levels of serum antibody (mainly IgG). Following subcutaneous or intradermal injection of the antigen a reaction develops at the injection site, sometimes with marked oedema and haemorrhage, depending on the amount of antigen injected. The reaction reaches a peak after 4–10 hours, then wanes and is usually minimal by 48 hours (*Fig. 24.9*). Immunofluorescence studies have shown that initial deposition of antigen, antibody and complement in the vessel wall is followed by neutrophil infiltration and intravascular clumping of platelets (*Fig. 24.10*). This platelet reaction can lead to vascular occlusion and necrosis in severe cases. After 24–48 hours the neutrophils are replaced by mononuclear cells and eventually some plasma cells appear.

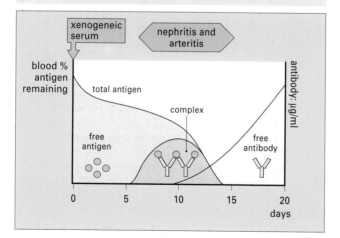

Time course of experimental serum sickness

Fig. 24.7 Following an injection of xenogeneic serum there is a lag period of approximately five days, in which only free antigen is detectable in serum. After this time, antibodies are produced to the foreign proteins and immune complexes are formed in serum; it is during this period that the symptoms of nephritis and arteritis appear. To begin with, small soluble complexes are found in antigen excess; with increasing antibody titres, larger complexes are formed which are deposited and subsequently cleared. At this stage the symptoms disappear.

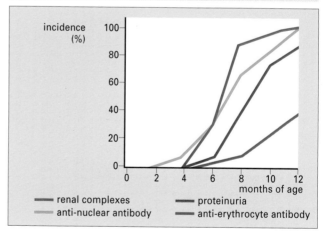

Autoimmune disease in NZB/NZW mice

Fig. 24.8 The graph shows the onset of autoimmune disease in female NZB/NZW mice with advancing age. Incidence refers to the percentage of mice with the features identified. Immune complexes were detected by immunofluorescent staining of a kidney section. Anti-nuclear antibodies were detected in serum by indirect immunofluorescence. Proteinuria reflects kidney damage. Autoantibodies to erythrocytes develop later in the disease and so are less likely to relate to kidney pathology. Onset of autoimmune disease is delayed in male mice by approximately three months.

Complement activation via either the classical or alternative pathways is essential for the Arthus reaction to develop. Without complement, neutrophils are not attracted to the site and the reaction will not proceed beyond a mild oedema.

TNFα enhances cell-mediated immune responses in various ways (see Chapter 9). Treatment with antibodies to TNF can reduce severity in the Arthus reaction. Anti-TNF has also been reported to be useful in treating rheumatoid arthritis.

The ratio of antibody to antigen is directly related to the severity of the ensuing reaction. Complexes formed in either antigen or antibody excess are much less toxic than those formed at equivalence.

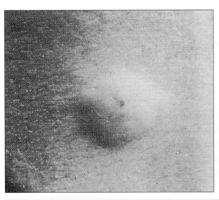
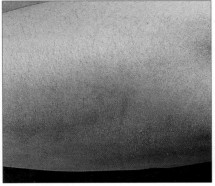
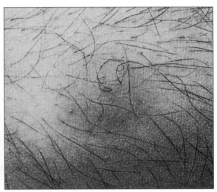

Fig. 24.9 The appearance of the three main skin test reactions. A Type I hypersensitivity reaction (**left**) produces a raised wheal, 5–7mm in diameter and with a well defined edge after about 15 minutes. A Type III hypersensitivity Arthus reaction (**centre**) produces a reaction after 5–12 hours that is larger (50mm or more), and which has a less well defined edge. A Type IV (delayed) hypersensitivity reaction shows as a red indurated lesion, about 5mm in diameter, at 24–48 hours.

The Arthus reaction

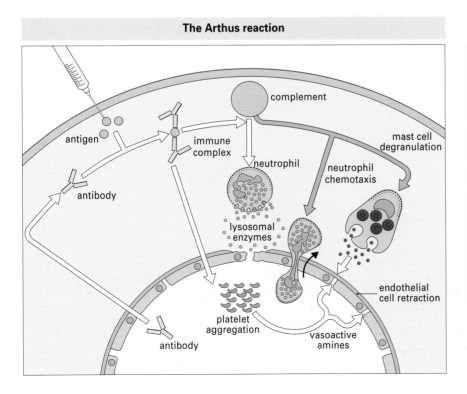

Fig. 24.10 Antigen injected intradermally combines with specific antibody from the blood to form immune complexes. The complexes activate complement and act on platelets, which release vasoactive amines. Immune complexes also induce macrophages to release TNF and IL-1 (not shown). Complement C3a and C5a fragments cause mast cell degranulation and attract neutrophils into the tissue. Mast cell products, including histamine and leukotrienes, induce increased blood flow and capillary permeability. The inflammatory reaction is potentiated by lysosomal enzymes released from the polymorphs. Furthermore, C3b deposited on the complexes opsonizes them for phagocytosis. The Arthus reaction can be seen in patients with precipitating antibodies, such as those with extrinsic allergic alveolitis associated with Farmer's lung disease.

■ PERSISTENCE OF COMPLEXES

Immune complexes are normally removed by the mononuclear phagocyte system

Immune complexes are opsonized with C3b following complement activation, and removed by the mononuclear phagocyte system, particularly in the liver and spleen. Removal is mediated by the complement C3b receptor, CR1: in primates, the bulk of CR1 in blood is found on erythrocytes. (Non-primates do not have erythrocyte CR1, and must therefore rely on platelet CR1.) There are about 700 receptors per erythrocyte, and their effectiveness is enhanced by the grouping of receptors in patches, allowing high-avidity binding to the large complexes. CR1 readily binds immune complexes that have fixed complement as has been shown by experiments with animals lacking complement (*Fig. 24.11*).

In normal primates the erythrocytes provide a buffer mechanism, binding complexes which have fixed complement and effectively removing them from the plasma. In small blood vessels 'streamline flow' allows the erythrocytes to travel in the centre of the vessel surrounded by the flowing plasma. Thus it is only the plasma that makes contact with the vessel wall (*Fig. 24.12*). Only in the sinusoids of the liver and spleen, or at sites of turbulence, do the erythrocytes make contact with the lining of the vessels.

The complexes are transported to the liver and spleen, where they are removed by fixed tissue macrophages (*Fig. 24.12*). Most of the CR1 is also removed in the process so, in situations of continuous immune-complex formation, the number of active receptors falls steadily, impairing the efficiency of immune complex handling. In patients with SLE, for example, the number of receptors may well be halved.

Complexes can also be released from erythrocytes in the circulation by the enzymatic action of Factor I, which cleaves C3b leaving a small fragment (C3dg) attached to the CR1 on the cell membrane. These soluble complexes are then removed by phagocytic cells bearing receptors for IgG Fc (*Fig. 24.13*).

Complement solubilization of immune complexes

It has been known since Heidelberger's work in the 1930s on the precipitin curve that complement delays precipitation of immune complexes, although this information was forgotten for a long time. The ability to keep immune complexes soluble is a function of the classical complement pathway. The complement components reduce the number of antigen epitopes that the antibodies can bind (i.e. they reduce the valency of the antigen) by intercalating into the lattice of the complex, resulting in smaller, soluble complexes. In primates these complement-bearing complexes are readily bound by the C3b receptor (CR1) on erythrocytes.

Complement can rapidly resolubilize precipitated complexes through the alternative pathway (*Fig. 24.14*). The solubilization appears to occur by the insertion of complement C3b and C3d fragments into the complexes.

It may be that complexes are continually being deposited in normal individuals, but are removed by solubilization. If this is the case, then the process will be inadequate in hypocomp-

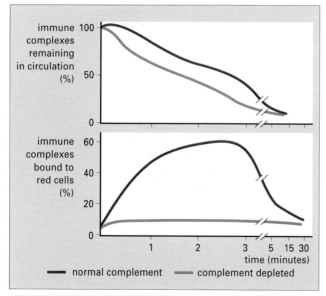

Effects of complement depletion on handling of immune complexes

Fig. 24.11 A bolus of immune complexes was infused into the circulation of a primate. In animals with a normal complement system the complexes were bound quickly by the CR1 on erythrocytes. In animals whose complement had been depleted by treatment with cobra venom factor, the erythrocytes hardly bound immune-complexes at all. Paradoxically, this results in slightly faster removal of complexes in the depleted animals, with the complexes being deposited in the tissues rather than being removed by the spleen. (Based on data from Waxman *et al.*)

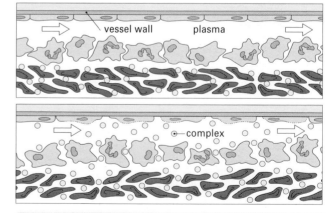

Role of erythrocytes in immune-complex disease

Fig. 24.12 Blood passes through blood vessels in a streamline flow, with erythrocytes in the centre, surrounded by white cells, and then a plasma sheath making contact with vessel walls. Immune complexes attached to erythrocytes via CR1 (**upper**) are kept away from vessel walls. Deficiencies in complement prevent attachment to erythrocytes and allow complexes to contact and bind to vessel walls (**lower**).

lementaemic patients and lead to prolonged complex deposition. Solubilization defects have indeed been observed in sera from patients with systemic immune-complex disease, but whether the defect is primary or secondary is not known.

Clearance of immune complexes in the liver

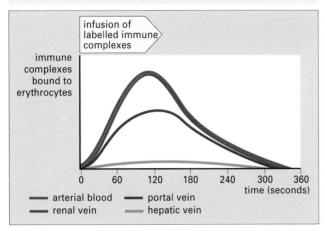

Fig. 24.13 ^{125}I-BSA/anti-BSA complexes were infused into a primate over a period of 120 seconds. Blood was sampled from renal, portal and hepatic veins, and the level of immune complexes bound to the erythrocytes was measured by radioactive counting. The levels of complexes in the renal and portal veins were similar to that in arterial blood. However, complexes were virtually absent from hepatic venous blood throughout, indicating that complexes bound to erythrocytes are removed during a single transit through the liver. (Based on data from Cornacoff *et al.*)

Solubilization of immune complexes by complement

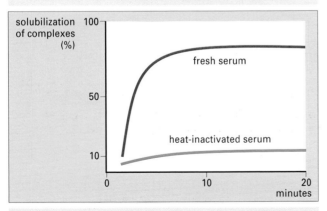

Fig. 24.14 Complement can solubilize precipitable complexes *in vitro*. Addition of fresh serum containing active complement to insoluble complexes induces solubilization over about 15 minutes at 37°C. Some of the complexes resist resolubilization. Heated serum (56°C for 30 minutes) lacks active complement and cannot resolubilize the complexes. Intercalation of complement components C3b and C3d into the complex causes their solubilization by disrupting antigen–antibody bonds. Complexes that have been artificially connected by covalent bonds cannot be solubilized by complement.

Complement deficiency impairs clearance of complexes

In patients with low levels of classical pathway components there is poor binding of immune complexes to erythrocytes. The complement deficiency may be due to depletion, caused by immune-complex disease, or could be due to a hereditary disorder, as is the case in C2 deficiency. This might be expected to result in persistent immune complexes in the circulation but in fact the reverse occurs, with the complexes disappearing rapidly from the circulation. These non-erythrocyte-bound complexes are taken up rapidly by the liver (but not the spleen) and are then released to be deposited in tissues such as skin, kidney and muscle, where they can set up inflammatory reactions (*Fig. 24.15*).

Infusion of fresh plasma, containing complement, restores the clearance patterns to normal, illustrating the importance of complement in clearance of immune complexes. Failure to localize in the spleen not only results in immune-complex disease, but may also have important implications for the development of appropriate immune responses. This is because the spleen plays a vital role in antigen processing and induction of immune responses (see Chapter 3).

The size of immune complexes affects their deposition

In general, larger immune complexes are rapidly removed by the liver within a few minutes, whereas smaller complexes circulate for longer periods (*Fig. 24.16*). This is because larger complexes are more effective at fixing complement and thus bind better to erythrocytes. Also, larger complexes are released more slowly from the erythrocytes by the action of

Immune-complex transport and removal

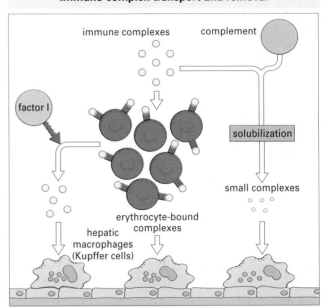

Fig. 24.15 In primates, complexes are bound by CR1 on erythrocytes and transported to the liver where they are removed by hepatic macrophages. Complexes released from erythrocytes by Factor I are taken up by cells (including macrophages) bearing receptors for Fc and complement. Complement solubilization of large complexes produces small soluble complexes which may be taken up directly by tissue macrophages.

Factor I. Anything that affects the size of complexes is therefore likely to influence clearance. (It has been suggested that a genetic defect which favours production of low-affinity antibody could well lead to formation of smaller complexes, and so to immune-complex disease.) Antibodies to self-antigens may have low affinity and recognize only a few epitopes. This results in small complexes and long clearance times, because the formation of large, cross-linked lattices is restricted.

Immunoglobulin classes affect the rate of immune complex clearance

Striking differences have been observed in the clearance of complexes with different immunoglobulin classes. IgG complexes are bound by erythrocytes and are gradually removed from the circulation, whereas IgA complexes bind poorly to erythrocytes but disappear rapidly from the circulation, with increased deposition in the kidney, lung and brain.

Phagocyte defects allow complexes to persist

Opsonized immune complexes are normally removed by the mononuclear phagocyte system, mainly in the liver and spleen. However, when large amounts of complex are present, the mononuclear phagocyte system may become overloaded, leading to a rise in the level of circulating complex and increased deposition in the glomerulus and elsewhere. Defective mononuclear phagocytes have been observed in human immune-complex disease, but this may well be the result of overload rather than a primary defect.

Carbohydrate on antibodies affects complex clearance

Carbohydrate groups on immunoglobulin molecules have been shown to be important for the efficient removal of immune complexes by phagocytic cells. Abnormalities of these carbohydrates occur in immune-complex diseases such as rheumatoid arthritis, thus aggravating the disease process. IgFc oligosaccharides lack the normally terminating galactose residue, enhancing rheumatoid-factor binding. Recently, mannan binding protein has been shown to bind a galactosyl IgG and subsequently activate complement.

■ DEPOSITION OF COMPLEXES IN TISSUES

Immune complexes may persist in the circulation for prolonged periods of time. However, simple persistence is not usually harmful in itself; the problems only start when complexes are deposited in the tissues.

Two questions are relevant to tissue deposition:
- Why are complexes deposited?
- Why do complexes show affinity for particular tissues in different diseases?

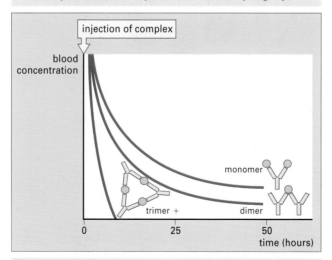

Complex clearance by the mononuclear phagocyte

Fig. 24.16 Large immune complexes are cleared most quickly because they present an IgG–Fc lattice to reticuloendothelial cells with Fc receptors, permitting higher avidity binding to these cells. They also fix complement better than small complexes.

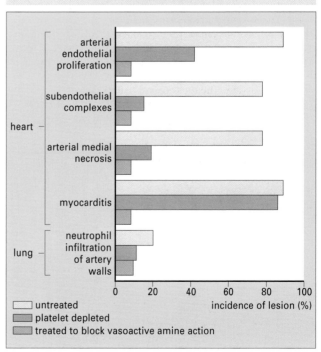

Effect of a vasoactive amine antagonist on immune-complex disease

Fig. 24.17 Serum sickness was induced in rabbits with a single injection of bovine serum albumin. The animals were either untreated, platelet depleted or treated with drugs to block vasoactive amine action. The incidence of serum sickness lesions in the heart and lung was scored. Drug treatment considerably reduced the signs of disease by lowering vascular permeability and thus minimizing immune complex deposition.

The most important trigger for tissue deposition of immune complexes is probably an increase in vascular permeability

Animal experiments have shown that inert substances such as colloidal carbon will be deposited in vessel walls following administration of vasoactive substances, such as histamine or serotonin. Circulating immune complexes are deposited in a similar way following the infusion of agents that cause liberation of mast cell vasoactive amines (including histamine). Pretreatment with antihistamines blocks this effect.

In studies of experimental immune-complex disease in rabbits, long-term administration of vasoactive amine antagonists, such as chlorpheniramine and methysergide, has been shown considerably to reduce immune complex deposition (*Fig. 24.17*). More importantly (from the point of view of disease prevention), young NZB/NZW mice treated with methysergide show less renal pathology than controls (*Fig. 24.18*).

Increases in vascular permeability can be initiated by a range of mechanisms which vary in importance, depending on the diseases and species concerned. This variability makes interpretation of some of the animal models difficult. In general, however, complement, mast cells, basophils and platelets must all be considered as potential producers of vasoactive amines.

Immune complex deposition is most likely where there is high blood pressure and turbulence

Many macromolecules deposit in the glomerular capillaries, where the blood pressure is approximately four times that of most other capillaries (*Fig. 24.19*). If the glomerular blood pressure of a rabbit is reduced by partially constricting the renal artery or by ligating the ureter, deposition is also reduced. If the glomerular blood pressure is increased by experimentally induced hypertension, immune complex deposition is also enhanced as shown by the development of serum sickness. Elsewhere, the most severe lesions also occur at sites of turbulence. They occur at turns or bifurcations of arteries,

and in vascular filters such as the choroid plexus, and the ciliary body of the eye.

Affinity of antigens for specific tissues can direct complexes to particular sites

Local high blood pressure explains the tendency for deposits to form in certain organs, but does not explain why complexes are deposited on specific organs in certain diseases. In SLE, the kidney is a particular target, whereas in rheumatoid arthritis, although circulating complexes are present, the kidney is usually spared and the joints are the principal target.

It is possible that the antigen in the complex provides the organ specificity, and a convincing model has been established to support this hypothesis. In the model, mice are given endotoxin causing cell damage and release of DNA, which then binds to healthy glomerular basement membrane. Anti-DNA is then produced by polyclonal activation of B cells, and is bound by the fixed DNA leading to local immune complex formation (*Fig. 24.20*). The production of rheumatoid factor IgM anti-IgG allows further immune complex formation to occur *in situ*. It is possible that in other diseases antigens will be identified with affinity for particular organs.

The charge of the antigen and antibody may be important in some systems. For example, positively charged antigens and antibodies are more likely to be deposited in the negatively charged glomerular basement membrane. The degree of glycosylation also affects the fate of complexes containing glycoprotein antigens because certain clearance mechanisms are activated by recognition of sugar molecules, e.g. mannan binding protein.

In certain diseases the antibodies and antigens are both produced within the target organ. The extreme of this is reached in rheumatoid arthritis, where IgG anti-IgG rheumatoid factor is produced by plasma cells within the synovium; these antibodies then combine with each other (self-association), so setting up an inflammatory reaction.

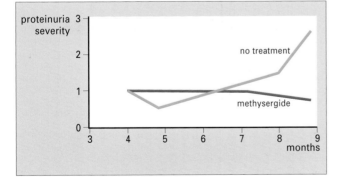

Effect of the vasoactive amine antagonist methysergide on kidney damage

Fig. 24.18 Kidney damage, assessed by proteinuria, was measured in NZB/NZW mice over five months. Untreated animals developed severe proteinuria, while methysergide-treated animals did not. Methysergide blocks formation of the vasoactive amine, 5-HT, and thus blocks a variety of inflammatory events, e.g. deposition of complexes, neutrophil infiltration of capillary walls and endothelial proliferation, all of which produce the glomerular pathology.

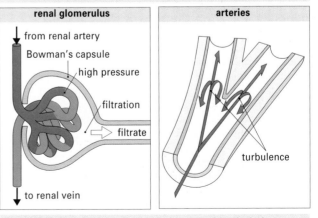

Haemodynamic factors affecting complex deposition

Fig. 24.19 Factors that affect complex deposition include filtration and high blood pressure, both of which occur in the formation of ultrafiltrate in the renal glomerulus (**left**). Turbulence at curves or bifurcations of arteries (**right**) also favours depostion of immune complexes.

Tissue binding of antigen with local immune-complex formation

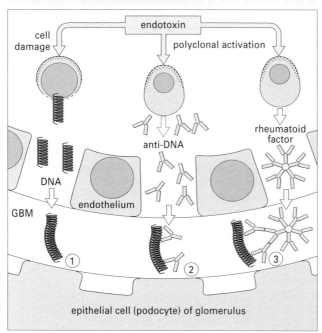

Fig. 24.20 Endotoxin, injected into mice, increases vascular permeability and induces cell damage and release of DNA. The DNA can then become deposited (1) on the collagen of the glomerular basement membrane (GBM) in the kidney. Endotoxin can also induce a polyclonal stimulation of B cells, some of which produce autoantibodies such as anti-DNA and anti-IgG – the latter are known as rheumatoid factors (RFs). Anti-DNA antibody can then bind to the deposited DNA forming a local immune complex (2). RFs have a low affinity for monomeric IgG, but bind with high avidity to the assembled DNA–anti-DNA complex (3). Thus further immune complex formation occurs *in situ*.

The site of immune-complex deposition depends partly on the size of the complex

This is exemplified in the kidney: small immune complexes can pass through the glomerular basement membrane, and end up on the epithelial side of the membrane; large complexes are unable to cross the membrane and generally accumulate between the endothelium and the basement membrane or the mesangium (*Fig. 24.21*). The size of immune complexes depends on the valency of the antigen, and on the titre and affinity of the antibody.

The class of immunoglobulin in an immune complex can also influence its deposition

There are marked age- and sex-related variations in the class and subclass of anti-DNA antibodies seen in SLE. Similarly, as NZB/NZW mice grow older there is a class switch, from predominantly IgM to IgG2a. This occurs earlier in females than in males and coincides with the onset of renal disease, indicating the importance of antibody class in the tissue deposition of complexes (*Fig. 24.22*).

Immune-complex deposition in the kidney

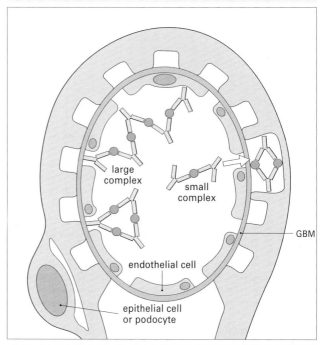

Fig. 24.21 The site of complex deposition in the kidney is dependent on the size of the complexes in the circulation. Large complexes become deposited on the glomerular basement membrane, while small complexes pass through the basement membrane and are seen on the epithelial side of the glomerulus.

■ DETECTION OF IMMUNE COMPLEXES

Deposited immune complexes can be visualized using immunofluorescence

The ideal place to look for complexes is in the affected organ. Tissue samples may be examined by immunofluorescence for the presence of immunoglobulin and complement. The composition, pattern and particular area of tissue affected all provide useful information on the severity and prognosis of the disease. For example, patients with the continuous, granular, sub-epithelial deposits of IgG found in membranous glomerulonephritis have a poor prognosis. In contrast, those whose complexes are localized in the mesangium have a good prognosis. Not all tissue-bound complexes give rise to an inflammatory response; for example in SLE, complexes are frequently found in skin biopsies from normal-looking skin, as well as from inflamed skin.

Assays for circulating immune complexes

Circulating complexes are found in two separate compartments: bound to erythrocytes and free in plasma. Erythrocyte-bound complexes are less likely to be damaging, so it is of more interest to determine the level of free complexes. Care is required when collecting the sample: bound complexes can easily be released during clotting by the action of Factor I. To obtain accurate assays of free complexes, the erythrocytes should be rapidly separated from

Antibody classes in immune-complex disease

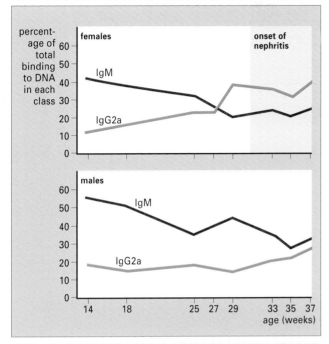

Fig. 24.22 Immune-complex disease is automatic in the NZB/NZW mouse and follows a class switch during early development, from IgM to IgG2a. The graphs show the proportions of anti-DNA antibodies of the IgM and IgG2a isotypes in females and males. Both the class switch and fatal renal disease occur earlier in the female mice of this strain.

An assay for immune complexes based on polyethylene glycol (PEG)

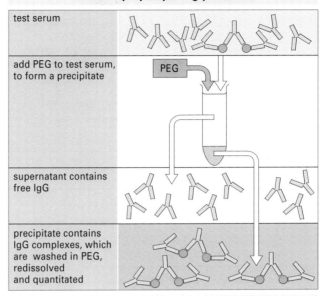

Fig. 24.23 Polyethylene glycol (PEG) is added to the test serum containing IgG complexes and IgG monomer. When the concentration of PEG reaches 2%, complexes are selectively precipitated; the free antibody remains in solution. The test tube is then centrifuged and the complexes form a pellet at the bottom. The supernatant containing free antibody is removed. The precipitate is washed and redissolved so that the amount of complexed IgG can be measured (e.g. by single radial immunodiffusion, nephelometry or radioimmunoassay).

Radioimmunoassay for immune complexes

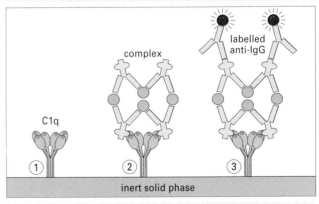

Fig. 24.24 A three-layer radioimmunoassay for immune complexes based on the use of C1q.
1. C1q is linked to an inert solid phase support, usually a polystyrene tube or plate.
2. Serum containing complexes is added. The complexes bind to the solid phase C1q by means of the array of Fc regions presented to the C1q.
3. Radiolabelled anti-IgG antibody is added. The amount of radioactivity remaining on the solid phase after washing is measured in a gamma-counter, and is used to calculate the amount of complex bound to the C1q.

the plasma to prevent the release of bound complexes.

Precipitation of the immune complex with polyethylene glycol (PEG) and estimation of the precipitated IgG is frequently used to identify high molecular weight IgG, and forms the basis for one of the commercial assays (*Fig. 24.23*).

Circulating complexes are often identified by their affinity for complement C1q, using either radiolabelled C1q or solid phase C1q (C1q linked to a solid support) (*Fig. 24.24*).

Other receptors may be used to bind immune complexes for measurement, such as the C3 receptor on RAJI (a B-cell tumour) cells or the Fc receptor on platelets.

However, care must be taken when determining complexes from patients with autoimmune diseases; these patients may have autoantibodies to components of the test system itself. In SLE, for example, patients produce anti-lymphocyte and anti-DNA antibodies that bind to the RAJI cells, giving a false positive for immune complexes. Similarly, anti-C1q antibodies have been found in a number of connective tissue diseases (C1q has a structure similar to collagen), raising the possibility of false-positive results in C1q-based assays.

In all these assays, it is important to check that what is thought to be an immune complex is actually of higher molecular weight than monomeric IgG. Finally, note that evaluation of the importance of circulating complexes requires even more care than the interpretation of tissue complexes. Many circulating complexes will not in themselves be harmful. Damage only occurs if they are deposited in the tissue.

Critical Thinking

■ What factors are likely to lead to persistence of immune complexes?

■ Why are immune complexes deposited in some organs and not in others?

■ What novel therapeutic manipulations of the immune system might help in the treatment of immune-complex diseases?

■ Does complement activation by immune complexes harm or help the individual?

■ In what ways does the class of antibody affect the handling of immune complexes?

■ Why is it difficult to determine immune complexes in the laboratory?

FURTHER READING

Agnello V. Immune complex assays in rheumatic diseases. *Hum Pathol* 1983;**14**:343.

Arthus M. Injections répétées de sérum de cheval chez le lapin. *C R Seances Soc Biol Filiales* 1903;**55**:817.

Birmingham DJ, Herbert LA, Cosio FG, Van Aman ME. Immune complex erythrocyte complement receptor interactions *in vivo* during induction of glomerulonephritis in non-human primates. *J Lab Clin Med* 1990;**116**:242.

Cornacoff JB, Hobart LA, Smead WL, Vanaman ME, Birmingham DJ, Waxman FJ. Primate erythrocyte immune complex clearing mechanism. *J Clin Invest* 1983;**71**:236.

Czop J, Nussenzweig V. Studies on the mechanism of solubilization of immune precipitates by serum. *J Exp Med* 1976;**143**:615.

Davies KA, Erlendsson K, Beynon HLC, *et al.* Splenic uptake of immune complexes in man is complement-dependent. *J Immunol* 1993;**151**:3866.

Davies KA, Hird V, Stewart S, *et al.* A study of *in vivo* immune complex formation and clearing in man. *J Immunol* 1990;**144**:4613.

Dixon FJ, Feldman JD, Vazquez JJ. Experimental glomerulonephritis: the pathogenesis of a laboratory model resembling the spectrum of human glomerulonephritis. *J Exp Med* 1961;**113**:899.

Dixon FJ, Vazquez JJ, Weigle WO, Cochrane CG. Pathogenesis of serum sickness. *Arch Pathol* 1958;**65**:18.

Emlen W, Burdick CG. Mechanism of transfer of immune complexes from red blood cell CR1 to monocytes. *Clin Exp Immunol* 1992;**89**:8.

Finbloom DS, Magilvary DB, Harford JB, Rifai A, Plotz PH. Influence of antigen on immune complex behaviour in mice. *J Clin Invest* 1981;**68**:214.

Heidelberger M. Quantitative chemical studies on complement or alexin. *J Exp Med* 1941;**73**:681.

Inman RD. Immune complexes in SLE. *Clin Res Dis* 1982;**8**:49.

Johnston A, Auda GR, Kerr MA, *et al.* Dissociation of primary antigen-antibody bonds is essential for complement mediated solubilization of immune complexes. *Mol Immunol* 1992;**29**:659.

Kjilstra H, Van Es LA, Daha MR. The role of complement in the binding and degradation of immunoglobulin aggregates by macrophages. *J Immunol* 1979;**123**:2488.

Lachman PJ. Complement deficiency and the pathogenesis of autoimmune complex disease. *Chem Immunol* 1980;**49**:245.

Lucisano YM, Lachmann PJ. The effects of antibody isotype and antigenic epitope density on the complement-fixing activity of immune complexes: a systematic study using chimaeric anti-NIP antibodies with human Fc regions. *Clin Exp Immunol* 1991;**84**:1.

Miller GW, Nussenzweig V. A new complement function: solubilization of antigen–antibody aggregates. *Proc Natl Acad Sci* 1975;**72**:418.

Qiao J-H, Castellani LW, Fishbein MC, *et al.* Immune-complex-mediated vasculitis increases coronary artery lipid accumulation in autoimmune-prone MRL mice. *Arteriosclerosis Thromb* 1993;**13**:932.

Schifferli JA, Ng YC, Peters DK. The role of complement and its receptor in the elimination of immune complexes. *N Engl J Med* 1986;**315**:488.

Takata Y, Tamura N, Fujita T. Interaction of C3 with antigen–antibody complexes in the process of solubilisation of immune precipitates. *J Immunol* 1984;**132**:2531.

Theofilopoulos AN, Dixon FJ. The biology and detection of immune complexes. *Adv Immunol* 1979;**28**:89.

Warren JS, Yabroff KR, Remick DG, *et al.* Tumour necrosis factor participates in the pathogenesis of acute immune complex alveolitis in the rat. *J Clin Invest* 1989;**84**:1873.

Waxman FJ, Hebert LE, Cornacoff JB, Van Aman ME, *et al.* Complement depletion accelerates the clearance of immune complexes from the circulation of primates. *J Clin Invest* 1984;**74**:1329.

Whaley K. Complement and immune complex diseases. In: Whaley K, ed. *Complement in Health and Disease*. Lancaster: MTP Press Ltd, 1987.

Williams RC. *Immune Complexes in Clinical and Experimental Medicine*. Massachusetts: Harvard University Press, 1980.

World Health Organization Scientific Group. *Technical Report 606. The Role of Immune Complexes in Disease*. Geneva: WHO, 1977.

There are three varieties of Type IV hypersensitivity: contact, tuberculin, and granulomatous.

Langerhans' cells internalize and process epicutaneously applied hapten and present it to antigen-specific T cells.

Cytokines produced by immune-competent skin cells (e.g. keratinocytes, Langerhans' cells, T cells) recruit antigen non-specific T cells and macrophages.

Tuberculin-type hypersensitivity is useful as a diagnostic test for exposure to a number of infectious agents.

In granulomatous reactions there is a balance between protective immunity and T-cell mediated tissue damage to insoluble antigen. A good example of this is seen in tuberculoid leprosy.

Persistence of antigen leads to differentiation of macrophages to epithelioid cells, and fusion to form giant cells. The whole pathological response is termed a granulomatous reaction and it results in tissue damage.

Granuloma formation is driven by T-cell activation of macrophages, and is dependent on TNF.

According to the Coombs & Gell classification, Type IV (delayed) hypersensitivity reactions take more than 12 hours to develop, and involve cell-mediated immune reactions rather than humoral immune reactions. However, it is now recognized that some hypersensitivity reactions straddle this definition. For example, the late-phase IgE-mediated reaction may peak 12–24 hours after contact with an allergen. Although an IgE-mediated mechanism is primarily involved, it also involves T-helper cells, and so the picture becomes more complicated. Other reactions (such as Jones–Mote hypersensitivity, which may be analogous to cutaneous basophil reactions in guinea-pigs) have also been included as Type IV hypersensitivity reactions in the past, although their mechanisms and clinical significance remain obscure: these reactions will not be discussed further in this chapter.

Unlike other forms of hypersensitivity, Type IV hypersensitivity cannot be transferred from one animal to another by serum, but can be transferred by T cells (TH1 cells in mice). It is obviously associated with T-cell protective immunity but does not necessarily run parallel with it – there is not always a complete correlation between Type IV hypersensitivity and protective immunity. The T cells responsible for the delayed response have been specifically sensitized by a previous encounter, and act by recruiting other cell types to the site of the reaction.

Three variants of Type IV hypersensitivity reaction are recognized (*Fig. 25.1*). Contact hypersensitivity and tuberculin-type hypersensitivity both occur within 72 hours of antigen challenge. Granulomatous hypersensitivity reactions develop over a period of 21–28 days; the granulomas are formed by the aggregation and proliferation of macrophages, and may persist for weeks. In terms of its clinical consequences, this is by far the most serious type of Type IV hypersensitivity response. Note that more than one type of reaction may follow a single antigenic challenge, and that the reactions may overlap.

The three types of delayed hypersensitivity were originally distinguished according to the reaction they produced when antigen was applied directly to the skin (epicutaneously) or injected intradermally. The degree of the response is usually assessed in animals by measuring thickening of the skin. This local response can also be followed by a variety of systemic immune reactions.

■ CONTACT HYPERSENSITIVITY

Contact hypersensitivity is characterized by an eczematous reaction at the point of contact with an allergen (*Fig. 25.2*). It is often seen following contact with agents such as nickel, chromate, rubber accelerators and pentadecacatechol (found in poison ivy). Contact with irritants that damage skin by toxic

The variants of delayed hypersensitivity

delayed reaction	maximal reaction time
contact	48–72 hours
tuberculin	48–72 hours
granulomatous	21–28 days

Fig. 25.1 Contact and tuberculin-type hypersensitivity have a similar time course and are maximal at 48–72 hours. In certain circumstances (e.g. with insoluble antigen) granulomatous reactions also develop at 21–28 days (e.g. skin testing in leprosy).

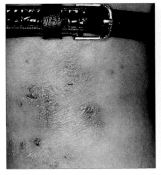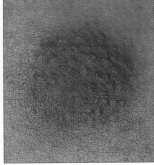

Fig. 25.2 Clinical and patch-test appearances of contact hypersensitivity. Left: The eczematous area at the wrist is due to sensitivity to nickel in the watch-strap buckle. **Right:** The suspected allergy may be confirmed by applying potential allergens, in the relevant concentrations and vehicles, to the patient's upper back (patch testing). A positive reaction causes a localized area of eczema at the site of the offending allergen, 2–4 days after application.

mechanisms not mediated by hypersensitivity can also produce eczema. Although the initial reactions are different, the immunological events following application of irritants and allergens show similarities.

The immunologically active portions of the agents listed above are called haptens. Haptens are too small to be antigenic by themselves, having a molecular weight often less than 1 kDa. They penetrate the epidermis and conjugate, most often covalently, to body proteins. The sensitizing potential of a hapten cannot reliably be predicted from its chemical structure, although there is some correlation with the number of haptens attached to the carrier and the ability of the molecule to penetrate the skin. Also, certain contact allergens have unsaturated carbon bonds and are easily oxidized. Some haptens, such as dinitrochlorobenzene (DNCB), sensitize nearly all individuals and can be used to assess cell-mediated immunity. Epicutaneously applied DNCB binds to epidermal proteins through the -NH$_2$ groups of lysine.

Langerhans' cells and keratinocytes have key roles in contact hypersensitivity

The Langerhans' cell is the principal antigen-presenting cell

Contact hypersensitivity is primarily an epidermal reaction, and the dendritic Langerhans' cell, located in the suprabasal epidermis, is the principal antigen-presenting cell (APC) involved (*Fig. 25.3*). Langerhans' cells are derived from bone marrow and express CD1, MHC class II antigens and surface receptors for Fc and complement (see Chapter 2). Electron microscopy shows Birbeck granules, organelles derived from cell membrane and specific for the cell. Langerhans' cells are inactivated by ultraviolet B, which can thus prevent or alleviate the effects of contact hypersensitivity.

In vitro, Langerhans' cells act as APCs and are more potent in this regard than monocytes. However, the mechanism by which Langerhans' cells process antigens is unknown. Antigens in association with MHC class II molecules may be internalized by receptor-mediated endocytosis, in a mechanism involving Birbeck granules.

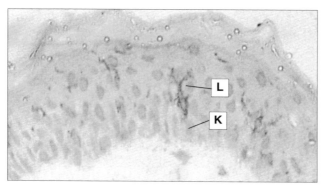

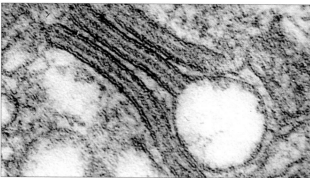

Fig. 25.3 The Langerhans' cell. Upper: These dendritic cells constitute 3% of all cells in the epidermis. They express a variety of surface markers which allow them to be visualized. Here they have been revealed in a section of normal skin using a monoclonal antibody which reacts with the CD1 antigen (counterstained with Mayer's haemalum). L = Langerhans' cell; K = keratinocyte. ×312.

Lower: Electron micrograph of a Langerhans' cell showing the characteristic 'Birbeck granule'. This organelle is a plate-like structure with a distinct central striation and often has a bleb-like extension at one end. ×132 000.

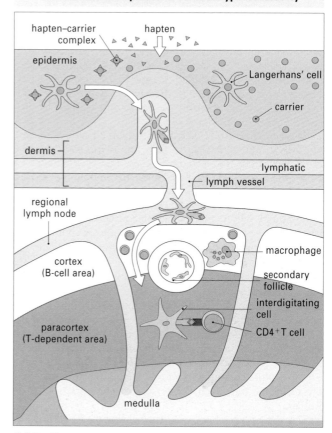

The sensitization phase of contact hypersensitivity

Fig. 25.4 The hapten forms a hapten–carrier complex in the epidermis. Langerhans' cells internalize the antigen and migrate via afferent lymphatics to the paracortical area of the regional lymph node where, as interdigitating cells, they present antigen to CD4$^+$ T cells.

Keratinocytes produce a range of cytokines important to the contact hypersensitivity response

Keratinocytes provide the structural integrity of the epidermis and have a central role in epidermal immunology. They may express MHC class II molecules and ICAM-1 in the cell membrane. They can also release cytokines including IL-1, IL-3, IL-6, IL-8, GM-CSF, M-CSF, TNFα, TGFα, and TGFβ. IL-3 can activate Langerhans' cells, co-stimulate proliferative responses and recruit mast cells, and induce the secretion of immunosuppressive cytokines (e.g. IL-10 and TGFβ) which dampen the immune response and induce clonal anergy (immunological unresponsiveness) in TH1 cells.

Keratinocytes can be activated by a number of stimuli, including allergens and irritants. Activated keratinocytes produce immunostimulatory cytokines such as TNFα and GM-CSF, which activate Langerhans' cells. Some antigens, such as urushiol in poison ivy, may directly induce TNFα and IL-8.

A contact hypersensitivity reaction has two stages: sensitization and elicitation

Sensitization produces a population of memory T cells

Sensitization takes 10–14 days in humans. Once absorbed, the hapten combines with a protein and is internalized by epidermal Langerhans' cells, which leave the epidermis and migrate as veiled cells, via efferent lymphatics, to the paracortical areas of regional lymph nodes. Here they present processed hapten–protein conjugates (in association with MHC class II

molecules) to CD4+ lymphocytes, producing a population of memory CD4+ T cells (*Fig. 25.4*). Human studies using DNCB show that dose of hapten per unit area of skin, rather than total dose or total area, is the main determinant of sensitization.

The elicitation phase involves recruitment of CD4+ lymphocytes and monocytes

The application of an allergen generally causes a modest decrease in Langerhans' cell numbers in the epidermis within hours of application. Antigen presentation by Langerhans' cells then occurs in skin and lymph nodes. Degranulation and cytokine release by mast cells follows soon after contact with an allergen. TNFα and IL-1 from many cell types, and from macrophages in particular, are potent inducers of endothelial cell adhesion molecules. These locally released cytokines produce a gradient signal for movement of mononuclear cells towards the dermo-epidermal junction and epidermis. For the elicitation phase of contact hypersensitivity, see *Figure 25.5*.

The earliest histological change, seen after 4–8 hours, is the appearance of mononuclear cells around adnexae and blood vessels, with subsequent epidermal infiltration. Macrophages invade the dermis and epidermis by 48 hours. The number of cells infiltrating the epidermis and dermis peaks At 48–72 hours (*Fig. 25.6*). Most infiltrating lymphocytes are CD4+, with a few CD8+. Less than 1% of infiltrating cells are of a single clonal lineage (i.e. antigen-specific memory CD4+ TH1 cells). The main mechanism for T cell recruitment is antigen independent.

The elicitation phase of contact hypersensitivity

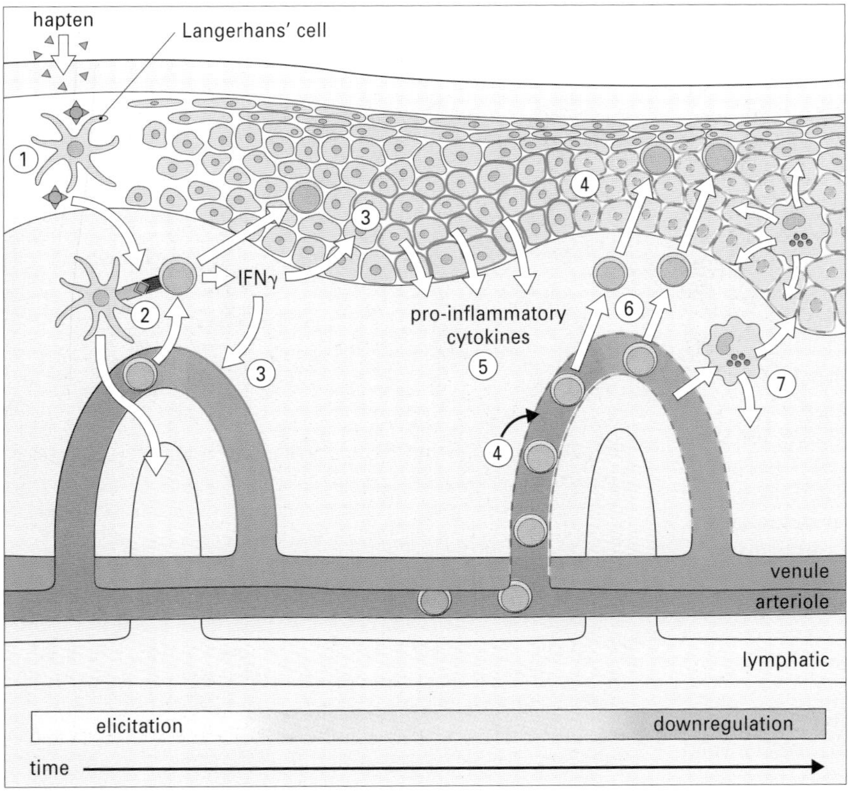

Fig. 25.5 Langerhans' cells carrying the hapten–carrier complex (1) move from the epidermis to the dermis, where they present the hapten–carrier complex to memory CD4+ T cells (2). Activated CD4+ T cells release IFNγ, which induces expression of ICAM-1 (3) and, later, MHC class II molecules (4) on the surface of keratinocytes and on endothelial cells of dermal capillaries and activates keratinocytes which release proinflammatory cytokines such as IL-1, IL-6 and GM-CSF (5). Non-antigen specific CD4+ T cells are attracted to the site by cytokines (6) and may bind to keratinocytes via ICAM-1 and class II molecules. Activated macrophages are also attracted to the skin, but this occurs later. Thereafter the reaction starts to downregulate. This downregulation may be influenced by eicosanoids such as PGE, produced by activated keratinocytes and macrophages (7).

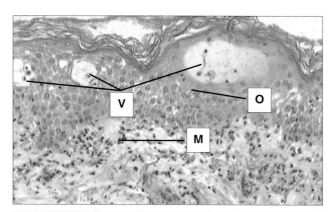

Fig. 25.6 Histological appearance of the lesion in contact hypersensitivity. Mononuclear cells (M) infiltrate both dermis and epidermis. The epidermis is pushed outwards and microvesicles (V) form within it due to oedema (O). H&E stain, ×130.

The mechanisms of reactions to allergens and irritants share some features

Allergens and irritants may damage Langerhans' cells and induce cytokines, stimulating Langerhans' cells to mature into potent APCs which migrate to lymph nodes, and initiate immune responses. TNFα, IFNγ and GM-CSF mRNA signals are induced within 30 minutes of topical application of either an antigen or irritant, and a tenfold increase in mRNA expression is found in 2–4 hours. Certain changes in mRNA transcription occur only after application of a hapten. These include an increase in the IL-1β mRNA signal by Langerhans' cells at 15 minutes, and upregulation of transcription by keratinocytes of IL-1α, macrophage inflammatory protein 2 (MIP-2), and interferon-induced protein 10 (IP-10) (*Fig. 25.7*).

Chemical reagents applied to the epidermis can result in increased expression of ELAM-1 and VCAM-1 within 2 hours, and ICAM-1 within 8 hours, regardless of whether the individual is sensitive or not. ICAM-1 is more prominent than VCAM-1 or ELAM-1: it is the ligand for LFA-1, found on lymphoid and myeloid cells, and is important for localizing these cells to the skin. Chemotactic cytokines and the 'beacon effect' of in-transit Langerhans' cells attract TH1 cells. Memory T cells reside in dermal capillaries where they can trigger the reaction and recruit in a non-antigen specific manner.

Suppression of the inflammatory reaction is mediated by a range of cytokines

The reaction wanes after 48–72 hours; macrophages and keratinocytes produce PGE, which inhibits IL-1 and IL-2 production; T cells bind to activated keratinocytes and the hapten conjugate undergoes enzymatic and cellular degradation. Down-regulation is assisted by the following mechanisms:
- Migration-inhibitory lymphokines prevent spread of the inflammatory reaction.
- TGFβ, from dermal mast cells, activated keratinocytes and lymphocytes, inhibits inflammation and blocks the proliferative effects of IL-1 and IL-2.
- IL-1, synthesized by keratinocytes following contact with allergens, inhibits oxidative metabolism in macrophages and depresses their production of pro-inflammatory mediators.
- IL-10 downregulates class II molecule expression,

Cytokines, prostaglandins and cellular interactions in contact hypersensitivity

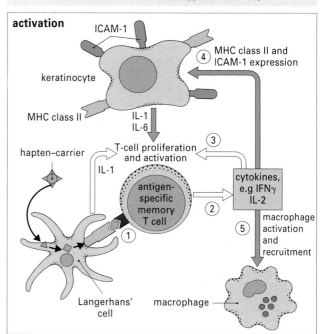

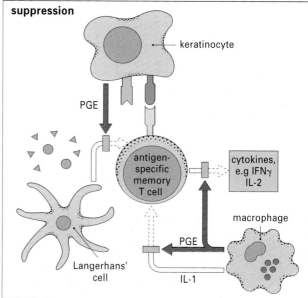

Fig. 25.7 Cytokines and prostaglandins are central to the complex interactions between Langerhans' cells, CD4+ T cells, keratinocytes, macrophages and endothelial cells in contact hypersensitivity. The act of antigen presentation (1) causes the release of a cascade of cytokines (2). This cascade initially results in the activation and proliferation of CD4+ T cells (3), the induction of expression of ICAM-1 and MHC class II molecules on keratinocytes and endothelial cells (4), and the attraction of T cells and macrophages to the skin (3, 5). Subsequent PGE production by keratinocytes and macrophages may have an inhibitory effect on IL-1 and IL-2 production. Production of PGE, binding of activated T cells to keratinocytes and enzymatic and cellular degradation of the hapten–carrier complex all contribute to the downregulation of the reaction.

suppresses cytokine production and antigen-specific proliferation by TH1 cells.

• External factors may also be involved: in mice UV light has been shown to induce a specific inhibitor of IL-1 activity.

• Keratinocytes expressing class II molecules without co-stimulatory molecules cannot act as APCs but, when haptenated and incubated with TH1 cells, can induce clonal anergy.

■ TUBERCULIN-TYPE HYPERSENSITIVITY

This form of hypersensitivity was originally described by Koch. He observed that if patients with tuberculosis were injected subcutaneously with a tuberculin culture filtrate (antigens derived from the tubercle bacillus) they reacted with fever and generalized sickness. An area of hardening and swelling developed at the site of injection. Soluble antigens from a number of organisms, including *Mycobacterium tuberculosis*, *M. leprae* and *Leishmania tropica*, induce similar reactions in sensitive people. The skin reaction is frequently used to test for sensitivity to the organisms following previous exposure (*Fig. 25.8*). This form of hypersensitivity may also be induced by non-microbial antigens, such as beryllium and zirconium.

The tuberculin skin test reaction principally involves monocytes

The tuberculin skin test is an example of the recall response to soluble antigen previously encountered during infection. Following intradermal tuberculin challenge in a sensitized individual, antigen-specific T cells are activated to secrete cytokines that mediate the hypersensitivity reaction. T cell-derived TNFα and lymphotoxin (TNFβ) act on endothelial cells in dermal blood vessels to induce the sequential expression of the adhesion molecules E-selectin, ICAM-1 and VCAM-1. These molecules bind receptors on leucocytes and recruit them to the site of the reaction. The initial influx at four hours is of neutrophils, but this is replaced at 12 hours by monocytes and T cells. This infiltrate, which extends outwards and disrupts the collagen bundles of the dermis,

increases to a peak at 48 hours. CD4⁺ T cells outnumber CD8⁺ cells by about 2:1. CD1⁺ cells (Langerhans'-like cells, but lacking Birbeck granules) are also found in the dermal infiltrate at 24 and 48 hours, and a few CD4⁺ cells infiltrate the epidermis between 24 and 48 hours.

Monocytes constitute 80–90% of the total cellular infiltrate. Both infiltrating lymphocytes and macrophages express MHC class II molecules, and this increases the efficiency of activated macrophages as APCs. Overlying keratinocytes express HLA-DR molecules 48–96 hours after the appearance of the lymphocytic infiltrate. These events are summarized in *Figure 25.9*.

Macrophages are probably the main APCs in the tuberculin hypersensitivity reaction. However, there are CD1⁺ cells in the dermal infiltrate, which suggests that Langerhans' cells or indeterminate dendritic cells may also participate. The circulation of immune cells to and from the regional lymph nodes is thought to be similar to that for contact hypersensitivity.

The tuberculin lesion normally resolves within 5–7 days, but if there is persistence of antigen in the tissues it may develop into a granulomatous reaction. Subepidermal infiltration with basophils is not a characteristic of this reaction, but can be seen in some contact hypersensitivity reactions and skin tests with heterologous proteins, as in the Jones–Mote reaction.

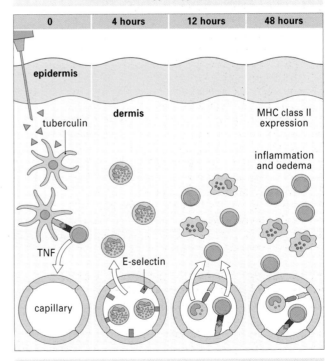

Tubererculin-type hypersensitivity

Fig. 25.9 This diagram illustrates cellular movements following intradermal injection of tuberculin. Within 1–2 hours there is expression of E-selectin on capillary endothelium leading to a brief influx of neutrophil leucocytes. By 12 hours ICAM-1 and VCAM-1 on endothelium bind the integrins LFA-1 and VLA-4 on monocytes and lymphocytes, leading to accumulation of both cell types in the dermis. This peaks at 48 hours and is followed by expression of the HLA class II molecules on keratinocytes. There is no oedema of the epidermis.

 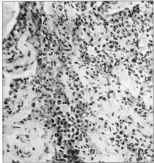

Fig. 25.8 Clinical and histological appearances of tuberculin-type sensitivity. The response to an injection of leprosy bacillus into a sensitized individual is known as the Fernandez reaction. The reaction is characterized by an area of firm red swelling of the skin and is maximal 48–72 hours after challenge (left). Histologically (right), there is a dense dermal infiltrate of leucocytes and macrophages. H&E stain, ×80.

■ GRANULOMATOUS HYPERSENSITIVITY

Granulomatous hypersensitivity is clinically the most important form of Type IV hypersensitivity, and causes many of the pathological effects in diseases that involve T-cell mediated immunity. It usually results from the persistence within macrophages of intracellular microorganisms or other particles that the cell is unable to destroy. On occasion it may also be caused by persistent immune complexes, for example in allergic alveolitis. This process results in epithelioid cell granuloma formation.

The histological appearance of the granuloma reaction is quite different from that of the tuberculin-type reaction. However, they often result from sensitization to similar microbial antigens, for example the antigens of *M. tuberculosis* and *M. leprae* (*Fig. 25.10*). Immunological granuloma formation also occurs in the sensitivity reactions to zirconium and beryl-

lium, and in sarcoidosis, although in the latter the antigen is unknown. Foreign-body granuloma formation occurs with talc, silica and a variety of other particulate agents. In this case macrophages are unable to digest the inorganic matter. These non-immunological granulomas may be distinguished by the absence of lymphocytes in the lesion.

Epithelioid cells and giant cells are typical of granulomatous hypersensitivity

Epithelioid cells – These cells are large and flattened with increased endoplasmic reticulum (*Fig. 25.11*). They are derived from activated macrophages under the chronic stimulation of cytokines; they continue to secrete TNF and thus potentiate continuing inflammation.

Giant cells – Epithelioid cells may fuse to form multinucleate giant cells (*Fig. 25.12*), sometimes referred to as Langhans'

Role of the T_{DTH} lymphocyte in Type IV hypersensitivity

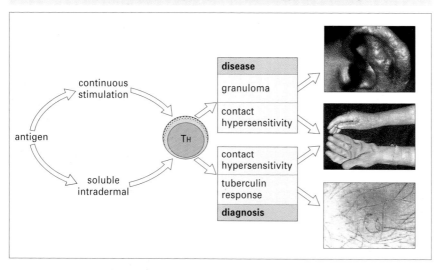

Fig. 25.10 The tuberculin skin reaction (**lower:** courtesy of Professor JHL Playfair) is the classic diagnostic test for cell-mediated immunity in tuberculosis. If there is continuous antigenic stimulation instead of a single injection of soluble antigen, a granulomatous reaction (**upper:** courtesy of Dr A du Vivier) or contact hypersensitivity (**middle:** courtesy Dr D Sharvill) follows. This can also occur if the macrophages cannot destroy the antigen.

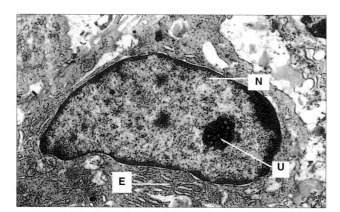

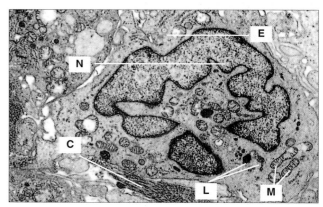

Fig. 25.11 Electron micrograph of an epithelioid cell. This is the characteristic cell of granulomatous hypersensitivity. Compare the extent of the endoplasmic reticulum (E) in the epithelioid cell

(left, ×4800) with that of a tissue macrophage (right, ×4800). (Courtesy of M. J. Spencer.) U = nucleolus; N = nucleus; C = collagen; L = lysosomes; M = mitochondria.

giant cells (not to be confused with the Langerhans' cell discussed earlier). Giant cells have several nuclei, but these are not at the centre of the cell. There is little endoplasmic reticulum, and the mitochondria and lysosomes appear to be undergoing degeneration. The giant cell may therefore be a terminal differentiation stage of the monocyte/macrophage line.

The granuloma contains epithelioid cells, macrophages, and lymphocytes

An immunological granuloma typically has a core of epithelioid cells and macrophages, sometimes with giant cells. In some diseases, such as tuberculosis, this central area may have a zone of necrosis, with complete destruction of all cellular architecture. The macrophage/epithelioid core is surrounded by a cuff of lymphocytes, and there may also be considerable fibrosis (deposition of collagen fibres) caused by proliferation of fibroblasts and increased collagen synthesis. Examples of granulomatous reactions are the Mitsuda reaction to *M. leprae* antigens (see *Fig. 25.12*) or the Kveim test, where patients suffering from sarcoidosis react to (unknown) splenic antigens derived from other sarcoid patients. The three types of delayed hypersensitivity are summarized in *Figure 25.13*.

■ CELLULAR REACTIONS IN TYPE IV HYPERSENSITIVITY

Experiments with gene knock-out (gko) mice have confirmed that T cells bearing αβ TCR rather than γδ TCR are essential for initiating delayed hypersensitivity reactions in response to infection with intracellular bacteria. Sensitized αβ T cells, stimulated with the appropriate antigen and APCs, undergo lymphoblastoid transformation prior to cell division (*Fig. 25.14*). This forms the basis of the lymphocyte stimulation test (see Chapter 28). Lymphocyte stimulation is accompanied by DNA synthesis and this can be measured by assaying the uptake of radiolabelled thymidine, a nucleoside that is required for DNA synthesis. Lymphocytes from a patient are cultured with the suspect antigen to determine whether it induces transformation. It is important to stress that this is a test for T-cell memory only, and does not necessarily imply the presence of protective immunity.

Delayed hypersensitivity reactions

type	reaction time	clinical appearance	histology	antigen
contact	48–72 hr	eczema	lymphocytes, later macrophages, oedema of epidermis	epidermal e.g. nickel rubber poison ivy
tuberculin	48–72 hr	local induration	lymphocytes monocytes, macrophages	intradermal e.g. tuberculin
granuloma	21–28 days	hardening e.g. skin or lung	macrophages, epithelioid cells, giant cells fibrosis	persistent Ag/Ab complexes or non-immunoglobin stimuli e.g. talc

Fig. 25.13 Characteristics of Type IV reactions.

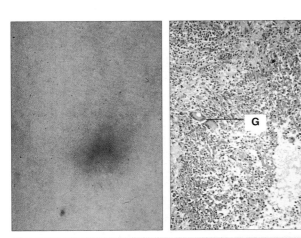

Fig. 25.12 Clinical and histological appearances of the Mitsuda reaction in leprosy seen at 28 days. Left: The resultant skin swelling (which may be ulcerated) is much harder and better defined than at 48 hours. Right: Histology shows a typical epithelioid-cell granuloma (H&E stain, ×60). Giant cells (G) are visible in the centre of the lesion, which is surrounded by a cuff of lymphocytes. This response is more akin to the pathological processes in delayed hypersensitivity diseases than the self-resolving tuberculin-type reaction. The reaction is due to the continued presence of mycobacterial antigen.

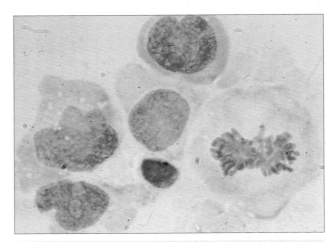

Fig. 25.14 Transformed lymphocytes. Following stimulation with appropriate antigen, T cells undergo lymphoblastoid transformation prior to cell division. Blast cells with expanded nuclei and cytoplasm (as well as one lymphocyte in the metaphase of cell division) are shown.

Following activation by APCs, T cells release a number of pro-inflammatory cytokines which attract and activate macrophages. These include IFNγ, lymphotoxin, IL-3 and GM-CSF. This TH1-like pattern of cytokines is enhanced by activation of the T cells in the presence of IL-12, which is released by macrophages on exposure to bacterial products. IL-12 suppresses the cytokine response of TH2 cells. The role of individual cytokines can be analysed in gko mice deficient for a single cytokine. For example, IFNγ gko mice are unable to activate macrophages and control infection with *M. tuberculosis* (*Fig. 25.15*). In granulomatous reactions the activated macrophages become a major source of TNF and the granulomas develop by auto-amplification, with differentiation of macrophages into epithelioid cells (*Figs 25.16* and *25.17*). These secrete more TNF, stimulating further epithelioid cell formation, with the fusion of epithelioid cells resulting in the formation of giant cells (*Fig. 25.18*).

■ DISEASES MANIFESTING TYPE IV GRANULOMATOUS HYPERSENSITIVITY

There are many chronic diseases in man that manifest Type IV hypersensitivity. Most are due to infectious agents such as mycobacteria, protozoa and fungi, although in other granu-lomatous diseases such as sarcoidosis and Crohn's disease, no infectious agent has been established.

Important diseases in this respect include the following:
- Leprosy
- Tuberculosis
- Schistosomiasis
- Sarcoidosis
- Crohn's disease

A common feature of these infections is that the pathogen presents a persistent, chronic antigenic stimulus. Activation of macrophages by lymphocytes may limit the infection, but continuing stimulation may lead to tissue damage through the release of macrophage products including reactive oxygen intermediates and hydrolases. Although delayed hypersensitivity is a measure of T cell activation, the infection is not always controlled, with the result that protective immunity and delayed hypersensitivity do not necessarily coincide. Therefore some subjects showing delayed hypersensitivity may not be protected against disease in the future.

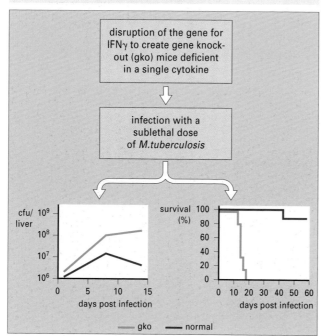

The importance of IFNγ in the activation of macrophages

disruption of the gene for IFNγ to create gene knock-out (gko) mice deficient in a single cytokine

⬇

infection with a sublethal dose of *M.tuberculosis*

gko ——— normal

Fig. 25.15 Mice deficient in IFNγ (gko mice) are unable to activate macrophages in response to infection with an intracellular bacterium. Macrophages initially accumulate at the site of infection but do not form typical granulomas. Uncontrolled infection (graph, left) causes widespread tissue necrosis and death (graph, right).

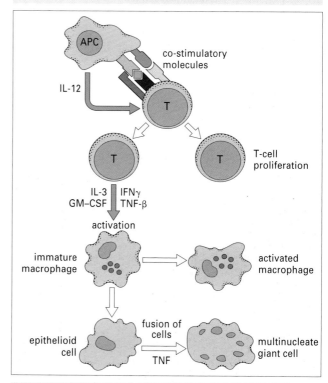

Macrophage differentiation

Fig. 25.16 Bacterial products stimulate macrophages to secrete IL-12. Activation of T cells in the presence of IL-12 leads to the release of IFNγ and other cytokines, TNFβ, IL-3 and GM-CSF. These cytokines activate macrophages to kill intracellular parasites. Failure to eradicate the antigenic stimulus causes persistent cytokine release and promotes differentiation of macrophages into epithelioid cells which secrete large amounts of TNFα. Some fuse to form multinucleate giant cells.

Leprosy – Leprosy is divided clinically into three main types: tuberculoid, borderline and lepromatous. In tuberculoid leprosy, the skin may have a few well-defined hypopigmented patches that show an intense lymphocytic and epithelioid infiltrate and no micro-organisms. In contrast, the polar reaction of lepromatous leprosy shows multiple confluent skin lesions characterized by numerous bacilli, 'foamy' macrophages and a paucity of lymphocytes. Borderline leprosy has characteristics of both (*Fig. 25.19*). In leprosy, pro-

tective immunity is usually associated with cell-mediated immunity, but this declines across the leprosy spectrum towards the lepromatous pole with a rise in non-protective anti-*M. leprae* antibodies.

The borderline leprosy reaction is a dramatic example of delayed hypersensitivity. Borderline reactions occur either naturally or following drug treatment. In these reactions, hypopigmented skin lesions containing *M. leprae* become swollen and inflamed (*Fig. 25.20*), because the patient is now

The importance of TNF in the formation of granulomas

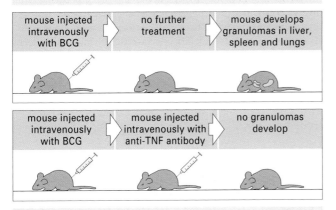

Fig. 25.17 TNF is essential for the development of epithelioid cell granulomas. If BCG-injected mice are injected with anti-TNFα antibodies, they do not develop granulomas.

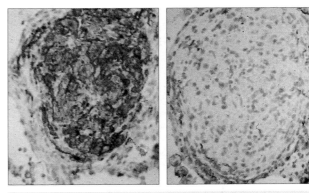

Fig. 25.18 Epithelioid cells in a granuloma from the lung of a patient with sarcoidosis. Left: The epithelioid cells and giant cells in the centre have been stained with the specific antibody RFD-9. Right: Mature tissue macrophages surrounding the granuloma are stained with the specific antibody RFD-7. (Courtesy of CS Munro.)

The immunological spectrum of leprosy

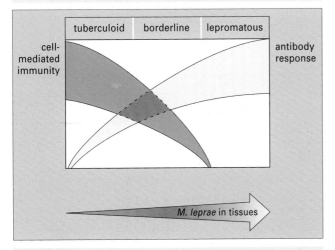

Fig. 25.19 The clinical spectrum of leprosy ranges from tuberculoid disease, with few lesions and bacteria, to lepromatous leprosy, with multiple lesions and uncontrolled bacterial proliferation. This range reflects host immunity as measured by specific cellular and antibody responses to *M. leprae*, and the tissue expression of cytokines.

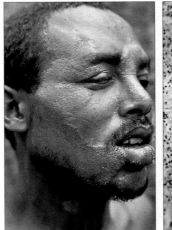
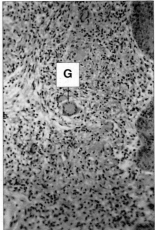

Fig. 25.20 A borderline leprosy reaction. Left: The previously hypopigmented skin lesions have become swollen and inflamed following sensitization to antigens of *M. leprae*. Right: The histological appearance is typical of granulomatous hypersensitivity. Note the giant cell (G) and infiltration by monocytes and lymphocytes. H&E stain, ×140.

Lymphocyte stimulation test in leprosy

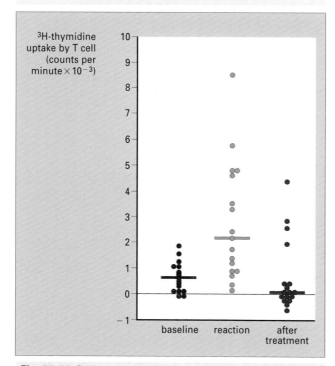

Fig. 25.21 During a borderline leprosy reaction, the lymphocyte stimulation response to *M. leprae* rises. There is a fall in response when the reaction is treated successfully with corticosteroids. The lymphocyte stimulation responses to sonicated *M. leprae* (measured by uptake of ^{3}H-thymidine) are shown for 17 patients who developed such reactions: (a) before starting treatment with anti-leprosy drugs (baseline); (b) during the reaction; and (c) following successful treatment with steroids. Medians are indicated by horizontal bars.

able to mount a delayed-type hypersensitivity reaction. The histological appearance shows a more tuberculoid pattern with an infiltrate of IFNγ-secreting lymphocytes. The process may occur in peripheral nerves, where Schwann cells contain *M. leprae*; this is the most important cause of nerve destruction in this disease. The lesion in borderline leprosy is typical of granulomatous hypersensitivity (*Fig. 25.20*). In patients with a tuberculoid type reaction, T-cell sensitization may be assessed *in vitro* by the lymphocyte stimulation test (see Chapter 28), using either whole or sonicated *M. leprae* as antigen (*Fig. 25.21*).

Tuberculosis – In tuberculosis there is a balance between the effects of activated macrophages controlling the infection on the one hand, and causing tissue damage in infected organs on the other. In the lung, granulomatous reactions lead to cavitation and spread of bacteria. The reactions are frequently accompanied by extensive fibrosis and the lesions may be seen in the chest radiographs of affected patients (*Fig. 25.22*). The histological appearance of the lesion is typical of a granulomatous reaction, with central caseous (cheesy) necrosis (*Fig. 25.23*). This is surrounded by an area of epithelioid cells, with a few giant cells. Mononuclear cell infiltration occurs around the edge.

Schistosomiasis – In schistosomiasis, caused by parasitic trematode worms (schistosomes), the host becomes sensitized to the ova of the worms, leading to a typical granulomatous reaction in the parasitized tissue (*Fig. 25.24*; see also Chapter 18).

Sarcoidosis – Sarcoidosis is a chronic disease of unknown aetiology in which activated macrophages and granuloma accumulate in many tissues, frequently accompanied by fibrosis (*Fig. 25.25*). The disease particularly affects lymphoid tissue, and enlarged lymph nodes may be detected in chest radiographs of affected patients (*Fig. 25.26*). No infectious agent has been isolated, although mycobacteria have been implicated because of the similarities in the pathology.

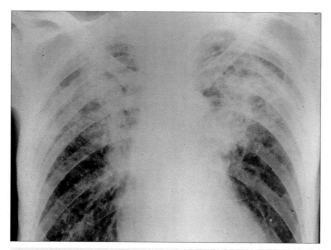

Fig. 25.22 **Chest radiograph of a patient with pulmonary tuberculosis.** There is extensive parenchymal streaking, predominantly in the upper fields of the lungs. These changes are typical of chronic bilateral pulmonary tuberculosis. Some enlargement of the heart is also evident.

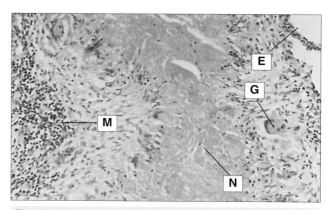

Fig. 25.23 **Histological appearance of a tuberculous section of lung.** This shows an epithelioid cell granuloma (E) with giant cells (G). Mononuclear cell infiltration can be seen (M). There is also marked caseation and necrosis (N) within the granuloma. H&E stain, ×75.

One of the paradoxes of clinical immunology is that this disease is usually associated with depression of delayed hypersensitivity both *in vivo* and *in vitro*. Patients with sarcoidosis are anergic on testing with tuberculin; however, when cortisone is injected with tuberculin antigen the skin tests are positive, suggesting that cortisone-sensitive T-suppressor cells are responsible for the anergy. Cortisone would normally suppress delayed hypersensitivity.

In sarcoidosis, granulomas develop in a variety of organs, most commonly the lungs, lymph nodes, bone, nervous tissue and skin. Patients may present acutely with fever and malaise, although in the longer term those with pulmonary involvement develop shortness of breath caused by lung fibrosis. The diagnosis is often suggested by the clinical pattern and radiographic changes and confirmed by tissue biopsy. Angiotensin converting enzyme (ACE) and serum calcium are sometimes elevated, as activated macrophages are a source of both ACE and 1,25-dihydroxy-cholecalciferol (the active metabolite of vitamin D_3).

Crohn's Disease – This is another non-infectious disease in which granulomas are prominent. In Crohn's disease, a chronic inflammatory disease of the ileum and colon, lymphocytes and macrophages accumulate in all layers of the bowel. The granulomatous reaction and fibrosis cause stricture of the bowel and penetrating fistulas into other organs. The natures of the antigens or infectious agents initiating and perpetuating this granulomatous reaction are unknown.

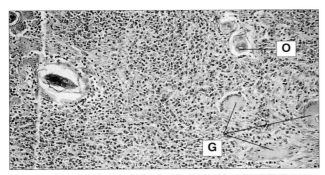

Fig. 25.24 Histological appearance of the liver in schistosomiasis. The epithelioid-cell granuloma surrounds the schistosome ovum (O). Note also the giant cells (G). H&E stain, ×100.

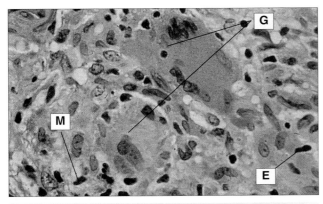

Fig. 25.25 Histological appearance of sarcoidosis in a lymph node biopsy. The granuloma of sarcoidosis is typically composed of epithelioid cells (E) and multinucleate giant cells (G), but without caseous necrosis. There is only a sparse mononuclear cell infiltrate (M) evident at the periphery of the granuloma. H&E stain, ×240.

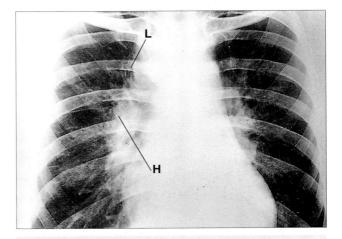

Fig. 25.26 The chest radiograph of a patient with sarcoidosis. There is enlargement of the lymph nodes adjacent to the hilar (H) and paratracheal (L) areas of the lungs, with diffuse pulmonary infiltration characteristic of the disease.

Critical Thinking

- How can the same cytokines that activate a macrophage to kill intracellular parasites also induce tissue damage?

- What other immunological reactions might be blocked by anti-cytokine antibodies?

- How do irritants and contact hypersensitivity produce the same reaction in the skin?

- What form of Type IV hypersensitivity produces the most damage to tissues?

- How can the late-phase IgE-mediated reaction be distinguished from Type IV hypersensitivity reactions?

- How does the number and function of T cells influence the expression of tuberculin-type hypersensitivity?

- Can borderline leprosy reactions be exacerbated by other immune mechanisms?

- Can the concept of UVB exposure of the skin be used to determine mechanisms of Type IV hypersensitivity?

FURTHER READING

Baadsgaard O, Wang T. Immune regulation in allergic and irritant skin reactions. *Int J Dermatol* 1991;**30**:161–72.

Bevilacqua MP. Endothelial-leukocyte adhesion molecules. *Ann Rev Immunol* 1993;**11**:767–804.

Bjune G, Barnetson RStC, Ridley DS, Kronvall G. Lymphocyte transformation test in leprosy: correlation of the response with inflammation of lesions. *Clin Exp Immunol* 1976;**25**:85–94.

Britton WJ. Immunology of leprosy. *Trans Roy Soc Trop Med Hyg* 1993;**87**:508–14.

Flynn JL, Chan J, Triebold KJ, Datton DK, Stewart TA, Bloom BR. An essential role for interferon-γ in resistance to *Mycobacterium tuberculosis* infection. *J Exp Med* 1993;**178**:2249–54.

Friedmann PS. The immunology of allergic contact dermatitis: the DNCB story. *Adv Dermatol* 1991;**5**:175–96.

Gaspari AA. Advances in the understanding of contact hypersensitivity. *Am J Cont Derm* 1993;**4**:138–49.

Gawkrodger DJ, McVittie E, Carr MM, Ross JA, Hunter JAA. Phenotypic characterisation of the early cellular responses in allergic and irritant contact dermatitis. *Clin Exp Immunol* 1986;**66**:590–98.

Gawkrodger DJ, Carr MM, McVittie E, Guy K, Hunter JAA. Keratinocyte expression of MHC class II antigens in allergic sensitisation and challenge reactions and in irritant contact dermatitis. *J Invest Dermatol* 1987;**88**:11–16.

Kaufmann SHE. Bacterial and protozoal infection in genetically disrupted mice. *Curr Op Immunol* 1994;**6**:518–25.

Kindler V, Sappino A-P, Gran GE, Pignet P-F, Vassalli P. The inducing role of tumour necrosis factor in the development of bactericidal granulomas during BCG infection. *Cell* 1989;**56**:731–40.

Lowes J, Jewell D. Immunology of inflammatory bowel disease. Vol 12. *Springer Seminars in Immunopathology* 1990;**180**:251–68.

Munro CS, Campbell DA, Collings LA, Poulter LW. Monoclonal antibodies distinguish macrophages and epithelioid cells in sarcoidosis and leprosy. *Clin Exp Immunol* 1987;**68**,282–87.

Sauder DN. Allergic contact dermatitis. In: Thiers BH, Dobson RL, eds. *Pathogenesis of Skin Diseases*. New York: Churchill Livingstone, 1986:3–12.

Trinchieri G. Interleukin-12 and its role in the generation of Th1 cells. *Immunol Today* 1993;**14**:335–38.

Yamamura M, Uyemura K, Deans RJ, *et al.* Defining protective immune responses to pathogens: cytokine profiles in leprosy lesions. *Science* 1991;**254**:277–279.

Rejection of transplanted tissues occurs because the immune system of the recipient recognizes and responds to foreign (tissue) histocompatibility antigens expressed on the graft.

The histocompatibility antigens that are most important are those encoded by the major histocompatibility complex (MHC).

T lymphocytes can directly recognize and respond to foreign MHC molecules.

Activated T-helper cells make lymphokines which drive the activation of many different effector mechanisms of graft destruction.

Lymphokines also act upon the graft to increase the expression of MHC molecules and adhesion molecules, making the graft more susceptible to rejection.

Graft rejection responses can be reduced by the matching of donor and recipient MHC molecules, especially for MHC class II molecules.

Non-specific immunosuppressive agents can be used to block transplant rejection, but these may also reduce resistance to infections.

Specific immunosuppression will be used in the future inactivating only those lymphocyte clones which cause graft rejection.

The immunobiology of transplantation is important for many reasons, both in terms of its impact on our understanding of immunological processes as well as its application in the development of clinical transplantation. It was the study of mouse skin-graft rejection that led to the discovery of the major histocompatibility complex (MHC) molecules (see Chapter 5), which function in the presentation of antigens to T cells (see Chapter 7). T cells are pivotal in transplant rejection, and much of our knowledge of T-cell physiology and function, of self tolerance and autoimmunity, and of the role of the thymus in T-cell education, is derived from studies of transplantation. Last, but not least, transplantation of tissues is very important clinically. The need to prevent transplantation rejection has led to the development and use of new immunomodulatory drugs and a search for ways to induce tolerance of the grafted tissues. These approaches also have a more general application in the treatment of various immune disorders, such as immune-mediated tissue-damage in hypersensitivity and autoimmunity.

In clinical practice, organs are transplanted to make good a functional deficit (*Fig. 26.1*). Unless the donor and recipient are genetically identical, the graft antigens will elicit an immunological rejection response. Transplantation can stimulate all of the various active mechanisms of humoral and cellular immunity, both specific and non-specific. This is a consequence of the recognition by the recipient's T cells of foreign peptide antigens associated with the foreign MHC molecules on the grafted cells. In this context, the peptide antigens are usually derived from normal constituents of donor cells, but they may also come from viruses within the cells, or from other microbes. By the same token, a transplant can activate all of the regulatory mechanisms that control immune responses (see Chapter 11). Hence, transplantation immunobiology encompasses virtually all aspects of immune function.

■ BARRIERS TO TRANSPLANTATION

Transplantation barriers can be described in terms of the genetic disparity between the donor and the recipient: grafts can be categorized as autografts, isografts, allografts or xenografts (*Fig. 26.2*). Autografts from one part of the body to another are not foreign and therefore do not elicit rejection. Similarly, isografts between isogeneic (genetically identical) individuals, such as monozygotic (identical) twins or mice of the same inbred strain, do not express antigens foreign to the recipient and so do not activate a rejection response. The allograft is the common clinical transplant, where one person donates an organ to a genetically different individual. In this case the graft is allogeneic (i.e. between members of the same species, having allelic variants of certain genes). The cells of the allograft will express alloantigens which are recognized as foreign by the recipient.

The maximal genetic disparity is between members of different species, and a xenograft across such a xenogeneic barrier is generally rapidly rejected, either by naturally occurring IgM antibodies in the recipient or by a rapid cell-mediated

Clinical transplantation

organ transplanted	examples of disease
kidney	end-stage renal failure
heart	terminal cardiac failure
lung or heart/lung	pulmonary hypertension, cystic fibrosis
liver	cirrhosis, cancer, biliary atresia
cornea	dystrophy, keratitis
pancreas or islets	diabetes
bone marrow	immunodeficiency, leukaemia
small bowel	cancer
skin	burns

Fig. 26.1 Organs and tissues are transplanted to treat various conditions. Each type of transplant has its own particular medical and surgical difficulties.

Genetic barriers to transplantation

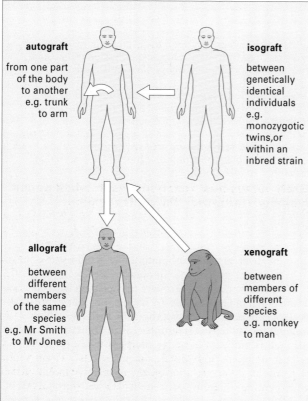

Fig. 26.2 The genetic relationship between the donor and recipient determines whether or not rejection will occur. Autografts or isografts are usually accepted, while allografts and xenografts are not.

Mouse histocompatibility antigens and graft survival

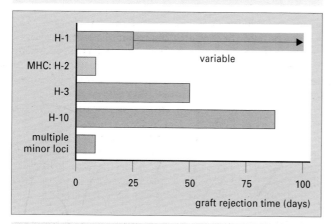

Fig. 26.3 This chart gives the rejection times for skin grafts between mice differing at the minor histocompatibility loci (red) or at the major histocompatibility H-2 locus (green). Grafts which differ at multiple minor loci are rejected as quickly as those that differ at H-2. (Data from Graff and Bailey.)

rejection (see below). If they are treated to reduce their immunogenicity, tissue xenografts that would otherwise be non-viable, such as pig skin, blood vessels or valves, can be grafted to man. Despite this, attempts to transplant whole organs from animal to man have been spectacularly unsuccessful, although some success has been achieved in xenografting between animal species. If the immunological problems of xenografting can be overcome, the use of animal donors could alleviate the world-wide shortage of human organs for transplantation. Nevertheless, various non-immunological problems remain, including donor organ size, transmission of animal diseases and the ethics of xenografting.

■ HISTOCOMPATIBILITY ANTIGENS

Histocompatibility antigens are the targets for rejection

The antigens primarily responsible for rejection of genetically different tissues are known as histocompatibility (i.e. tissue compatibility) antigens and the genes coding for these antigens are referred to as histocompatibility genes. There are more than 30 histocompatibility gene loci, and they cause rejection at different rates. Of these, alloantigens encoded by the genes of the MHC induce particularly strong reactions; these are the molecules that present antigens in a form recognizable to T cells – all vertebrate species have an MHC. In mice the MHC is called H-2, while in man it is known as the human leucocyte antigen (HLA) system (see Chapter 5). The products of allelic variants of the other histocompatibility genes individually cause weaker rejection responses and are consequently known as minor histocompatibility antigens; these antigens are normal cellular constituents. None the less, combinations of several minor antigens can elicit strong rejection responses (*Fig. 26.3*).

MHC haplotypes are inherited from both parents and are co-dominantly expressed

The genes of the MHC are subject to simple Mendelian inheritance and are co-dominantly expressed. In other words, each individual has two 'half-sets' (haplotypes) of genes, one haplotype inherited from each parent (*Fig. 26.4*); both of these haplotypes are expressed equally so that each cell in the offspring has both maternal and paternal MHC molecules on its surface (*Fig. 26.5*).

MHC molecules are expressed on transplanted tissues and induced by cytokines

MHC molecules are not equally distributed on all cells of the body. Class I molecules are normally expressed on most nucleated cells (and on erythrocytes and platelets in some species), while class II molecules are restricted to antigen-presenting cells (APCs, e.g. dendritic cells and activated macrophages), B cells and, in some species, activated T cells and vascular endothelial cells. The expression of MHC on cells is controlled by cytokines: Interferon-γ (IFNγ) and tumour necrosis factor (TNF) are powerful inducers of MHC expression on many cell types which would otherwise express MHC molecules only weakly. As will be seen, this is important in graft rejection (see p. 26.5).

Haplotype inheritance of MHC antigens

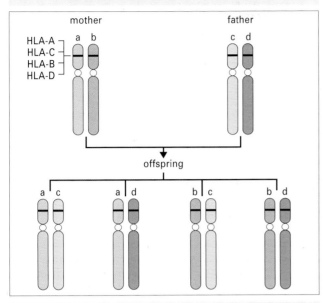

Fig. 26.4 The human MHC (HLA) is located on the short arm of chromosome 6. One set (haplotype) of the MHC class I (HLA-A, B and C) and class II (HLA-D) antigens are inherited en bloc from each parent according to simple Mendelian inheritance.

Co-dominant expression of MHC antigens

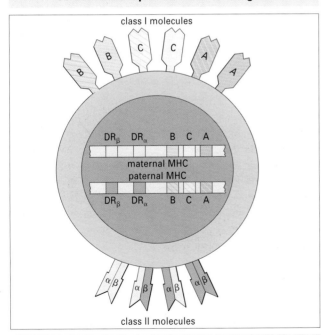

Fig. 26.5 Inherited MHC genes are all expressed on the cell surface. For each maternal and paternal class I gene there are class I molecules on the membrane. For each class II α and β gene there are α and β chains on the cell surface, but these can associate to form four different molecules. Note that there are other class II α and β genes coding for DP and DQ antigens as well. B cells have 23×10^5 class I molecules and the same number of class II molecules per cell.

■ THE LAWS OF TRANSPLANTATION

The transplant situation is unique in that foreign MHC molecules can directly activate T cells. Conventional T cell responses against foreign proteins require that such antigens are processed into peptides and presented on the surface of the recipient's APCs in association with MHC molecules.

Host-versus-graft responses cause transplant rejection

The overriding consideration for organ allograft rejection is whether the graft carries any antigens that are not present in the recipient. This principle of host-versus-graft reactions is illustrated in *Figure 26.6*.

Graft-versus-host reactions result when donor lymphocytes attack the graft recipient

A special situation occurs in bone marrow transplantation, in which graft-versus-host disease (GVHD) is induced by immunologically competent T cells being transplanted into allogeneic recipients which are unable to reject them. This inability may be due to the genetic differences between the donor and recipient, or because of a lack of immunocompetence (through immaturity or immunosuppression) of the recipient. In this situation, the immunocompetent T cells transplanted with the bone marrow can attack the recipient (*Fig. 26.7*). GVHD is a major complication of bone marrow transplantation, causing severe damage, particularly to the skin and intestine, and is avoided by careful typing, removal of mature T cells from the graft and the use of immunosuppressive drugs.

■ THE ROLE OF T LYMPHOCYTES IN REJECTION

T cells are pivotal in graft rejection

Rodents born without a thymus (congenitally athymic or 'nude') have no mature T cells and cannot reject transplants. The same is true of normal rats or mice whose thymus is removed in the neonatal period, before mature T cells are released to the periphery. Likewise, adult thymectomy (AT) of rats or mice (to stop the production of T cells), followed by irradiation (to remove existing mature T cells) and bone marrow (BM) transplantation (to restore haematopoiesis) produces 'ATx.BM recipients' which have no T cells and cannot reject grafts.

In any of these animals (nudes, neonatally thymectomized or ATx.BM), the ability to reject grafts is restored by the injection of T cells from a normal animal of the same strain. Thus, T cells are necessary for rejection. This does not imply that antibodies, B cells or other cells play no part. Indeed, antibodies cause graft damage and macrophages may be involved in inflammatory reactions in grafted tissue.

Rejection responses have a molecular basis in the TCR–MHC interaction

Via their T-cell receptors (TCRs), the T cells involved in rejection recognize donor-derived peptides in association with the MHC antigens expressed on the graft. As we already know, the structure of the T-cell receptor (TCR) (see Chapter 5) is such that T cells can only 'see' peptide antigens when they are associated with MHC molecules, and this MHC restriction is imposed by positive selection in the thymus (see Chapters 10 and 12 and *Fig. 26.8*). So to understand the involvement of T cells in rejection, we need to examine the differences between recipient and graft MHC molecules and how such differences affect the range of antigens presented to the recipient's TCR.

Different MHC molecules have similar structures but different peptide-binding grooves

The structures of different MHC molecules are almost identical, with the overall shape consisting of two α helices lying on a β-pleated sheet atop two immunoglobulin-like domains which sit on the cell membrane (see Chapter 5). Between the α helices is a deep groove into which peptides can be bound. The part of the MHC molecule that is important in T-cell recognition is the outer surface of these α helices, which is highly conserved between different MHC molecules.

The significant amino-acid sequence differences between two MHC molecules – comparing the example, A2 and Aw68 allelic variants of the HLA-A antigen – lie deep in the groove between the α helices, not on the outer surface contacted by the TCR (see Chapter 5). Hence, for T-cell recognition, the principal difference between MHC molecules is in the shape and charge of the peptide-binding groove (see Chapter 5), and this governs which peptides can be bound and in what orientation they are presented to TCRs (see Chapter 7).

Graft and host MHC molecules present different peptides

In the normal physiological situation, the MHC groove is occupied by peptides derived from normal cellular constituents by intracellular degradative pathways. Thymic tolerance mechanisms (clonal deletion of self-reactive T cells – see Chapter 12) ensure that T-cell recognition of these self-peptide–self-MHC complexes, which would lead to autoimmunity, does not occur. However, when cells are infected (with virus, for example), the normal cell-derived peptides are replaced by peptides of foreign origin, as in the case in 'professional' APCs. T cells then respond to these foreign peptides in association with self-MHC molecules.

However, in the case of a genetically distinct transplanted tissue, a third situation arises. A different array of peptides is presented on the cell surface because of the different shape and charge of the groove in the graft's MHC molecules. In addition, the graft may have different allelic forms of the normal cellular constituents (determined by minor histocompatibility loci), giving rise to an altogether new and foreign selection of peptides. In this way differences between graft donor and recipient in their MHC molecules (differently shaped and charged grooves) or in their minor histocompatibility antigens (different peptides) leads to the expression on transplanted tissues of a very large number of foreign novel antigens which can be recognized by recipient T cells. Up to 10% of an individual's T cells may respond to these antigens on the tissues from an allogeneic donor.

Host-versus-graft reactions

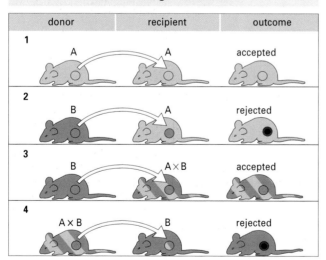

Fig. 26.6 Grafts between genetically identical animals are accepted. Grafts between genetically non-identical animals are rejected with a speed which is dependent on where the genetic differences lie. For example syngeneic animals, which are identical at the MHC locus, accept grafts from each other (1). Animals that differ at the MHC locus reject grafts from each other (2). The ability to accept a graft is dependent on the recipient sharing all the donor's histocompatibility genes: this is illustrated by the difference between grafting from parental to (A × B)F1 animals (3) and vice versa (4). Animals that differ at loci other than the MHC reject grafts from each other, but much more slowly.

Graft-versus-host disease

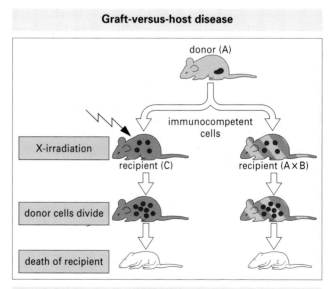

Fig. 26.7 Immunocompetent cells from a donor of type A are injected into an immunosuppressed (X-irradiated) host of type C, or a normal (A × B)F1 recipient. The immunosuppressed individual is unable to reject the cells and the F1 animal is fully tolerant to parental type A cells. In both cases the donor cells recognize the foreign tissue types B or C of the recipient. They divide and react against the recipient tissue cells and recruit large numbers of host cells to inflammatory sites. Very often the process leads to the death of the recipient.

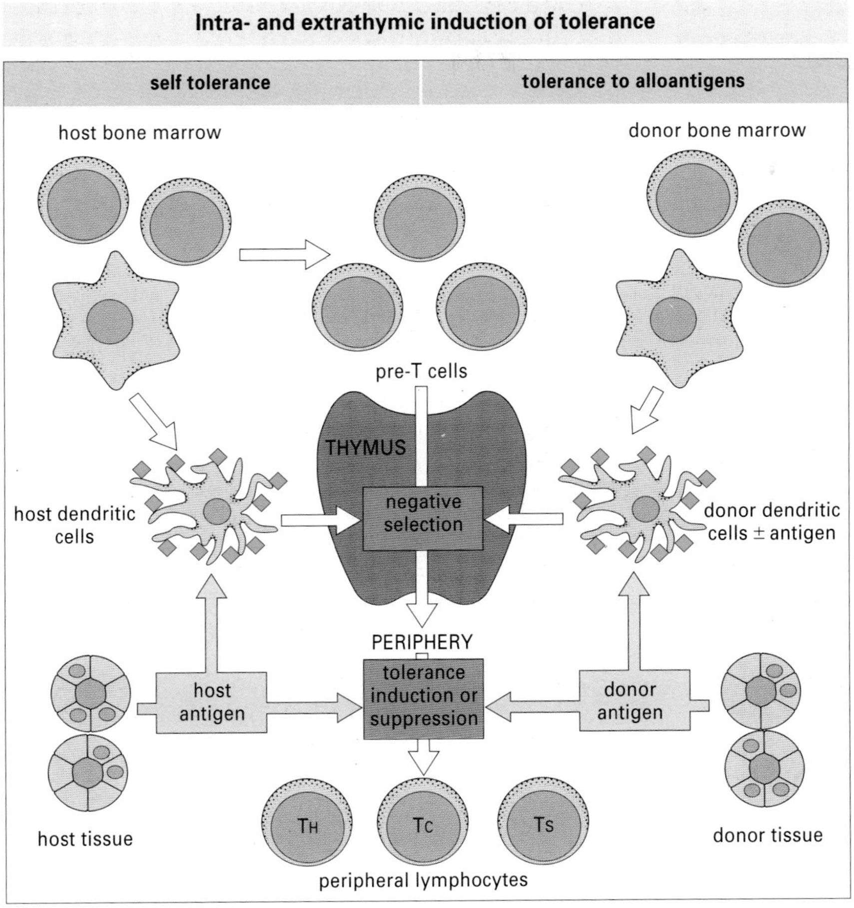

Intra- and extrathymic induction of tolerance

Fig. 26.8 Under normal physiological conditions bone marrow-derived pre-T cells enter the thymus and undergo positive selection for interaction with self MHC (rescue from programmed cell death) when they meet epithelial cells in the cortex and negative selection (deletion of self-reactive clones) when they contact dendritic cells at the corticomedullary junction. Newly derived self-reactive T cells can still be inactivated outside the thymus (but not necessarily eliminated) by antigen in the periphery; alternatively, they can become activated suppressor cells.

In allotolerant animals, foreign antigen may be present in the thymic medulla (as donor-type dendritic cells, i.e. 'passenger cells' or as donor antigen presented by recipient dendritic cells) where, performing the same function as self antigen, it can cause tolerance by negative selection of T cells that react with it (clonal deletion). Alternatively, foreign antigen in the periphery may cause clonal anergy (unresponsiveness – tolerance induction) or stimulate active suppression in allotolerant animals.

T Helper (TH) cells and lymphokines are involved in rejection

The role of T helper (TH) cells in rejection

Injecting T cells of the CD4$^+$ subpopulation (TH cells) into nude or ATx.BM recipients leads to acute skin-graft rejection. Naive, unsensitized CD8$^+$ T cells (TC cells) are unable to do this, but when CD8$^+$ T cells are mixed with a very low number of CD4$^+$ T cells, or are pre-sensitized to graft antigens (i.e. taken from animals which have already rejected a graft), rapid graft destruction is then seen. Treating recipients with monoclonal anti-CD4$^+$ antibodies (*Fig. 26.9*) confirms the importance of TH cells in rejection.

TH cells are activated by APCs derived from bone marrow and carrying MHC class II molecules. The APCs activating rejection can come from either the donor or the recipient. Those of donor origin are present in the graft as 'passenger leucocytes' (interstitial dendritic cells) and they cause 'direct' activation of the recipient's TH cells. Those of recipient origin are located in draining lymphoid tissues and acquire antigen that is shed from the transplant, and present it to the recipient's TH cells to cause 'indirect' activation. Direct activation is a more powerful stimulus to rejection than the so-called indirect route. Thus, passenger cells may have a strong influence on graft survival (*Fig. 26.10*).

The role of lymphokines in rejection

In addition to the role of CD4$^+$ TH cells, a multiplicity of immunological mechanisms including lymphokines are involved in the process of rejection. The overall picture is shown in *Figure 26.11*.

The most important lymphokines in cellular rejection are interleukin-2 (IL-2), which is required for activation of TC cells, and IFNγ, which induces MHC expression, increases APC activity, activates large granular lymphocytes and, in concert with TNFβ (lymphotoxin), activates macrophages. (Note: the mixture of IFNγ and TNFβ was formerly known as macrophage activating factor or MAF.)

Lymphokines (IL-4, 5 and 6) are also required for B-cell activation, leading to the production of anti-graft antibodies. These antibodies fix complement and cause damage to the vascular endothelium, resulting in haemorrhage, platelet aggregation within the vessels, graft thrombosis, lytic damage to cells of the transplant, and the release of the pro-inflammatory complement components C3a and C5a.

Not all parts of the graft need to be attacked for rejection to occur. The critical targets are the vascular endothelium of the microvasculature and the specialized parenchymal cells of the organ, such as renal tubules, pancreatic islets of Langerhans or cardiac myocytes.

IFNγ can cause vascular endothelial cells to express high levels of class II MHC molecules, and can induce the expression of class I and II molecules on parenchymal cells, which usually express little or none of these. This upregulation of MHC expression on cells of the graft can provoke greater stimulation of the rejection response and provide a greater number of target molecules within the graft for antibodies and activated cells.

TNFβ and IFNγ also upregulate the expression of adhesion molecules on vascular endothelium. These are required for the adhesion of blood-borne leucocytes to the walls of blood vessels prior to their migration across the endothelium into the tissues.

■ THE TEMPO OF REJECTION

The rate of rejection depends in part on the underlying effector mechanisms (*Fig. 26.12*).

Hyperacute rejection – This occurs very rapidly in patients who already have antibodies against a graft. Anti-HLA antibodies are induced by prior blood transfusions, multiple pregnancies or the rejection of a previous transplant. In addition, antibodies against the ABO blood group system can cause hyperacute rejection. Pre-formed antibodies fix complement, damaging the endothelial cell-lining of the blood vessels. This damage allows the leakage of cells and fluids and causes aggre-

gation of platelets which then block the microvasculature depriving the graft of a blood supply (*Fig. 26.13*; see also p. 23.5). Hyperacute rejection can be avoided by ABO matching and by performing cross-matching, in which serum from a prospective recipient is tested for the presence of cytotoxic anti-donor antibodies.

Because humans have pre-formed IgM and IgG natural antibodies to animal cells, hyperacute rejection prevents transplantation of animal organs to man. Various approaches to overcoming this – by removing the antibodies, depleting complement or genetically engineering donor animals whose tissues are less susceptible to hyperacute rejection – are under active investigation.

Acute rejection – This takes days or weeks to become manifest and is due to the primary activation of T cells and the consequent triggering of various effector mechanisms (*Figs 26.14–26.16*). If a transplant is given to someone who has been pre-sensitized to antigens on the graft, a secondary reactivation of T cells occurs, leading to an accelerated cell-mediated rejection response. Accelerated or 'second-set' rejection of skin grafts is particularly dramatic, the so-called 'white graft rejection' in which the graft is rejected before it has time to heal (*Fig. 26.17*).

Chronic rejection – Depending on the genetic disparity between donor and recipient and the use of immunosuppressive treatment, graft rejection can be a slow process tak-

---

Role of T cells in graft rejection

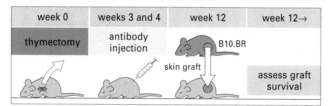

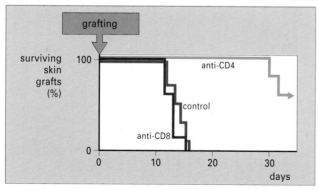

Fig. 26.9 Thymectomized CBA mice were treated with cytotoxic monoclonal antibodies to CD4 or CD8, to selectively deplete TH and TC cell populations, respectively. They were then grafted with skin from B10.BR mice, which differ at minor histocompatibility loci. The survival of the grafts was assessed. Animals treated with anti-CD4 had greatly extended graft survival by comparison with untreated animals (control) or those treated with anti-CD8. This emphasizes the importance of the CD4+ (TH) population in graft rejection. (Based on data of Cobbold and colleagues.)

The role of passenger cells in graft destruction

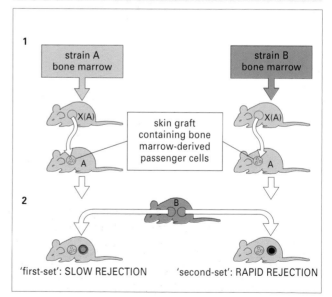

Fig. 26.10 Strain A mice were X-irradiated (X(A)) and then reconstituted with bone marrow cells of either strain A or strain B. Skin grafts from these mice were accepted by strain A mice (1). The recipients subsequently received strain B skin grafts. Animals whose first graft came from an animal reconstituted with strain A cells rejected the strain B graft more slowly than animals whose first graft came from a mouse reconstituted with strain B cells (2). This implies that strain B bone marrow cells, carried as passengers in the first graft, primed the recipient to strain B alloantigen.

Immunological components of rejection

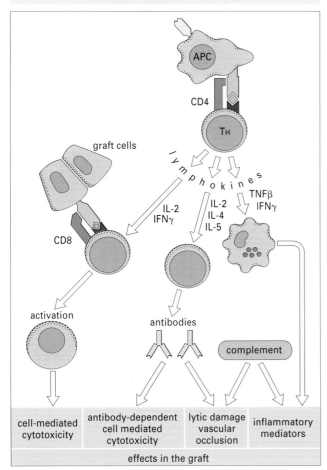

Fig. 26.11 Tн cells are activated by APCs to release lymphokines. IL-2 and IFNγ are required for Tc-cell activation; IL-2, IL-4 and IL-5 are involved in B-cell activation; a mixture of TNFβ (lymphotoxin) and IFNγ acts as macrophage-activating factor (MAF). These cells reject the graft by specific cell-mediated and antibody-mediated immune pathways, or by non-specific inflammatory reactions.

Tempo of rejection reactions

type of rejection	time taken	cause
hyperacute	minutes–hours	pre-formed anti-donor antibodies and complement
accelerated	days	reactivation of sensitized T cells
acute	days–weeks	primary activation of T cells
chronic	months–years	causes are unclear: antibodies, immune complexes, slow cellular reaction, recurrence of disease

Fig. 26.12 Much can be determined about the mechanisms of rejection by observing the speed of graft damage. Pre-formed antibodies and presensitized lymphocytes cause rapid rejection compared with primary and slowly evolving responses.

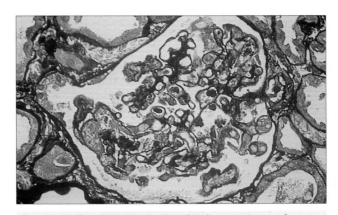

Fig. 26.13 Renal histology showing hyperacute graft rejection. There is extensive necrosis of the glomerular capillary associated with massive interstitial haemorrhage. This extensive necrosis is preceded by an intense polymorphonuclear infiltration which occurs within the first hour of the graft's revascularization. The changes shown here occurred 24–48 hours after this. H&E stain, × 200.

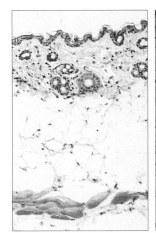
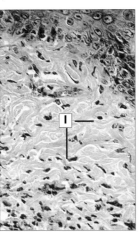
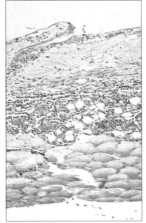

Fig. 26.14 Sections of strain A mouse skin showing the normal appearance (left) and the allograft 5 days (middle) and 12 days (right) after transplantation to a CBA host.
At 5 days there is a substantial infiltration (I) of the allograft area by host mononuclear cells. At 12 days the epithelium has been totally destroyed and is lifting off the dermis, which is now free of cells; the infiltrating host cells have been destroyed by anoxia but there is still a brisk cellular traffic in the graft bed between the dermis and the panniculus carnosus. (Courtesy of Professor L. Brent.)

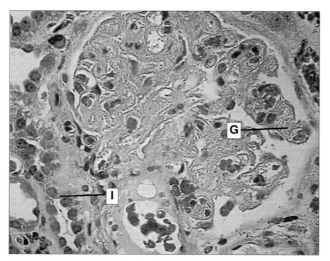

Fig. 26.15 Renal histology showing acute graft rejection – I.
Small lymphocytes and other cells are accumulating in the
interstitium of the graft. Such infiltration (I) is characteristic of
acute rejection and occurs before the appearance of any clinical
signs. (G = glomerulus.) H&E stain, × 200.

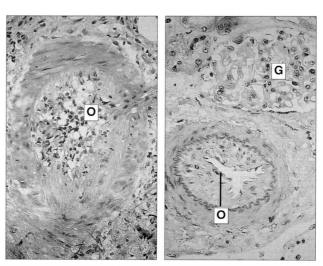

Fig. 26.16 Renal histology showing acute graft rejection – II.
The section of acutely rejecting kidney on the left (H&E stain)
shows vascular obstruction (o) and that on the right (van Gieson's
stain) the end stage of this process (g = glomerulus). × 140.

ing months or years. The walls of the blood vessels in the graft
thicken and eventually become blocked. This is called chronic rejection and may be due to several different causes, such
as a low-grade cell-mediated rejection or the deposition of
antibodies or antigen–antibody complexes in the grafted tissue, which damage or activate the endothelial cells lining the
vessel and trigger inappropriate repair responses. Grafts may
also be damaged by the recurrence of the disease process that
originally necessitated the original transplant.

■ PREVENTION OF REJECTION

The rejection response can be reduced by tissue matching

The perfectly matched donor and recipient would be isogeneic, for example monozygotic twins. However, this situation is rare, and in all other cases there will be major and/or
minor histocompatibility differences between the donor and

recipient. Only the major (MHC, i.e. HLA) antigens can be
practicably matched. This can be done by serology (*Fig.
26.18*), which takes only a few hours and can therefore be performed while the donor organ is preserved on ice. Recently,
sensitive and accurate typing has been achieved using the polymerase chain reaction (PCR) (see Chapter 28) to identify
HLA genes in the DNA of donors and recipients.

Matching for all known HLA antigens is practically impossible, but good organ graft survival is obtained when the
donor and recipient share only the same MHC class II antigens, especially HLA-DR (*Fig. 26.19*), because these are the
antigens that directly activate the recipient's TH cells.

The lists of known class I (HLA-A, HLA-B and HLA-C)
and class II (HLA-DP, HLA-DQ and HLA-DR) antigens
are long (*Fig. 26.20*), and the chances of completely matching two individuals at random are extremely remote.

The mixed lymphocyte reaction (MLR) can also be used
to test the responsiveness of recipient lymphocytes to
antigens expressed on donor cells (*Fig. 26.21*). Low recipient

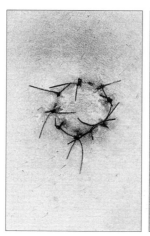
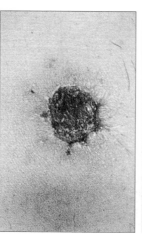
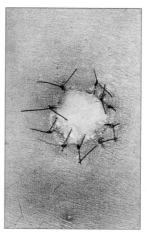

**Fig. 26.17 Graft rejection displays
immunological memory.** A human
skin allograft at day 5 (left) is fully
vascularized and the cells are dividing,
but by day 12 (middle) it is totally
destroyed. A second graft ('second-set'
graft) from the same donor shown here
on day 7 (right) does not become
vascularized and is destroyed rapidly.
This indicates that sensitization to the
first graft produces immunological
memory.

anti-donor MLR responses are associated with excellent transplant survival. However, the 4–5 days required for the MLR test precludes its use in most clinical organ transplantation, because organs from dead or brain-dead donors cannot be preserved for more than 24–48 hours. In cases where living donors (e.g. relatives) are to be used, it can be used. The MLR is especially important in bone-marrow transplantation to assess whether the donor bone marrow cells can respond to recipient antigens and cause GVHD (see p. 26.4).

Non-specific immunosuppression can control rejection reactions

There are two main categories of immunosuppressive treatment, antigen non-specific and antigen specific immunosuppression. Non-specific immunosuppression blunts or abolishes the activity of the immune system regardless of the antigen. This can leave a graft recipient very vulnerable to infections.

For instance, a large dose of X-rays prevents rejection but also has many deleterious effects, as well as abolishing antimicrobial immunity. Most non-specific treatments used today are selective for the immune system, or are used in a way which creates some selectivity. The very best treatment would take this further and inactivate only those clones of lymphocytes with specificity for donor antigens, leaving other clones intact, so that the patient does not suffer infections or side effects. Such highly specific immunosuppression remains the 'Holy Grail' of transplantation immunobiology and is described later (see p. 26.11).

The three non-specific agents that are most widely used in current clinical practice are steroids, cyclosporin and azathioprine (*Fig. 26.22*).

Steroids have anti-inflammatory properties and suppress activated macrophages, interfere with APC function and reduce the expression of MHC antigens. In effect, steroids reverse many of the actions of IFNγ on macrophages and transplanted tissues.

Cyclosporin is a fungal macrolide (see *Fig. 26.23*) produced by soil organisms, and has interesting and potent immunosuppressive properties. Its principal action is to suppress lymphokine production by Tн cells by interfering with

Serological tissue typing

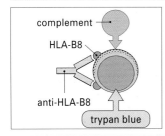

Fig. 26.18 Tissue typing is performed serologically by adding typing antisera of defined specificity (e.g. anti-HLA-B8), complement and trypan blue stain to test cells on a microassay plate. Cell death, as assessed by trypan blue staining, confirms that the test cell carried the antigen in question (HLA–B8). Dead, trypan blue-stained cells (dark staining) are shown on the right.

Kidney graft survival and HLA matching

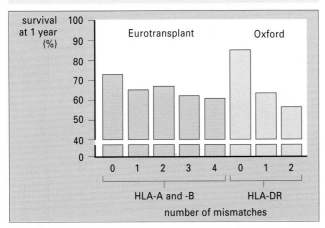

Fig. 26.19 The bar chart shows the percentage survival of cadaver kidney grafts at 1 year in humans in two separate studies. In the first study (Eurotransplant), donors were matched for HLA-A and -B (class I). In the second study (Oxford) donors were matched for HLA-DR (class II).

Serologically detected HLA specificities

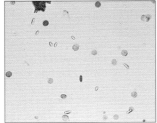

locus	class I			class II		
	A	B	C	DR	DQ	DP
antigens	1	5	w50	w1	1	w1	w1
	2	7	51	w2	2	w2	w2
	3	8	w52	w3	3	w3	w3
	9	12	w53	w4	4	w4	w4
	10	13	w54	w5	5	w5	w5
	11	14	w55	w6	w6	w6	w6
	w19	15	w56	w7	7	w7	
	23	16	w57	w8	w8	w8	
	24	17	w58	w9	w9	w9	
	25	18	w59	w10	w10		
	26	21	w60	w11	w11		
	28	w22	w61		w12		
	29	27	w62		w13		
	30	35	w63		w14		
	31	37	w64		w15		
	32	38	w65		w16		
	w33	39	w67		w17		
	w34	40	w70		w18		
	w36	w41	w71		w52		
	w43	w42	w72		w53		
	w66	44	w73				
	w68	45	w75				
	w69	w46	w76				
	w74	w47	w4				
		w48	w6				
		49					

Fig. 26.20 Approximately 80 different class I (HLA-A, B and C) molecules and over 35 different class II (HLA-DP, DQ and DR) molecules are recognized in humans. The techniques of molecular genetics are leading to the discovery of many more variants. Not all of these newly discovered variants, however, are serologically distinguishable.

the activation of lymphokine genes and, directly or indirectly, to reduce the expression of the receptors for IL-2 on lymphocytes undergoing activation. Other macrolides such as FK506 and Rapamycin also have immunosuppressive properties. FK506 suppresses lymphokine production by TH cells in a way similar to cyclosporin. Rapamycin interferes with the intracellular signalling pathways of the IL-2 receptor and therefore prevents IL-2-dependent lymphocyte activation.

The rejection response involves the rapid division and differentiation – proliferation – of lymphocytes. Azathioprine is an anti-proliferative drug, an analogue of 6-mercaptopurine. Its incorporation into the DNA of dividing cells prevents further proliferation. New anti-proliferative drugs, such as mycophenolic acid derivatives, are under investigation.

These agents can be effective used alone, although high doses are usually required and the likelihood of adverse toxic effects is increased. Used together in various combinations they work in synergy because they interfere with different stages of the same immune pathway. The doses of individual agents can thus be reduced and the adverse effects minimized. The clinical results obtained since the introduction of cyclosporin are very good (85–90% graft acceptance at 1 year for kidneys, hearts and livers). However, the expected half-life of a kidney transplant is 7–8 years because of the problem of chronic rejection, and long-term use of drugs is still associated with adverse effects. Further improvements might be obtained with the introduction of new drugs.

New non-specific but more selective agents are under development (*Fig. 26.24*). Monoclonal antibodies against lymphocyte surface molecules, especially CD3, CD4, CD8 and the IL-2 receptor can be used to eliminate cells or to block their function. Cytotoxic drugs can be attached to these antibodies to increase their effectiveness. A related approach is to attach a toxin to IL-2 so that cells undergoing activation in response to graft antigens and expressing receptors for IL-2 take up the IL-2–toxin conjugate and are selectively poisoned.

Specific immunosuppression reduces anti-graft responses without increasing susceptibility to infection

The immune system is regulated by various feedback mechanisms that control the magnitude, type and specificity of immunological reactions (see Chapter 11). It is possible, in experimental models, to harness these feedback systems to prevent transplant rejection. There are three classical procedures which can be used: neonatally-induced tolerance, active enhancement and passive enhancement.

Neonatal exposure to donor antigen can induce unresponsiveness to transplants in animals

Neonatal rodents (unlike humans) are born just before mature T cells are first exported from the thymus (the equivalent stage of human development is 16–20 weeks' gestation). If a persistent source of antigen, for instance viable cells with potential for growth or repeated injections of antigen, is given to the neonate rodents, the development of mature T cells that react with that antigen is suppressed. Classically, bone marrow cells from an (A × B) F$_1$ mouse are injected into a B-strain neonate. (The donor cells used are (A × B) F$_1$ to obviate the A-strain anti-B GVH reaction that occurs if A donor

Tissue typing – mixed lymphocyte reaction

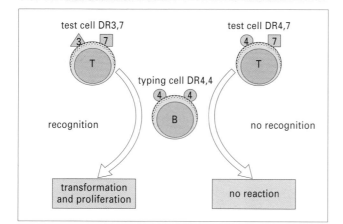

Fig. 26.21 In the mixed lymphocyte reaction, the cells being tested are incubated with 'typing' cells of known HLA specificity (DR4,4 in this case). The DR3,7 cells recognize the typing cell as foreign; this is revealed by the test cells transforming and proliferating (the typing cells are treated to stop them dividing in response to test cells). Conversely, DR4,7, which carries the typing cell's specificity (DR4), does not recognize the typing cell and so does not react to it.

Immunosuppression with drugs

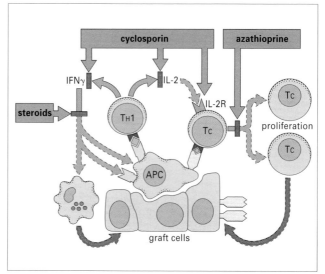

Fig. 26.22 The agents in common clinical use, steroids, cyclosporin and azathioprine, suppress the rejection response at different points. Steroids are anti-inflammatory and suppress activated macrophages, decrease APC function, and reduce MHC expression. Cyclosporin interferes with lymphokine production. Azathioprine prevents the proliferation of activated cells.

cells are used). The bone marrow inoculum produces cells that provide a continuous source of antigen. When the B-strain mouse grows to adulthood it is unresponsive to the A antigens to which it has been exposed neonatally and is tolerant of the A antigens on skin grafts and other tissues from A or $(A \times B)F_1$ strain donors. Mechanisms to account for neonatal tolerance are outlined in *Figure 26.8* and detailed in Chapter 10.

Antigen may selectively activate certain subpopulations of lymphocytes. It is currently proposed that there are two major types of TH cell, known as TH1 and TH2 cells (see Chapter 8). Neonatally tolerized mice can have a deficit of donor-spe-

cific TH1 cells and an increased number of donor-specific TH2 cells. TH1 cells make IFNγ and IL-2 and are the TH cells illustrated in *Figure 26.22*, which are involved in rejection. In contrast, TH2 cells make other lymphokines including IL-10 or cytokine synthesis inhibitory factor (CSIF), which interferes with the synthesis of lymphokines by TH1 cells. For neonatally tolerized mice, fewer donor-specific TH1 cells and more donor-specific TH2 cells mean a shift in the balance between rejection and acceptance, leading to tolerance of the graft. This form of tolerance is not strictly unresponsiveness *per se* but, rather, a deviated response. Interestingly, cyclosporin may have a preferential effect on TH1 cells and spare TH2 cells.

Finally, antigen can activate suppressor T cells (Ts cells). The precise identity of these T cells is still shrouded in mystery. What is known is that, when transferred to another animal, T cells from an animal tolerant of a graft from donor A can prevent rejection of a graft carrying A antigens. This is referred to as the adoptive transfer of suppression and the cells responsible can be TH or Ts cells. Much controversy still exists concerning Ts cells and their mode of action, but experimental data provide a clear indication that functional Ts cells do exist. They are resistant to cyclosporin and may contribute to this agent's mode of action and mediate tolerance by active suppression.

Equivalents in man – A direct equivalent of neonatally-induced tolerance is not possible in humans. However, procedures such as total lymphoid irradiation (TLI), in which mature lymphocytes are severely depleted by radiation while the bone marrow is shielded and therefore remains intact, may create in adults a situation analogous to that in the neonatal rodent. Indeed, TLI followed by antigen exposure induces

The structure of immunosuppressive fungal macrolides

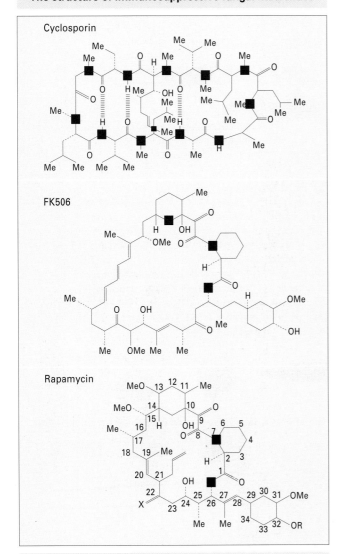

Fig. 26.23 The immunosuppressive fungal macrolides, cyclosporin, FK506 and Rapamycin, have quite different structures. They act on lymphocytes in different ways, cyclosporin and FK506 affecting lymphokine production and Rapamycin interfering with signalling through the IL-2 receptor (IL-2R).

Selective approaches to immunosuppression

agent		target
heterologous antisera/ antibodies	anti-lymphocyte serum (ALS) anti-thymocyte globulin (ATG)	all lymphocytes selective for T cells
monoclonal antibodies	anti-CD3 anti-CD4 anti-CD25 (IL-2R)	mature T cells TH cells activated T cells
antibody–toxin conjugates	anti-CD5 coupled to the A chain of ricin toxin	activated (CD5+) T cells
lymphokine–toxin conjugates	IL-2 coupled to diphtheria toxin	activated T cells (which express IL-2r)
complement inactivating molecules	DAF/MCP CD59 transfected into donor cells (especially of xenografts)	complement-mediated damage via the classical and alternative pathways

Fig. 26.24 Antibodies and lymphokines can be targeted to cells of the immune system. By contrast, drugs can have adverse effects on non-lymphoid tissue, e.g. nephrotoxicity and hepatotoxicity. The efficacy of biological agents can be increased by coupling drugs or toxins to them.

profound tolerance. However, TLI is rather hazardous for routine clinical use. Anti-lymphocyte serum (ALS), made by immunizing animals with human lymphocytes, is widely used in heart transplant recipients to deplete circulating T cells. The use of monoclonal antibodies to mature T cells may achieve their depletion in a much safer but equally effective way, and anti-CD3 antibodies are in clinical use.

Unresponsiveness to transplants can be induced in humans by blood transfusions

In some cases, prior exposure to donor antigens can cause prolonged or indefinite graft survival (*Fig. 26.25*). This is, of course, contrary to expectation since one might expect accelerated or hyperacute rejection. The phenomenon is called active enhancement of graft survival. The route of exposure to antigen is important, possibly because it impinges on particular lymphoid tissues. It has been shown in a rat kidney-graft model that a transfusion of donor blood given intravenously to the recipient 1 week before kidney transplantation leads to long-term organ graft acceptance, while the same dose of blood given subcutaneously causes accelerated rejection. The effect is immunologically specific, so the blood donor and the kidney donor must share at least some antigens.

An active enhancement effect has been employed clinically using donor-specific transfusions (DST). For example, if a parent is about to donate a kidney to a child, the recipient can be treated with blood transfusions from the parent before transplantation. Unfortunately, about 20% of patients receiving DST develop anti-donor antibodies and cannot then receive the kidney as planned, for fear of hyperacute rejection. However, of the remaining 80% the transplant success rate is 95–100%.

The beneficial effect of pre-transplant blood transfusion, known as the blood transfusion effect, has also been documented in patients receiving random transfusions, perhaps because of the chance exposure to antigens which happen to be on their transplant (*Fig. 26.26*). Indeed, the blood transfusion effect increases with the number of random transfusions, and for a time most transplant centres adopted the policy of deliberately transfusing prospective recipients. However, there is always a risk of sensitization of the patient, as well as the transmission of AIDS, and improvements in the availability and use of immunosuppressive drugs have largely made this practice redundant.

Active enhancement requires an active response by the recipient to the injected donor antigen. The mechanism could be induction of anergy, selective activation of TH2 cells, or activation of Ts cells by the blood transfusion, as described for neonatally-induced tolerance. Alternatively, the mechanism might involve the production of 'enhancing antibodies' which block recognition of specific donor antigens, thus interfering with the graft rejection process, or by destroying highly immunogenic passenger leucocytes within the graft. Enhancing antibodies may also be formed to antigen receptors, thus eliminating donor reactive cells or affecting antigen presentation so that, for instance, TH2 and Ts cells are selectively activated after transplantation.

Antibody can play a feedback role in transplanted individuals. Injection of anti-donor antibody (passive enhancement) into a rat kidney graft recipient at the time of grafting can cause long-term graft acceptance (see *Fig. 26.25*).

Immunological enhancement of graft survival

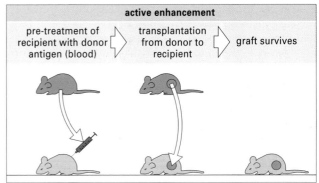

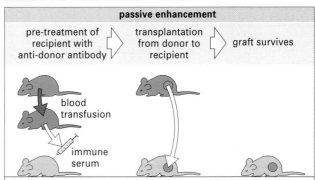

Fig. 26.25 Pre-treatment of recipients with donor antigen given intravenously can prolong the survival of a subsequent allograft. This is known as active enhancement of graft survival because the effect requires an active response on the part of the recipient. (Note that the same blood, given by a different route, can result in rapid rejection.) Alternatively, anti-donor antibody given to the recipient at the time of transplantation can cause passive enhancement of graft survival. Both active and passive enhancement are immunologically specific since only the response to the particular donor is suppressed and the survival of 'third-party' unrelated grafts is not enhanced.

The effect of blood transfusion on kidney transplantation

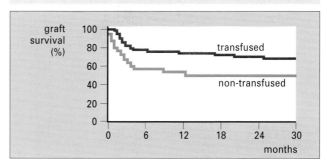

Fig. 26.26 Survival of kidney grafts is higher in transfused patients (102 patients) than in non-transfused patients (71 patients).

Critical Thinking

■ In what ways do the responses induced by direct activation of recipient T cells by donor peptide-donor MHC complexes differ from those induced by indirect activation by donor peptide-recipient MHC complexes

■ What methods might be used to limit rejection of endocrine tissue, for example, Islets of Langerhans?

■ Blood transfusion before a kidney graft enhances survival. How might development of anti-donor antibodies be prevented?

■ Would a kidney graft to a pregnant women lead to enhanced graft survival or an increased rate of rejection?

■ How do both routes of immunization contribute to graft rejection?

■ What combination of treatment with drugs, antibodies or antigens do you think would be most effective in inducing the acceptance of a histoincompatible transplant?

FURTHER READING

Alexandre GPJ, Latime D, Gianello P, Squiflet JP. Preformed cytotoxic antibodies and ABO-incompatible grafts. *Clin Transplant* 1991;**5**:583.

Bach FH. Xerotransplantation: problems for consideration.*Clin Transplant* 1991;**5**:595.

Bjorkman PJ, Saper MA, Samaouri B, Bennett WS, Strominger JL, Wiley DC. The foreign antigen binding site and T cell recognition regions of class I histocompatibility antigens. *Nature* 1987;**329**:512.

Burdick JF. Chronic rejection. *Clin Transplant* 1991;**5**:489.

Concar D. The organ factory of the future? *New Scientist* 1994;**1930**:24–29.

Dallman MJ, Clark GJ. Cytokines and their receptors in transplantation. *Curr Opin Immunol* 1991;**3**:729.

Hall BM, Dorsch S, Roser B. The cellular basis of allograft rejection *in vivo*. I. The cellular requirements for first set rejection of heart grafts. *J Exp Med* 1978;**148**:878.

Halloran PF, Broski AP, Batiuk TD, Madrenas J. The molecular immunology of acute rejection: an overview. *Transplant Immunol* 1993;**1**:3–27.

Hunt S, Billingham M. Long-term results of cardiac transplantation. *Ann Rev Med* 1991;**42**:437.

Hutchinson IV. Cellular mechanisms of allograft rejection. *Curr Opin Immunol* 1991;**3**:722.

Lechler RI, Lombardi G, Batchelor JR, Reinsmoen N, Bach FH. The molecular basis of alloreactivity. *Immunol Today* 1990;**11**:83.

Mason DW, Morris PJ. Effector mechanisms in allograft rejection. *Ann Rev Immunol* 1986;**4**:119.

Masoor S, Schroeder TJ, Michler RE, Alexander JW, First MR. Monoclonal antibodies in organ transplantation: an overview. *Transplant Immunol* 1986;**4**:176–189.

Opelz G. Effect of HLA matching in heart transplantation. *Transplant Proc* 1989;**21**:794.

Platt JL, Bach FH. The barrier to xenotransplantation. *Transplantation* 1991;**52**:937.

Sablinski T, Hancock WW, Tilney NL, Kupiec-Weglinski JW. CD4 monoclonal antibodies in organ transplantation. A review of progress. *Transplantation* 1991;**52**:579.

Sachs DH, Bach FH. Immunology of xenograft rejection. *Human Immunol* 1990;**28**:245.

Steinmuller D. Which T cells mediate allograft rejection? *Transplantion* 1985;**40**:229.

Thomson AW. Immunosuppressive drugs and the induction of transplantation tolerance. *Transplant Immunol* 1994;**2**:263–270.

Waldmann H. Manipulation of T-cell responses with monoclonal antibodies. *Ann Rev Immunol* 1989;**7**:407.

Wood KJ. Transplantation tolerance. *Curr Opin Immunol* 1991;**3**:710.

Autoimmune mechanisms underly many diseases, some organ-specific, others systemic in distribution.

Autoimmune disorders can overlap: an individual may have more than one organ-specific disorder; or more than one systemic disease.

Genetic factors such as HLA type are important in autoimmune disease, and it is probable that each disease involves several factors.

Autoimmune mechanisms are pathogenic in experimental and spontaneous animal models associated with the development of autoimmunity.

Human autoantibodies can be directly pathogenic.

Immune complexes are often associated with systemic autoimmune disease.

Autoreactive B and T cells persist in normal subjects but in disease are selected by autoantigen in the production of autoimmune responses.

Microbial cross-reacting antigens and cytokine dysregulation can lead to autoimmunity.

Autoantibody tests are valuable for diagnosis and sometimes for prognosis.

Treatment of organ-specific diseases usually involves metabolic control.

Treatment of systemic diseases includes the use of anti-inflammatory and immunosuppressive drugs.

Future treatment will probably focus on manipulation of the pivotal autoreactive T cells by antigens or peptides, by anti CD4 and possibly T-cell vaccination.

■ THE ASSOCIATION OF AUTOIMMUNITY WITH DISEASE

The immune system has tremendous diversity and because the repertoire of specificities expressed by the B- and T-cell populations is generated randomly, it is bound to include many which are specific for self components. Thus, the body must establish self-tolerance mechanisms, to distinguish between self and non-self determinants, so as to avoid autoreactivity (see Chapter 12). However, all mechanisms have a risk of breakdown. The self-recognition mechanisms are no exception, and a number of diseases have been identified in which there is autoimmunity, due to copious production of autoantibodies and autoreactive T cells.

One of the earliest examples in which the production of autoantibodies was associated with disease in a given organ is Hashimoto's thyroiditis. Among the autoimmune diseases, thyroiditis has been particularly well-studied, and many of the aspects discussed in this chapter will draw upon our knowledge of it. It is a disease of the thyroid which is most common in middle-aged women and often leads to formation of a goitre and hypothyroidism. The gland is infiltrated, sometimes to an extraordinary extent, with inflammatory lymphoid cells. These are predominantly mononuclear phagocytes, lymphocytes and plasma cells, and secondary lymphoid follicles are common (*Fig. 27.1*). In Hashimoto's disease, the gland often shows regenerating thyroid follicles but this is not a feature of the thyroid in the related condition, primary myxoedema, in which comparable immunological features are seen and where the gland undergoes almost complete destruction and shrinks.

The serum of patients with Hashimoto's disease usually contains antibodies to thyroglobulin. These antibodies are demonstrable by agglutination and by precipitin reactions when present in high titre. Many patients also have antibodies

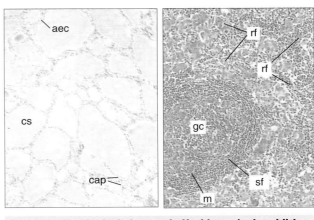

Fig. 27.1 Histological changes in Hashimoto's thyroiditis. In the normal thyroid gland (left), the follicular cells or acinar epithelial cells (aec) line the colloid space (cs) into which they secrete thyroglobulin, which is broken down on demand to provide thyroid hormones (cap = capillaries containing red blood cells). In the Hashimoto gland (right), the normal architecture is virtually destroyed and replaced by invading cells (ic), which consist essentially of lymphocytes, macrophages and plasma cells. A secondary lymphoid follicle (sf), with a germinal centre (gc) and a mantle of small lymphocytes (m), and small regenerating thyroid follicles (rf) are present. H&E stain, × 80.

directed against a cytoplasmic or microsomal antigen, also present on the apical surface of the folliculai epithelial cells (*Fig. 27.2*), and now known to be thyroid peroxidase, the enzyme which iodinates thyroglobulin.

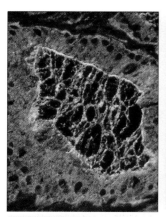
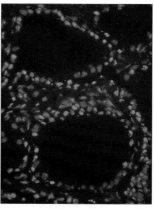

Fig. 27.2 Autoantibodies to thyroid. Healthy, unfixed human thyroid sections were treated with patients' serum, and then with fluoresceinated rabbit anti-human Ig. The acinar epithelial cells of the follicles are stained by antibodies from a patient with Hashimoto's disease, which react with the cells' cytoplasm but not the nuclei (left). Colloid remains in the unfixed section, so some thyroglobulin staining is seen within the colloid/acinar space (left). In contrast, serum from a patient with SLE (right) contains antibodies which react only with the nuclei of acinar epithelial cells and leave the cytoplasm unstained (right). (Courtesy Mr. G. Swana.)

■ THE SPECTRUM OF AUTOIMMUNE DISEASES

The antibodies associated with Hashimoto's thyroiditis and primary myxoedema react only with the thyroid, so the resulting lesion is highly localized. In contrast, the serum from patients with diseases such as systemic lupus erythematosus (SLE) reacts with many, if not all, of the tissues in the body. In SLE, one of the dominant antibodies is directed against the cell nucleus (*Fig. 27.2*). These two diseases represent the extremes of the autoimmune spectrum (*Fig. 27.3*).

The common target organs in organ-specific disease include the thyroid, adrenals, stomach and pancreas. The non-organ-specific diseases, which include the rheumatological disorders, characteristically involve the skin, kidney, joints and muscle (*Fig. 27.4*).

An individual may have more than one autoimmune disease

Interestingly, there are remarkable overlaps at each end of the spectrum. Thyroid antibodies occur with a high frequency in pernicious anaemia patients who have gastic autoimmunity, and these patients have a higher incidence of thyroid autoimmune disease than the normal population. Similarly, patients with thyroid autoimmunity have a high incidence of

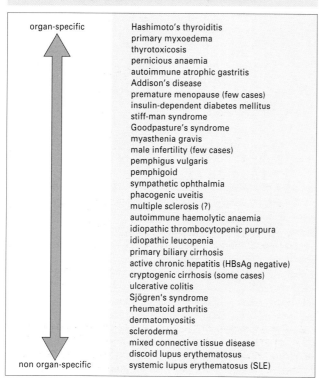

The spectrum of autoimmune diseases

organ-specific

Hashimoto's thyroiditis
primary myxoedema
thyrotoxicosis
pernicious anaemia
autoimmune atrophic gastritis
Addison's disease
premature menopause (few cases)
insulin-dependent diabetes mellitus
stiff-man syndrome
Goodpasture's syndrome
myasthenia gravis
male infertility (few cases)
pemphigus vulgaris
pemphigoid
sympathetic ophthalmia
phacogenic uveitis
multiple sclerosis (?)
autoimmune haemolytic anaemia
idiopathic thrombocytopenic purpura
idiopathic leucopenia
primary biliary cirrhosis
active chronic hepatitis (HBsAg negative)
cryptogenic cirrhosis (some cases)
ulcerative colitis
Sjögren's syndrome
rheumatoid arthritis
dermatomyositis
scleroderma
mixed connective tissue disease
discoid lupus erythematosus

non organ-specific
systemic lupus erythematosus (SLE)

Fig. 27.3 Autoimmune diseases may be classified as organ-specific or non-organ-specific depending on whether the response is primarily against antigens localized to particular organs, or against widespread antigens.

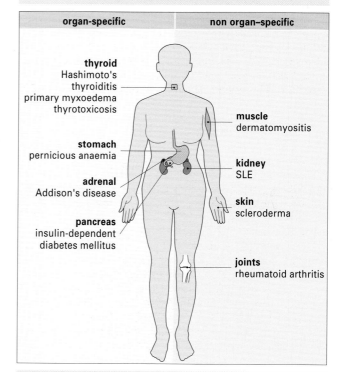

Two types of autoimmune disease

organ-specific	non organ–specific

thyroid
Hashimoto's
thyroiditis
primary myxoedema
thyrotoxicosis

muscle
dermatomyositis

stomach
pernicious anaemia

kidney
SLE

adrenal
Addison's disease

skin
scleroderma

pancreas
insulin-dependent
diabetes mellitus

joints
rheumatoid arthritis

Fig. 27.4 Although the non-organ-specific diseases characteristically produce symptoms in the skin, joints, kidney and muscle, particular organs are more markedly affected by particular diseases, for example the kidney in systemic lupus erythematosus (SLE) and the joints in rheumatoid arthritis.

stomach autoantibodies and, to a lesser extent, the clinical disease itself, namely pernicious anaemia.

The cluster of rheumatological disorders at the other end of the spectrum also shows considerable overlap. Features of rheumatoid arthritis, for example, are often associated with the clinical picture of SLE. In these diseases immune complexes are deposited systemically, particularly in the kidney, joints and skin, giving rise to widespread lesions. In contrast, overlap of diseases from the two ends of the spectrum is relatively rare (*Fig. 27.5*).

The mechanisms of immunopathological damage vary depending on where the disease lies in the spectrum. Where the antigen is localized in a particular organ, Type II hypersensitivity and cell-mediated reactions are most important (see Chapters 23 and 25). In non-organ-specific autoimmunity, immune complex deposition leads to inflammation through a variety of mechanisms, including complement activation and phagocyte recruitment (see Chapter 24).

■ GENETIC FACTORS

Autoimmune disease can occur in families

There is an undoubted familial incidence of autoimmunity, a remarkable example of which is shown in *Fig. 27.6*. This is largely genetic rather than environmental, as may be seen from studies of identical and non-identical twins, and from the association of thyroid autoantibodies with abnormalities of the X-chromosome.

Autoimmunity within families often shows a bias towards organ-specific reactivity. As well as a general predisposition to develop organ-specific antibodies, it is clear that there are other genetically controlled factors which tend to select the organ that is mainly affected. It is interesting to note that relatives of Hashimoto patients and relatives of pernicious

anaemia patients both have a higher than normal incidence and titre of thyroid autoantibodies, whereas relatives of pernicious anaemia patients have a far higher frequency of gastric autoantibodies, indicating that there are genetic factors which differentially select the stomach as the target within this group of organ-specific autoimmune disorders.

Certain HLA haplotypes predispose to autoimmunity

Further evidence for the operation of genetic factors in autoimmune disease comes from their tendency to be associated with particular HLA specificities (*Fig. 27.7*). The haplotype B8,DR3 is particularly common in the organ-specific diseases, though Hashimoto's thyroiditis tends to be associated more with DR5. Rheumatoid arthritis shows no associations with the HLA-A and -B loci haplotypes but is associated with a nucleotide sequence that is common to DR1 and major subtypes of DR4 (encoding amino acids 66–75 in the DRβ chain). It is notable that for insulin-dependent (Type 1) diabetes mellitus, DR3/4 heterozygotes have a greatly increased risk of developing the disease (see *Fig. 27.7*). This supports the concept of several genetic factors being involved in the development of autoimmune diseases: genes predisposing individuals to develop autoimmunity, either organ-specific or non-organ-specific, and others determining the particular antigen or antigens involved.

Confirmation of these views comes from the animal models of autoimmunity, which we will discuss in the next section.

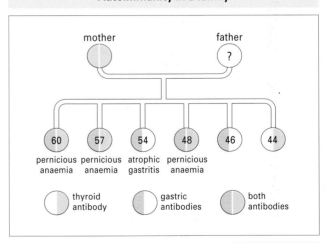

Autoimmunity in a family

Fig. 27.6 This family chart shows the incidence of organ-specific abnormalities affecting the thyroid and stomach. (At the time of study, the father was dead, and his antibody status unknown.) The siblings all presented with gastric autoimmune disease, unlike the mother who had primary myxoedema. However, there was a striking overlap with thyroid autoimmunity at the serological level, although the siblings lacked clinical symptoms of thyroid disease. Autoantibodies were more prevalent with increasing age (the ages given are those at which autoantibodies were detected).

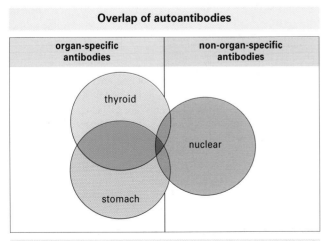

Overlap of autoantibodies

Fig. 27.5 The organ-specific autoantibodies directed against thyroid and stomach often occur together in the same individual, but there is little overlap with non-organ-specific antibodies such as those with reactivity for DNA and nucleoproteins.

HLA associations in autoimmune disease

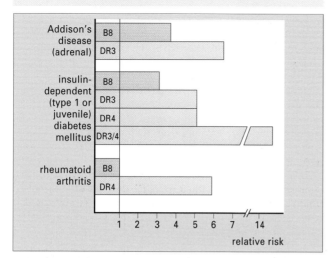

relative risk

Fig. 27.7 The relative risk is a measure of the increased chance of contracting the disease for individuals bearing the HLA antigen, relative to those lacking it. Virtually all autoimmune diseases studied have shown an association with some HLA specificity. The greater relative risk for Addison's disease associated with HLA-DR3, as compared with HLA-B8, suggests that DR3 is closely linked to or even identical with the 'disease susceptibility gene'. In this case it is not surprising that B8 has a relative risk greater than 1, because it is known to occur with DR3 more often than expected by chance in the general population, a phenomenon termed linkage disequilibrium. Both DR3 and DR4 are associated with Type 1 diabetes mellitus, and when a gene for both is present, in the the DR3/4 heterozygote, there is a greatly increased risk, supporting the concept of multiple, additive genetic factors. Rheumatoid arthritis is linked to HLA-DR but not to any HLA-A or HLA-B alleles.

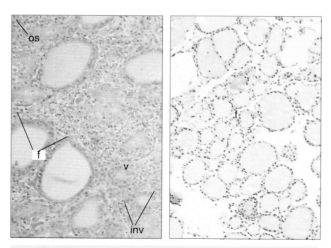

Fig. 27.8 The histological appearance of experimental autoallergic thyroiditis. In the section from a thyroglobulin-injected animal (left) there is gross destruction of the follicular architecture with only isolated intact follicles (f), extensive invasion by mononuclear inflammatory cells (inv), associated with distended blood vessels (v), oedema (os = oedematous space) and fibrosis. A control section, showing normal thyroid follicles (f) with colloid, is seen on the right. H&E stain, × 200.

■ PATHOGENESIS

Autoimmune processes are often pathogenic. When autoantibodies are found in association with a particular disease there are three possible inferences:

- The autoimmunity is responsible for producing the lesions of the disease.
- There is a disease process which, through the production of tissue damage, leads to the development of autoantibodies.
- There is a factor which produces both the lesions and the autoimmunity.

Autoantibodies secondary to a lesion (the second possibility) are sometimes found. For example, cardiac autoantibodies may develop after myocardial infarction. However, autoantibodies are rarely induced following the release of autoantigens by simple trauma. In most diseases associated with autoimmunity, the evidence supports the first possibility, that the autoimmune process produces the lesions.

The pathogenic role of autoimmunity can be demonstrated in experimental models
Examples of induced autoimmunity
The most direct test of whether autoimmunity is responsible for the lesions of disease is to induce autoimmunity deliberately in an experimental animal and see if this leads to the production of the lesions. Autoimmunity can be induced in experimental animals by injecting autoantigen (self antigen) together with complete Freund's adjuvant (see Chapter 17), and this does indeed produce organ-specific disease in certain organs. For example, thyroglobulin injection can induce an inflammatory disease of the thyroid while myelin basic protein can cause encephalomyelitis. In the case of thyroglobulin-injected animals, not only are thyroid autoantibodies produced, but the gland becomes infiltrated with mononuclear cells and the acinar architecture crumbles (*Fig. 27.8*). Although this response is not identical in every respect to Hashimoto's thyroiditis, the thyroiditis produced bears a remarkable overall similarity to the human condition.

The ability to induce experimental autoimmune disease depends on the strain of animal used. For example, it is found that the susceptibility of rats and mice to myelin basic protein-induced encephalomyelitis depends on a small number of gene loci, of which the most important are the MHC class II genes. It is also possible to induce autoallergic encephalomyelitis in susceptible strains by injecting T cells specific for myelin basic protein. These T-helper (TH) cells are CD4+ and it has been found that induction of disease can be prevented by treating the recipients with antibody to CD4 just before the expected time of disease onset, blocking the interaction of the TH cells' CD4 with the class II MHC of antigen-presenting cells (APCs) (see Chapter 8). The results indicate the importance of class II restricted autoreactive TH cells in the development of these conditions, and emphasize the prominent role of the MHC.

Examples of spontaneous autoimmunity
There is much that we can learn from spontaneous autoimmune disease in animals. One well-established example is the Obese strain (OS) chicken (*Fig. 27.9*) in which thyroid autoantibodies occur spontaneously and the thyroid undergoes the progressive destruction associated with chronic

inflammation. The sera of these animals contain thyroglobulin autoantibodies (*Fig. 27.10*). Furthermore, approximately 15% of the sera react by immunofluorescence with the stomach (proventriculus) of the normal chicken. This pattern is similar to that obtained when the same test is carried out with sera from patients with pernicious anaemia who have autoantibodies which react with inammalian parental cells.

The Obese strain chicken example parallels human autoimmune thyroid disease in terms of the lesion in the gland, the production of antibodies to different components in the thyroid, and the overlap with gastric autoimmunity. So it is of interest that when the immunological status of these animals is altered, quite dramatic effects on the outcome of the disease are seen. For example, if the bursa of Fabricius (in which B cells mature) is removed soon after hatching, the severity of the thyroiditis is greatly diminished, indicating that antibody contributes to the pathogenesis of the disease. However, removal of the thymus at birth appears to exacerbate the thyroiditis, suggesting that the thymus exerts a controlling effect on the disease (*Fig. 27.11*). Paradoxically, destruction of the entire T-cell population in adult animals, by massive injections of anti-chick T-cell serum, completely inhibits both autoantibody production and the attack on the thyroid. Thus, T cells clearly play a variety of pivotal roles as mediators and regulators of this disease.

Human autoantibodies can be directly pathogenic

When investigating human autoimmunity directly, rather than animal models, it is of course more difficult to carry out experiments. Nevertheless, there is much evidence to suggest that autoantibodies may be important in pathogenesis, and we will discuss the major examples here.

Thyrotoxicosis – A number of diseases have been recognized in which autoantibodies to hormone receptors may actually mimic the function of the normal hormone concerned and produce disease. Thyrotoxicosis was the first disorder in which such anti-receptor antibodies were clearly recognized (*Fig. 27.12*). The phenomenon of neonatal thyrotoxicosis provides us with a natural 'passive transfer' study, because the IgG antibodies from the thyrotoxic mother cross the placenta. Many babies born to thyrotoxic mothers and showing thyroid hyperactivity have been reported, but the problem spontaneously resolves as the antibodies derived from the mother are catabolized in the baby over several weeks.

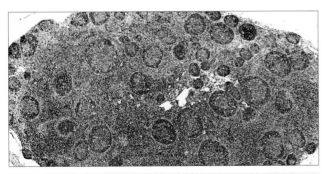

Fig. 27.9 Obese strain (OS) chicken. Chickens of this strain are afficted with a spontaneously occurring autoimmune Hashimoto-like thyroiditis. They are much smaller (**right**) than age-matched normal controls and also show additional symptoms of *hypo*thyroidism, such as cold sensitivity (ruffled feathers), skin abnormalities (long silky feathers), poor reproduction, subcutaneous and abdominal fat deposits (hence the name), lipid serum, etc. These symptoms can be prevented by early thyroxine supplementation. (Courtesy Professor G. Wick.)

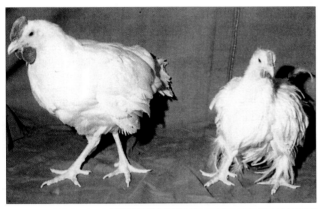

Fig. 27.10 Histopathological appearance of the thyroid gland of a six-week old OS chicken showing severe destruction by a mononuclear cell infiltrate with very few colloid-containing thyroid follicules left. Note the well-developed germinal centres similar to the hallmark of Hashimoto thyroiditis. Original magnification ×200. (Courtesy Professor G. Wick.)

Modification of thyroiditis in OS chicken by neonatal bursectomy and thymectomy

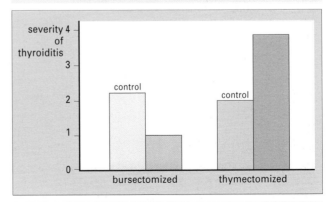

Fig. 27.11 The severity of thyroiditis is assessed by lymphocyte infiltration. Neonatal bursectomy reduces thyroiditis, suggesting an important role for antibody in pathogenesis. Removal of the thymus at birth exacerbates the disease, indicating a controlling effect of T-suppressor (Ts) cells.

Myasthenia gravis – A similar phenomenon has been observed with mothers suffering from myasthenia gravis, where antibodies to acetylcholine receptors cross the placenta into the fetus and cause transient muscle weakness in the newborn baby.

Other receptor diseases – Somewhat rarely, autoantibodies to insulin receptors and to β-adrenergic receptors can be found, the latter associated with bronchial asthma.

Male infertility – Yet another example of autoimmune disease is seen in rare cases of male infertility where antibodies to spermatozoa lead to clumping of spermatozoa, either by their heads or by their tails, in the semen (*Fig. 27.13*).

Pernicious anaemia – In this disease an autoantibody interferes with the normal uptake of vitamin B_{12}. Vitamin B_{12} is not absorbed directly, but must first associate with a protein called intrinsic factor; the vitamin–protein complex is then transported across the intestinal mucosa. Early passive transfer studies demonstrated that serum from a patient with pernicious anaemia, if fed to a healthy individual together with intrinsic factor–B_{12} complex, inhibited uptake of the vitamin. Subsequently, the factor in the serum which blocked vitamin uptake was identified as antibody against intrinsic factor. It is now known that plasma cells in the gastric mucosa of patients with pernicious anaemia secrete this antibody into the lumen of the stomach (*Fig. 27.14*).

Goodpasture's syndrome – In Goodpasture's syndrome, antibodies to the glomerular capillary basement membrane bind to the kidney *in vivo* (see *Fig. 24.3*). To demonstrate that the antibodies can have a pathological effect, a passive transfer experiment was performed. The antibodies were eluted from the kidney of a patient who had died with this disease, and injected into primates whose kidney antigens were sufficiently similar for the injected antibodies to localize on the glomerular basement membrane. The injected monkeys subsequently died with glomerulonephritis.

Autoimmunity to cell surface receptors

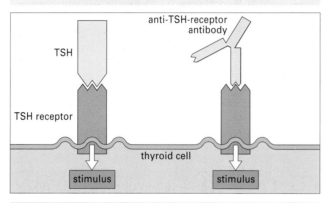

Fig. 27.12 The thyroid cell is stimulated when thyroid stimulating hormone (TSH) binds to its receptors (left). Antibody to the TSH receptor, present in the serum of a patient with thyrotoxicosis (Graves' or Basedow's disease), combines with the receptor in a similar fashion, thereby delivering a comparable stimulus to the thyroid cell (right) and resulting in overproduction of thyroid hormones.

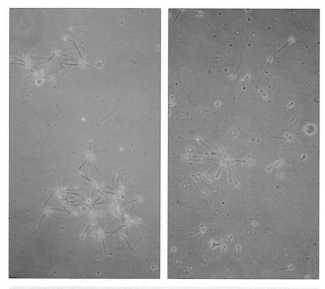

Fig. 27.13 Sperm agglutination. The presence of sperm autoantibodies produces either head-to-head (left) or tail-to-tail (right) agglutination.

Failure of vitamin B_{12} absorption in pernicious anaemia

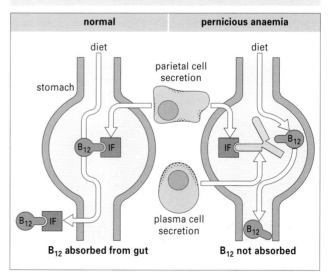

Fig. 27.14 Normally, dietary vitamin B_{12} is absorbed by the small intestine as a complex with intrinsic factor (IF), which is synthesized by parietal cells in gastric mucosa. In pernicious anaemia, locally synthesized autoantibodies, specific for intrinsic factor, combine with intrinsic factor to inhibit its role as a carrier for vitamin B_{12}.

Immune complexes appear to be pathogenic in systemic autoimmunity

In the case of SLE, it can be shown that immune complexes containing autoantigen and antibody, which are deposited in the kidney of patients, produce the Type III hypersensitivity reactions outlined in Chapter 24. Glomerulonephritis and proteinuria are kown to be induced by repeated injections of high doses of antigen, which lead to chronic immune complex disease and deposition in the kidney. Even a single large dose of antigen can produce acute damage.

Turning to experimental animals, the hybrid of the New Zealand Black and New Zealand White strains of mice spontaneously develops murine SLE in which immune-complex glomerulonephritis and anti-DNA autoantibodies are major features. The fact that measures which suppress the immune response in these animals (e.g. treatment with anti-CD4) also suppress the disease and prolong survival, adds to the evidence for autoimmune reactions causing such disease (*Fig. 27.15*).

■ AETIOLOGY

Self-reactive B and T cells persist even in normal subjects

Despite the complex selection mechanisms operating to establish self-tolerance during lymphocyte development, the body contains large numbers of lymphocytes which are potentially autoreactive. This is particularly true of developing thymic T cells (thymocytes) that fail to be eliminated by a subset of self peptides (self epitopes). Normally, thymic APCs carrying self epitope delivers the negative selection that prompts the death of autoreactive T cells. But cryptic self epitopes are present in relatively low concentrations on APCs, because of either inefficient processing or low affinity for the MHC groove, or both, and are therefore unable to tolerize the autoreactive T cells (*Fig. 27.16*).

Many autoantigens, when injected with adjuvants, make autoantibodies in normal animals, demonstrating the presence of autoreactive B cells, and it is possible to identify a small number of autoreactive B cells (e.g. anti-thyroglobulin) in the normal population. Autoreactive T cells are also present in normal individuals, as shown by the fact that it is possible to produce autoimmune lines of T cells by stimulation

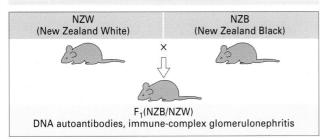

Suppression of autoimmune disease

NZW (New Zealand White) × NZB (New Zealand Black)

F₁(NZB/NZW)
DNA autoantibodies, immune-complex glomerulonephritis

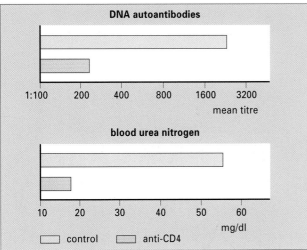

DNA autoantibodies

1:100   200   400   800   1600   3200
mean titre

blood urea nitrogen

10   20   30   40   50   60
mg/dl

☐ control   ☐ anti-CD4

Fig. 27.15 The New Zealand Black mouse spontaneously develops autoimmune haemolytic anaemia. The hybrid between this and the New Zealand White strain develops DNA autoantibodies and immune-complex glomerulonephritis, like patients with SLE. Immunosuppression with monoclonal antibodies to the TH cell marker CD4 considerably reduced the severity of the glomerulonephritis and the titre of double-stranded DNA autoantibodies at 8 months of age, showing the relevance of the immune processes to the generation of the disease. (Based on data from Wofsy D, *et al., J Exp Med,* 1985;**161**:378.)

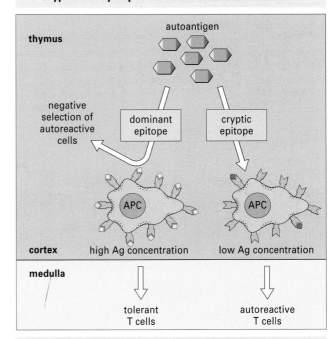

Cryptic self epitopes do not induce T-cell tolerance

thymus — autoantigen

negative selection of autoreactive cells

dominant epitope   cryptic epitope

APC   APC

cortex   high Ag concentration   low Ag concentration

medulla

tolerant T cells   autoreactive T cells

Fig. 27.16 Self epitopes which, after processing, appear in a high concentration on the surface of APCs in association with MHC are called dominant epitopes and are powerful stimulants which will delete or anergize developing autoreactive T cells, so that only tolerant T cells leave the thymus. In contrast, self epitopes which appear in a very low concentration on the APC are termed cryptic in the sense that they do not delete autoreactive T cells, which can then join the peripheral adult T-cell repertoire.

of normal circulating T cells with the appropriate autoantigen (e.g. myelin basic protein) and IL-2.

Autoimmunity is antigen driven

Given that autoreactive B cells exist, the question remains whether they are stimulated to proliferate and produce autoantibodies by interaction with autoantigens or by some other means, such as non-specific polyclonal activators or idiotypic interactions (see *Fig. 24.18*). Evidence that B cells are selected by antigen comes from the existence of high affinity autoantibodies which arise through somatic mutation, a process which requires both T cells and autoantigen. Additionally, autoantibodies occur to antigen clusters, which consist of several epitopes on the same autoantigenic molecule. Apart from the presence of autoantigen itself, it is very difficult to envisage a mechanism that could account for the co-existence of antibody responses to different epitopes on the same molecule. Similarly to autoantigen clusters, different molecular components of intracellular organelles (e.g. nucleosomes) or antigens linked within the same organ (e.g. thyroglobulin and thyroid peroxidase) can induce autoantibodies in one individual.

The most direct evidence for autoimmunity being antigen driven comes from studies of the Obese strain chicken which, as described earlier, spontaneously develops thyroid autoimmunity. If the thyroid gland (the source of antigen) is removed at birth, the chickens mature without developing thyroid autoantibodies (*Fig. 27.17*). Furthermore, once thyroid autoimmunity has developed, later removal of the thyroid leads to a gross decline of thyroid autoantibodies, usually to undetectable levels.

T cells are utterly pivotal for the development of autoimmune disease. The high affinity and somatic mutations which are characteristic of the IgG autoantibodies are dependent on the cooperative action of TH cells. Direct evidence for an involvement of T cells comes from animal models of autoimmune disease (see pp. 27.4–5), but is more difficult to obtain in human disorders. However, thyroid-specific T-cell clones have been isolated from the glands of patients with thyrotoxicosis and anti-CD4 therapy can be beneficial in rheumatoid arthritis (as in autoimmune disease in animals – see p. 27.4). Furthermore, associations between autoimmune diseases and certain MHC types (see *Fig. 27.7*) are probably related to the role of MHC molecules in presentation of antigen to T cells.

In organ-specific disorders, there is ample evidence for T cells responding to antigens present in the organs under attack. But in non-organ-specific autoimmunity, we have very little idea which antigens are recognized by the T cells. One possibility is that the T cells do not see conventional peptide antigen (possibly true of anti-DNA responses) but instead recognize an antibody's idiotype (an antigenic determinant on the V region of antibody). In this view SLE, for example, would be an 'idiotype disease', like the model presented in *Fig. 27.18*. In this scheme, autoantibodies are produced normally at low levels by B cells using germ-line genes. If these then form complexes with the autoantigen, the complexes can be taken up by APCs (including B cells) and

Effect of neonatal thyroidectomy on Obese chickens

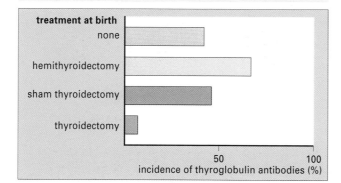

Fig. 27.17 Because removal of the thyroid at birth prevents the development of thyroid autoantibodies, it would appear that the autoimmune process is driven by the autoantigen in the thyroid gland. (Based on data from de Carvalho LCP *et al.*, *J Exp Med* 1982;**155**:1255.)

Model of T-cell help via processing of intermolecular complexes in the induction of autoimmunity

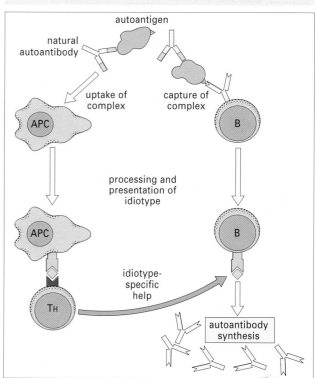

Fig. 27.18 An immune complex consisting of autoantigen (e.g. DNA) and a naturally occurring (germ-line) autoantibody is taken up by an APC, and peptides derived by processing of the idiotypic segment of the antibody (Id) are presented to TH cells. B cells that express the 'pathogenic' autoantibody can capture the complex and so can receive T-cell help via presentation of the processed Id to the TH cell.

components of the complex, including the antibody idiotype, presented to T cells. Idiotype-specific T cells would then help the autoantibody-producing B cells.

Controls on the development of autoimmunity can be bypassed in a number of ways

Molecular mimicry by cross-reactive microbial antigens can stimulate autoreactive B and T cells

Normally, naive autoreactive T cells recognizing cryptic self epitopes are not switched on because the antigen is only presented at low concentrations on 'professional' APCs or it may be presented on 'non-professional' APCs such as pancreatic β-islet cells or thyroid epithelial cells, which lack B7 or other co-stimulator molecules. However, infection with a microbe bearing antigens that cross-react with the cryptic self epitopes (i.e. have shared epitopes) will load the professional APCs with levels of processed peptides that are sufficient to activate the naive autoreactive T cells. Once primed, these T cells are able to recognize and react with the self epitope on the non-professional APCs since they no longer require a co-stimulatory signal and have a higher avidity for the target, due to upregulation of accessory adhesion molecules (*Fig. 27.19*).

Cross-reactive antigens which share B-cell epitopes with self molecules can also break tolerance but by a different mechanism. Many autoreactive B cells cannot be activated because the CD4$^+$ T cells which could provide help have been selectively tolerized since T cells are rendered unresponsive at lower concentrations of autoantigens than are B cells.

However, these 'helpless' B cells can be stimulated if the cross-reacting antigen bears a 'foreign' carrier epitope to which the T cells have not been tolerized (*Fig. 27.20*).

A disease in which such molecular mimicry operates is rheumatic fever, in which autoantibodies to heart valve antigens can be detected. These develop in a small proportion of individuals several weeks after a streptococcal infection of the throat. Carbohydrate antigens on the streptococci cross-react with an antigen on heart valves, so the infection may bypass T-cell self-tolerance to heart valve antigens. There may also be cross-reactivity between HLA-B27 and certain strains of *Klebsiella* in connection with ankylosing spondylitis, and cross-reactivity between *Proteus mirabilis* and DR4 in relationship to rheumatoid arthritis. Close similarities between the highly conserved heat shock proteins of mycobacteria and those of humans might also be a contributory factor in rheumatoid arthritis.

In some cases foreign antigen can directly stimulate autoreactive cells

Another mechanism to bypass the tolerant autoreactive TH cell is where antigen or another stimulator directly triggers the autoreactive effector cells. For example, lipopolysaccharide or Epstein–Barr virus causes direct B-cell stimulation and some of the clones of activated cells will produce autoantibodies, although in the absence of T-cell help these are normally of low titre and affinity.

Cytokine dysregulation, inappropriate MHC expression and failure of suppression may induce autoimmunity

It appears that dysregulation of the cytokine network can also lead to activation of autoreactive T cells. One experi-

Cross-reactive antigens induce autoimmune TH cells

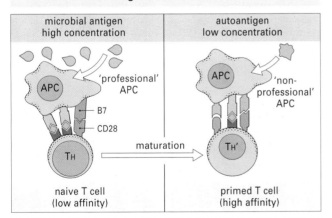

Fig. 27.19 The inability of naive TH cells to recognize autoantigen on a tissue cell, whether because of low concentration or low affinity, can be circumvented by a cross-reacting microbial antigen at higher concentration or with higher innate affinity, together with a co-stimulator such as B7 on a 'professional' APC; this primes the TH cells (left). Due to increased expression of accessory molecules (e.g. LFA-1 and CD2) the primed TH cells now have high affinity and because they do not require a co-stimulatory signal, they can interact with autoantigen on 'non-professional' APCs such as organ-specific epithelial cells to produce autoimmune disease (right).

Induction of autoimmunity by cross-reactive antigens

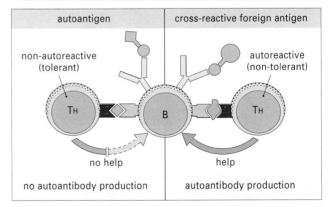

Fig. 27.20 The B cell recognizes an epitope present on autoantigen, but coincidentally present also on a foreign antigen. Normally the B cell presents the autoantigen but receives no help from autoreactive TH cells, which are functionally deleted. If a cross-reacting foreign antigen is encountered, the B cell can present peptides of this molecule to non-autoreactive T cells and thus be driven to proliferate, differentiate and secrete autoantibodies.

mental demonstration of this is the introduction of a transgene for interferon-γ (IFNγ) into pancreatic β-islet cells. If the transgene for IFNγ is fully expressed in the cells, MHC class II genes are upregulated and autoimmune destruction of the islet cells results (*Fig. 27.21*). This is not simply a result of a non-specific chaotic IFNγ-induced local inflammatory milieu since normal islets grafted at a separate site are rejected, implying clearly that T-cell autoreactivity to the pancreas has been established.

The surface expression of MHC class II in itself is not sufficient to activate the naive autoreactive T cells: animals bearing a transgene of MHC class II on an insulin promoter (but no IFNγ transgene) express surface class II molecules on their β-islets but do not provoke autoimmunity. Nonetheless, surface expression of class II may be necessary for the islet cell to act as a target for the primed autoreactive TH cells, and it was therefore most exciting when cells in thyrotoxic thyroiditis were found to be actively synthesizing class II MHC molecules (*Fig. 27.22*) and so were able to be recognized by CD4⁺ T cells (T cells). In this context it is interesting that several animal strains that are susceptible to autoimmunity are also more readily induced by IFNγ to express MHC class II on cell types which would not do so in non-susceptible strains. These include the Lewis rat (experimental autoimmune encephalomyelitis), the Obese strain chicken (thyroiditis) and the BB rat (susceptible to autoimmune diabetes).

The argument that imbalanced cytokine production may also contribute to autoimmunity receives further support from the unexpected finding that tumour necrosis factor (by introduction of a TNF transgene) ameliorates autoimmune disease in NZB/NZW hybrid mice.

Aside from the normal 'ignorance' of cryptic self epitopes, other regulatory factors may include Ts cells, the suppressive action of hormones (e.g. steroids) and cytokines (e.g. TGFβ), and products of macrophages (*Fig. 27.23*). Deficiencies in any of them may increase susceptibility to autoimmunity. Thus, apparently healthy relatives of patients with SLE show a defect in the generation of non-specific Ts cells (as in the patients themselves), suggesting that this defect is just one factor contributing towards SLE. It is possible that more than one element of the suppressor network has to fail for an autoimmune response to develop and in SLE patients, there may be further abnormalities in either antigen- or idiotype-specific regulatory T cells.

Pre-existing defects in the target organ may increase susceptibility to autoimmunity.

We have already alluded to the undue sensitivity of target cells to upregulation of MHC class II by IFNγ in animals susceptible to certain autoimmune diseases. Other evidence also favours the view that there may be a pre-existing defect in the target organ. In the Obese strain chicken model of spontaneous thyroid autoimmunity (see p. 27.5), it has been shown that, when endogenous TSH is suppressed by thyroxine treatment, the uptake of iodine into the thyroid glands is far higher in the Obese strain than in a variety of normal strains. Furthermore, this is not due to any stimulating effect of the autoimmunity, because immunosuppressed animals show even higher uptakes of iodine (*Fig. 27.24*). Interestingly, the Cornell strain (from which the Obese strain was derived by breeding) shows even higher uptakes of iodine, yet these animals do not develop spontaneous thyroiditis. This could

Autoimmunity due to cytokine dysregulation

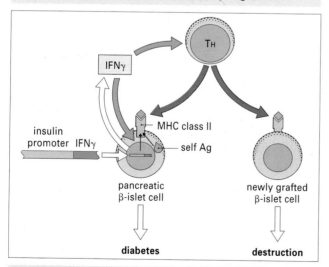

Fig. 27.21 Introduction of a transgene comprising IFNγ on an insulin promoter leads to copious pancreatic expression and secretion of IFNγ. This leads to upregulation of surface MHC class II and activation of autoreactive T cells by an as yet unexplained mechanism but possibly mediated via 'professional' APCs. The primed T cells now initiate autoimmune destruction of the β cells. That this is a true autoaggression is shown by the prompt destruction of newly grafted normal syngeneic islet cells (genetically indentical cells lacking the transgene).

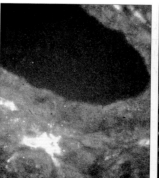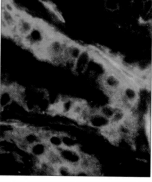

Fig. 27.22 Human thyroid sections stained for MHC class II. **Left:** Normal thyroid with unstained follicular cells, and an isolated dendritic cell that is strongly positive for MHC class II. **Right:** thyrotoxic (Graves' disease) thyroid with abundant MHC class II molecules in the cytoplasm, indicating that rapid synthesis of MHC class II is occurring.

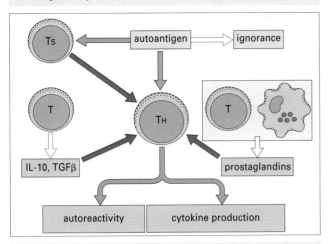

Regulatory mechanisms controlling autoimmunity

Fig. 27.23 Autoreactive TH cells are not normally stimulated by cryptic epitopes ('ignorance') but should they become activated, they would usually be held in check by a network of suppressive signals including antigen-specific suppression by T cells, which may be mediated directly or via suppressive cytokines such as IL-10 and TGFβ. Non-specific suppression (e.g. mediated by prostaglandins) also limits the capacity of the TH cell to respond. Should the TH cell show an enhanced capacity to respond, e.g. increased levels of IL-2 receptor, or the suppressive influences fail, the balance would be shifted towards autoimmune disease.

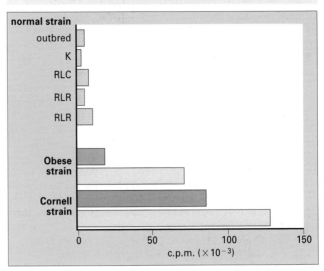

Thyroid ^{131}I uptake in TSH-suppressed chickens

Fig. 27.24 Thyroid ^{131}I uptake in Obese strain chickens and in the related Cornell strain is abnormally high compared with normal strains. Endogenous TSH production was suppressed by administration of thyroxine; therefore the experiment measured TSH-independent ^{131}I uptake. Values were far higher than normal in Obese strain chickens, which spontaneously develop thyroid autoimmunity, and even higher in the non-autoimmune Cornell strain from which the Obese strain was bred. That this abnormality was not due to immune mechanisms was shown by the finding that immunosuppression (blue bars) actually increased ^{131}I uptake into the thyroid gland.

be indicative of a type of abnormal thyroid behaviour which in itself is insufficient to induce autoimmune disease but does contribute to susceptibility in the Obese strain. Confirmation of this comes from experiments in which lymphoid cells from older Obese strain chickens with thyroid disease were transferred to other chickens. These cells induced thyroiditis in young Obese strain chickens and the Cornell strain, but not in other histocompatible strains, which must lack the pre-existing defect that makes the Obese and Cornell strains susceptible to autoimmunity. These experiments re-emphasize the considerable importance of multiple factors in the establishment of prolonged autoimmunity.

■ DIAGNOSTIC AND PROGNOSTIC VALUE OF AUTOANTIBODIES

Whatever the relationship of autoantibodies to the disease process, they frequently provide valuable markers for diagnostic purposes. A particularly good example is the test for mitochondrial antibodies, used in diagnosing primary biliary cirrhosis (*Fig. 27.25*). Exploratory laparotomy was previously needed to obtain this diagnosis, and was often hazardous because of the age and condition of the patients concerned.

Autoantibodies, especially to pancreatic β-islet cells, may also have a predictive value, as shown in *Fig. 27.26*.

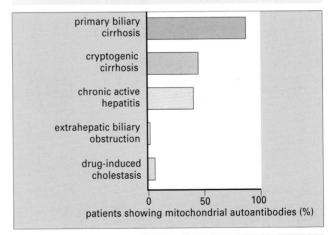

Diagnostic value of anti-mitochondrial antibodies

Fig. 27.25 Mitochondrial antibody tests using indirect immunofluorescence, together with percutaneous liver biopsy, can be used to assist in the differential diagnosis of these diseases. A large proportion of patients with primary biliary cirrhosis but less than half of patients with cryptogenic cirrhosis or chronic active hepatitis have anti-mitochondrial antibodies; the antibodies are rare in the other diseases.

■ TREATMENT

Often, in organ-specific autoimmune disorders, the symptoms can be corrected by metabolic control. For example, hypothyroidism can be controlled by administration of thyroxine, and thyrotoxicosis by antithyroid drugs. In pernicious anaemia, metabolic correction is achieved by injection of vitamin B_{12}, and in myasthenia gravis by administration of cholinesterase inhibitors. Where function is lost and cannot be substituted by hormones, as may occur in lupus nephritis or chronic rheumatoid arthritis, tissue grafts or mechanical substitutes may be appropriate. In the case of tissue grafts, protection from the immunological processes which necessitated the transplant may be required.

Conventional immunosuppressive therapy with antimitotic drugs can be used to damp down the immune response but, because of the dangers involved, tends to be used only in life-threatening disorders such as SLE and dermatomyositis. The potential of cyclosporin and related drugs has yet to be fully realized, but quite dramatic results have been reported in the treatment of Type I diabetes mellitus. Anti-inflammatory drugs are, of course, prescribed for rheumatoid diseases.

As we understand more about the precise defects, and learn how to manipulate the immunological status of the patient, some less well-established approaches may become practicable (*Fig. 27.27*). In particular, some experimental autoimmune diseases have been treated successfully with autoantigenic peptides and thier analogues, and by 'vaccination' with autoreactive T-cells. This suggests that stimulating normally suppressive functions, including the idiotype network, could be promising.

The predictive value of autoantibodies

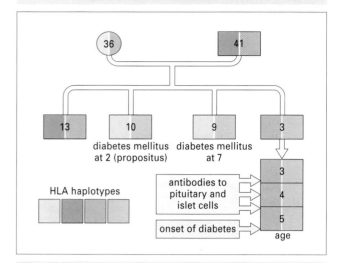

Fig. 27.26 Prospective study of a family with insulin-dependent diabetes mellitus (ages of each family member at the start of the study are given). The sibling sharing a haplotype with the propositus, and having complement-fixing islet-cell antibodies, became diabetic over 2 years later.

Current and potential treatment of autoimmune disease

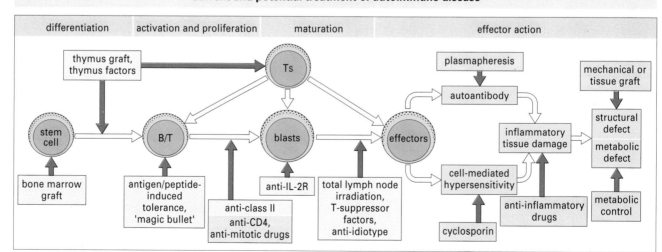

Fig. 27.27 Current treatments for arresting the pathological developments in autoimmune disease are given in blue boxes, and those that may become practicable in green boxes. Antimitotic drugs are given in severe cases of SLE or chronic active hepatitis, and anti-inflammatory drugs are widely prescribed in rheumatoid arthritis. Organ-specific disorders (e.g. primary myxoedema), can be treated by supplying the defective component (e.g. thyroid hormone). When a live graft is necessary, immunosuppressive therapy can protect the tissue from damage.

Critical Thinking

■ Why is it unlikely that DNA is a thymus-dependent autoantigen and by what mechanisms could it become so?

■ What evidence is there to support a pathogenic role for autoantibodies in disease?

■ Transgenes consisting of (1) a viral glycoprotein from lymphocytic chonomeningitis (LCM) virus on an insulin promoter and (2) the TCR of a T-cell clone cytotoxic for cells infected with LCM virus, are introduced into a mouse. Diabetes only results when the mouse is infected with LCM virus. What is happening?

■ How might particular MHC haplotypes predispose to certain autoimmune diseases?

■ Of what value has the Obese strain chicken been in helping our understanding of autoimmune disease?

■ How would you try to manipulate T cells to treat autoimmune disease?

FURTHER READING

Brostoff J, Scadding GK, Male D, Roitt IM. *Clinical Immunology.* London: Gower Medical Publishing, 1991.

Campbell RD, Milner CM. MHC genes in autoimmunity. *Curr Opin Immunol* 1993;**5**:887–893 (and several other critical essays on autoimmunity in each annual volume).

Chapel HM, Haeney M. *Essentials of Clinical Immunology.* 3rd ed. Oxford: Blackwell Scientific Publications, 1992.

Lachmann PJ, Peters DK, Rosen FS, Walport MJ, eds. *Clinical Aspects of Immunology.* 5th ed. Oxford: Blackwell Scientific Publications, 1992.

Lanzavecchia A. Identifying strategies for immune intervention. *Science* 1993;**260**:937.

Roitt IM, Hutchings PR, Dawe KI, Sumar N, Bodman KB, Cooke AJ. The forces driving autoimmune disease. *J Autoimmun* 1992;**5(Suppl A)**:11–26.

Schoenfeld Y, Isenberg D. *The Mosaic of Autoimmunity (Factors Associated with Autoimmune Disease).* Amsterdam: Elsevier, 1989.

Shin E, *et al.* Variable regions of Ig heavy chains encoding antithyrotropin receptor antibodies of patients with Graves' disease. *J Immunol* 1994;**152**:1485–92.

For recognizing and quantifying antigens in tissues or fluids many immunological techniques utilize the exquisite specificity of the antigen–antibody bond.

Cell populations can be identified and characterized by their surface markers, using the techniques of immunofluorescence or immunohistochemistry.

Cell populations can be isolated according to their surface markers, by techniques which include fluorescence-activated cell sorting (FACS), panning and density-dependent centrifugations.

The principal assays for lymphocyte function are by antibody or cytokine production, by proliferation in response to antigen, or by cytotoxicity.

Immunologists employ a number of techniques which are common to other biological sciences. For example, the methods used to isolate antigens and antibodies are those of biochemistry and protein fractionation, while the gene sequences of immunologically important molecules have been elucidated by the standard techniques of molecular genetics. Immunology has, however, developed a number of its own techniques, particularly those based on the antigen–antibody interaction. These have found many uses in other biological sciences. For example, any molecule that acts as antigen can be identified in tissues by immunocytochemical methods. Very low concentrations of such molecules can be quantified by radioimmunoassay (RIA) and enzyme-linked immunosorbent assay (ELISA). There are hundreds of different immunological methods now being used, and some of the most common are outlined in this chapter.

◼ ANTIGEN–ANTIBODY INTERACTIONS

Precipitation reactions

One of the first observations of antigen–antibody reactions was their ability to precipitate when combined in proportions at or near equivalence. This is seen in the classic precipitin reaction, where antigen and antibody are mixed in solution (*Fig. 28.1*). By performing these reactions in agar gels it is possible to distinguish separate antigen–antibody reactions produced by different populations of antibody which are present in a serum – the immuno-double-diffusion technique. This technique has been extended to the examination of the relationship between different antigens (*Fig. 28.2*).

Some antigen mixtures, however, are too complex to be resolved by simple diffusion and precipitation and so the technique of immunoelectrophoresis was developed – antigens are separated on the basis of their charge before being visualized by precipitation (*Fig. 28.3*).

These gel techniques only identify antigens and antibodies qualitatively, but by further modification, using the technique of single radial immunodiffusion, they can be made quantitative (*Fig. 28.4*).

By applying a voltage across the gels to move the antigens and antibodies together, immunodiffusion becomes counter-current electrophoresis, and single radial immunodiffusion becomes rocket electrophoresis (*Fig. 28.5*).

These techniques operate in the range of 20 µg/ml to 2 mg/ml of antigen or antibody.

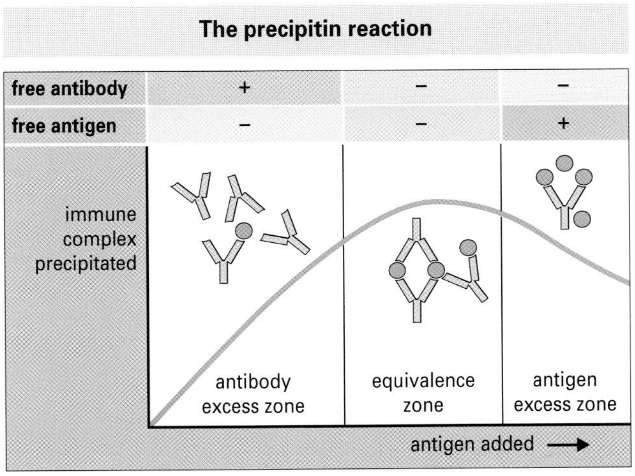

The precipitin reaction

free antibody	+	–	–
free antigen	–	–	+

immune complex precipitated

antibody excess zone | equivalence zone | antigen excess zone

antigen added ⟶

Fig. 28.1 The classical illustration of the antigen–antibody reaction *in vitro* is the precipitin reaction. As increasing concentrations of antigen are added to a constant amount of antibody, the amount of immune complex precipitated rises and then falls. The precipitin curve generated in this way has three zones:
Antibody excess zone: the amount of antigen is insufficient to react with and precipitate all the antibody present; thus free antibody can be detected in the supernatant.
Equivalence zone: the added antigen is sufficient to combine with and precipitate all the antibody present and neither free antigen nor antibody can be detected in the supernatant.
Antigen excess zone (prozone): the amount of antigen exceeds that required to bind all the antibody, and this leads to a reduction in the amount of antibody precipitated. This fall is due to the solubilization of the antigen–antibody complexes by the excess antigen. The extent to which this phenomenon occurs varies with different antibodies and with the species from which the antibody is derived.

Haemagglutination and complement fixation

Antibody may be detected and measured by haemagglutination at lower concentrations than those detectable by countercurrent electrophoresis and rocket electrophoresis. This relies on the ability of antibody to cross-link red blood cells by interacting with the antigens on their surface (*Fig. 28.6*).

Precipitin reactions in gels: immuno-double-diffusion

a. identity

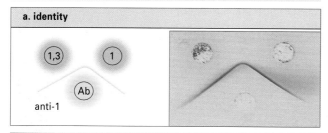

anti-1

b. non-identity

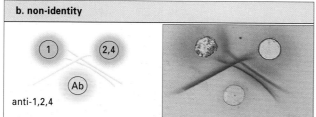

anti-1,2,4

c. partial identity

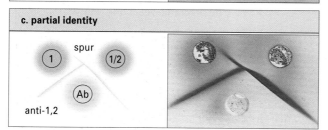

anti-1,2

Fig. 28.2 In immuno-double-diffusion, agar gels are poured onto slides and allowed to set; wells are then punched in the gel and the test solutions of antigen (Ag) and antibody (Ab) are added. The solutions diffuse out and where Ag and Ab meet they bind to each other, cross-link and precipitate leaving a line of precipitation. The precipitin bands can be visualized by washing the gel to remove soluble proteins and then staining the precipitin arcs with a protein stain such as Coomassie blue. This technique may be used to determine the relationship between antigens (blue) and a particular test antibody (yellow). Three basic patterns appear. The numbers in the blue wells refer to the epitopes present on the test antigen. In reaction (a) the precipitin arcs formed between the antibody and the two test antigens fuse, indicating that the antibody is precipitating identical epitopes in each preparation (epitope 1). This does not mean that the antigens are necessarily identical; they are only identical in as far as the antibody cannot distinguish a difference. In reaction (b) the antibody preparation distinguishes the three different antigens, which form independent precipitin arcs. In reaction (c) the antigens share epitope 1 but one antigen also has epitope 2. This is the same situation as in (a), but in this case the antibody can distinguish them, by virtue of being able to react against both epitopes. A line of identity forms with anti-epitope 1, with the addition of a 'spur' where the anti-epitope 2 has reacted with the second epitope, thus indicating partial rather than total identity between the antigen preparations.

Immunoelectrophoresis

1. separation of antigens

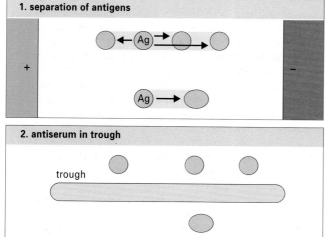

2. antiserum in trough

trough

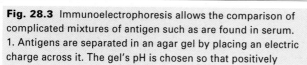

3. diffusion and precipitation

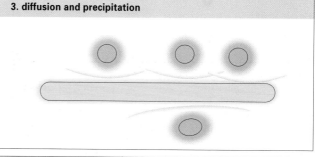

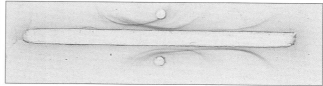

Fig. 28.3 Immunoelectrophoresis allows the comparison of complicated mixtures of antigen such as are found in serum. 1. Antigens are separated in an agar gel by placing an electric charge across it. The gel's pH is chosen so that positively charged proteins move to the negative electrode and negatively charged proteins to the positive. 2. A trough is then cut between the wells and filled with the antibody, which is left to diffuse. 3. The antigens and antibody form precipitin arcs.

Antigen–antibody reactions lead to immune complex formation which produces complement fixation via the classical pathway, and this may be exploited to determine the amount of antigen or antibody present (*Fig. 28.7*). Haemagglutination and complement fixation can detect antibody at levels of less than 1 μg/ml.

Direct and indirect immunofluorescence

Immunofluorescence is used extensively to detect autoantibodies and antibodies to tissue and cellular antigens (*Fig. 28.8*). Although these techniques are more cumbersome than those described earlier if a quantitative measure of antibody concentration is required, they do have advantages. By using tissue sections (which contain a large number of antigens), antibodies to several different antigens can be identified on a

---

Single radial immunodiffusion

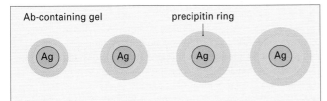

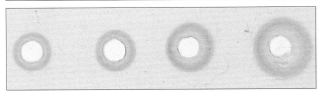

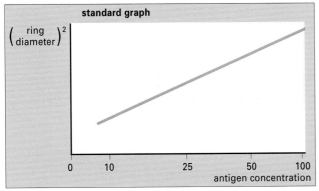

Fig. 28.4 Single radial immunodiffusion allows quantitation of antigens. Antibody is added to the agar gel which is then poured onto slides and allowed to set. Wells are punched in the agar and standard volumes of test antigen of different concentration are put in the wells. The plates are left for at least 24 hours, during which time the antigen diffuses out of the wells to form soluble complexes (in antigen excess) with the antibody. These continue to diffuse outwards, binding more antibody until an equivalence point is reached and the complexes precipitate in a ring. The area within the precipitin ring, measured as ring diameter squared, is proportional to the antigen concentration. Unknowns are derived by interpolation from the standard curve (graph). The whole process may be reversed using an antigen-containing gel to determine unknown concentrations of antibody.

Countercurrent electrophoresis and rocket electrophoresis

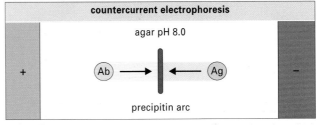

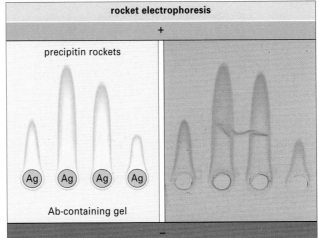

Fig. 28.5 Countercurrent electrophoresis is performed in agar gels where the pH is chosen so that the antibody is positively charged and the antigen being tested is negatively charged. By applying a voltage across the gel the antigen and antibody move towards each other and precipitate. The principle is the same as for immuno-double-diffusion but the sensitivity is increased 10–20-fold. Antigens may be quantitated by electrophoresing them into an antibody-containing gel in the technique termed rocket electrophoresis. The pH of the gel is chosen so that the antibodies are immobile and the antigen is negatively charged. Precipitin rockets form; the height of the rocket is proportional to antigen concentration, and unknowns are determined by interpolation from standards. The appearance of stained rockets is shown on the right. Both techniques rely on the antigen and antibody having different charges at the selected pH; this is true for most antigens since antibodies have a relatively high isoelectric point (i.e. they are neutrally charged at a more alkaline pH than most antigens). If the charges on the antigen and antibody do not differ sufficiently, the antibody or antigen can be chemically modified to alter its isoelectric point. Rocket electrophoresis can be reversed to estimate antibody concentration if a suitable pH gel can be found to immobilize the antigen, without damaging it or preventing the antigen–antibody reaction.

Haemagglutination

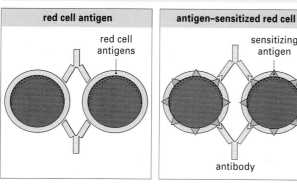

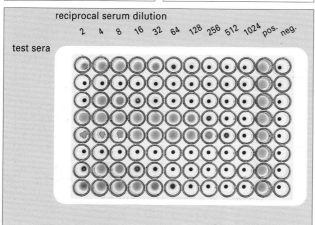

Fig. 28.6 The active haemagglutination test (upper panel, left) detects antibodies to red blood-cell antigens. The antibody is serially diluted (usually in doubling dilutions) in physiological saline and placed in the wells (columns 1–10, lower panel read left to right) of the haemagglutination plate. Positive controls (column 11) and negative controls (column 12) are included. In this example, eight different antisera (rows A–H) are being tested. A suspension of red cells (containing a protein to prevent the red cells agglutinating non-specifically) is added to each well to give a final concentration of about 1% cells. If sufficient antibody is present to agglutinate (cross-link) the cells, they sink as a mat to the bottom of the well. If insufficient antibody is present, the cells roll down the sloping sides of the plate to form a red pellet at the bottom. Some antibodies do not agglutinate red cells very effectively and may be detected in the indirect agglutination test by the addition of a second antibody which binds to the non-agglutinating antibody already bound on the red cell. By binding different antigens onto the red-cell surface, covalently or non-covalently, the test can be extended to detect antibodies to antigens other than those found on red cells (upper right panel). Chromic chloride, tannic acid, glutaraldehyde and a number of other chemicals are used to cross-link the antigen to the cells.

Complement fixation

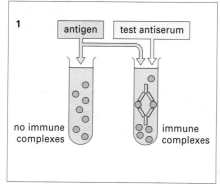

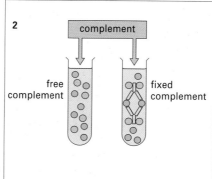

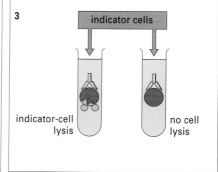

Fig. 28.7 The complement fixation test detects antibody. 1. A test antiserum is titred in doubling dilutions and a fixed amount of antigen is added to each tube or well. If antibody is present in the test serum, immune complexes will form. 2. Complement is then added to the mixture. If complexes are present, they will fix complement and 'consume' it. 3. In the final step, indicator cells (red cells) together with a subagglutinating amount of antibody (erythrocyte antibody) are added to the mixture. If there is any complement remaining these cells will be lysed; if it was consumed by immune complexes in stage 2, there will be insufficient to lyse the red cells. A quantity of complement is used that is just enough to lyse the indicator cells if none is consumed by the complexes. The assay is often performed on plastic plates. By using constant amounts of antibody and titrations of antigen, the assay can be applied to testing for antigens. Appropriate controls are most important in this assay because some antibody preparations consume complement without the addition of antigen, for example if the antibody preparation is serum that already contains immune complexes. Some antigens can also have anti-complement activity. The controls should therefore include antibody alone and antigen alone to check that neither fix complement by themselves.

single slide according to their distribution between cells or in different subcellular compartments.

Furthermore, the immunofluorescence tests can be used to identify particular cells in suspension, that is, to identify antigens on live cells. When a live stained-cell suspension is put through a fluorescence-activated cell sorter (FACS), the machine measures the fluorescence intensity of each cell and then the cells are separated according to their particular fluorescent brightness. This technique permits the isolation of different cell populations with different surface antigens stained with different fluorescent antibodies (*Fig. 28.9*). Chapter 11 gives a demonstration of how this technique is used to identify different populations of developing thymocytes (see Fig. 11.19).

Direct and indirect immunofluorescence

direct	indirect	indirect complement amplified
fluoresceinated antibody — tissue section	antibody	antibody
wash	wash	wash
	add fluoresceinated anti-Ig	add complement
	wash	wash
		add fluoresceinated anti-C3 antibody
		wash

Fig. 28.8 Immunofluorescence detects antigen *in situ*. A section is cut on a cryostat from a deep-frozen tissue block. This ensures that labile antigens are not damaged by fixatives.

Direct: the test solution of fluoresceinated antibody is applied to the section in a drop, incubated and washed off. Any bound antibody is then revealed under the microscope; UV light is directed onto the section through the objective, thus the field is dark and areas with bound fluorescent antibody fluoresce green. The pattern of fluorescence is characteristic for each tissue antigen.

Indirect: antibody applied to the section as a solution is visualized using fluoresceinated anti-immunoglobulin.

Indirect complement amplified: this is an elaboration of the indirect method for the detection of complement-fixing antibody (see *Fig. 28.7*). In the second step fresh complement is added which becomes fixed around the site of antibody binding. Due to the amplification steps in the classical complement pathway (see Chapter 13) one antibody molecule can cause many C3b molecules to bind to the section; these are then visualized with fluoresceinated anti-C3.

Fluorescence-activated cell sorter (FACS)

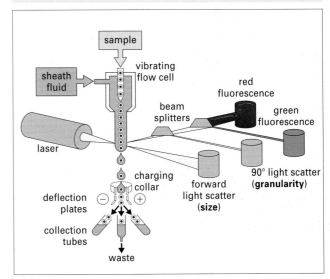

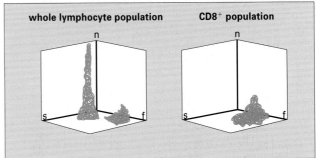

whole lymphocyte population   **CD8⁺ population**

Fig. 28.9 Cells in the sample are stained with specific fluorescent reagents to detect surface molecules and are then introduced into the vibrating flow chamber of the FACS. The cell stream passing out of the chamber is encased in a sheath of buffer fluid. The stream is illuminated by laser light and each cell is measured for size (forward light scatter) and granularity (90° light scatter), as well as for red and green fluorescence, to detect two different surface markers. The vibration in the cell stream causes it to break into droplets which are charged and may then be steered by deflection plates under computer control to collect different cell populations according to the parameters measured. The 3-dimensional graphs plot size (s), number (n) and fluorescence (f) for a whole lymphocyte population and a CD8⁺ population obtained by cell sorting, both stained with anti-CD8.

Immunoassay

The techniques of immunoassay using labelled reagents for detecting antigens and antibodies are exquisitely sensitive and extremely economical in the use of reagents (*Fig. 28.10*). Solid-phase assays for antibodies employing ligands labelled with radioisotopes or enzymes (enzyme-linked immunosorbent

test; ELISA, *Fig. 28.11*) are probably the most widely used of all immunological assays because large numbers can be performed in a relatively short time, although fluorescent or chemiluminescent markers are tending to replace radioisotopes for labelling. Antigen may be measured by either the two-site capture assay or the competitive assay, which may be carried out using any of the labels for detection (*Fig. 28.12*).

Immunoblotting and immunoprecipitation

The methods described so far are particularly useful for measuring levels of certain known antigens or antibodies, but often

Immunoassay for antibody

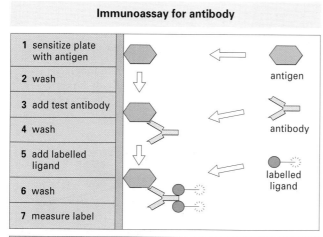

typical titration curve

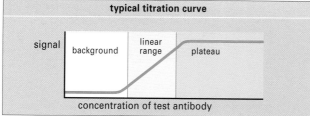

Fig. 28.10 Immunoassay for antibody. 1. Antigen in saline is incubated on a plastic plate or tube, and small quantities become absorbed onto the plastic surface. 2. Free antigen is washed away. (The plate may then be blocked with excess of an irrelevant protein to prevent any subsequent non-specific binding of proteins.) 3. Test antibody is added, which binds to the antigen. 4. Unbound proteins are washed away. 5. The antibody is detected by a labelled ligand. The ligand may be a molecule such as staphylococcal protein A which binds to the Fc region of IgG – more often it is another antibody specific for the test antibody. By using a ligand which binds to particular classes or subclasses of test antibody it is possible to distinguish isotypes. 6. Unbound ligand is washed away. 7. The label bound to the plate is measured. A typical titration curve is shown in the graph above. With increasing amounts of test antibody the signal rises from a background level through a linear range to a plateau. Antibody titres can only be detected correctly within the linear range. Typically the plateau binding is 20–100 times the background. The sensitivity of the technique is usually about 1–50 ng/ml of specific antibody. Specificity of the assay may be checked by adding increasing concentrations of free test antigen to the test antibody at step 3; this binds to the antibody and blocks it from binding to the antigen on the plate. Addition of increasing amounts of free antigen reduces the signal.

Enzyme-linked immunosorbent assay (ELISA)

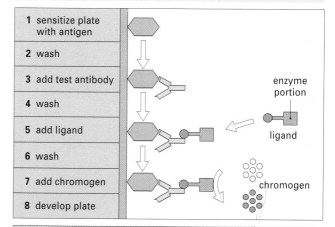

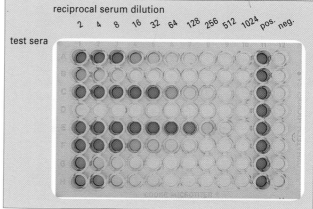

Fig. 28.11 The ELISA plate is prepared in the same way as the assay in *Figure 28.10* up to step 4. In this system, ligand is a molecule which can detect the antibody and is covalently coupled to an enzyme such as peroxidase. This binds the test antibody and after free ligand is washed away (6) the bound ligand is visualized by the addition of chromogen (7) – a colourless substrate which is acted on by the enzyme portion of the ligand to produce a coloured end-product. A developed plate is shown in the lower panel. The amount of test antibody is measured by assessing the amount of coloured end-product by optical density scanning of the plate.

Assay of antigen

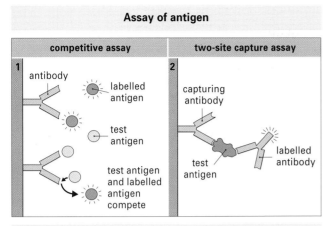

competitive assay	two-site capture assay

Fig. 28.12 1. Competitive assay. The test antigen is placed together with labelled antigen onto a plate coated with specific antibody. The more test antigen is present, the less of the labelled standard antigen binds. This type of assay is often used to measure antigens at relatively high concentrations or hormones which only have a single site available for combination with antibody. 2. Two-site capture assay. The assay plate is coated with specific antibody, the test solution then applied and any antigen present captured by the bound antibody. After washing away unbound material, the captured antigen is detected using a labelled antibody against another epitope on the antigen. Since the antigen is detected by two different antibodies, the second in excess, such assays are both highly specific and sensitive.

it is necessary to identify and characterize previously unknown antigens from a complex mixture, in which case immunoblotting is very useful.

In immunoblotting, complex mixtures are resolved in analytical separation gels and then the molecules are transferred to membranes (blots) for the identification of individual antigens by specific antisera. By using sodium dodecyl sulphate (SDS) gels, isoelectric focusing gels or peptide mapping gels in the initial separation, it is possible to obtain data on the size, isoelectric point and molecular relationships of the antigens which are under investigation (*Fig. 28.13*).

In some cases an antigen becomes so denatured by the gel separations and blotting procedures that some of its epitopes are destroyed and it can no longer bind to particular antibodies. In this case it is necessary to use immunoprecipitation instead to identify which antigen an antibody binds to. The technique can be used either with soluble antigens or with cell-surface antigens (*Fig. 28.14*).

■ ISOLATION OF PURE ANTIBODIES

Immunologists often need to isolate pure antibodies, which may be either antigen-specific or non-specific immunoglobulin. Isolation of non-specific immunoglobulin from serum is usually carried out by sequential protein fractionation steps which may include:

Immunoblotting

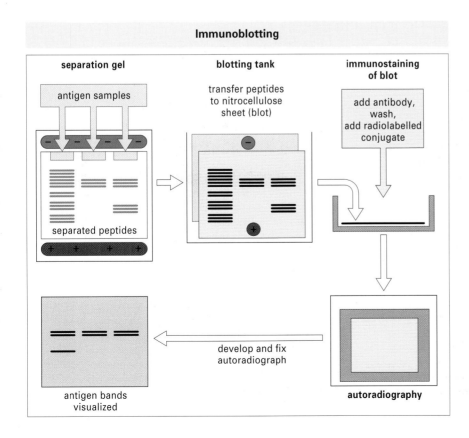

Fig. 28.13 In immunoblotting, antigen samples are first separated in an analytical gel, for example an SDS polyacrylamide gel or an isoelectric focusing gel. The resolved molecules are transferred electrophoretically to a nitrocelluose membrane in a blotting tank. The blot is then treated with antibody to the specific antigen, washed, and a radiolabelled conjugate to detect antibodies is bound to the blot. The principle is similar to that of a RIA or ELISA. After washing again, the blot is placed in contact with X-ray film in a cassette; the autoradiograph is developed and the antigen bands which have bound the antibody are visible. The technique can be modified for use with a chemiluminescent label or an enzyme-coupled conjugate (as in ELISA), where the bound material can be detected by treatment with a chromogen which deposits an insoluble reagent directly onto the blot.

- **Precipitation of the gammaglobulins** in 30–50% ammonium sulphate.
- **Gel filtration** to obtain molecules of the correct size.
- **Ion exchange chromatography** to isolate molecules which are positively charged at neutral pH.
- **Affinity chromatography** on natural ligands for immunoglobulin, such as protein A (protein A is a component of staphylococcal cell walls which binds to a region in Cγ2 and Cγ3 of most IgG subclasses, i.e. IgG1, IgG2 and IgG4).

Isolation of antigen-specific immunoglobulin is carried out by affinity chromatography using antigen coupled to Sepharose; pure antibody is eluted from the immunoabsorbent with chaotropic agents such as sodium thiocyanate, or glycine–HCl buffer, or diethylamine buffer. Affinity chromatography is the technique used where the isolation of pure antibody or pure antigen is the objective (*Fig. 28.15*).

Monoclonal antibody production

Another way of obtaining pure antibody of a defined specificity is to produce monoclonal antibodies from cells in culture. By creating an immortal clone of cells which manufacture a single antibody of defined specificity, production can

Immunoprecipitation

add specific antibody   add co-precipitating reagents   spin down precipitate

labelled antigen mixture   complexed antigen   resolubilize

autoradiograph   SDS gel sample   separated proteins of the immune complex

Fig. 28.14 In immunoprecipitation the antigens being tested are labelled with ^{125}I, and antibody is added, which binds only to its specific antigen. The complexes are precipitated by the addition of co-precipitating agents, such as anti-immunoglobulin antibodies or staphylococcal protein A. The insoluble complexes are spun down and washed to remove any unbound labelled antigens. Then the precipitate is resolubilized, for example in SDS, and the components separated on analytical gels. After running, the fixed gels are autoradiographed, to show the position of the specific labelled antigen. Frequently the antigens are derived from the surface of radiolabelled cells, which are solubilized with detergents before the immunoprecipitation. It is also possible to label the antigens with biotin, and detect them at the end chromatographically using streptavidin (binds biotin) coupled to an enzyme such as peroxidase (cf. ELISA technique).

Affinity chromatography

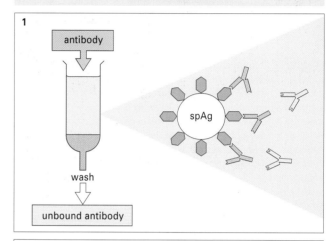

antibody

spAg

wash

unbound antibody

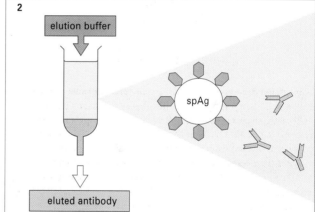

elution buffer

spAg

eluted antibody

Fig. 28.15 By using affinity chromatography a pure population of antibodies may be isolated. 1. A solid-phase immunoabsorbent is prepared (spAg); this is an antigen covalently coupled to an inert support (e.g. cross-linked dextran beads). The immunoabsorbent is placed in a column and the antibody mixture is run in under physiological conditions. Antibody to the antigen binds to the column while unbound antibody washes through. 2. In the second step the column is eluted to obtain the bound antibody using elution buffer (e.g. acetate pH 3.0, diethylamine pH 11.5, 3M guanidine HCl), which dissociates the antigen–antibody bond. By placing antibody on the column the process can be reversed to obtain pure antigen. The technique can also be used to obtain other types of molecule. For example, a lectin column will absorb all molecules with particular sugar residues and these can be eluted in buffer containing the free sugar molecules, which competes with the bound protein for the attachment site on the lectin.

be maintained indefinitely (*Fig. 28.16*), obviating the vagaries of antiserum production (lack of uniformity). Monoclonal antibodies have found widespread use in many biological sciences, where the antibody is used as a highly specific probe.

Monoclonal antibody production

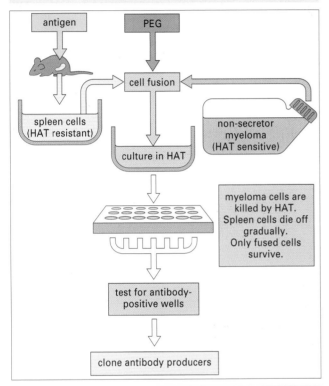

Fig. 28.16 Animals (usually mice or rats) are immunized with antigen. Once the animals are making a good antibody response their spleens are removed and a cell suspension is prepared (lymph node cells may also be used). These cells are fused with a myeloma cell line by the addition of polyethylene glycol (PEG) which promotes membrane fusion. Only a small proportion of the cells fuse successfully. The fusion mixture is then set up in culture with medium containing 'HAT'. HAT is a mixture of hypoxanthine, aminopterin and thymidine. Aminopterin is a powerful toxin which blocks a metabolic pathway. This pathway can be bypassed if the cell is provided with the intermediate metabolites hypoxanthine and thymidine. Thus spleen cells can grow in HAT medium, but the myeloma cells die in HAT medium because they have a metabolic defect and cannot use the bypass pathway. When the culture is set up in HAT medium it contains spleen cells, myeloma cells and fused cells. The spleen cells die in culture naturally after 1–2 weeks and the myeloma cells are killed by the HAT. Fused cells survive however, as they have the immortality of the myeloma and the metabolic bypass of the spleen cells. Some of them will also have the antibody-producing capacity of the spleen cells. Any wells containing growing cells are tested for the production of the desired antibody (often by solid-phase immunoassay) and if positive the cultures are cloned by plating out so that there is only one cell in each well. This produces a clone of cells derived from a single progenitor, which is both immortal and a producer of monoclonal antibody.

Since any particular B cell is effectively producing a monoclonal antibody, the requirement is to immortalize and propagate individual B cells. Most monoclonal antibodies are generated by the fusion of mouse splenocytes with a B-cell myeloma from the same strain which does not secrete its own antibody. It is also possible to produce interstrain or even interspecies hybrids, but these are often unstable. An alternative method is to transform B cells; for example, human B cells may be immortalized for monoclonal antibody production by infecting them with Epstein–Barr virus.

A new way of generating antibodies is by phage display. In this exciting technique it is possible to express antibody-variable regions (VH and VL) as part-molecules (Fv) of defined antigen-binding specificity and affinity on the surface of M13 filamentous phage so that they can be selected by antigen. In addition, if the phages are used to infect certain bacteria, the Fv protein is secreted in large amounts into the culture medium. This approach does not necessarily require the deliberate immunization of animals or humans (*Fig. 28.17*).

Production of Fv antibodies by phage display

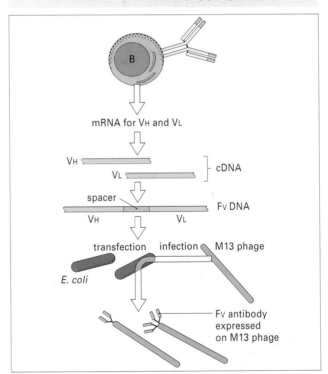

Fig. 28.17 To produce Fv antibodies by phage display, antibody VH and VL genes are first amplified from B cell mRNA by the polymerase chain reaction. The genes are joined together with a spacer to give a gene for an Fv fragment. Bacteria are then transfected with the gene in a phagemid vector containing a leader sequence, a fragment of the gene expressing phage coat protein 3 and an M13 origin of replication and then infected with M13 phage. The phages replicate and express the Fv on their tips. Phages displaying the right specificity are isolated by panning on antigen-coated plates and amplified. The antigen-specific phage can be used to infect strains of bacteria which allow the secretion of the Fv protein into the culture medium.

Although a monoclonal antibody is a well-defined reagent it does not have a greater specificity than a polyclonal antiserum which recognizes the antigen by means of a number of different epitopes.

■ ASSAYS FOR COMPLEMENT

The simplest measurement of complement activity is to determine the concentration of serum which will cause lysis of 50% of a standardized preparation of antibody-sensitized erythrocytes (EA). This is carried out in tubes or microwells. A simpler system, which provides a crude measure of complement activity is single-radial haemolysis. The technique is similar to that of single-radial immunodiffusion (see *Fig. 28.4*) except that the wells contain the test serum and the gel contains EA. A zone of haemolysis develops around wells containing active complement, and the size of the zone is proportional to the amount of complement in the well. This technique measures the total activity of the classical and lytic pathways (C1–C9), but if a serum is deficient in complement activity it cannot identify which complement protein is lacking.

Individual components may be measured separately to determine either their total level or their functional level. This is an important distinction, since a component may be present in normal quantities but be functionally inactive. Total levels of individual complement proteins are usually measured by RIA or by ELISA using antibody specific for the protein under investigation. Functional levels are measured in assays tailored to detect each individual complement protein by providing a cocktail of sensitized red cells plus all the components required for lysis, except the one under investigation (*Fig. 28.18*).

■ ISOLATION OF LYMPHOCYTE POPULATIONS

Many of the experiments performed by immunologists use populations of lymphocytes for work either *in vivo* or *in vitro*. The main sources of lymphocytes from experimental animals are the thymus, the spleen or the peripheral lymph nodes. Specialized studies may require isolation of cells from other areas such as Peyer's patches. Recirculating cells may be obtained by cannulating the thoracic duct and collecting the draining lymphocytes over a number of hours. In studies on humans, peripheral blood lymphocytes are the most readily available source of cells, but spleen, tonsil or lymph nodes may become available following surgical resection. However, problems can arise with surgical material due to the presence of infectious agents or tumour cells, depending on the circumstances that led to surgery. It should be emphasized that the cell populations derived from each of these tissues is quite distinct, with respect to the maturity of the lymphocytes and the proportions of different cell populations. The thymus is a source of fairly pure T cells but these are at varying stages of maturity. When working on lymphocytes from other sources, it is often desirable to separate the different cell populations so as to distinguish their effects.

Reference has already been made to the use of the fluorescence-activated cell sorter (FACS) for the isolation of

Assays for complement components

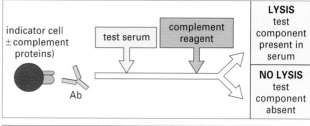

test	indicator	complement reagent
C1	EAC 4 (guinea-pig)	C1 reagent
C4	EA	C4-deficient guinea-pig serum
C2	EAC 4 (human) (antrypol)	C2 reagent
C3	EAC 142 (guinea-pig)	C5–9(NH$_3$ treated guinea-pig serum)
C5	EAC 14 oxy 23	C5-deficient mouse serum
C6	EAC 143 (human) (antrypol)	C6-deficient rabbit serum
FB	EA+EGTA+Mg^{2+}	B-deficient serum (50°C treated)
FD	EA+EGTA+Mg^{2+}	D-deficient serum (Sephadex G75 exclusion peak)

Fig. 28.18 These assays detect specific complement components in a test serum. The principle of the assay is to mix sensitized red cells with a 'complement reagent' so that the sensitized cells plus the reagent contain all the complement components needed to lyse the red cells except for the component being tested. For example, to test for C4, erythrocytes sensitized with antibody (EA) are placed with C4-deficient guinea-pig serum. The cells will be lysed if there is C4 in the test serum, but not if none is present. The table lists the combinations of reagents used for each test component. The red cells are prepared by blocking the reactions of EA with complement at a specific point. The complement reagents may be sera thought to be deficient in one component or sera treated physicochemically to remove or inactivate one component. In practice the assay would be performed quantitatively, for example, by single-radial haemolysis, or in tubes to determine the point at which 50% of the red cells are lysed.

lymphocyte populations, based on their surface markers. The number of cells isolated is, however, limited by the flow-through rate, which is slow because each cell is individually sorted. A number of bulk methods are also available for separating lymphocytes and the specific subpopulations. These include density-gradient separation, rosetting, panning and magnetic separations.

Density-gradient separation relies on lymphocytes being less dense than erythrocytes and granulocytes (*Fig. 28.19*), and is used to isolate the majority of blood lymphocytes.

Rosetting and panning (or plating) are used to isolate subpopulations (*Figs 28.20* and *28.21*). Lymphocyte panning is a type of affinity chromatography applied to lymphocytes. A related technique uses magnetic beads coated with specific antibodies (e.g. anti-CD4). The beads are mixed with the cell population and bind to those recognized by the antibody. These cells can then be removed or isolated by applying a magnetic field.

Another useful method for removing unwanted cell populations relies on antibody and complement. When a specific antibody (e.g. anti-CD8) is added to a mixture of cells, followed by complement, that subpopulation of cells will be lysed. Naturally this will only work with antibodies that fix complement, and where the target population of cells has sufficient surface antigens to fix a lytic dose of complement.

Another approach to the preparation of lymphocytes is to generate antigen-specific lines of T cells, and propagate them for an extended period (*Fig. 28.22*). This obviates the need for frequent isolation of primary cultures from animals.

■ EFFECTOR-CELL ASSAYS

Various methods have been developed for assaying lymphocyte-effector functions, including antibody production, cytotoxicity, and T-cell-mediated help and suppression.

Density-gradient separation of lymphocytes on Ficoll Isopaque

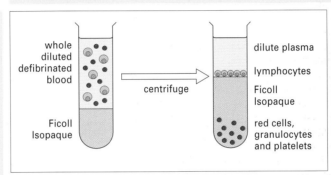

Fig. 28.19 Lymphocytes can be separated from whole blood using a density gradient. Whole blood is defibrinated by shaking with glass beads and the resulting clot removed. The blood is then diluted in tissue culture medium and layered on top of a tube half full of Ficoll. Ficoll has a density greater than that of lymphocytes but less than that of red cells and granulocytes (e.g. neutrophils). After centrifugation the red cells and polymorphonuclear neutrophils (PMNs) pass down through the Ficoll to form a pellet at the bottom of the tube while lymphocytes settle at the interface of the medium and Ficoll. The lymphocyte preparation can be further depleted of macrophages and residual PMNs by the addition of iron filings; these are taken up by phagocytes which can then be drawn away with a strong magnet. Macrophages can be removed by leaving the cell suspension to settle on a plastic dish. Macrophages adhere to plastic, whereas the lymphocytes can be washed off.

Isolation of lymphocyte subpopulations – rosetting

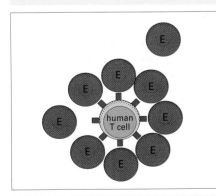
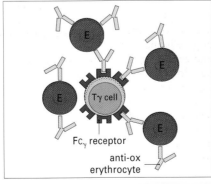
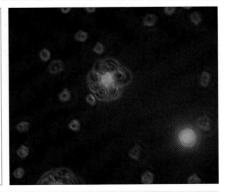

Fig. 28.20 Rosetting relies on the fact that some lymphocyte populations have receptors for erythrocytes. Human T cells have receptors for sheep erythrocytes (E); these are CD2 molecules (left). They are not present on mouse T cells in sufficient quantities, so mouse T cells cannot be isolated by this approach. When mixed together the T cells form rosettes with the erythrocytes and may be separated from non-rosetting B cells on Ficoll gradients. A modification of this technique to isolate cells with other receptors is also shown (middle). For example, some T cells (Tγ cells) have a receptor for the Fc of IγG (Fcγ). These cells may be identified and isolated by rosetting with ox erythrocytes sensitized with a subagglutinating amount of anti-ox erythrocyte. A rosetted lymphocyte is shown on the right. (Courtesy of Dr P. M. Lydyard.)

Isolation of lymphocyte subpopulations – panning

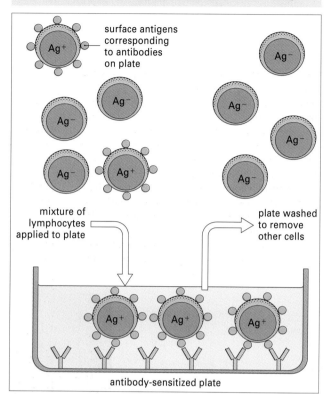

Fig. 28.21 Cell populations can be separated on antibody-sensitized plates. Antibody binds non-covalently to the plastic plate (as for solid-phase immunoassay) and the cell mixture is applied to the plate. Antigen-positive cells (Ag⁺) bind to the antibody and the antigen-negative cells (Ag⁻) can be carefully washed off. By changing the culture conditions or by enzyme-digestion of the cells on the plate it is sometimes possible to recover the cells bound to the plate. Often the cells that have bound to the plate are altered by their binding; for example, binding to the plate cross-links the antigen which can cause cell activation. Thus, the method is most satisfactory for removing a subpopulation from the population, rather than isolating it. Examples of the application of this method include separating T_H and T_C cell populations using antibodies to CD4 or CD8, and separating T cells from B cells using anti-Ig (which binds to the surface antibody of the B cell). In reverse, by sensitizing the plate with antigen, antigen-binding cells can be separated from non-binding cells.

Antibody-forming cells are measured by plaque-forming cell assay (*Fig. 28.23*), which can detect IgG- or IgM-producing cells. Another way of detecting antibody-producing cells is by the ELISPOT enzymatic test assay (*Fig. 28.24*). A development of this assay allows the detection of functional T cells according to the soluble mediators they release, i.e. cytokines. In this assay the plate is sensitized with an antibody to the specific cytokine (e.g. anti-IFN). This captures the specific cytokine released in a spot around the active T cell.

T-cell lines

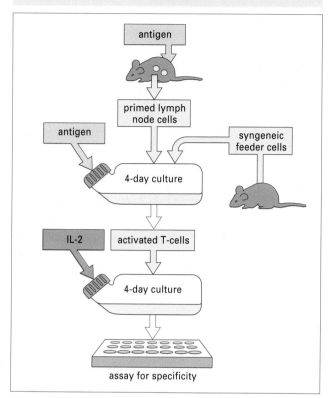

Fig. 28.22 The figure illustrates one protocol for the preparation of T-cell lines, although many other protocols are used. Mice are primed with antigen (usually subcutaneously in the rear foot pad), and the draining lymph nodes (in this case the popliteal and inguinal) are removed 1 week later and set up in co-culture with the antigen and with syngeneic feeder cells, i.e. cells from mice of the same inbred line (e.g. normal thymocytes or splenocytes). After 4 days the lymphoblasts are isolated and induced to proliferate with interleukin-2 (IL-2). When the population of cells has expanded sufficiently they are checked for antigen and MHC specificity in a lymphocyte transformation test, and are maintained by alternate cycles of culture on antigen-treated feeder cells and culture in IL-2-containing medium.

Antigen-specific T cells are often detected by the lymphocyte stimulation test, which measures their response to antigen as shown by their entering the cell cycle and incorporating precursors of DNA synthesis (*Fig. 28.25*). The cytotoxic activity of cell populations is usually detected by their ability to lyse target cells (e.g. virally infected cells, tumour cells, allogeneic tissue cells). Target-cell lysis is determined in the chromium-release assay (*Fig. 28.26*).

Lymphocyte migration

Experiments for the detection of lymphocyte migration *in vivo* usually involve tracking of labelled lymphocytes to particular tissues after intravenous infusion. The cells may be radiolabelled or marked with stable fluorescent dyes.

Plaque-forming cell assay

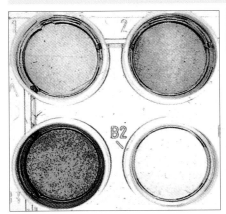

Fig. 28.23 Antibody-forming cells are measured by mixing the test population with antigen-sensitized red cells. Following incubation, the red cells surrounding the cells secreting specific antibody become coated with the antibody and so may be lysed by complement. Two types of plaque can be identified:

Direct plaques: antigen-specific IgM antibodies produced by antibody-forming cells are able to directly cause complement-mediated lysis of antigen-sensitized red cells, because of their excellent complement-fixing ability.

Indirect plaques: antigen-specific IgG antibodies do not fix complement so efficiently and so anti-IgG antibodies must be added to enhance the ability of IgG-producing cells to lyse the target red cells.

By carrying out the assay with or without the anti-IgG step, it is possible to distinguish the number of IgM-producing B cells from the IgG-producing B cells.

ELISPOT assays

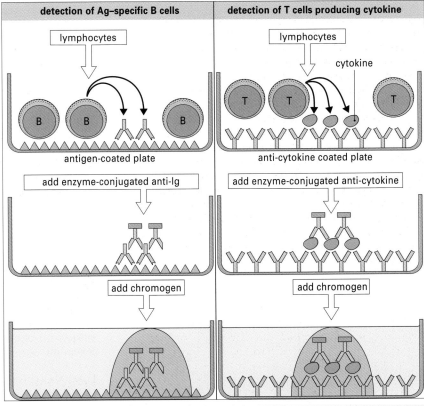

Fig. 28.24 Individual B cells producing specific antibody or individual T cells secreting particular cytokines may be detected by ELISPOT assay. For detection of antibody-producing cells, the lymphocytes are plated onto an antigen-sensitized plate. Secreted antibody binds antigen in the immediate vicinity of cells producing the specific antibody. The spots of bound antibody are then detected chromatographically using enzyme coupled to anti-immunoglobulin and a chromogen. For detection of cytokine-producing cells the plates are coated with anti-cytokine and the captured cytokine is detected with enzyme-coupled antibody to a different epitope on the cytokine. The appearance of a developed plate is shown top left.

(Photograph courtesy of P. Hutchings and Blackwell Scientific Publications.)

The lymphocyte stimulation test

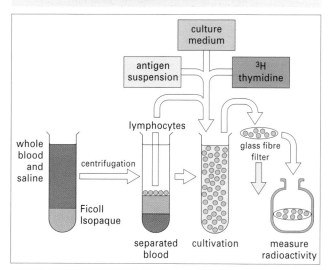

Fig. 28.25 In the lymphocyte stimulation test whole blood in saline solution is first layered on Ficoll Isopaque (which has a density between, and therefore separates, white cells and red cells) and centrifuged (400 × G). This separates the lymphocytes from the other cell and serum constituents (*see Fig. 28.19*). The cells are washed (to remove contaminants such as antigen) and then put into test tubes with a suspension of antigen and culture medium. Tritiated thymidine (^{3}H-thymidine) is added 16 hours before the cells are harvested. The cells are harvested on a glass-fibre filter disc and their radioactivity measured by placing the disc in a liquid scintillation counter. A high count indicates that the lymphocytes have undergone transformation and confirms their responsiveness to the antigen. This test can also be used for cells from lymphoid tissue.

Cytotoxicity assay by chromium release

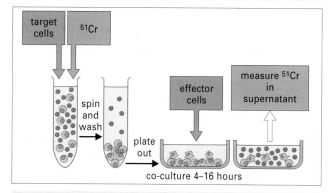

Fig. 28.26 To assay the cytotoxity of effector cells, target cells are incubated with ^{51}Cr, which is taken up into the cells and binds to protein. After incubation the free ^{51}Cr is washed away and the target cells are plated out. They are then co-cultured with the effector cells for 4–16 hours and the supernatant is removed and counted to detect chromium released from target cells lysed by the effector cells.

Radiolabelled cells are used for quantitative measurements of cell migration. Localization patterns within organs can be seen by autoradiography of labelled cells, or by direct visualization of fluorescent cells by microscopy under ultraviolet illumination.

Analysis of the adhesion molecules involved in lympho-cyte migration has mostly been carried out *in vitro*. In the Stamper–Woodroofe assay, the direct binding of lymphocytes to high endothelial venules is measured by allowing the lymphocytes to adhere to tissue sections of lymph node, Peyer's patch or other tissues containing high endothelial venules. Adherent cells are counted under the microscope. Antibodies to intercellular adhesion molecules will reduce the level of binding, provided that the antibodies attach to the adhesion molecules near their active sites. The adhesion of lymphocytes to endothelial-cell monolayers can also be blocked *in vitro*. The identity of the adhesion molecules may then be confirmed by labelling the lymphocytes or endothelial cells and using the antibodies which block adhesion, to immunoprecipitate the specific adhesion molecules.

■ GENE TARGETING AND TRANSGENIC ANIMALS

Transgenic animals

One way of investigating the function of a particular molecule is to produce a transgenic animal in which the gene for that molecule is deleted, over-expressed, or expressed in a mutated form. The original way of producing transgenic mice was to inject about 100 copies of the gene in question directly into the pronucleus of a fertilized oocyte. This is then transferred to the oviduct of a pseudopregnant female mouse, and the embryo left to develop. A variety of animals develop from such implantations. In a minority of embryos, one or more copies of the gene become incorporated into one of the chromosomes, before the first cell division occurs; these animals are heterozygous for the transgene. In another minority of the animals, the transgene becomes incorporated after the first division, and these are chimeras of normal cells and cells containing the transgene. In the majority of animals, no genes are incorporated. The status of each animal is established by taking some cells and establishing whether the gene is present by Southern blotting. Once heterozygous transgenics have been identified, these can be used in a programme of inbreeding to create a homozygous transgenic line.

Usually the transgenes become incorporated into a chromosome at random as a block. The number of transgenes incorporated is referred to as the copy number. It is important that this block does not disrupt another essential gene. How the transgenes are expressed depends on a number of factors. Sometimes the genes will be under the control of general promotors, and will be expressed in most tissues. Sometimes they will be linked with tissue-specific promotors so that they will only be expressed in some tissues (e.g. only in lymphocytes) or at particular stages of development. Care must be taken when interpreting the phenotype of transgenic animals, since it is unphysiological to express high quantities of transgenes in the wrong tissue.

Gene targeting

A more subtle approach is to use gene targeting. In this technique, a gene is transferred which interacts or recombines with the endogenous gene causing it to be altered in some way. For example the endogenous gene could be deleted (so-called 'knockout mice') or point mutated, or an exon could be removed. The altered gene in this case is injected into a pluripotent embryonic stem cell, where it recombines with the endogenous gene. The stem cell is then injected into a blastocyst and implanted as above (*Figure 28.27*).

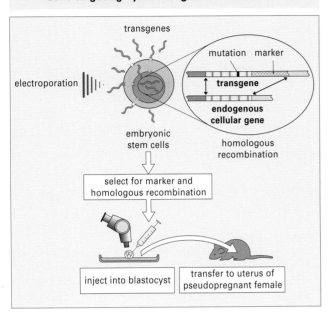

Gene targeting by homologous recombination

Fig. 28.27 Transgenic animals can be produced by gene targeting by homologous recombination. A gene segment is used which contains a sequence homologous to a cellular gene but with a mutation, for example, and with a ligated marker gene. These are electroporated into embryonic stem cells, which are then selected, using the marker gene, for cells which have taken up the exogenous gene. The cells are further selected for those which have recombined the exogenous gene with the endogenous gene. These cells are now injected into blastocysts, which are implanted into the uteri of pseudopregnant mice. The transgenic embryos are then left to develop and to be born normally.

Critical Thinking

■ You have identified a molecule present on the surface of T lymphocytes using a new monoclonal antibody and immunofluorescence. Select a combination of techniques which answer the following questions:

■ If you culture T cells in the presence of concanavalin-A (mitogen) and different amounts of the antibody, does the antibody reduce their ability to proliferate? Does it reduce the number of T cells which produce IL-2?

■ What is the molecular weight of the molecule?

■ Is the molecule present on both CD4+ T cells and CD8+ T cells?

■ What is the concentration of the antibody in the supernatant of the hybridoma cells which produce it?

FURTHER READING

Coligan JE, Kruisbeck AM, Margulies DH, Shevach EM, Shober W. (eds). *Current Protocols in Immunology*, Greene Publishing Associates & Wiley-Interscience, New York. 1991-continually updated.

Hudson L, Hay FC. *Practical Immunology*. 3rd ed. Oxford: Blackwell Scientific Publications, 1989.

Johnstone A, Thorpe R. *Immunochemistry in Practice*. 2nd ed. Oxford: Blackwell Scientific Publications, 1987.

Nairn RC, ed. *Practical Methods in Clinical Immunology*. Series. Edinburgh: Churchill Livingstone, 1980–1984.

Weir DM. *Handbook of Experimental Immunology*. Vols I & II. 4th ed. Oxford: Blackwell Scientific Publications, 1986.

Appendix I: HLA specifications

Allele	Specificity
DPA1*0101	-
DPA1*0102	-
DPA1*0103	-
DPA1*0201	-
DPA1*02021	-
DPA1*02022	-
DPA1*0301	-
DPA1*0401	-
DPB1*01011c	DPw1
DPB1*01012	DPw1
DPB1*0201d	DPw2
DPB1*02011	DPw2
DPB1*02012	DPw2
DPB1*0202	DPw2
DPB1*0301	DPw3
DPB1*0401	DPw4
DPB1*0402	DPw4
DPB1*0501	DPw5
DPB1*0601	DPw6
DPB1*0801	-
DPB1*0901	-
DPB1*1001	-
DPB1*11011c	-
DPB1*11012	-
DPB1*1301	-
DPB1*1401	-
DPB1*1501	-
DPB1*1601	-
DPB1*1701	-
DPB1*1801	-
DPB1*1901	-
DPB1*20011c	-
DPB1*20012	-
DPB1*2101	-
DPB1*2201	-
DPB1*2301	-
DPB1*2401	-
DPB1*2501	-
DPB1*26011c	-
DPB1*26012	-
DPB1*2701	-
DPB1*2801	-
DPB1*2901	-
DPB1*3001	-
DPB1*3101	-
DPB1*3201	-
DPB1*3301	-
DPB1*3401	-
DPB1*3501	-
DPB1*3601	-
DPB1*3701	-
DPB1*3801	-
DPB1*3901	-
DPB1*4001	-
DPB1*4101	-
DPB1*4401	-
DPB1*4501	-
DPB1*4601	-
DPB1*4701	-
DPB1*4801	-
DPB1*4901	-
DPB1*5001	-
DPB1*5101	-
DPB1*5201	-
DPB1*5301	-
DPB1*5401	-
DPB1*5501	-

Allele	Specificity
DQA1*0101	-
DQA1*0102	-
DQA1*0103	-
DQA1*0104	-
DQA1*0201	-
DQA1*03011	-
DQA1*03012	-
DQA1*0302	-
DQA1*0401	-
DQA1*0501e	-
DQA1*05011	-
DQA1*05012	-
DQA1*05013	-
DQA1*0502	-
DQA1*0601	-
DQB1*0501	DQ5(1)
DQB1*0502	DQ5(1)
DQB1*05031	DQ5(1)
DQB1*05032	DQ5(1)
DQB1*0504	-
DQB1*06011c	DQ6(1)
DQB1*06012	DQ6(1)
DQB1*0602	DQ6(1)
DQB1*0603	DQ6(1)
DQB1*0604	DQ6(1)
DQB1*06051c	DQ6(1)
DQB1*06052	DQ6(1)
DQB1*0606	-
DQB1*0607	-
DQB1-0608	-
DQB1*0609	-
DQB1*0201	DQ2
DQB1*0202	DQ2
DQB1*0301	DQ7(3)
DQB1*0302	DQ8(3)
DQB1*03031	DQ9(3)
DQB1*03032	DQ9(3)
DQB1*0304	DQ7(3)
DQB1*0305	-
DQB1*0401	DQ4
DQB1*0402	DQ4

Allele	Specificity
DMA*0101	
DMA*0102	
DMA*0103	
DMA*0104	
DMB*0101	
DMB*0102	
DMB*0103	
DMB*0104	

Allele	Specificity
DRA*0101	-
DRA*0102	-
DRB1*0101	DR1
DRB1*0102	DR1
DRB1*0103	DR103
DRB1*0104	DR1
DRB1*1501	DR15(2)
DRB1*15021c	DR15(2)
DRB1*15022	DR15(2)
DRB1*1503	DR15(2)
DRB1*1504	DR15(2)
DRB1*1601	DR16(2)
DRB1*1602	DR16(2)

Allele	Specificity
DRB1*1603	-
DRB1*1604	DR16(2)
DRB1*1605	-
DRB1*1606	DR2
DRB1*03011c	DR17(3)
DRB1*03012	DR17(3)
DRB1*0302	DR18(3)
DRB1*0303	DR18(3)
DRB1*0304	DR3
DRB1*0401	DR4
DRB1*0402	DR4
DRB1*0403	DR4
DRB1*0404	DR4
DRB1*0405	DR4
DRB1*0406	DR4
DRB1*0407	DR4
DRB1*0408	DR4
DRB1*0409	DR4
DRB1*0410	DR4
DRB1*0411	DR4
DRB1*0412	DR4
DRB1*0413	DR4
DRB1*0414	DR4
DRB1*0415	DR4
DRB1*0416	DR4
DRB1*0417	DR4
DRB1*0418	DR4
DRB1*0419	DR4
DRB1*11011	DR11(5)
DRB1*11012	DR11(5)
DRB1*1102	DR11(5)
DRB1*1103	DR11(5)
DRB1*11041	DR11(5)
DRB1*11042	DR11(5)
DRB1*1105	DR11(5)
DRB1*1106	DR11(5)
DRB1*1107	-
DRB1*11081	DR11(5)
DRB1*11082	DR11(5)
DRB1*1109	DR11(5)
DRB1*1110	-
DRB1*1111	-
DRB1*1112	-
DRB1*1113	-
DRB1*1201	DR12(5)
DRB1*1202	DR12(5)
DRB1*1203	DR12(5)
DRB1*1301	DR12(6)
DRB1*1302	DR13(6)
DRB1*1303	DR13(6)
DRB1*1304	DR13(6)
DRB1*1305	DR13(6)
DRB1*1306	DR13(6)
DRB1*1307	-
DRB1*1308	DR13(6)
DRB1*1309	-
DRB1*1310	DR13(6)
DRB1*1311	DR13(6)
DRB1*1312	-
DRB1*1313	-
DRB1*1401	DR14(6)
DRB1*1402	DR14(6)
DRB1*1403	DR1403
DRB1*1404	DR1404
DRB1*1405	DR14(6)
DRB1*1406	DR14(6)
DRB1*1407	DR14(6)
DRB1*1408	DR14(6)
DRB1*1409	DR14(6)

Allele	Specificity
DRB1*1410	-
DRB1*1411	-
DRB1*1412	-
DRB1*1413	-
DRB1*1414	-
DRB1*1415	-
DRB1*1416	-
DRB1*1417	-
DRB1*0701	DR7
DRB1*0801	DR8
DRB1*08021	DR8
DRB1*08022	DR8
DRB1*08031	DR8
DRB1*08032	DR8
DRB1*08041c	DR8
DRB1*08042	DR8
DRB1*0805	DR8
DRB1*0806	DR8
DRB1*0807	DR8
DRB1*0808	DR8
DRB1*0809	DR8
DRB1*0810	DR8
DRB1*0811	DR8
DRB1*09011	DR9
DRB1*09012	DR9
DRB1*1001	DR10
DRB3*0101	DR52
DRB3*0201	DR52
DRB3*0202	DR52
DRB3*0301	DR52
DRB4*01f	DR53
DRB4*01011c	DR53
DRB4*01012N	DR53
DRB4*0102	DR53
DRB4*0103	DR53
DRB5*0101	DR51
DRB5*0102	DR51
DRB5*0201	DR51
DRB5*0202	DR51
DRB5*0203	DR51
DRB6*0101	-
DRB6*0201	-
DRB6*0202	-
DRB7*01011	-
DRB7*01012	-

Allele	Specificity
B*0701	B7
B*0702	B7
B*0703	B703
B*0704	B7
B*0801	B8
B*0802	B8
B*1301	B13
B*1302	B13
B*1401	B64(14)
B*1402	B65(14)
B*1501	B62(15)
B*1502	B75(15)
B*1503	B72(15)
B*1504	B62(15)
B*1505	B62(15)
B*1506	B62(15)
B*1507	B62(15)
B*1508	B62(15)
B*1509	B70
B*1510	B7(70)
B*1511	B15
B*1512	B76(15)

Allele	Specificity
B*1513	B77(15)
B*1514	B76(15)
B*1515	B62(15)
B*1516	B63(15)
B*1517	B63(15)
B*1518	-
B*1519	B76(15)
B*1520	B62(15)
B*1801	B18
B*1802	B18
B*2701	B27
B*2702	B27
B*2703	B27
B*2704	B27
B*27051c	B27
B*27052	B27
B*2706	B27
B*2707	B27
B*2708	-
B*3501	B35
B*3502	B35
B*3503	B35
B*3504	B35
B*3505	B35
B*3506	B35
B*3507	B35
B*3508	B35
B*3701	B37
B*3801	B38(16)
B*3802	B38(16)
B*39011c	B3901
B*39013	B3901
B*39021c	B3902
B*39022	B3902
B*3903	B39(16)
B*3904	B39(16)
B*40011c	B60(40)
B*40012	B60(40)
B*4002	B61(40)
B*4003	B40
B*4004	B40
B*4005	B4005
B*4006	B61(40)
B*4101	B41
B*4201	B42
B*4402	B44(12)
B*4403	B44(12)
B*4404	B44(12)
B*4501	B45(12)
B*4601	B46
B*4701	B47
B*4801	B48
B*4802	B48
B*4901	B49(21)
B*5001	B50(21)
B*5101	B51(5)
B*5102	B5102
B*5103	B5103
B*5104	B51(5)
B*5105	B51(5)
B*52011d	B52(5)
B*52012	B52(5)
B*5301	B53
B*5401	B54(22)
B*5502	B55(22)
B*5601	B56(22)
B*5602	B56(22)
B*5701	B57(17)

Allele	Specificity
B*5702	B57(17)
B*5801	B58(17)
B*5901	B59
B*6701	B67
B*7301	B73
B*7801	B7801

Allele	Specificity
Cw*0101	Cw1
Cw*0102	Cw1
Cw*0201	Cw2
Cw*02021	Cw2
Cw*02022	Cw2
Cw*0301	Cw3
Cw*0302	Cw3
Cw*0303	Cw3
Cw*0304	Cw3
Cw*0401	Cw4
Cw*0402	Cw4
Cw*0501	Cw5
Cw*0601	Cw6
Cw*0602	Cw6
Cw*0701	Cw7
Cw*0702	Cw7
Cw*0703	Cw7
Cw*0801	Cw8
Cw*0802	Cw8
Cw*0803	Cw8
Cw*1201	-
Cw*12021c	-
Cw*12022	-
Cw*1203	-
Cw*1301	-
Cw*1401	-
Cw*1402	-
Cw*1501	-
Cw*1502	-
Cw*1503	-
Cw*1504	-
Cw*1601	-
Cw*1602	-
Cw*1701	-
E*0101	-
E*0102	-
E*0103	-
E*0104	-
G*01011	-
G*01012	-
G*0102	-
G*0103	-

Allele	Specificity
A*0101	A1
A*0102	A1
A*0201	A2
A*0202	A2
A*0203	A203
A*0204	A2
A*0205	A2
A*0206	A2
A*0207	A2
A*0208	A2
A*0209	A2
A*0210	A210
A*0211	A2
A*0212	A2
A*0213	A2
A*0301	A3

Allele	Specificity
A*0302	A3
A*1101	A11
A*1102	A11
A*2301	A23(9)
A*2401	A24(9)
A*2402	A24(9)
A*2403	A2403
A*2501	A25(10)
A*2601	A26(10)
A*2602	A26(10)
A*2603	A26(10)
A*2604	A26(10)
A*2901	A29(19)
A*2902	A29(19)
A*3001	A30(19)
A*3002	A30(19)
A*3003	A30(19)
A*31011	A31(19)
A*31012	A31(19)
A*3201	A32(19)
A*3301	A33(19)
A*3302	A33(19)
A*3401	A34(10)
A*3402	A34(10)
A*3601	A36
A4301	A43
A6601	A66(10)
A*6602	A66(10)
A*68011c	A68(28)
A*68012	A68(28)
A*6802	A68(28)
A*6901	A69(28)
A*7401	A74(19)
A*8001	-

Allele	Specificity
TAP1*0101	
TAP1*02011	
TAP1*02012	
TAP1*0301	
TAP1*0401	
TAP2*0101	
TAP2*0102	
TAP2*0201	

The right-hand column of each subregion lists the distinct antigenic specificities detected serologically. HLA-D specificities are also detected in the MLR. Specificities not yet sufficiently defined are designated by 'w' (workshop). Allelic variants of MHC genes at each locus are also shown. (Based on data from Bodmer JG, Marsh SGE, Parham P, et al. Nomenclature for factors of the HLA system. 1994. *Tissue Antigens* 1994;**44**: 1–18.)

Appendix II: CD markers

CD	identity/function	mol. wt (× 10³)	T cell	B cell	NK/non-lineage	monocyte	macrophage	granulocyte	platelet	Langerhans cell/dendritic cell	stem cell
CD1a		49	Thy								
CD1b		45	Thy							LC	
CD1c		43	Thy							DC	
CD2	LFA-3 receptor	50									
CD2R		50	★								
CD3	TCR subunit (γ,δ,ε,ζ,η)	25,20,19,16,22									
CD4	MHC class II receptor	55									
CD5		67									
CD6		100									
CD7		40			●				●		
CD8	MHC class I receptor	36/32									
CD9		24		pre-B							
CD10	CALLA, neutral endopeptidase	100		pre-B							Lymph
CD11a	LFA-1 (α chain)	180									
CD11b	CR3 (α chain)	165									
CD11c	CR4 (α chain)	150									
CDw12		90–120							●		
CD13	Aminopeptidase N	150									
CD14	LPS-binding protein	55						●		● (LC)	
CD15	sLeˣ				●						
CD16	FcγRIIIA/FcγRIIIB	50–65									
CD16b	FcγRIIIB	48									
CDw17	Lactosylceramide										
CD18	(β chain of CD11)	95									
CD19		95									
CD20	ion channel?	37/35									
CD21	CR2	140		Mat						FDC	
CD22		135									
CD23	FcεRII	45–50		Mat, ★		★	E				
CD24		41/38									
CD25	IL-2 receptor (β)	55	★	★		★					
CD26	Dipeptidylpeptidase IV	120	★								
CD27		55									
CD28		44		★							
CD29	VLA (β chain)	130									
CD30		120	★	★							
CD31	PECAM-1	140									
CD32	FcγRII	40									
CD33		67									BM
CD34		105–120									BM
CD35	CR1	160–260									
CD36		90		●							
CD37		40–52	●	Mat			●				
CD38		45	Thy, ★	PC							Lymph
CD39		70–100		Mat		●				FDC	
CD40		50								FDC	
CD41		120/25									
CD42a	GPIX	23									
CD42b	GPIB–α	135,23									
CD42c	GPIB–β	22									
CD42d	GP V	85									
CD43	Leukosialin	95									
CD44		80–95									
CD45	Leucocyte common antigen(LCA)	T200									

CD	identity/function	mol. wt (× 10³)	T cell	B cell	NK/non-lineage	monocyte	macrophage	granulocyte	platelet	Langerhans cell/dendritic cell	stem cell
CD45RA	Restricted LCA	220			●			●			
CD45RB	Restricted LCA	190/205/220									
CD45RO	Restricted LCA	190									
CD46	MCP(membrane cofactor protein)	66/56									
CD47		47–52									
CD48		41									
CD49a	VLA-1 α_1 integrin	210	★								
CD49b	VLA-2 α_2 integrin	160	+	+	+	+	+	+			
CD49c	VLA-3 α_3 integrin	125									
CD49d	VLA-4 α_4 integrin	150,80,70	+	+		+				LC	
CD49e	VLA-5 α_5 integrin	135,25									
CD49f	VLA-6 α_6 integrin	120,25	●						+		
CD50	ICAM-3	124	+	+	+	+	+	+			
CD51	Vitronectin receptor α	120/24									
CDw52	Campath-1	21–28									
CD53		32–40									BM
CD54	ICAM-1										
CD55	DAF(Decay accelerating factor)	70									
CD56	NKH1 = NCAM	220/135	●								
CD57		110		●							
CD58	LFA-3	40–65									
CD59	TAP, protectin	18–20									
CDw60	NeuAc–NeuAc–Gal										
CD61	Vitronectin receptor β	105							+		
CD62P	P-selectin	150							+		
CD62E	E-selectin	115									
CD62L	L-selectin	75-80	+			+		+			
CD63		53	●	●				●			
CD64	FcγRI	70									
CDw65	Ceramide dodecasaccharide										
CD66a	BGP	180–200						+			
CD66b	Previously CD67	95-100						+			
CD66c	NCA	90-95						+			
CD66d	CGMI	30						+			
CD66e	Carcinoembryonic antigen (CEA)	180-200						+			
CD68		110									
CD69		32/28	★	★							
CD70	CD27-ligand	55,75.95,110.170	★	★							
CD71	Transferrin receptor	95	★	★	★	★					
CD72		43/39									
CD73	Ecto-5'-nucleotidase	69									
CD74	MHC class II invariant chain	41/35/33									
CDw75	α 2,6 sialyltransferase	53		Mat							
CD76				Mat							
CD77	Globotriaosylceramide										
CDw78											
CD79a	Igα	33,40		+							
CD79b	Igβ	33,40		+							
CD80	B7,BBI	60		+							

This table shows the recognized CD markers of haemopoietic cells and their distribution. Thy = thymocytes; DC = dendritic cells; LC = Langerhans' cells; N = neutrophils; E = eosinophils; GC = germinal centre B cell; FDC = follicular dendritic cell; PC = plasma cell; BM = bone-marrow cell. A filled rectangle or + = cell population present; a half-filled rectangle = subpopulation. ● = subject to further analysis; ★ = activated cells only; Rest = resting cells only; Lymph = lymphoid cells; Mat = mature cells only.

Appendix II: CD markers

designation	identity	cells which express marker
CD81	TAPA-1	B cells
CD82		B cells
CD83		B cells
CDw84		B cells
CD85		B cells
CD86		B cells
CD87		Myeloid cells
CD88	C5a receptor	Monocytes/Neutrophils
CD89	Fcα receptor	Myeloid cells
CDw90	Thy –1.	T Cells - Monocytes
CD91	α2 -macroglobulin receptor	Myeloid cells
CDw92		Myeloid cells
CD93		Myeloid cells
CD94		NK Cells
CD95	APO-1 Fas	Activated Tc cells
CD96	TACTILE	Activated cells
CD97		Activated cells
CD98		T cells
CD99		T cells
CD100		T cells
CDw101		T cells
CD102	ICAM-2	Endothelium
CD103		
CD104	ß4 - integrin	Lymphocytes
CD105	Endoglin	Endothelium
CD106	VCAM-1	Activated Endothelium
CD107a	LAMP-1	Platelet
CD107b	LAMP-2	Platelet
CDw108		Endothelium
CDw109		
CD115	M-CSF receptor	Monocytes/Macrophages ⎤
CDw116	GM-CSF receptor	Myeloid precursors
CD117	cKIT	
CDw119	IFNα receptor	
CD120a	TNF receptor (55 KDa)	
CD120b	TNF receptor (75 KDa)	
CDw121a	IL-1 receptor (Type 1)	
CDw121b	IL-1 receptor (Type 2)	⎬ cytokine receptors
CD122	IL-2 receptor (ß) (75 KDa)	
CDW124	IL-4 receptor	
CD126	IL-6 receptor	
CDw127	IL-7 receptor	
CDw128	IL-8 receptor	
CDw130	IL-6 receptor - gp 130 S1g	⎦

Cells which express CD markers.

Appendix III: The major cytokines

cytokine	immune system source	other cells	principal targets	principal effects
IL-1α IL-1β	macrophages, LGLs, B cells	endothelium, fibroblasts, astrocytes, etc.	T cells, B cells, macrophages, endothelium, tissue cells	lymphocyte activation, macrophage stimulation, ↑ leucocyte/endothelial adhesion, pyrexia, acute phase proteins
IL-2	T cells		T cells	T-cell proliferation and differentiation, activation of cytotoxic lymphocytes and macrophages
IL-3	T cells		stem cells	multilineage colony stimulating factor
IL-4	T cells		B cells, T cells	B-cell growth factor, isotype selection, IgE, IgG1
IL-5	T cells		B cells	B-cell growth and differentiation, IgA selection
IL-6	T cells, B cells, macrophages	fibroblasts	B cells, hepatocytes	B-cell differentiation, induces acute phase proteins
IL-7		bone marrow stromal cells	pre-B cells, T cells	B-cell and T-cell proliferation
IL-8	monocytes		neutrophils, basophils	chemotaxis
IL-10	T cells		TH1 cells	inhibition of cytokine synthesis
IL-12	monocytes		T cells	induction of TH1 cells
IL-13	activated T cells		monocytes, B cells	adhesion blocks IL-12 production proliferation
IL-15	monocytes	epithelium muscles	T cells, activated B cells	proliferation
TNFα	macrophages, lymphocytes, mast cells		macrophages, granulocytes, tissue cells	activation of macrophages, granulocytes and cytotoxic cells, ↑leucocyte/endothelial cell adhesion, cachexia, pyrexia, induction of
TNFβ(LT)	T cells			acute phase protein, stimulation of angiogenesis, enhanced MHC class I production
IFNα IFNβ	leucocytes	epithelia, fibroblasts	tissue cells	MHC class I induction, antiviral effect, stimulation of NK cells
IFNγ	T cells, NK cells	epithelia, fibroblasts	leucocytes, tissue cells, TH2 cells	MHC class I and II induction, macro- phage activation,↑ endothelial cell/lymphocyte adhesion, ↓ cytokine synthesis
M–CSF	monocytes	endothelium, fibroblasts		proliferation of macrophage precursors
G–CSF	macrophages	fibroblasts	stem cells	stimulate division and differentiation
GM–CSF	T cells, macrophages	endothelium, fibroblasts		proliferation of granulocyte and macrophage precursors and activators
MIF	T cells		macrophages	migration inhibition

The cytokines in this list have all been identified as distinct by genomic cloning. Note that only the principal sources, targets and effects have been included in this table. Most cytokines act in concert with others to produce their biological effects *in vivo*.

GLOSSARY

Acute phase proteins. Serum proteins whose levels increase during infection or inflammatory reactions.

ADCC (antibody-dependent cell-mediated cytotoxicity). A cytotoxic reaction in which Fc receptor-bearing killer cells recognize target cells via specific antibodies.

Adjuvant. A substance that non-specifically enhances the immune response to an antigen.

AFCs (antibody-forming cells). Functionally equivalent to plasma cells.

Affinity. A measure of the binding strength between an antigenic determinant (epitope) and an antibody-combining site (paratope).

Affinity maturation. The increase in average antibody affinity frequently seen during a secondary immune response.

Allele. Interspecies variance at a particular gene locus.

Allergen. An agent, e.g. pollen, dust, animal dander, that causes IgE-mediated hypersensitivity reactions.

Allergy. Originally defined as altered reactivity on second contact with antigen; now usually refers to a Type I hypersensitivity reaction.

Allogeneic. Refers to interspecies genetic variations.

Allotype. The protein of an allele which may be detectable as an antigen by another member of the same species.

Alternative pathway. The activation pathways of the complement system involving C3 and factors B, D, P, H and I, which interact in the vicinity of an activator surface to form an alternative pathway C3 convertase.

Amplification loop. The alternative complement activation pathway, which acts as a positive feedback loop when C3 is split in the presence of an activator surface.

Anaphylatoxins. Complement peptides (C3a and C5a) which cause mast cell degranulation and smooth muscle contraction.

Anaphylaxis. An antigen-specific immune reaction mediated primarily by IgE which results in vasodilation and constriction of smooth muscles, including those of the bronchus, and which may result in death of the animal.

Antibody. A molecule produced by animals in response to antigen which has the particular property of combining specifically with the antigen which induced its formation.

Antigen. A molecule which reacts with preformed antibody at the specific receptors on T and B cells.

Antigen presentation. The process by which certain cells in the body (antigen-presenting cells) express antigen on their cell surface in a form recognizable by lymphocytes.

Antigen processing. The conversion of an antigen into a form in which it can be recognized by lymphocytes.

APCs (antigen-presenting cells). A variety of cell types which carry antigen in a form that can stimulate lymphocytes.

Atopy. The clinical manifestation of Type I hypersensitivity reactions including eczema, asthma and rhinitis.

Autologous. Part of the same individual.

Autosomes. Chromosomes other than the X or Y sex chromosomes.

Avidity. The functional combining strength of an antibody with its antigen which is related to both the affinity of the reaction between the epitopes and paratopes, and the valencies of the antibody and antigen.

β_2-microglobulin. A polypeptide which constitutes part of some membrane proteins including the Class I MHC molecules.

BCG (Bacille Calmette Guérin). An attenuated strain of *Mycobacterium tuberculosis* used as a vaccine, an adjuvant or a biological response modifier in different circumstances.

Biozzi mice. Lines of mice bidirectionally bred to produce low or high antibody responses to a variety of antigens (originally sheep erythrocytes).

Bradykinin. A vasoactive nonapeptide which is the most important mediator generated by the kinin system.

Bursa of Fabricius. A lymphoepithelial organ found at the junction of the hind gut and cloaca in birds which is the site of B cell maturation.

Bystander lysis. Complement-mediated lysis of cells in the immediate vicinity of a complement activation site, which are not themselves responsible for the activation.

C domains. The constant domains of antibody and the T-cell receptor. These domains do not contribute to the antigen-binding site and show relatively little variability between receptor molecules.

C genes. The gene segments which encode the constant portion of the immunoglobulin heavy and light chains and the α, β, γ and δ chains of the T-cell antigen receptor.

C1–C9. The components of the complement classical and lytic pathways which are responsible for mediating inflamatory reactions, opsonization of particles and lysis of cell membranes.

Capping. A process by which cell surface molecules are caused to aggregate (usually using antibody) on the cell membrane.

Carrier. An immunogenic molecule, or part of a molecule that is recognized by T cells in an antibody response.

CD markers. Cell surface molecules of leucocytes and platelets that are distinguishable with monoclonal antibodies and may be used to differentiate different cell populations.

CDRs (complementary-determining regions). The sections of an antibody or T-cell receptor V region responsible for antigen or antigen-MHC binding.

Cell adhesion molecules (CAMs). A group of proteins of the immunoglobulin supergene family involved in intercellular adhesion, including ICAM-1, ICAM-2, ICAM-3, VCAM-1, MAdCAM-1 and PECAM.

Cell cycle. The process of cell division which is divisible into four phases G1, S, G2 and M. DNA replicates during the S phase and the cell divides in the M (mitotic) phase.

Chemokinesis. Increased random migratory activity of cells.

Chemotaxis. Increased directional migration of cells particularly in response to concentration gradients of certain chemotactic factors.

Chimaerism. The situation in which cells from genetically different individuals coexist in one body.

Class I/II/III MHC molecules. Three major classes of molecule are coded within the MHC. Class I molecules have one MHC-encoded peptide complexed with β_2-microglobulin, class II molecules have two MHC-encoded peptides which are non-covalently associated, and class III molecules are other molecules including complement components.

Class I/II restriction. The observation that immunologically active cells will only cooperate effectively when they share MHC haplotypes at either the class I or class II loci.

Classical pathway. The pathway by which antigen-antibody complexes can activate the complement system, involving components C1, C2 and C4, and generating a classical pathway C3 convertase.

Class switching. The process by which an individual B cell can link immunoglobulin heavy chain C genes to its recombined V gene to produce a different class of antibody with the same specificity. This process is also reflected in the overall class switch seen during the maturation of an immune response.

Clonal selection. The fundamental basis of lymphocyte activation in which antigen selectively causes activation, division and differentiation only in those cells which express receptors with which it can combine.

Clone. A family of cells or organisms having a genetically identical constitution.

CMI (cell-mediated immunity). A term used to refer to immune reactions that are mediated by cells rather than by antibody or other humoral factors.

Cobra venom factor. A cobra complement component equivalent to mammalian C3b.

Complement. A group of serum proteins involved in the control of inflammation, the activation of phagocytes and the lytic attack on cell membranes. The system can be activated by interaction with the immune system (classical) .

Complement control protein (CCP) domains (also called short consensus repeats). A domain structure found in many proteins of the complement classical and alternative pathways and in some complement receptors and control proteins,

Complement receptors (CR1-CR4). A set of four cell surface receptors for fragments of complement C3. CR1 and CR2 have numerous CCP domains, while CR3 and CR4 are integrins.

Costimulation. The signals required for the activation of a lymphocyte, in addition to the antigen-specific signal delivered via their antigen-receptors.

ConA (concanavalin A). A mitogen for T cells.

Congenic. Animals which are genetically constructed to differ at one particular locus.

Conjugate. A reagent which is formed by covalently coupling two molecules together, such as fluorescein coupled to an immunoglobulin molecule.

Constant regions. The relatively invariant parts of immunoglobulin heavy and light chains, and the α, β, γ and δ chains of the T-cell receptor.

CR1 CR2 CR3. Receptors for activated C3 fragments.

CSFs (colony stimulating factors). A group of cytokines which control the differentiation of haemopoietic stem cells.

Cyclophosphamide. A cytotoxic drug frequently used as an immunosuppressive.

Cyclosporin. A T cell suppressive drug that is particularly useful in suppression of graft rejection.

Cytokines. A generic term for soluble molecules which mediate interactions between cells.

Cytophilic. Having a propensity to bind to cells.

Cytostatic. Having the ability to stop cell growth.

Cytotoxic. Having the ability to kill cells.

D genes. Sets of gene segments lying between the V and J genes in the immunoglobulin heavy chain genes, and in the T-cell receptor β and δ chain genes which are recombined with V and J genes during ontogeny.

Degranulation. Exocytosis of granules from cells such as mast cells and basophils.

Dendritic cells. A set of cells present in tissues, which capture antigens and migrate to the lymph nodes and spleen, where they are particularly active in presenting the processed antigen to T cells.

DTH (delayed type hypersentivity). This term includes the delayed skin reactions associated with Type IV hypersensitivity.

DNP (dinitrophenol). A commonly used hapten.

Domain. A region of a peptide having a coherent tertiary structure. Both immunoglobulins and MHC Class I and Class II molecules have domains.

Dominant idiotypes. Individual idiotypes which are present on a large proportion of the antibodies generated by a particular antigen.

dsDNA. Double-stranded DNA.

Epstein–Barr virus (EBV). Causal agent of Burkitt's lymphoma and infectious mononucleosis, which has the ability to transform human B cells into stable cell lines.

Effector cells. A functional concept which in context means those lymphocytes or phagocytes which produce the end effect.

Endogenous. Originating within the organism.

Endothelium. Cells lining blood vessels and lymphatics.

Enhancement. Prolongation of graft survival by treatment with antibodies directed towards the graft alloantigens.

Epitope. A single antigenic determinant. Functionally it is the portion of an antigen which combines with the antibody paratope.

Exon. Gene segment encoding protein.

Fab. The part of an antibody molecule which contains the antigen-combining site, consisting of a light chain and part of the heavy chain; it is produced by enzymatic digestion.

Factors B, P, D, H, and I. Components of the alternative complement pathway.

Fc. The portion of an antibody that is responsible for binding to antibody receptors on cells and the C1q component of complement.

Framework segments. Sections of antibody V regions which lie between the hypervariable regions.

Freund's adjuvant. An emulsion of aqueous antigen in oil. Complete Freund's adjuvant contains killed *Mycobacterium tuberculosis*, while incomplete Freund's adjuvant does not.

GALT (gut-associated lymphoid tissue). Refers to the accumulations of lymphoid tissue associated with the gastrointestinal tract.

Genetic association. A term used to describe the condition where particular genotypes are associated with other phenomena, such as particular diseases.

Genetic restriction. The term used to describe the observation that lymphocytes and antigen-presenting cells cooperate most effectively when they share particular MHC haplotypes.

Genome. The total genetic material contained within the cell.

Genotype. The genetic material inherited from parents; not all of it is necessarily expressed in the individual.

Germ line. The genetic material which is passed down through the gametes before it is modified by somatic recombination or maturation.

Giant cells. Large multinucleated cells sometimes seen in granulomatous reactions and thought to result from the fusion of macrophages.

GVH (graft versus host) disease. A condition caused by allogeneic donor lymphocytes reacting against host tissue in an immunologically compromised recipient.

H–2. The mouse major histocompatibility complex.

Haplotype. A set of genetic determinants located on a single chromosome.

Hapten. A small molecule which can act as an epitope but is incapable by itself of eliciting an antibody response.

Helper (T$_H$) cells. A functional subclass of T cells which can help to generate cytotoxic T cells and cooperate with B cells in the production of antibody responses. Helper cells recognize antigen in association with class II MHC molecules.

Heterologous. Refers to interspecies antigenic differences.

HEV (high endothelial venule). An area of venule from which lymphocytes migrate into lymph nodes.

Hinge. The portion of an immunoglobulin heavy chain between the Fc and Fab regions which permits flexibility within the molecule and allows the two combining sites to operate independently. The hinge region is usually encoded by a separate exon.

Histamine. A major vasoactive amine released from mast cell and basophil granules.

Histocompatibility. The ability to accept grafts between individuals.

HLA. The human major histocompatibility complex.

Homologous. The same species.

hnRNA (heteronuclear RNA). The fraction of nuclear RNA which contains primary transcripts of the DNA prior to processing to form messenger RNA.

Humoral. Pertaining to the extracellular fluids, including the serum and lymph.

Hybridoma. Cell line created *in vitro* by fusing two different cell types, usually lymphocytes, one of which is a tumour cell.

5-hydroxytryptamine. A vasoactive amine present in platelets and a major mediator of inflammation in rodents.

Hypervariable region. The most variable areas (3) of the V domains of immunoglobulin and T-cell receptor chains. These regions are clustered at the distal portion of the V domain and contribute to the antigen-binding site.

ICAM-1 and ICAM-2 (intercellular adhesion molecules). Cell surface molecules found on a variety of leucocytes and non-haematogenous cells which interact with LFA-1.

Idiotope. A single antigenic determinant on an antibody V region.

Idiotype. The antigenic characteristic of the V region of an antibody.

Immune-complex. The product of an antigen-antibody reaction which may also contain components of the complement system.

Immunofluorescence. A technique used to identify particular antigens microscopically in tissues or on cells by the binding of a fluorescent antibody conjugate.

Immunogenic. Having the ability to evoke B and/or T cell mediated immune reactions.

Integrins. A large family of cell surface adhesion molecules, some of which interact with CAMs, others with complement fragments, and others with components of the extracellular matrix.

Interferons (IFNs). A group of molecules involved in signalling between cells of the immune system.

Interleukins (IL-1–IL-15). A group of molecules involved in signalling between cells of the immune system.

Intron. Gene segment between exons not encoding protein.

Ir gene. A group of immune response (Ir) genes determining the level of an immune response to a particularly antigen or foreign stimulus. A number of them are found in the major histocompatibility complex.

Isoelectric focusing. Separation of molecules on the basis of charge. Each molecule will migrate to the point in a pH gradient where it has not net charge.

Isologous. Of identical genetic constitution.

Isotype. Refers to genetic variation within a family of proteins or peptides such that every member of the species will have each isotype of the family represented in its genome (e.g. immunoglobulin classes).

J chain. A monomorphic polypeptide present in polymeric IgA and IgM, and essential to their formation.

J genes. Sets of gene segments in the immunoglobulin heavy and light chain genes, and in the genes for the chains of the T-cell receptor, which are recombined during lymphocyte ontogeny and contribute towards the genes for variable domains.

K cell. A group of lymphocytes which are able to destroy their target by antibody-dependent cell-mediated cytotoxicity. They have Fc receptors.

κ (kappa) chains. One of the immunoglobulin light chain isotypes.

Karyotype. The chromosomal constitution of a cell which may vary between individuals of a single species, depending on the presence or absence of particular sex chromosomes or on the incidence of translocations between sections of different chromosomes.

Kinins. A group of vasoactive mediators produced following tissue injury.

Knockout. An animal whose endogenous gene for a particular protein has been deleted or mutated to be non-functional.

Kupffer cells. Phagocytic cells which line the liver sinusoids.

λ (lambda) cells. One of the immunoglobulin light chain isotypes.

Langerhans' cells. Antigen-presenting cells of the skin which emigrate to local lymph nodes to become dendritic cells; they are very active in presenting antigen to T cells.

Large granular lymphocytes (LGLs). A group of morphologically defined lymphocytes containing the majority of K cell and NK cell activity. They have both lymphocyte and monocyte/macrophage markers.

Lectin pathway. A recently defined pathway of complement activation, initiated by mannan-binding protein, which intersects the classical pathway,

Leukotrienes. A collection of metabolites of arachidonic acid which have powerful pharmacological effects.

LFAs (leucocyte functional antigens). A group of three molecules which mediate intercellular adhesion between leucocytes and other cells in an antigen non-specific fashion.

Ligand. A linking (or binding) molecule.

Line. A collection of cells produced by continuously growing a particular cell culture *in vitro*. Such cell line will usually contain a number of individual clones.

Linkage. The condition where two genes are both present in close proximity on a single chromosome and are usually inherited together.

Linkage disequilibrium. A condition where two genes are found together in a population at a greater frequency than that predicted simply by the product of their individual gene frequencies.

Locus. The position on a chromosome at which a particular gene is found.

LPR (lymphoproliferation gene). A gene found in MRL mice which is involved in the generation of autoimmune phenomena.

LPS (lipopolysaccharide). A product of some Gram-negative bacterial cell walls which can act as a B-cell mitogen.

Lymphokines. A generic term for molecules other than antibodies which are involved in signalling between cells of the immune system and are produced by lymphocytes (*cf.* interleukins).

Ly antigens. A group of cell surface markers found on murine T cells which relate to the differentiation of T cell subpopulations.

Lytic pathway. The complement pathway effected by components C5–C9 that is responsible for lysis of sensitized cell plasma membranes.

MALT (mucosa-associated lymphoid tissue). Generic term for lymphoid tissue associated with the gastrointestinal tract, bronchial tree and other mucosa.

Membrane attack complex (MAC). The assembled terminal complement components C5b–C9 of the lytic pathway which becomes inserted into cell membranes.

MHC (major histocompatibility complex). A genetic region found in all mammals whose products are primarily responsible for the rapid rejection of grafts between individuals, and function in signalling between lymphocytes and cells expressing antigen.

MHC restriction. A characteristic of many immune reactions in which cells cooperate most effectively with other cells sharing an MHC haplotype.

MIF (migration inhibition factor). A group of peptides produced by lymphocytes which are capable of inhibiting macrophage migration.

MLR/MLC (mixed lymphocyte reaction/mixed lymphocyte culture). Assay system for T cell recognition of allogenic cells in which response is measured by proliferation in the presence of the stimulating cells.

Mitogens. Substances which cause cells, particularly lymphocytes, to undergo cell division.

Monoclonal. Derived from a single clone, for example, monoclonal antibodies, which are produced by a single clone and are homogenous.

Myeloma. A lymphoma produced from cells of the B cell lineage.

Neoplasm. A synonym for cancerous tissue.

Network theory. A proposal first put forward by Jerne (since developed) which states that T cells and B cells mutually inter-regulate by recognizing idiotypes on their antigen receptors.

NIP (4-hydroxy, 5-iodo, 3-nitrophenylacetyl). A commonly used hapten.

NK (natural killer) cells. A group of lymphocytes which have the intrinsic ability to recognize and destroy some virally infected cells and some tumour cells.

NP (4-hydroxy, 3-nitrophenylacetyl). A hapten which partially cross-reacts with NIP.

Nude mouse. A genetically athymic mouse which also carries a closely linked gene producing a defect in hair production.

NZB/W. An F_1 strain of mouse which is a model for systemic lupus erythematosus. The parental NZB strain also suffers from autoimmunity.

Opsonization. A process by which phagocytosis is facilitated by the deposition of opsonins (e.g. antibody and C3b) on the antigen.

PAF (platelet activating factor). A factor released by basophils which causes platelets to aggregate.

PALS (periarteriolar lymphatic sheath). The accumulations of lymphoid tissue constituting the white pulp of the spleen.

Pathogen. An organism which causes disease.

PC (phosphorylcholine). A commonly used hapten which is also found on the surface of a number of microorganisms.

PCA (passive cutaneous anaphylaxis). The technique used to detect antigen-specific IgE, in which the test animal is injected intravenously with the antigen and dye, the skin having previously been sensitized with antibody.

PFC (plaque forming cell). An antibody-producing cell detected *in vitro* by its ability to lyse antigen-sensitized erythrocytes in the presence of complement.

PHA (phytohaemagglutin). A mitogen for T cells.

Phagocytosis. The process by which cells engulf material and enclose it within a vacuole (phagosome) in the cytoplasm.

Phenotype. The expressed characteristics of an individual (*cf.* genotype).

Pinocytosis. The process by which liquids or very small particles are taken into the cell.

Plasma cell. An antibody-producing B cell which has reached the end of its differentiation pathway.

Pokeweed mitogen. A mitogen for B and T cells.

Polyclonal. A term which describes the products of a number of different cell types (*cf.* monoclonal).

Primary lymphoid tissues. Lymphoid organs in which lymphocytes complete their initial maturation steps; they include the fetal liver, adult bone marrow and thymus, and bursa of Fabricius in birds.

Primary response. The immune response (cellular or humoral) following an initial encounter with a particular antigen.

Prime. To give an initial sensitization to antigen.

Prostaglandins. Pharmacologically active derivatives of arachidonic acid. Different prostaglandins are capable of modulating cell mobility and immune responses.

Pseudoalleles. Tandem variants of a gene: they do not occupy a homologous position on the chromosome (e.g. C4).

Pseudogenes. Genes which have homologous structures to other genes but which are incapable of being expressed, e.g. *Jk3* in the mouse.

Radioimmunoassay (RIA). A number of different, sensitive techniques for measuring antigen or antibody titres, using radiolabelled reagents.

Receptor. A cell surface molecule which binds specifically to particular extracellular molecules.

Recombination. A process by which genetic information is rearranged during meiosis. This process also occurs during the somatic rearrangements of DNA which occur in the formation of genes encoding antibody molecules and T-cell antigen receptors.

Recurrent idiotype. An idiotype present in the immune response of different animals or strains to a particular antigen.

Respiratory burst. Increase in oxidative metabolism of phagocytes following uptake of opsonized particles.

Reticuloendothelial system. A diffuse system of phagocytic cells derived from the bone marrow stem cells which are associated with the connective tissue framework of the liver, spleen, lymph nodes and other serous cavities. An old-fashioned term, rarely used, mononuclear phagocyte system being preferred.

Rosetting. A technique for identifying or isolating cells by mixing them with particles or cells to which they bind (e.g. sheep erythrocytes to human T cells). The rosettes consist of a central cell surrounded by bound cells.

Secondary response. The immune response which follows a second or subsequent encounter with a particular antigen.

Secretory component. A polypeptide produced by cells of some secretory epithelia which is involved in transporting secreted polymeric IgA across the cell and protecting it from digestion in the gastrointestinal tract.

Skin test. A reaction in the skin following injection or contact with an antigen/allergen.

SLE (systemic lupus erythematosus). An autoimmune disease of humans usually involving anti-nuclear antibodies.

Somatic mutation. A process occurring during B cell maturation and affecting the antibody gene region, which permits refinement of antibody specificity.

Suppressor (Ts) cell. Functionally defined populations of T cells which reduce the immune responses of other T cells or B cells, or switch the response into a different pathway to that under investigation.

Synergism. Cooperative interaction.

Syngeneic. Strains of animals produced by repeated inbreeding so that each pair of autosomes within an individual is identical.

T15. An idiotype associated with anti-phosphorylcholine antibodies, named after the TEPC15 myeloma prototype sequence.

T-cell receptor (TCR). The T-cell antigen receptor consisting of either and $\alpha\beta$ dimer (TCR-2) or a $\gamma\delta$ dimer (TCR-1) associated with the CD3 molecular complex.

T-dependent/T-independent antigens. T-dependent antigens require immune recognition by both T and B cells to produce an immune response. T-independent antigens can directly stimulate B cells to produce specific antibody.

Thy. A cell surface antigen of mouse T cells which has allotypic variants.

TNF (tumour necrosis factor). A cytokine released by activated macrophages that is structurally related to lymphotoxin released by activated T cells.

Tolerance. A state of specific immunological unresponsiveness.

Transformation. Morphological changes in a lymphocyte associated with the onset of division. Also used to denote the change to the autonomously dividing state of a cancer cell.

Transgenic animal. An animal in which one or more new genes have been incorporated. These are often placed under specific promotors so that they are only expressed in particular tissues for limited periods.

V domains. The N-terminal domains of antibody heavy and light chains and the α, β, γ and δ chains of the T-cell receptor, and become recombined with appropriate sets of D and J genes during lymphocyte ontogeny.

Vasoactive amines. Products such as histamine and 5-hydroxytryptamine released by basophils, mast cells and platelets which act on the endothelium and smooth muscle of the local vasculature.

White pulp. The lymphoid component of spleen, consisting of periarteriolar sheaths of lymphocytes and antigen-presenting cells.

Xenogeneic. Referring to interspecies antigenic differences (*cf.* heterologous).

INDEX